Principles and Practice of Clinical Trials

Steven Piantadosi · Curtis L. Meinert
Editors

Principles and Practice of Clinical Trials

Volume 1

With 241 Figures and 191 Tables

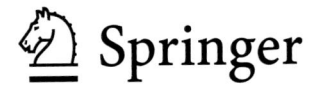 Springer

Editors
Steven Piantadosi
Department of Surgery
Division of Surgical Oncology
Brigham and Women's Hospital
Harvard Medical School
Boston, MA, USA

Curtis L. Meinert
Department of Epidemiology
School of Public Health
Johns Hopkins University
Baltimore, MD, USA

ISBN 978-3-319-52635-5   ISBN 978-3-319-52636-2 (eBook)
https://doi.org/10.1007/978-3-319-52636-2

This Springer imprint is published by the registered company Springer Nature Switzerland AG.
The registered company address is: Gewerbestrasse 11, 6330 Cham, Switzerland

In memory of
Lulu, Champ, and Dudley

A Foreword to the Principles and Practice of Clinical Trials

Trying to identify the effects of treatments is not new. The *Book of Daniel* (verses 12–15) describes a test of the effects King Nebuchadnezzar's meat:

> *Prove thy servants, I beseech thee, ten days; and let them give us pulse to eat, and water to drink. Then let our countenances be looked upon before thee, and the countenance of the children that eat of the portion of the King's meat: and as thou seest, deal with thy servants. So he consented to them in this matter, and proved them ten days. And at the end of ten days their countenances appeared fairer and fatter in flesh than all the children which did eat the portion of the King's meat.*

The requirement of comparison in identifying treatment effects was recognized in the tenth century by Abu Bakr Muhammad ibn Zakariya al-Razi (Persian physician):

> *When the dullness (thiqal) and the pain in the head and neck continue for three and four and five days or more, and the vision shuns light, and watering of the eyes is abundant, yawning and stretching are great, insomnia is severe, and extreme exhaustion occurs, then the patient after that will progress to meningitis (sirsâm). . . If the dullness in the head is greater than the pain, and there is no insomnia, but rather sleep, then the fever will abate, but the throbbing will be immense but not frequent and he will progress into a stupor (lîthûrghas). So when you see these symptoms, then proceed with bloodletting. For I once saved one group [of patients] by it, while I intentionally neglected [to bleed] another group. By doing that, I wished to reach a conclusion (ra'y). And so all of these [latter] contracted meningitis.* (Tibi 2006)

But it was not until the beginning of the eighteenth century before the importance of treatment comparisons was broadly acknowledged, for example, as in chances of contracting smallpox among people inoculated with smallpox lymph versus those who caught smallpox disease naturally (Bird 2018).

By the middle of the eighteenth century there were examples of tests with comparison groups, for example, as described by James Lind in relation to his scurvy experiment on board the HMS Salisbury at sea:

> *On the 20th of May 1747, I took twelve patients in the scurvy, on board the Salisbury at sea. Their cases were as similar as I could have them. They all in general had putrid gums, the spots and lassitude, with weakness of their knees. They lay together in one place, being a proper apartment for the sick in the fore-hold; and had one diet common to all, viz., watergruel sweetened with sugar in the morning; fresh mutton-broth often times for dinner;*

at other times puddings, boiled biscuit with sugar, etc; and for supper, barley and raisins, rice and currants, sago and wine, or the like. Two of these were ordered each a quart of cyder a-day. Two others took twenty-five gutts of elixir vitriol three times a day, upon an empty stomach; using a gargle strongly acidulated with it for their mouths. Two others took two spoonfuls of vinegar three times a day, upon an empty stomach; having their gruels and their other food well acidulated with it, as also the gargle for their mouth. Two of the worst patients, with the tendons in the ham rigid, (a symptom none of the rest had), were put under a course of seawater. Of this they drank half a pint every day, and sometimes more or less as it operated, by way of gentle physic. Two others had each two oranges and one lemon given them every day. These they eat with greediness, at different times, upon an empty stomach. They continued but six days under this course, having consumed the quantity that could be spared. The two remaining patients, took the bigness of a nutmeg three times a-day, of an electuary recommended by an hospital surgeon, made of garlic, mustard-seed, rad raphan, balsam of Peru, and gum myrrh; using for common drink, barley-water well acidulated with tamarinds; by a decoction of which, with the addition of cremor tartar, they were gently purged three or four times during the course.

    * * *

The consequence was, that the most sudden and visible good effects were perceived from the use of the oranges and lemons; one of those who had taken them, being at the end of six days fit for duty. (Lind 1753)

Lind did not make clear how his 12 sailors were assigned to the treatments in his experiment. During the late nineteenth and early twentieth century, alternation (and sometimes randomization) became used to create study comparison groups that differed only by chance (Chalmers et al. 2011).

In 1937 assignment was discussed in Hill's book, *Principles of Medical Statistics*, in which he emphasized the importance of strictly observing the allocation schedule. Implementation of this principle was reflected in concealment of allocation schedules in two important clinical trials designed for the UK Medical Research Council in the 1940s (Medical Research Council 1944; 1948). Sir Austin Bradford Hill's 1937 book went into 12 editions, and his other writings, such as *Statistical Methods in Clinical and Preventive Medicine*, helped propel the upward methodological progression.

The United States Congress passed the Kefauver-Harris Amendments to the Food, Drug, and Cosmetic Act of 1938 in 1962. The amendments revolutionized drug development by requiring drug manufacturers to prove that a drug was safe and effective. A feature of the amendments was language spelling out the nature of scientific evidence required for a drug to be approved:

The term "substantial evidence" means evidence consisting of adequate and well-controlled investigations, including clinical investigations, by experts qualified by scientific training and experience to evaluate the effectiveness of the drug involved, on the basis of which it could fairly and responsibly be concluded by such experts that the drug will have the effect it purports or is represented to have under the conditions of its use prescribed, recommended, or suggested in the labeling or proposed labeling thereof. (United States Congress 1962)

Post World War II prosperity brought sizeable increases in government funding for training and research. The National Institutes of Health played a major role in training biostatisticians in the 1960s and 1970s with its fellowship programs. By the

1980s clinical trial courses started showing up in syllabi of academic institutions. By the 1990s academic institutions started offering PhDs focused on design and conduct of trials with a few now offering PhD training in clinical trials.

The clinical trial enterprise is huge. There were over 25,000 trials registered on CT.gov starting in 2019. That number, assuming CT.gov registrations account for 70% of all registered trials, translates to 38,000 trials. That amounts to 2.3 million people studied when those trials are finished assuming a median sample size of 60 per trial.

Lind did his trial before IRBs and consents, before requirements for written protocols, before investigator certifications, before the Health Insurance Portability and Accountability Act (HIPAA), before data sharing, before data monitoring committees, before site visiting, and before requirements for posting results within 1 year of completion. Trials moved from the backroom of obscurity to front and center with trials seen as forms of public trust.

The act of trying progressed from efforts involving a single investigator to efforts involving cadres of investigators with training in medicine, biostatistics, epidemiology, programming, data processing, and in regulations and ethics underlying trials.

The size of the research team increases with the size and complexities of the trials. Multicenter trials may involve investigatorships numbering in the hundreds.

Enter trialists – persons with training and experience in the design, organization, conduct, and analysis of trials. Presently trialists are scattered, located in various departments in medical schools and schools of public health. They have no academic home.

The scattering works to the disadvantage of the art and science of trials in that it stymies communications and development of curricula relevant to trials. One of our motivations in undertaking this work is hope of speeding development of such homes.

The blessing of online publications is that works can be updated at will. The curse is that the work is never done. We hope to advance the science of trials by providing the trials world with a comprehensive work from leaders in the field covering the waterfront of clinical trials serving as a reference resource for novices and experts in trials for use in designing, conducting, and analyzing them.

13 May 2020   Steven Piantadosi and Curtis L. Meinert
                                                                      Editors

Postscript

When we started this effort, there was no COVID-19. Now we are living through a pandemic caused by the virus leading us to proclaim in regard to trials, as Charles Dickens did in his *A Tale of Two Cities* in a different context, "the best of times, the worst of times."

"The best of times" because never before has there been more interest and attention directed to trials, even from the President. Everybody wants to know when there will be a vaccine to protect us from COVID-19.

"The worst of times" because of the chaos caused by the pandemic in mounting and doing trials and the impact of "social distancing" on the way trials are done now.

It is a given that the pandemic will change how we do trials, but whatever those changes will be, trials will remain humankind's best and most enduring answer to addressing the conditions and maladies that affect us.

Acknowledgment

We are indebted to Sir Iain Chalmers for his review and critical input in reviewing this piece. Dr. Chalmers is founder of the Cochrane Collaboration and first coordinator of the James Lind Library.

Events in the Development of Clinical Trials

Date	Author/source	Event
1747	Lind	Experiment with untreated control group (Lind 1953)
1799	Haygarth	Use of sham procedure (Haggard 1932)
1800	Waterhouse	Smallpox trial (Waterhouse 1802, 1800)
1863	Gull	Use of placebo treatment (Sutton 1865)
1918		First department of biostatistics; Johns Hopkins University, https://www.jhsph.edu/departments/biostatistics/about-us/history/
1923	Fisher	Application of randomization to experimentation (Fisher and MacKenzie 1923)
1931		Committee on clinical trials created by the Medical Research Council of Great Britain (Medical Research Council 1931)
1931	Amberson	Random assignment of treatment to groups of patients (Amberson et al. 1931)
1937	NIH	Start of NIH grant support with creation of the National Cancer Institute (National Institutes of Health 1981)
1944		Publication of multicenter trial on treatment for common cold (Patulin Clinical Trials Committee 1944)
1946		Nüremberg Code for Human Experimentation (Curran and Shapiro 1970) https://history.nih.gov/research/downloads/nuremberg.pdf
1948	MRC	Streptomycin TB multicenter trial published; BMJ: 30 Oct, 1948 (Medical Research Council 1948)
1962	Hill	Book: *Statistical Methods in Clinical and Preventive Medicine* (Hill 1962)
1962	Kefauver, Harris	Amendments to the Food, Drug, and Cosmetic Act of 1938 (United States Congress 1962)

Date	Author/source	Event
1964	NLM	MEDLARS® (MEDical Literature Analysis and Retrieval System) of the National Library of Medicine initiated
1966; 8 Feb	USPHS	Memo from Surgeon General of USPHS informing recipients of NIH funding of requirement for informed consent as condition for funding henceforth (Stewart 1966), https://history.nih.gov/research/downloads/surgeongeneraldirective1966.pdf
1966	Levine	Publication of U.S. Public Health Service regulations leading to creation of Institutional Review Boards for research involving humans (Levine 1988)
1966; 6 Sep	US govt	Freedom of Information Act (FOIA) signed into law by Lyndon Johnson 6 September 1966 (Public Law 89-554, 80 Statue 383); Act specifies US Governmental Agencies records subject to disclosure under the Act; amended and extended in 1996, 2002, and 2007, https://www.justice.gov/oip/foia_guide09/foia-final.pdf; 5 September 2009
1967	Tom Chalmers	Structure for separating the treatment monitoring and treatment administration process (Coronary Drug Project Research Group: 1973)
1974; 12 July	US govt	Creation of U.S. National Commission for the Protection of Human Subjects of Biomedical and Behavioral Research; part of the National Research Act (Public Law No. 93-348, § 202, 88 Stat. 342)
1974	US govt	US Code of Federal Regulations promulgated establishing Institutional Review Boards, https://www.hhs.gov/ohrp/humansubjects/guidance/45cfr46
1979	OPRR	Belmont Report (Ethical Principles and Guidelines for the Protection of Human Subjects of Research); product of the National Commission for the Protection of Human Subjects of Biomedical and Behavioral Research (Office for Protection from Research Risks Belmont Report 1979)
1979	Gorden	NIH Clinical Trials Committee (chaired by Robert Gorden) recommends that "every clinical trial should have provisions for data and safety monitoring" (National Institutes of Health 1979)
1979		Society for Clinical Trials established
1980		First issue of *Controlled Clinical Trials* (Meinert and Tonascia 1998)
1981	Friedman	Book: *Fundamentals of Clinical Trials* (Friedman et al. 1981)

Date	Author/source	Event
1983	Pocock	Book: *Clinical Trials: A Practical Approach* (Pocock 1983)
1986	Meinert	Book: *Clinical Trials: Design, Conduct, and Analysis* (Meinert and Tonascia 1986)
1990	ICH	International Conference on Harmonisation (ICH) formed (European Union, Japan, and the United States) (Vozeh 1995)
1990		Initiation of PhD training program in clinical trials at Johns Hopkins University
1992	FDA	Prescription Drug User Fee Act (PDUFA) enacted; allows FDA to collect fees for review of New Drug Applications (Public Law 102-571; 102 Congress; https://www.fda.gov/ForIndustry/UserFees/PrescriptionDrugUserFee/ucm200361.htm; 2002)
1993	US govt	Mandate regarding valid analysis for gender and ethnic origin treatment interactions (United States Congress 1993)
1993	UK	Cochrane Collaboration founded under leadership of Iain Chalmers; developed in response to Archie Cochrane's call for up-to-date, systematic reviews of all relevant trials in the healthcare field
1996	HIPAA	Health Insurance Portability and Accountability Act (HIPAA) enacted (Public Law 104-191; 104th US Congress; https://aspe.hhs.gov/admnsimp/pL10419.htm)
1996	NLM	PubMed (search engine for MEDLINE) made free to public
1996		Consolidated Standards of Reporting Trials (CONSORT) (Begg et al. 1996)
1997	US govt	US public law calling for registration of trials; Food and Drug Administration Modernization Act of 1997; Public Law 105-115; Nov 21, 1997 (https://www.govinfo.gov/content/pkg/PLAW-105publ115/pdf/PLAW-105publ115.pdf)
1997	Piantadosi	Book: *Clinical Trials: A Methodologic Perspective* (Piantadosi 1997)
2000	NIH	ClinicalTrials.gov registration website launched (Zarin et al. 2007)
2003	NIH	NIH statement on data sharing (National Institutes of Health 2003)
2003	UK	Launch of James Lind Library; marking 250th anniversary of the publication of James Lind's Treatise of the Scurvy (https://www.jameslindlibrary.org/search/)

Date	Author/source	Event
2004	ICMJE	Requirement of registration of trials in public registries as condition for publication for trials starting enrollment after 1 July 2005 by member journals of the International Committee of Medical Journal Editors (ICMJE) (DeAngelis et al. 2004)
2004; 3 Sep	NIH	NIH notice NOT-OD-04-064 (Enhanced Public Access to NIH Research Information) required "its grantees and supported Principal Investigators provide the NIH with electronic copies of all final version manuscripts upon acceptance for publication if the research was supported in whole or in part by NIH funding" for deposit in PubMed Central within six months after publication
2006	WHO	World Health Organization (WHO) launch of International Clinical Trials Registry Platform (ICTRP) (https://www.who.int/ictrp/en/)
2007	FDA	Requirement for investigators to post tabular results of trials covered under FDA regulations on ClinicalTrials.gov within one year of completion [Food and Drug Administration Amendments Act of 2007 (FDAAA)]
2007		Wiley Encyclopedia of Clinical Trials (4 vols) (D'Agostino et al. 2007)
2013		Standard Protocol Items: Recommendations for Interventional Trials (SPIRIT) (Chan et al. 2013)
2016	NIH	Final NIH policy on single institutional review board for multi-site research (NOT-OD-16-094)
2017	FDA	2007 requirement for posting results extended to all trials, whether or not subject to FDA regulations (81 FR64983)
2017	ICMJE	ICMJE requirement for data sharing in clinical trials (Ann Intern Med doi: 10.7326/M17-1028) (Taichman et al. 2017)

References

Amberson JB Jr, McMahon BT, Pinner M (1931) A clinical trial of sanocrysin in pulmonary tuberculosis. Am Rev Tuberc 24:401–435

Begg C, Cho M, Eastwood S, Horton R, Moher D, Olkin I, Pitkin R, Rennie D, Schulz KF, Simel D, Stroup DF (1996) Improving the quality of reporting of randomized controlled trials. The CONSORT statement. JAMA 276(8):637–639

Bird A (2018) James Jurin and the avoidance of bias in collecting and assessing evidence on the effects of variolation. JLL Bulletin: Commentaries on the history of treatment evaluation. https://www.jameslindlibrary.org/articles/james-jurin-

and-the-avoidance-of-bias-in-collecting-and-assessing-evidence-on-the-effects-of-variolation/

Chalmers I, Dukan E, Podolsky SH, Davey Smith G (2011) The advent of fair treatment allocation schedules in clinical trials during the 19th and early 20th centuries. JLL Bulletin: Commentaries on the history of treatment evaluation. https://www.jameslindlibrary.org/articles/the-advent-of-fair-treatment-allocation-schedules-in-clinical-trials-during-the-19th-and-early-20th-centuries/

Chan AW, Tetzlaff JM, Altman DG, Laupacis A, Gøtzsche PC, Krleža-Jeric K, Hróbjartsson A, Mann H, Dickersin K, Berlin JA, Doré CJ, Parulekar WR, Summerskill WSM, Groves T, Schulz KF, Sox HC, Rockhold FW, Drummond R, Moher D (2013) SPIRIT 2013 statement: defining standard protocol items for clinical trials. Ann Intern Med 158(3):200–207

Coronary Drug Project Research Group (1973) The Coronary Drug Project: design, methods, and baseline results. Circulation 47(Suppl I):I-1-I-50

Curran WJ, Shapiro ED (1970) Law, medicine, and forensic science, 2nd edn. Little, Brown, Boston

D'Agostino R, Sullivan LM, Massaro J (eds) (2007) Wiley encyclopedia of clinical trials, 4 vols. Wiley, New York

DeAngelis CD, Drazen JM, Frizelle FA, Haug C, Hoey J, Horton R, Kotzin S, Laine C, Marusic A, Overbeke AJPM, Schroeder TV, Sox HC, Van Der Weyden MB (2004) Clinical Trial Registration: A statement from the International Committee of Medical Journal Editors. JAMA 292:1363–1364

Fisher RA, MacKenzie WA (1923) Studies in crop variation: II. The manurial response of different potato varieties. J Agric Sci 13:311–320

Friedman LM, Furberg CD, DeMets DR (1981) Fundamentals of clinical trials, 5th edn, [2015]. Springer, New York

Haggard HW (1932) The Lame, the Halt, and the Blind: the vital role of medicine in the history of civilization. Harper and Brothers, New York

Hill AB (1937) Principles of medical statistics. Lancet

Hill AB (1962) Statistical methods in clinical and preventive medicine. Oxford University Press, New York

Levine RJ (1988) Ethics and regulation of clinical research, 2nd edn. Yale University Press, New Haven

Lind J (1753) A treatise of the scurvy (reprinted in Lind's treatise on scurvy, edited by CP Stewart, D Guthrie, Edinburgh University Press, Edinburgh, 1953). Sands, Murray, Cochran, Edinburgh

Medical Research Council (1931) Clinical trials of new remedies (annotations). Lancet 2:304

Medical Research Council (1944) Clinical trial of patulin in the common cold. Lancet 16:373–375

Medical Research Council (1948) Streptomycin treatment of pulmonary tuberculosis: a Medical Research Council investigation. Br Med J 2:769–782

Meinert CL, Tonascia S (1986) Clinical trials: design, conduct, and analysis. Oxford University Press, New York (2nd edn, 2012)

Meinert CL, Tonascia S (1998) Controlled Clinical Trials. Encyclopedia of biostatistics, vol 1. Wiley, New York, pp 929–931

National Institutes of Health (1979) Clinical trials activity (NIH Clinical Trials Committee; RS Gordon Jr, Chair). NIH Guide Grants Contracts 8 (# 8):29

National Institutes of Health (1981) NIH Almanac. Publ no 81-5. Division of Public Information, Bethesda

National Institutes of Health (2003) NIH data sharing policy and implementation guidance. http://grants.nih.gov/grants/policy/data_sharing/data_sharing_ guidance.htm

Office for Protection from Research Risks (1979) The Belmont Report. Ethical principles and guidelines for the protection of human subjects of research, 18 April 1979

Patulin Clinical Trials Committee (of the Medical Research Council) (1944) Clinical trial of Patulin in the common cold. Lancet 2:373–375

Piantadosi S (1997) Clinical trials: a methodologic perspective. Wiley, Hoboken (3rd edn, 2017)

Pocock SJ (1983) Clinical trials: a practical approach. Wiley, New York

Stewart WH (1966) Surgeon general's directives on human experimentation. https:// history.nih.gov/research/downloads/surgeongeneraldirective1966.pdf

Sutton HG (1865) Cases of rheumatic fever. Guy's Hosp Rep 11:392–428

Taichman DB, Sahni P, Pinborg A, Peiperl L, Laine C, James A, Hong ST, Haileamlak A, Gollogly L, Godlee F, Frizelle FA, Florenzano F, Drazen JM, Bauchner H, Baethge C, Backus J (2017) Data sharing statements for clinical trials: a requirement of the International Committee of Medical Journal Editors. Ann Intern Med 167(1):63–65

Tibi S (2006) Al-Razi and Islamic medicine in the 9th century; J R Soc Med 99(4): 206–207

United States Congress (103rd; 1st session): NIH Revitalization Act of 1993, 42 USC § 131 (1993); Clinical research equity regarding women and minorities; part I: women and minorities as subjects in clinical research, 1993

United States Congress (87th): Drug Amendments of 1962, Public Law 87-781, S 1522. Washington, Oct 10, 1962

Vozeh S (1995) The International Conference on Harmonisation. Eur J Clin Pharmacol 48:173–175

Waterhouse B (1800) A prospect of exterminating the small pox. Cambridge Press, Cambridge

Waterhouse B (1802) A prospect of exterminating the small pox (part II). University Press, Cambridge

Zarin DA, Ide NC, Tse T, Harlan WR, West JC, Lindberg DAB (2007) Issues in the registration of clinical trials. JAMA 297:2112–2120

Preface

The two of us have spent our professional lives doing trials; writing textbooks on how to do them, teaching about them, and sitting on advisory groups responsible for trials. We are pleased to say that over our lifetime trials have moved up the scale of importance to now where people feel cheated if denied enrollment.

Clinical trials are admixtures of disciplines: Medicine, behavioral sciences, biostatistics, epidemiology, ethics, quality control, and regulatory sciences to name the principal ones, making it difficult to cover the field in any textbook on the subject. This reality is the reason we campaigned (principally SP) for a collective work designed to cover the waterfront of trials. We are pleased to have been able to do this in conjunction with Springer Nature, both as print and e-books.

There has long been a need for a comprehensive clinical trials text written at a level accessible to both technical and nontechnical readers. The perspective is the same as that in many other fields where the scope of a "principles and practice" textbook has been defining and instructive to those learning the discipline. Accordingly, the intent of *Principles and Practice of Clinical Trials* has been to cover, define, and explicate the field in ways that are approachable to trialists of all types. The work is intended to be comprehensive, but not encyclopedic.

Boston, USA
Baltimore, USA
April 2022

Steven Piantadosi
Curtis L. Meinert
Editors

Acknowledgments

The work involved nine subject sections and appendices.

Section	Section editor	Affiliation
1 Perspectives on clinical trials	Steven N. Goodman Karen A. Robinson	Stanford University; Professor Johns Hopkins University; Professor
2 Conduct and management	Eleanor McFadden	Managing Director; Frontier Science (Scotland)
3 Regulation and oversight	Winifred Werther	Amgen; Epidemiologist
4 Bias control and precision	O. Dale Williams	Florida International University; Retired
5 Basics of trial design	Christopher S. Coffey	University of Iowa; Professor
6 Advanced topics in trial design	Babak Choodari-Oskooei Mahesh K. B. Parmar	University College London; Senior Research Associate University College London; Professor
7 Analysis	Stephen L. George	Duke University; Professor Emeritus
8 Publication and related issues	Tianjing Li	University of Colorado; Associate Professor
9 Special topics	Lawrence Friedman Nancy L. Geller	NIH:NHLBI; Retired NIH:NHLBI; Director, Office of Biostatistics Research
10 Appendices	Gillian Gresham	Cedars-Sinai Medical Center (Los Angeles); Assistant Professor

We are most grateful to the section editors in producing this work.

Thanks to Springer Nature in making this work possible.

Thanks for the guidance and council provided by Alexa Steele, editor, Springer Nature, and for the help and guidance provided by Rukmani Parameswaran and Swetha Varadharajan in shepherding this work to completion.

A special thanks to Gillian Gresham for her production of the appendices and her efforts as Senior Associate Editor.

Steven Piantadosi and Curtis L. Meinert
Editors

Contents

Volume 2

Volume 3

About the Editors

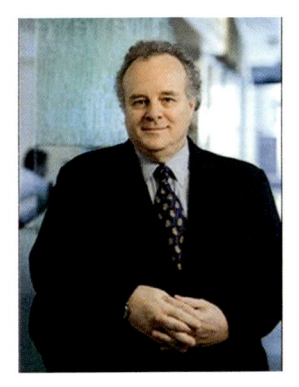

Steven Piantadosi, MD, PhD, is a clinical trialist with 40 years' experience in research, teaching, and healthcare leadership. He has worked on clinical trials of all types, including multicenter and international trials, academic portfolios, and regulatory trials. Most of his work has been in cancer; he also works in other disciplines such as neurodegenerative and cardiovascular diseases.

Dr. Piantadosi began his career in clinical trials early during an intramural Staff Fellowship at the National Cancer Institute's Clinical and Diagnostic Trials Section from 1982 to 1987. That group focused on theory, methodology, and applications with the NCI-sponsored *Lung Cancer Study Group*. Collaborative work included studies of bias induced by missing covariates, factorial clinical trials, and the ecological fallacy. In the latter years, the Branch was focused on Cancer Prevention, including design of the PLCO Trial, which would conclude 30 years later.

In 1987, Dr. Piantadosi joined the Johns Hopkins Oncology Center (now the Johns Hopkins Sidney Kimmel Comprehensive Cancer Center) as the first Director of Biostatistics and the CC Shared Resource. He also carried appointments in the Department of Biostatistics, and in the Johns Hopkins Center for Clinical Trials in the Department of Epidemiology in the School of Public Health (now the Johns Hopkins Bloomberg School). The division he founded became well diversified in cancer research and peer reviewed support, including the CCSG, 6 SPORE grants, PPGs, R01s, and many other grants. A program in Bioinformatics was begun jointly with the Biostatistics Department in Public Health, which would eventually develop into its own funded CCSG Shared Resource. The Biostatistics Division also had key responsibilities in Cancer Center teaching, the Protocol Review and Monitoring Committee, Clinical Research Office, Clinical Informatics, and Research Data Systems and Informatics.

From 1987 onward Dr. Piantadosi's work involved nearly every type of cancer, but especially bone marrow transplant, lung cancer, brain tumors, and drug development. In 1994, he helped to found the New Approaches to Brian Tumor Therapy Consortium (now the *Adult Brian Tumor Consortium*, ABTC), focused on early developmental trials of new agents. This group was funded by NCI for 25 years, was one of the first to accomplish multicenter phase I trials, and was an early implementer of the Continual Reassessment Method (CRM) for dose-finding.

Collaborations at Johns Hopkins extended well beyond the Oncology Department and included Epidemiology (Multi-Center AIDS Cohort Study), Biostatistics, Surgery, Medicine, Anesthesiology, Urology, and Neurosurgery. His work on design and analysis of brain tumor trials through the Department of Neurosurgery led to the FDA approval of BCNU-impregnated biodegradable polymers (Gliadel) for treatment of glioblastoma. He also maintained important external collaborations such as with the *Parkinson's Study Group*, based at the University of Rochester. He ran the Coordinating Center for the *National Emphysema Treatment Trial (NETT)* sponsored by NHLBI and CMS. Numerous important findings emerged from this trial, not the least of which was sharpened indications for risks, benefits, and efficacy of lung volume reduction surgery for emphysema. Dr. Piantadosi also participated actively in prevention trials such as the Alzheimer's Disease Anti-Inflammatory Prevention Trial (ADAPT) and the Chemoprevention for Barrett's Esophagus Trial, both employing NSAIDs and concluding that they were ineffective preventives. He worked with FDA, serving on the *Oncologic Drugs Advisory Committee*, and afterwards on various review panels, and as advisor to industry.

From 2007 to 2017, Dr. Piantadosi was the inaugural Director of the Samuel Oschin Cancer Institute at Cedars Sinai, a UCLA teaching hospital, Professor of Medicine, and Professor of Biomathematics and

Medicine at UCLA. Cedars is the largest hospital in the western USA and treats over 5000 new cancer cases each year, using full-time faculty, in-network oncologists, and private practitioners. Broadly applied work continued with activities in the *Long-Term Oxygen Treatment Trial* (LOTT), dose-finding designs for cancer drug combinations, neurodegenerative disease trial design, and support of the UCLA multi-campus CTSA. During this interval, numerous clinicians and researchers were recruited. Peer-reviewed funding increased from ~$1M to over $20M annually. A clinical trialist is an unusual choice for a Cancer Center director, but it represented an opportunity to improve cancer care in Los Angeles, strengthen the academics at the institution using the NCI P30 model, and serve as a role model for clinical trialists.

In 2018, Dr. Piantadosi joined the Division of Surgical Oncology at Brigham and Women's Hospital, as Professor in Residence, Harvard Medical School. Work at BWH, HMS, includes roles on the *Alliance* NCTN group Executive Committee as the Associate Group Chair for Strategic Initiatives and Innovation, as well as mentoring in the Alliance Statistics Office. He is currently course Co-director for Methods in Clinical Research at DFCI and Course Director for Advanced Clinical Trials (CI 726) in the Master of Medical Sciences in Clinical Investigation Program at Harvard Medical School.

Teaching and Education: In 1988, while at Hopkins Dr. Piantadosi began teaching Experimental Design followed by advanced Clinical Trials. This work formed the foundation for the textbook *Clinical Trials: A Methodologic Perspective*, first published in 1997 and now in its 3rd edition. His course was a staple for students in Biostatistics, Epidemiology, and the Graduate Training Program in Clinical Investigation, where he also taught a research seminar. Subsequently, he mentored numerous PhD graduate students and fellows and served on many doctoral committees. At UCLA, he continued to teach Clinical Trials in their Specialty Training and Research Program.

Dr. Piantadosi has also taught extensively in national workshops focused on training of clinical investigators in cancer, biostatistics, and neurologic disease. This began with the start of the well-known Vail Workshop, and similar venues in Europe and Australia. He was also the Director of several similarly structured courses solely for biostatisticians sponsored by AACR. Independent of those workshops, he taught extensively in Japan, Holland, and Italy.

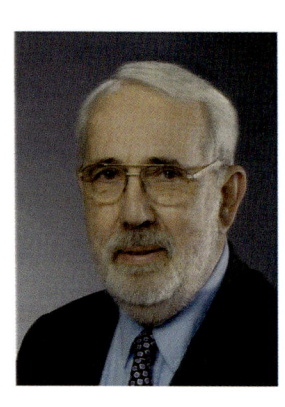

Curtis L. Meinert
Department of Epidemiology
School of Public Health
Johns Hopkins University
Baltimore, MD, USA

Professor Emeritus (Retired 30 June 2019)

I was born 30 June 1934 on a farm four miles west of Sleepy Eye, Minnesota.

My birthday was the first day of a three-day rampage orchestrated by Adolf Hitler known as the Night of the Long Knives. Ominous foreboding of events to come.

My first 6 years of schooling was in a country school located near the Chicago and Northwestern railroad line. There was no studying when freight trains got stuck making the grade past the school.

As was the custom of my parents, all four of us were sent to St John's Lutheran School in Sleepy Eye for our seventh and eighth years of schooling for modicums of religious training. After Lutheran School it was Sleepy Eye Public School, and after that it was the University of Minnesota.

Bachelor of Arts in psychology (1956)

Masters of Science in biostatistics (1959)

Doctor of Philosophy in biostatistics (1964) (Dissertation: Quantitation of the isotope displacement insulin immunoassay)

My sojourn in trials started when I was a graduate student at the University of Minnesota. It started when I signed on to work with Chris Klimt looking for someone to work with him developing what was to become the University Group Diabetes Program (UGDP).

Dr. Klimt decided to move to Baltimore in 1962 to take an appointment in the University of Maryland Medical School. He wanted me to move with him. I did, albeit reluctantly because I wanted to stay and finish my PhD dissertation.

Being Midwestern, Baltimore seemed foreign. People said we talked with an accent, but in our mind it was they who had the accents. A few days after we unpacked I told my wife we would stay a little while, but that I did not want to wake up dead in Baltimore. That surely now is my fate with all my daughters and grand children living here.

The UGDP begat the Coronary Drug Project (CDP; 1966) and it begat others.

I moved across town in 1979 to accept an appointment in the Department of Epidemiology, School of Public Health, Johns Hopkins University. The move led to classroom teaching, mentoring passels of doctoral students, several text books, and a blog site trialsmeinertsway.com.

It was Abe Lilienfeld, after I arrived at Hopkins, who rekindled my "textbook fire." I had taken a sabbatical a few years back while at Maryland to write a text on design and conduct of trials and produced nothing! The good news was that the "textbook bug" was gone – that is until Abe got a hold of me at Hopkins.

Trials became my life with the creation of the Center for Clinical Trials (now the Center for Clinical Trials and Evidence Synthesis) established in 1990 with the urging and help of Al Sommer, then dean of the school. The Center has done dozens and dozens of trials since its creation.

I lost my wife 20 February 2015. I met her at a Tupperware party on Washington's birthday in 1954. We married a year and half later. She was born and raised in Sioux Falls, South Dakota. Being 5′9″ inches tall she was happy to be able to wear her 3″ heels when we went out on the town and still be 6 in. shorter than her escort. Height has its advantages, but not when you are in the middle seat flying sardine!

I came to know Steve Piantadosi after he arrived at Hopkins in 1987. He started talking about a collective work as we are now involved in long before it had a name. For years I ignored his talk, but the "smooth talking North Carolinian" can be insidious and convincing.

So here I am, with Steve joined at the hip, trying to shepherd this work to the finish line.

About the Section Editors

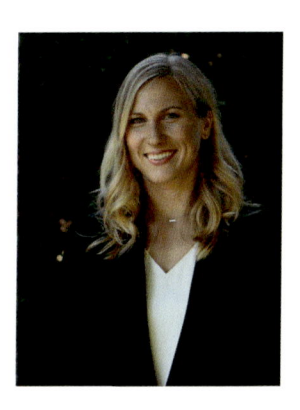

Gillian Gresham
Department of Medicine
Cedars-Sinai Medical Center
Los Angeles, CA, USA

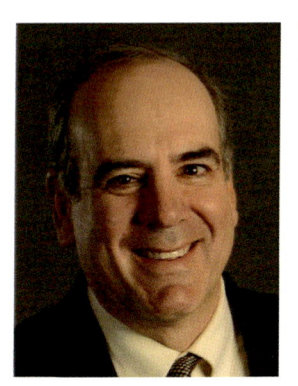

Steven N. Goodman
Stanford University School of Medicine
Stanford, CA, USA

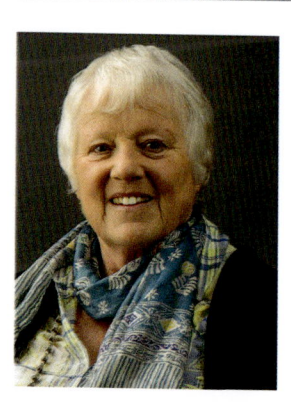

Eleanor McFadden
Frontier Science (Scotland) Ltd.
Kincraig, Scotland

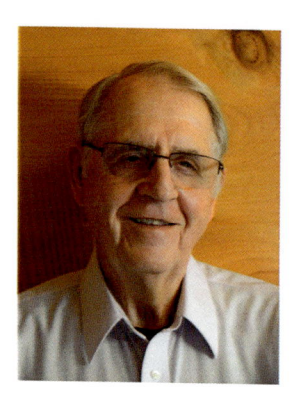

O. Dale Williams
University of North Carolina at Chapel Hill
Chapel Hill, NC, USA

University of Alabama at Birmingham
Birmingham, AL, USA

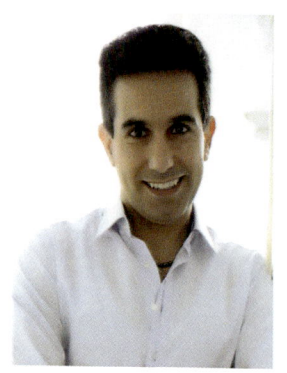

Babak Choodari-Oskooei
MRC Clinical Trials Unit at UCL
Institute of Clinical Trials and Methodology, UCL
London, UK

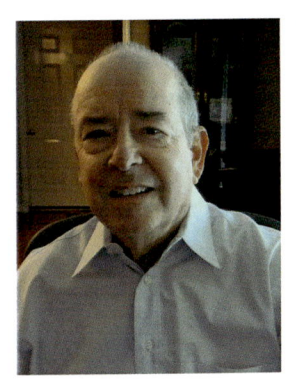

Stephen L. George
Department of Biostatistics and Bioinformatics
Duke University School of Medicine
Durham, NC, USA

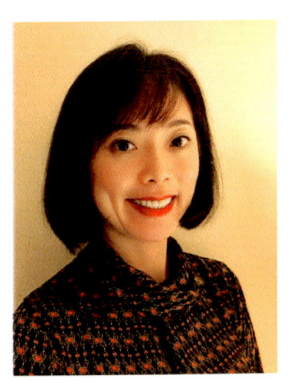

Tianjing Li
Department of Ophthalmology
School of Medicine
University of Colorado Anschutz Medical Campus
Colorado School of Public Health
Aurora, CO, USA

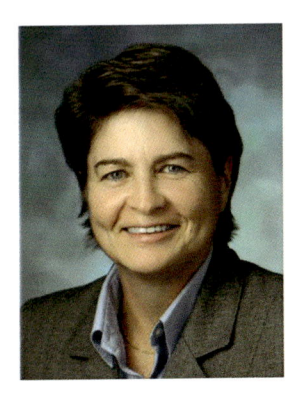

Karen A. Robinson
Johns Hopkins University
Baltimore, MD, USA

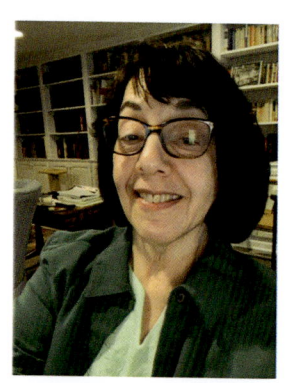

Nancy L. Geller
Office of Biostatistics Research
NHLBI
Bethesda, MD, USA

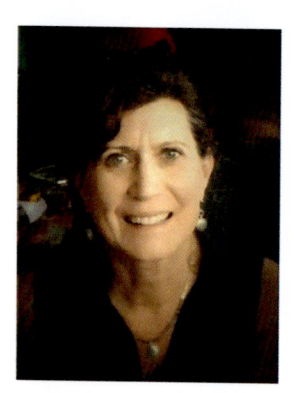

Winifred Werther
Amgen Inc.
South San Francisco, CA, USA

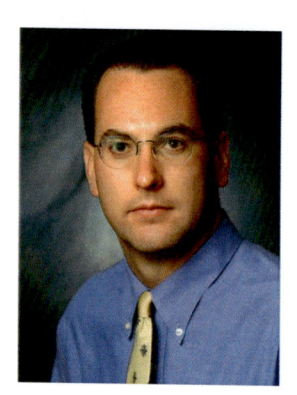

Christopher S. Coffey
University of Iowa
Iowa City, IA, USA

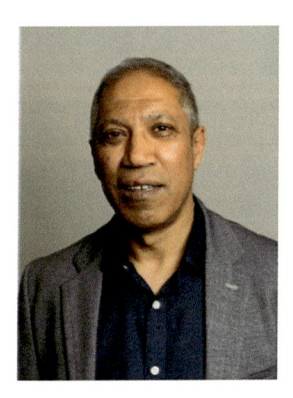

Mahesh K. B. Parmar
University College of London
London, England

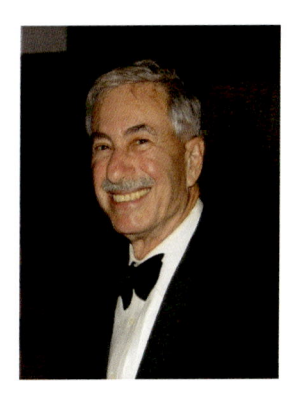

Lawrence Friedman
Rockville, MD, USA

Contributors

Inmaculada Aban Department of Biostatistics, University of Alabama at Birmingham, Birmingham, AL, USA

Trinidad Ajazi Alliance for Clinical Trials in Oncology, University of Chicago, Chicago, IL, USA

Andrew S. Allen Department of Biostatistics and Bioinformatics, Duke University, School of Medicine, Durham, NC, USA

Daniel Almirall University of Michigan, Ann Arbor, MI, USA

Suresh Ankolekar Cytel Inc, Cambridge, MA, USA
Maastricht School of Management, Maastricht, Netherlands

M. Antoniou F. Hoffmann-La Roche Ltd, Basel, Switzerland

Gillian Armstrong GSK, Slaoui Center for Vaccines Research, Rockville, MD, USA

Sheriza Baksh Johns Hopkins Bloomberg School of Public Health, Baltimore, MD, USA

Bruce A. Barton Department of Population and Quantitative Health Sciences, University of Massachusetts Medical School, Worcester, MA, USA

Emine O. Bayman University of Iowa, Iowa City, IA, USA

Vance W. Berger Biometry Research Group, National Cancer Institute, Rockville, MD, USA

Kate Bickett Emmes, Rockville, MD, USA

Lynette Blacher Frontier Science Amherst, Amherst, NY, USA

Gillian Booth Leeds Institute of Clinical Trials Research, University of Leeds, Leeds, UK

Laura E. Bothwell Worcester State University, Worcester, MA, USA

Anne-Laure Boulesteix Institute for Medical Information Processing, Biometry, and Epidemiology, LMU Munich, Munich, Germany

Isabelle Boutron Epidemiology and Biostatistics Research Center (CRESS), Inserm UMR1153, Université de Paris, Paris, France

Otis W. Brawley Johns Hopkins School of Medicine, and Johns Hopkins Bloomberg School of Public Health, Baltimore, MD, USA

L. C. Brown MRC Clinical Trials Unit, UCL Institute of Clinical Trials and Methodology, London, UK

Carolyn Burke The Emmes Company, LLC, Rockville, MD, USA

Kristin M. Burns National Heart, Lung, and Blood Institute, National Institutes of Health, Bethesda, MD, USA

Marc Buyse International Drug Development Institute (IDDI) Inc., San Francisco, CA, USA

CluePoints S.A., Louvain-la-Neuve, Belgium and I-BioStat, University of Hasselt, Louvain-la-Neuve, Belgium

Interuniversity Institute for Biostatistics and Statistical Bioinformatics (I-BioStat), Hasselt University, Hasselt, Belgium

Samantha-Jo Caetano Department of Mathematics and Statistics, McMaster University, Hamilton, ON, Canada

Steve Canham European Clinical Research Infrastructure Network (ECRIN), Paris, France

Ashley Case Emmes, Rockville, MD, USA

Anna Chaimani Université de Paris, Research Center of Epidemiology and Statistics (CRESS-U1153), INSERM, Paris, France

Cochrane France, Paris, France

Bingshu E. Chen Canadian Cancer Trials Group, Queen's University, Kingston, ON, Canada

Victoria Chia Amgen Inc., Thousand Oaks, CA, USA

Emmanuel Chigutsa Pharmacometrics, Eli Lilly and Company, Zionsville, IN, USA

Babak Choodari-Oskooei MRC Clinical Trials Unit at UCL, Institute of Clinical Trials and Methodology, London, UK

Joan B. Cobb Pettit Johns Hopkins Bloomberg School of Public Health, Baltimore, MD, USA

Graham A. Colditz Division of Public Health Sciences, Department of Surgery, Washington University School of Medicine, Saint Louis, MO, USA

Alan Colley Amgen, Ltd, Cambridge, UK

Julia Collins The Emmes Company, LLC, Rockville, MD, USA

Mark R. Conaway University of Virginia Health System, Charlottesville, VA, USA

David Couper Department of Biostatistics, Gillings School of Global Public Health, University of North Carolina, Chapel Hill, NC, USA

Gary R. Cutter Department of Biostatistics, University of Alabama at Birmingham, Birmingham, AL, USA

John J. DeBoy Covington & Burling LLP, Washington, DC, USA

James J. Dignam Department of Public Health Sciences, The University of Chicago, Chicago, IL, USA

Márcio A. Diniz Biostatistics and Bioinfomatics Research Center, Samuel Oschin Cancer Center, Cedars Sinai Medical Center, Los Angeles, CA, USA

Damien Drubay INSERM U1018, CESP, Paris-Saclay University, UVSQ, Villejuif, France
Gustave Roussy, Service de Biostatistique et d'Epidémiologie, Villejuif, France

Lea Drye Office of Clinical Affairs, Blue Cross Blue Shield Association, Chicago, IL, USA

Amylou C. Dueck Division of Biomedical Statistics and Informatics, Department of Health Sciences Research, Mayo Clinic, Scottsdale, AZ, USA

Keren R. Dunn Office of Research Compliance and Quality Improvement, Cedars-Sinai Medical Center, Los Angeles, CA, USA

Richard Emsley Department of Biostatistics and Health Informatics, King's College London, London, UK

Katrina Epnere WCG Statistics Collaborative, Washington, DC, USA

Ann-Margret Ervin Johns Hopkins Bloomberg School of Public Health, Baltimore, MD, USA
The Johns Hopkins Center for Clinical Trials and Evidence Synthesis, Johns Hopkins University, Baltimore, MD, USA

Theodoros Evrenoglou Université de Paris, Research Center of Epidemiology and Statistics (CRESS-U1153), INSERM, Paris, France

Valerii V. Fedorov ICON, North Wales, PA, USA

Bart Ferket Ichan School of Medicine at Mount Sinai, New York, NY, USA

Maria Figueroa The Emmes Company, LLC, Rockville, MD, USA

Jane Forrest Frontier Science (Scotland) Ltd, Grampian View, Kincraig, UK

Boris Freidlin Biometric Research Program, Division of Cancer Treatment and Diagnosis, National Cancer Institute, Bethesda, MD, USA

Patricia A. Ganz Jonsson Comprehensive Cancer Center, University of California at Los Angeles, Los Angeles, CA, USA

Elizabeth Garrett-Mayer American Society of Clinical Oncology, Alexandria, VA, USA

Jennifer J. Gassman Department of Quantitative Health Sciences, Cleveland Clinic, Cleveland, OH, USA

Nancy L. Geller National Heart, Lung and Blood Institute, National Institutes of Health, Bethesda, MD, USA

Stephen L. George Department of Biostatistics and Bioinformatics, Basic Science Division, Duke University School of Medicine, Durham, NC, USA

Bruce J. Giantonio The ECOG-ACRIN Cancer Research Group, Philadelphia, PA, USA

Massachusetts General Hospital, Boston, MA, USA

Department of Medical Oncology, University of Pretoria, Pretoria, South Africa

David V. Glidden Department of Epidemiology and Biostatistics, University of California San Francisco, San Francisco, CA, USA

Ekkehard Glimm Novartis Pharma AG, Basel, Switzerland

Jogarao V. Gobburu Center for Translational Medicine, University of Maryland School of Pharmacy, Baltimore, MD, USA

Judith D. Goldberg Department of Population Health and Environmental Medicine, New York University School of Medicine, New York, NY, USA

Benjamin A. Goldstein Department of Biostatistics and Bioinformatics, Duke Clinical Research Institute, Duke University Medical Center, Durham, NC, USA

Julie D. Gottlieb Johns Hopkins University School of Medicine, Baltimore, MD, USA

Stephen J. Greene Duke Clinical Research Institute, Durham, NC, USA

Division of Cardiology, Duke University School of Medicine, Durham, NC, USA

Gillian Gresham Samuel Oschin Comprehensive Cancer Institute, Cedars-Sinai Medical Center, Los Angeles, CA, USA

Jeff Jianfei Guo Division of Pharmacy Practice and Administrative Sciences, University of Cincinnati College of Pharmacy, Cincinnati, OH, USA

Gordon H. Guyatt McMaster University, Hamilton, ON, Canada

Olivia Hackworth University of Michigan, Ann Arbor, MI, USA

Tarek Haddad Medtronic Inc, Minneapolis, MN, USA

Susan Halabi Department of Biostatistics and Bioinformatics, Duke University Medical Center, Durham, NC, USA

Eric Hardter The Emmes Company, LLC, Rockville, MD, USA

Barbara S. Hawkins Johns Hopkins School of Medicine and Bloomberg School of Public Health, The Johns Hopkins University, Baltimore, MD, USA

Richard J. Hayes Faculty of Epidemiology and Population Health, London School of Hygiene and Tropical Medicine, London, UK

Adrian F. Hernandez Duke Clinical Research Institute, Durham, NC, USA

Division of Cardiology, Duke University School of Medicine, Durham, NC, USA

Sally Hopewell Centre for Statistics in Medicine, Nuffield Department of Orthopaedics, Rheumatology and Musculoskeletal Sciences, University of Oxford, Oxford, UK

George Howard Department of Biostatistics, University of Alabama at Birmingham, Birmingham, AL, USA

Asbjørn Hróbjartsson Cochrane Denmark and Centre for Evidence-Based Medicine Odense, University of Southern Denmark, Odense, Denmark

Sam Hsiao Cytel Inc, Cambridge, MA, USA

Jason C. Hsu Department of Statistics, The Ohio State University, Columbus, OH, USA

Julie Jackson Frontier Science (Scotland) Ltd, Grampian View, Kincraig, UK

Shu Jiang Division of Public Health Sciences, Department of Surgery, Washington University School of Medicine, Saint Louis, MO, USA

Byron Jones Novartis Pharma AG, Basel, Switzerland

David S. Jones Harvard University, Cambridge, MA, USA

A. L. Jorgensen Department of Health Data Science, University of Liverpool, Liverpool, UK

John A. Kairalla University of Florida, Gainesville, FL, USA

Eloise Kaizar The Ohio State University, Columbus, OH, USA

Shamir N. Kalaria Center for Translational Medicine, University of Maryland School of Pharmacy, Baltimore, MD, USA

Michael Kelsh Amgen Inc., Thousand Oaks, CA, USA

Siyoen Kil LSK Global Pharmaceutical Services, Seoul, Republic of Korea

Christopher Kim Amgen Inc., Thousand Oaks, CA, USA

Jonathan Kimmelman Biomedical Ethics Unit, McGill University, Montreal, QC, Canada

Kristin Knust Emmes, Rockville, MD, USA

Edward L. Korn Biometric Research Program, Division of Cancer Treatment and Diagnosis, National Cancer Institute, Bethesda, MD, USA

Richard Kravitz University of California Davis, Davis, CA, USA

Wen-Hua Kuo National Yang-Ming University, Taipei City, Taiwan

Sabine Landau Department of Biostatistics and Health Informatics, King's College London, London, UK

Jimmy Le National Eye Institute, Bethesda, MD, USA

Justin M. Leach Department of Biostatistics, University of Alabama at Birmingham, Birmingham, AL, USA

Michael LeBlanc SWOG Statistical Center, Fred Hutchinson Cancer Research Center, Seattle, WA, USA

J. Jack Lee Department of Biostatistics, University of Texas MD Anderson Cancer Center, Houston, TX, USA

Shing M. Lee Department of Biostatistics, Mailman School of Public Health, Columbia University, New York, NY, USA

Cheng-Shiun Leu Department of Biostatistics, Mailman School of Public Health, Columbia University, New York, NY, USA

Bruce Levin Department of Biostatistics, Mailman School of Public Health, Columbia University, New York, NY, USA

Fan Li Department of Biostatistics, Yale University, School of Public Health, New Haven, CT, USA

Heng Li Center for Devices and Radiological Health, U.S. Food and Drug Administration, Silver Spring, MD, USA

Liang Li Department of Biostatistics, The University of Texas MD Anderson Cancer Center, Houston, TX, USA

Tianjing Li Department of Ophthalmology, University of Colorado Anschutz Medical Campus, Aurora, CO, USA

Amanda Lilley-Kelly Clinical Trials Research Unit, Leeds Institute of Clinical Trials Research, University of Leeds, Leeds, UK

Yuliya Lokhnygina Department of Biostatistics and Bioinformatics, Duke University, Durham, NC, USA

James P. Long Department of Biostatistics, University of Texas MD Anderson Cancer Center, Houston, TX, USA

Anita M. Loughlin Corrona LLC, Waltham, MA, USA

Zheng Lu Clinical Pharmacology and Exploratory Development, Astellas Pharma, Northbrook, IL, USA

Tiago M. Magalhães Department of Statistics, Institute of Exact Sciences, Federal University of Juiz de Fora, Juiz de Fora, Minas Gerais, Brazil

Adrian P. Mander Centre for Trials Research, Cardiff University, Cardiff, UK

Linda Marillo Frontier Science Amherst, Amherst, NY, USA

Barbara K. Martin Administrative Director, Research Institute, Penn Medicine Lancaster General Health, Lancaster, PA, USA

J. Rosser Matthews General Dynamics Health Solutions, Defense and Veterans Brain Injury Center, Silver Spring, MD, USA

Madhu Mazumdar Director of Institute for Healthcare Delivery Science, Mount Sinai Health System, NY, USA

Gina L. Mazza Division of Biomedical Statistics and Informatics, Department of Health Sciences Research, Mayo Clinic, Scottsdale, AZ, USA

Michael P. McDermott Department of Biostatistics and Computational Biology, University of Rochester Medical Center, Rochester, NY, USA

Eleanor McFadden Frontier Science (Scotland) Ltd., Kincraig, Scotland, UK

Katie Meadmore University of Southampton, Southampton, UK

Cyrus Mehta Cytel Inc, Cambridge, MA, USA
Harvard T.H. Chan School of Public Health, Boston, MA, USA

Curtis L. Meinert Department of Epidemiology, School of Public Health, Johns Hopkins University, Baltimore, MD, USA

Catherine A. Meldrum University of Michigan, Ann Arbor, MI, USA

Sreelatha Meleth RTI International, Atlanta, GA, USA

Diana Merino Friends of Cancer Research, Washington, DC, USA

Peter Mesenbrink Novartis Pharmaceuticals Corporation, East Hannover, NJ, USA

Silvia Metelli Université de Paris, Research Center of Epidemiology and Statistics (CRESS-U1153), INSERM, Paris, France
Assistance Publique - Hôpitaux de Paris (APHP), Paris, France

Catherine M. Meyers Office of Clinical and Regulatory Affairs, National Institutes of Health, National Center for Complementary and Integrative Health, Bethesda, MD, USA

Stefan Michiels INSERM U1018, CESP, Paris-Saclay University, UVSQ, Villejuif, France

Gustave Roussy, Service de Biostatistique et d'Epidémiologie, Villejuif, France

Johanna Mielke Novartis Pharma AG, Basel, Switzerland

J. Philip Miller Division of Biostatistics, Washington University School of Medicine in St. Louis, St. Louis, MO, USA

Reza D. Mirza Department of Medicine, McMaster University, Hamilton, ON, Canada

David Moher Centre for Journaology, Clinical Epidemiology Program, Ottawa Hospital Research Institute, Canadian EQUATOR centre, Ottawa, ON, Canada

Lawrence H. Moulton Departments of International Health and Biostatistics, Johns Hopkins Bloomberg School of Public Health, Baltimore, MD, USA

Rajat Mukherjee Cytel Inc, Cambridge, MA, USA

Patrick Onghena Faculty of Psychology and Educational Sciences, KU Leuven, Leuven, Belgium

Jamie B. Oughton Clinical Trials Research Unit, Leeds Institute of Clinical Trials Research, University of Leeds, Leeds, UK

Matthew J. Page School of Public Health and Preventive Medicine, Monash University, Melbourne, VIC, Australia

Yuko Y. Palesch Data Coordination Unit, Department of Public Health Sciences, Medical University of South Carolina, Charleston, SC, USA

Olympia Papachristofi London School of Hygiene and Tropical Medicine, London, UK

Clinical Development and Analytics, Novartis Pharma AG, Basel, Switzerland

Mahesh K. B. Parmar MRC Clinical Trials Unit at UCL, Institute of Clinical Trials and Methodology, London, UK

Wendy R. Parulekar Canadian Cancer Trials Group, Queen's University, Kingston, ON, Canada

Gail D. Pearson National Heart, Lung, and Blood Institute, National Institutes of Health, Bethesda, MD, USA

Victoria L. Pemberton National Heart, Lung, and Blood Institute, National Institutes of Health, Bethesda, MD, USA

Michelle Pernice Dynavax Technologies Corporation, Emeryville, CA, USA

Julien Peron CNRS, UMR 5558, Laboratoire de Biométrie et Biologie Evolutive, Université Lyon 1, France

Departments of Biostatistics and Medical Oncology, Centre Hospitalier Lyon-Sud, Institut de Cancérologie des Hospices Civils de Lyon, Lyon, France

Gina R. Petroni Translational Research and Applied Statistics, Public Health Sciences, University of Virginia Health System, Charlottesville, VA, USA

David Petullo Division of Biometrics II, Office of Biostatistics Office of Translational Sciences, Center for Drug Evaluation and Research, U.S. Food and Drug Administration, Silver Spring, MD, USA

Patrick P. J. Phillips UCSF Center for Tuberculosis, University of California San Francisco, San Francisco, CA, USA

Department of Epidemiology and Biostatistics, University of California San Francisco, San Francisco, CA, USA

Steven Piantadosi Department of Surgery, Division of Surgical Oncology, Brigham and Women's Hospital, Harvard Medical School, Boston, MA, USA

Scott H. Podolsky Harvard Medical School, Boston, MA, USA

Gregory R. Pond Department of Oncology, McMaster University, Hamilton, ON, Canada

Ontario Institute for Cancer Research, Toronto, ON, Canada

Philip C. Prorok Division of Cancer Prevention, National Cancer Institute, Bethesda, MD, USA

Michael A. Proschan National Institute of Allergy and Infectious Diseases, Bethesda, MD, USA

Eric Riley Frontier Science (Scotland) Ltd., Kincraig, Scotland, UK

Karen A. Robinson Department of Medicine, Johns Hopkins University, Baltimore, MD, USA

Emily Robison Optum Labs, Las Vegas, NV, USA

Frank W. Rockhold Department of Biostatistics and Bioinformatics, Duke Clinical Research Institute, Duke University Medical Center, Durham, NC, USA

Sergei Romashkan National Institutes of Health, National Institute on Aging, Bethesda, MD, USA

Wayne Rosamond Department of Epidemiology, Gillings School of Global Public Health, University of North Carolina, Chapel Hill, NC, USA

William F. Rosenberger Biostatistics Center, The George Washington University, Rockville, MD, USA

Patrick Royston MRC Clinical Trials Unit at UCL, Institute of Clinical Trials and Methodology, London, UK

Estelle Russek-Cohen Office of Biostatistics, Center for Drug Evaluation and Research, U.S. Food and Drug Administration, Silver Spring, MD, USA

Laurie Ryan National Institutes of Health, National Institute on Aging, Bethesda, MD, USA

Anna Sadura Canadian Cancer Trials Group, Queen's University, Kingston, ON, Canada

Ian J. Saldanha Department of Health Services, Policy, and Practice and Department of Epidemiology, Brown University School of Public Health, Providence, RI, USA

Amber Salter Division of Biostatistics, Washington University School of Medicine in St. Louis, St. Louis, MO, USA

Marc D. Samsky Duke Clinical Research Institute, Durham, NC, USA
Division of Cardiology, Duke University School of Medicine, Durham, NC, USA

Frank J. Sasinowski University of Rochester School of Medicine, Department of Neurology, Rochester, NY, USA

Willi Sauerbrei Institute of Medical Biometry and Statistics, Faculty of Medicine and Medical Center - University of Freiburg, Freiburg, Germany

Roberta W. Scherer Department of Epidemiology, Johns Hopkins Bloomberg School of Public Health, Baltimore, MD, USA

Pamela E. Scott Office of the Commissioner, U.S. Food and Drug Administration, Silver Spring, MD, USA

Nicholas J. Seewald University of Michigan, Ann Arbor, MI, USA

Praharsh Shah University of Pennsylvania, Philadelphia, PA, USA

Linda Sharples London School of Hygiene and Tropical Medicine, London, UK

Pamela A. Shaw University of Pennsylvania Perelman School of Medicine, Philadelphia, PA, USA

Dikla Shmueli-Blumberg The Emmes Company, LLC, Rockville, MD, USA

Ellen Sigal Friends of Cancer Research, Washington, DC, USA

Ida Sim Division of General Internal Medicine, University of California San Francisco, San Francisco, CA, USA

Richard Simon R Simon Consulting, Potomac, MD, USA

Jennifer Smith Sunesis Pharmaceuticals Inc, San Francisco, CA, USA

Alfred Sommer Johns Hopkins Bloomberg School of Public Health, Baltimore, MD, USA

Mark Stewart Friends of Cancer Research, Washington, DC, USA

Inna Strakovsky University of Pennsylvania, Philadelphia, PA, USA

Oleksandr Sverdlov Novartis Pharmaceuticals Corporation, East Hannover, NJ, USA

Michael J. Sweeting Department of Health Sciences, University of Leicester, Leicester, UK

Department of Public Health and Primary Care, University of Cambridge, Cambridge, UK

Matthew R. Sydes MRC Clinical Trials Unit at UCL, Institute of Clinical Trials and Methodology, London, UK

Szu-Yu Tang Roche Tissue Diagnostics, Oro Valley, AZ, USA

Catherine Tangen SWOG Statistical Center, Fred Hutchinson Cancer Research Center, Seattle, WA, USA

Mourad Tighiouart Cedars-Sinai Medical Center, Los Angeles, CA, USA

Guangyu Tong Department of Sociology, Duke University, Durham, NC, USA

Xiao Tong Clinical Pharmacology, Biogen, Boston, MA, USA

Alison Urton Canadian Cancer Trials Group, Queen's University, Kingston, ON, Canada

Diane Uschner Department of Statistics, George Mason University, Fairfax, VA, USA

James E. Valentine University of Maryland Carey School of Law, Baltimore, MD, USA

Ben Van Calster Department of Development and Regeneration, KU Leuven, Leuven, Belgium

Department of Biomedical Data Sciences, Leiden University Medical Center, Leiden, The Netherlands

S. Swaroop Vedula Malone Center for Engineering in Healthcare, Whiting School of Engineering, The Johns Hopkins University, Baltimore, MD, USA

Jenifer H. Voeks Department of Neurology, Medical University of South Carolina, Charleston, SC, USA

Sunita Vohra University of Alberta, Edmonton, AB, Canada

Annie X. Wang Covington & Burling LLP, Washington, DC, USA

Hechuan Wang Center for Translational Medicine, University of Maryland School of Pharmacy, Baltimore, MD, USA

J. Wason Population Health Sciences Institute, Newcastle University, Newcastle upon Tyne, UK

MRC Biostatistics Unit, University of Cambridge, Cambridge, UK

Claire Weber Excellence Consulting, LLC, Moraga, CA, USA

Heidi L. Weiss Biostatistics and Bioinformatics Shared Resource Facility, Markey Cancer Center, University of Kentucky, Lexington, KY, USA

Pascale Wermuth Basel, Switzerland

Winifred Werther Center for Observational Research, Amgen Inc, South San Francisco, CA, USA

Matthew Westmore University of Southampton, Southampton, UK

Graham M. Wheeler Imperial Clinical Trials Unit, Imperial College London, London, UK

Cancer Research UK & UCL Cancer Trials Centre, University College London, London, UK

O. Dale Williams Department of Biostatistics, University of North Carolina, Chapel Hill, NC, USA

Department of Medicine, University of Alabama at Birmingham, Birmingham, AL, USA

Janet Wittes Statistics Collaborative, Inc, Washington, DC, USA

Jianrong Wu Biostatistics and Bioinformatics Shared Resource Facility, Markey Cancer Center, University of Kentucky, Lexington, KY, USA

Samuel S. Wu University of Florida, Gainesville, FL, USA

Sharon D. Yeatts Data Coordination Unit, Department of Public Health Sciences, Medical University of South Carolina, Charleston, SC, USA

Lauren Yesko Emmes, Rockville, MD, USA

Gui-Shuang Ying Center for Preventive Ophthalmology and Biostatistics, Department of Ophthalmology, Perelman School of Medicine, University of Pennsylvania, Philadelphia, PA, USA

Jessica L. Yoos University of Pennsylvania, Philadelphia, PA, USA

Qilu Yu Office of Clinical and Regulatory Affairs, National Institutes of Health, National Center for Complementary and Integrative Health, Bethesda, MD, USA

Fan-fan Yu Statistics Collaborative, Inc., Washington, DC, USA

Lilly Q. Yue Center for Devices and Radiological Health, U.S. Food and Drug Administration, Silver Spring, MD, USA

Rachel Zahigian Vertex Pharmaceuticals, Boston, MA, USA

Lijuan Zeng Statistics Collaborative, Inc., Washington, DC, USA

Xiaobo Zhong Ichan School of Medicine at Mount Sinai, New York, NY, USA

Tracy Ziolek University of Pennsylvania, Philadelphia, PA, USA

Part I

Perspectives on Clinical Trials

Social and Scientific History of Randomized Controlled Trials

1

Laura E. Bothwell, Wen-Hua Kuo, David S. Jones, and Scott H. Podolsky

Contents

L. E. Bothwell (✉)
Worcester State University, Worcester, MA, USA
e-mail: lbothwell@worcester.edu

W.-H. Kuo
National Yang-Ming University, Taipei City, Taiwan
e-mail: whkuo@ym.edu.tw

D. S. Jones
Harvard University, Cambridge, MA, USA
e-mail: dsjones@harvard.edu

S. H. Podolsky
Harvard Medical School, Boston, MA, USA
e-mail: scott_podolsky@hms.harvard.edu

© Springer Nature Switzerland AG 2022
S. Piantadosi, C. L. Meinert (eds.), *Principles and Practice of Clinical Trials*,
https://doi.org/10.1007/978-3-319-52636-2_196

Abstract

The practice and conceptual foundations of randomized controlled trials have been changed both by societal forces and by generations of investigators committed to applying rigorous research methods to therapeutic evaluation. This chapter briefly discusses the emergence of key trial elements such as control groups, alternate allocation, blinding, placebos, and finally randomization. We then explore how shifting intellectual, social, political, economic, regulatory, ethical, and technological forces have shaped the ways that RCTs have taken form, the types of therapies explored, the ethical standards that have been prioritized, and the populations included in studies. This history has not been a simple, linear march of progress. We also highlight key challenges in the historical use of RCTs and the more recent expansion of concerns regarding competing commercial interests that can influence trial design. As investigators continue to advance the rigor of controlled trials amid these challenges, exploring the influence of historical contexts on clinical trial development can help us to understand the forces that may impact trials today.

Keywords

History · Randomized controlled trial · Control groups · Fair allocation · Policy · Regulations · Ethics · Globalization · Ethnicity · Clinical trial

Introduction

Since the mid-twentieth century, clinical researchers have increasingly deployed randomized controlled trials (RCTs) in efforts to improve the reliability and objectivity of medical knowledge. RCTs have come to serve as authoritative standards of evidence for the evaluation of experimental drugs and therapies, the remuneration for medical interventions by insurance companies and governmental payers, and the evaluation of an increasingly diverse range of social and policy interventions, from educational programs to injury prevention campaigns. Yet, as researchers have increasingly relied on the RCT as an evidentiary "gold standard," critics have also identified myriad challenges. This chapter highlights and adds to historical explorations of how RCTs have come to serve such prominent roles in modern scientific (particularly clinical) knowledge, considering the intellectual, social, political, economic, regulatory, ethical, and technological contexts of this history. We also examine the history of the enduring social and scientific challenges in the conduct, interpretation, and application of RCTs.

Early History of Clinical Trials

Trials comparing intervention and control groups are as old as the historical record itself, appearing in the Hebrew Bible and in texts from various societies around the world, albeit sporadically, for centuries (Lilienfeld 1982).The tenth century

Persian physician, Abu Bakr Muhammad ibn Zakariyyaal-Razi, has been celebrated for conducting empirical experiments with control and intervention groups testing contemporaneous medical practices such as bloodletting as a prevention for meningitis (Tibi 2006). In the eighteenth century, Scottish surgeon James Lind demonstrated the efficacy of citrus fruits over five alternative treatments for scurvy among groups of sailors by following their responses to the ingested substances under controlled conditions (Milne 2012). Loosely controlled trials, often conducted by skeptics, increasingly appeared in the eighteenth and nineteenth centuries to test therapies ranging from mesmerism to homeopathy to venesection (Tröhler 2000).

These trials remained relatively scattered and dwarfed in the literature by case reports that doctors published of their experiences with individual patients. Early controlled trials had little apparent impact on therapeutic practice. Indeed, medical epistemology through the nineteenth century tended to privilege the belief that patients should be treated on an individual basis and that disease experiences were not easily comparable among different patients (Warner 1986).

However, major shifts in the social and scientific structure of medicine in the late nineteenth and early twentieth centuries created new opportunities and demands for more rigorous clinical research methods. Hospitals expanded, providing settings for more clinical researchers to compare treatment effects among numerous patients simultaneously. Germ theory and developments in physiology and chemistry provided the stimulus for researchers to produce new vaccines and drugs that had never been tested in patients. Charlatans also sought to capitalize from this wave of discovery and innovation by marketing a host of poorly tested proprietary drugs of dubious effectiveness. All these factors motivated scrupulous or skeptical clinical investigators to pursue more sophisticated approaches to evaluate experimental therapies. Simultaneously, public health researchers expanded their use of statistics, bolstering empiricism in health research overall (Bothwell and Podolsky 2016; Bothwell et al. 2016).

Among those interested in empirically testing the efficacy of remedies, the question of controlling for the bias or enthusiasm of the individual arose, along with related concerns about basing scientific knowledge on clinicians' reports of experiences with individual patients. In response, by the end of the nineteenth century, several medical societies launched "collective investigations" that amalgamated numerous practitioners' experiences using remedies among different patients. The method was employed, for example, by the American Pediatric Society in its 1896 evaluation of diphtheria antiserum, which incorporated input from 613 clinicians in 114 cities and towns and 3384 cases. The study demonstrated a 13% mortality rate among treated patients (4.9% when treated on the first day of symptoms), far below the expected mortality baseline. This contributed to the uptake of the remedy (Marks 2006). Still, some within the medical profession critiqued "collective investigation" as an insufficiently standardized research method, while numerous practicing clinicians complained that the method was a potentially elitist infringement upon their patient care prerogatives. This dynamic would prove to be an enduring tension between the clinical art of individualized patient care and an aspiration to a generalizable medical science (Warner 1991).

Refining Trial Methods in the Early Twentieth Century

As medical research overall continued to become more empirical and scientific in the early twentieth century, some researchers began to test remedies in humans much as they would in the laboratory. They began to employ "alternate allocation" studies, treating every other patient with a novel remedy, withholding it from the others, and comparing outcomes. Dozens of alternate allocation studies appeared in the medical literature in the early twentieth century (Chalmers et al. 2012; Podolsky 2015). Reflecting the major threat of infectious diseases during this era, the majority of alternate allocation trials assessed anti-infective therapies. For example, Waldemar Haffkine, Nasarwanji Hormusji Choksy, and their colleagues conducted investigations of plague remedies in India in the 1900s, German Adolf Bingel performed a double-blinded study of anti-diphtheria antiserum in the 1910s, and a series of American researchers investigated anti-pneumococcal antiserum in the 1920s. The researchers who conducted these alternate allocation trials also introduced varying degrees of statistical sophistication in their assessments of outcomes, ranging from simple quantitative comparisons and impressionistic judgments to the far rarer use of complex biometric evaluations and tests of statistical significance (Podolsky 2006, 2009).

Many researchers espoused ethical hesitations toward designating control groups in trials, as they often had more faith in the experimental treatment than the control treatment, and therefore felt that it was unethical to allocate patients to a control group. This was exemplified by Rufus Cole and his colleagues at the Hospital of the Rockefeller Institute during the development of anti-pneumococcal antiserum. After convincing themselves of the utility of antiserum based on early case series, the researchers "did not feel justified as physicians in withholding a remedy that in our opinion definitely increased the patient's chances of recovery" (Cole, as cited in Podolsky 2006). Amid a culture in medicine that tended to give clinical experimentation less emphasis than physicians' beliefs, values, and individual experiences regarding treatment efficacy, clinical trials remained overshadowed in the pre-World War II era by research based on a priori mechanistic justifications and case series, as well as laboratory and animal studies.

Despite the minimal uptake of clinical trials with control groups, however, those who saw trials as the optimal means of adjudicating therapeutic efficacy became more sophisticated in their attempts to minimize biased assessments and ensure fair allocation of patients to active versus control groups. Regarding bias, *patient* suggestibility had long been acknowledged, with numerous researchers employing sham treatments in the assessments of eighteenth- and nineteenth-century unorthodox interventions like mesmerism (in France) and homeopathy (in America, as well as in Europe) (Kaptchuk 1998; Podolsky et al. 2016). By the early decades of the twentieth century, investigators began to increasingly use sham control groups in their assessments of conventional pharmaceuticals, with Cornell's Harry Gold and colleagues using the existing clinical term "placebo" to describe such sham control remedies in their assessment of xanthines for the chest pain characteristic of angina pectoris in the 1930s (Gabriel 2014; Podolsky et al. 2016; Shapiro and Shapiro 1997).

Attempts to minimize *researcher* bias were grounded in the recognition that researchers were apt to see what they hoped or expected to find. Researchers in the late nineteenth and early twentieth century often acknowledged the presence of this "personal equation" in clinical research (Podolsky et al. 2016). Such concerns led to periodic efforts to "blind" or mask research observers as to whether or not a given subject had been exposed to an experimental agent, with the term "blinding" first appearing in the medical literature in the 1910s (Shapiro and Shapiro 1997). By the 1950s, Harry Gold formally placed concerns over both research subject suggestibility and research observer enthusiasm into the same phrase, coining the term "double-blind" and stating that "the whole history of therapeutics, especially that having to do with the action of drugs on subjective symptoms, demonstrates that the verdict of one study is frequently reversed by another unless one takes measures to rule out the psychic effect of a medication on the patient and the unconscious bias of the doctor" (Gold, as cited in Podolsky et al. 2016).

Attempts to further ensure *fair allocation* of patients to active experimental groups versus control groups with placebos or existing methods of care captured international attention. Among investigators in the United States who had conducted alternate allocation studies of anti-pneumococcal antiserum, some felt that the bias of well-intended researchers could lead to their cheating the alternation scheme (e.g., by assigning sicker patients to the active treatment group). Britain's Medical Research Council (MRC), aware of such US studies, conducted its own assessment of anti-pneumococcal antiserum by the early 1930s. And when the statistician Austin Bradford Hill was asked to evaluate this series of trials, he likewise grew suspicious of such cheating. In designing a major, groundbreaking RCT – the 1948 MRC assessment of streptomycin for tuberculosis – Bradford Hill thus replaced alternate allocation with the strictly concealed randomization of patients to treatment or control groups in order to prevent researchers from interfering with the allocation of patients. This was not the first use of randomization in a clinical trial, but it represented a turning point at which the RCT began to emerge as a major method of clinical investigation (Bothwell and Podolsky 2016; Chalmers 2005).

By the 1950s, Bradford Hill and his contemporaries implemented a number of large-scale RCTs, particularly evaluating therapies for tuberculosis. Moreover, as the post-World War II pharmaceutical industry began to produce and market a widening array of remedies ranging from antibiotics and antipsychotics to steroids and minor tranquilizers, pioneering clinical pharmacologists like Harry Gold, Henry Beecher, and Louis Lasagna joined statisticians like Bradford Hill and Donald Mainland in advocating for the need for clinical investigative rigor. They argued in multiple settings that the emerging controlled clinical trial methodology provided the best way to distinguish useful from useless novel drugs (Marks 1997, 2000).Throughout the 1950s and 1960s, formal involvement of statisticians and statistical input into design and analysis became a larger part of major pharmaceutical and clinical investigations, a key component of the "triumph of statistics" in medicine (Porter 1996; Marks 1997).

The Role of Governments in the Institutionalization of Randomized Controlled Trials

In the 1950s and 1960s, the British and US governments alike spearheaded heavy investments in academic medical research institutions. The British MRC, for instance, played a key role in the institutionalization of the controlled clinical trial (Lewontin 2008; Timmermann 2008). Academic clinical trials expanded substantially in these countries in part through this support and a political culture of investment in scientific research and institution-building in medicine (Bothwell 2014). Jonas Salk's polio vaccine trial drew broad scientific interest, as did the National Cancer Institute's clinical trial expansion (Meldrum 1998; Keating and Cambrosio 2012). As the 1950s also witnessed strong growth in industrial drug research and development, some companies collaborated with public sector researchers in devising clinical trials (Gaudilliere and Lowy 1998; Marks 1997). Some surgeons also adopted the technique, initiating a series of randomized controlled trials in the 1950s (Bothwell and Jones 2019).

Still, without a regulatory mandate to conduct rigorous trials, seemingly "well-controlled" clinical studies remained a small proportion of clinical investigations in the 1950s. For example, a 1951 study by Otho Ross of 100 articles entailing therapeutic assessment in 5 leading American medical journals found that only 27% were "well controlled," with 45% employing no controls at all (Ross 1951).

Within two decades of Ross' evaluation, however, the US Food and Drug Administration (FDA) established regulations that would dramatically shape the subsequent history of RCTs (Carpenter 2010). The US federal government had been gradually building and clarifying the FDA's power to regulate drug safety and efficacy since requiring accurate drug labeling with the Pure Food and Drug Act of 1906. As the pharmaceutical industry burgeoned in the 1950s, the scientific community and regulators observed with troubling frequency the use of unproven, ineffective, and sometimes dangerous drugs that had not been adequately tested before companies promoted their benefits. Yet the FDA lacked the necessary statutory authority to strengthen testing requirements for drug efficacy and safety. This changed following an international drug safety crisis in 1961 in which the inadequately vetted sedative thalidomide was found to cause stillbirths or devastating limb malformations among infants of women who had taken the drug for morning sickness during pregnancy (Carpenter 2010). This took place just as Senator Estes Kefauver was in the midst of extensive hearings and legislative negotiating regarding the excesses of pharmaceutical marketing and the inability of the FDA to formally adjudicate drug efficacy. Broad public concern galvanized the political support necessary in 1962 for the passage of the Kefauver-Harris amendments to the Federal Food, Drug, and Cosmetic Act. These established a legal mandate for the FDA to require drug producers to evaluate their products in "adequate and well-controlled investigations, including clinical investigations, by experts qualified by scientific training and experience to evaluate the effectiveness of the drug involved" (FDA 1963).

By 1970, after prevailing in a legal battle with Upjohn Pharmaceuticals over the methodological requirements of drug safety and efficacy studies, the FDA established that RCTs (ideally, double-blinded, placebo-controlled) should be carried out to fulfill the mandate of "adequate and well-controlled" drug studies. With this decision, the FDA formally placed RCTs at the regulatory and conceptual center of drug evaluation in America (Carpenter 2010; Podolsky 2015). While the FDA seems to have spearheaded this regulatory specification for RCTs in part as a result of a litigious culture in the American pharmaceutical industry, the global scientific and regulatory community had come to a general consensus on the public health benefits of high standards for drug trials. Regulators in Japan and the European Union soon established similar trial requirements. As it worked to comply with these regulations, the pharmaceutical industry, which had grown substantially since World War II, became a major international sponsor of RCTs (Bothwell et al. 2016). By the 1990s, industry replaced national governments as the leading funder of RCTs: governments continued to fund substantial numbers of RCTs, but the sheer volume of pharmaceutical studies led to a larger proportion of overall published RCTs reporting drug company funding than any other source. Pharmaceutical research grew more rigorous in this process, but critics also raised concerns about conflicts of interest and the shaping of biomedical knowledge through industry-sponsored trials, a problem that has persisted in different manifestations in ensuing decades (as described later in this chapter) (Bothwell 2014).

Historical Trial Ethics

New governmental policies also substantively influenced the ethical standards commonly held for RCTs. The thalidomide crisis was among a series of debacles drawing public ire over patient safety and protections in medical research. In the early to mid-1960s, Maurice Pappworth in the United Kingdom and Henry Beecher in the United States shed light on numerous ethically scandalous studies that had apparently been conducted without the informed consent of research subjects. Broad societal dismay about the lack of patient protections in clinical research prompted legislators to empower regulatory, ethical, and scientific leaders to create new policies to govern the ethics of research (Bothwell 2014; Jones et al. 2016).

For instance, in 1964, the World Medical Association, an international confederation of medical associations founded after World War II, had established the Declaration of Helsinki, including principles of informed consent and research subject protections previously outlined in the 1948 Nuremberg Code. But this Declaration lacked any enforcement mechanism. As the field of bioethics developed in the late 1960s and 1970s, growing numbers of philosophers, social scientists, and other non-clinical researchers drew further attention to ethical concerns in trials, such as reliance on vulnerable populations in research, including children, the elderly and infirm, racial minorities, prisoners, and people with disabilities. Ethicists argued that informed consent was insufficient in protecting the rights of vulnerable groups whose consent was often provided under social, economic, or physiological constraints that impeded their ability to either fully understand or freely and independently elect to participate in trials. They contended that external review of research was thus crucial to ensure that study designs were fair and informed consent would be meaningfully achieved (Bothwell 2014). Clinical research directors and investigators themselves also increasingly recognized the legal and ethical need for expanded policies on peer review of study protocol ethics (Stark 2011).

All of these concerns escalated in the early 1970s as more research scandals came to public light. Scientists, ethicists, and the public reeled when news broke of the 40-year Tuskegee study of untreated syphilis among African American men. Investigators deceived study participants and withheld treatment long after antibiotics had become available to cure the disease. In response to outcry over this tragedy, the US Department of Health and Human Services passed Title 45 Code of Federal Regulations, Part 46, in 1974, clarifying new ethical guidelines, formalizing institutional review boards, and expanding their use in clinical trials and other human subjects research. Since the United States was a leading global sponsor of RCTs at this time, these ethical requirements had a sizable impact on the conduct of RCTs overall (Bothwell 2014).

As RCT use expanded, ethicists began to clarify core challenges specifically related to randomized allocation of patients to treatments. Critics continued to raise concerns that withholding a promising treatment from patients simply in the name of methodological rigor prioritized scientific advancement over patient care. They argued that RCTs were not necessarily in the best short-term interests of patients, since patient allocation to control and intervention arms could prevent clinicians from fulfilling their obligations to administer what they believed to be promising experimental therapies to all patients (Bothwell and Podolsky 2016). Proponents of RCTs countered that randomized allocation to experimental and control groups was essential to determine whether promising experimental treatments would live up to the hopes of their proponents, or whether they would prove less effective or be accompanied by unacceptable adverse events (Bradford Hill 1963). Growing numbers of researchers favored the latter stance, and in subsequent decades, the notion was formalized as the principle of equipoise. This principle stipulated that in situations of genuine uncertainty over whether a new treatment is superior to the existing treatment, it is ethically acceptable for physicians to randomly assign patients to either control or intervention arms (Freedman 1987).

Critics of the principle of equipoise noted that investigators often did not possess a state of genuine uncertainty regarding whether an experimental treatment was preferable to an existing treatment. Rather, researchers often had a sense that the experimental treatment was favorable based on early case series or pilot studies. Responding to this ethical confusion, Benjamin Freedman proposed the more specific principle of "clinical equipoise" in 1987, stipulating that investigators may continue to randomly allocate patients to different arms in trials only when there is genuine uncertainty or honest professional disagreement among a *community* of expert practitioners as to which treatment in a trial is preferable. According to this interpretation, carefully conducted RCTs often would be necessary to determine the actual efficacy and adverse events associated with medical interventions (Freedman

1987). Most researchers now accept the rationale of clinical equipoise. Yet, among each new generation of investigators there are those with ethical hesitations about allocating trial participants to arms thought to be inferior.

RCTs and Evidence-Based Medicine

RCTs continued to expand in the closing decades of the twentieth century as part of broader trends toward more quantitative and empirical research methods in medicine. New technologies continuously broadened the evidentiary foundation from which medical knowledge could be developed. The introduction of computers into medical investigations in the 1960s and 1970s increased researchers' efficiency in collecting and processing large quantities of data from multiple study sites, facilitating the conduct of RCTs and the dissemination of trial results. Alongside the growing availability of data, critics increasingly questioned medical epistemology for relying too heavily on theory and expert opinion without evidence from controlled clinical experiments on statistically significant numbers of patients. In all fields of medicine, critics deployed RCTs to assess both new, experimental treatments and existing therapies that had become widespread despite never having been rigorously tested. Numerous RCTs revealed that popular medical interventions were ineffective or even harmful, leading to their discontinuation (Cochrane 1972).

By the early 1980s, scientists widely considered RCTs the "gold standard" of clinical research (Jones and Podolsky 2015). Large-scale multi-site RCTs grew exponentially in the published literature and were highly influential in medical knowledge and clinical research methodologies (Bothwell 2014). Academic programs also developed to explore and critique empirical research methods. In the 1990s, Canadian medical researchers Gordon Guyatt and David Sackett coined the term "evidence-based medicine" to refer to the application of current best evidence to decisions about individual patient care. Advocates of evidence-based medicine developed a pyramid illustrating a general hierarchy of research design quality, with expert opinion and case reports at the lowest level, various observational designs at intermediate levels, and RCTs at the pinnacle as the optimal study design. RCTs, in turn, could be incorporated into meta-analyses and systematic reviews. In 1993, Iain Chalmers led in the creation of the Cochrane Collaboration (now called Cochrane), an international organization designed to conduct systematic reviews by synthesizing large quantities of medical research evidence in order to inform clinical decision-making (Daly 2005). Internet expansion also facilitated wider access to information on evidence-based medicine. In 2000, the NIH established ClinicalTrials.gov, a publicly accessible online registry of clinical trials, with concomitant and now legal requirements to register trials before initiation. Recent legislation also requires the reporting of results from all registered trials on the site, regardless of outcome, so that physicians, scientists, and patients can access more complete data from unpublished trials. This has provided a counterpoint to publication bias while also allowing valuable comparisons between predefined and published trial endpoints.

The database has been a powerful tool to shift the power imbalance between those who conduct RCTs and those who use their results.

The Globalization of RCTs and the Challenges of Similarities and Differences in Global Populations

The recent history of RCTs and evidence-based medicine has been characterized in part by expanded trial globalization. This has often reflected commercial interests and has raised new ethical, political, and regulatory questions. Pharmaceutical companies want to complete increasingly demanding and complicated RCTs as quickly as possible. They have realized that they can do so by recruiting sufficient numbers of subjects on an international scale (Kuo 2008). Since the late 1970s, contract research organizations (CROs), now a multibillion-dollar annual industry, have grown to serve this demand. As for-profit entities, CROs have been broadly critiqued for questionable practices such as offshoring growing numbers of trials to middle-income countries, oftentimes studying fairly homogenous demographic groups, a move which has raised skepticism regarding their ability to measure treatment effects among diverse patients. CROs have also targeted research settings with looser regulatory oversights and weaker systems of institutional ethical review, raising concerns about the rights of research subjects. Access to a tested treatment after a trial ends has also been a critical ethical concern (Petryna 2009).

At the same time, health policymakers hope to create a harmonized regulatory platform to reduce redundant clinical trials and broaden accessibility to the latest medications for the people who need them. Policy initiatives arose in the early 1980s to address this from different perspectives and on different levels. The World Health Organization's (WHO) International Conference of Drug Regulatory Authorities (ICDRA) was the first attempt to establish common regulations to help drug regulatory authorities of WHO member states strengthen collaboration and exchange information. Other regional and bilateral harmonization efforts were motivated by commercial concerns. For example, pharmaceuticals were selected as a topic for trade negotiation at the first US-Japan Market-Oriented-Sector Selective talk in 1986 for the potential for higher sales of pharmaceuticals in Japan, then the second-largest national market in the world. It was followed by expert meetings on the technical requirements for drug approval, including RCT designs (Kuo 2005).

The International Conference on Harmonisation of Technical Requirements for Registration of Pharmaceuticals for Human Use (ICH) was created in 1990. Initially designed to incorporate Japan into global pharmaceutical markets with fewer regulatory hurdles, the ICH is a communication platform to accelerate the harmonization of pharmaceutical regulations. It started with only members from the United States, the European Union (EU), and Japan and carefully limited its working scope to technical issues. The outcomes were guidelines for safety, efficacy, quality, and drug labeling integrated into the regulations of each participating country/region after the ICH reached consensus. ICH guidelines thus further established global recognition for RCTs and helped to standardize approaches for the generation of medical evidence (Kuo 2005).

Following Japan, other East Asian states quickly recognized the importance of the ICH and began following ICH guidelines. Korea and Taiwan aggressively established sizable regulatory agencies and national centers for clinical trials. Even Japan made infrastructural changes to reform clinical trial protocols and use common technical documents (Chikenkokusaikakenkyukai [study group on the globalization of clinical trials] 2013). In 1999, the ICH founded the Global Cooperation Group (GCG) to serve as a liaison to other countries affected by these guidelines, but it did not permit policy contributions from non-ICH member regions. It was not until 2010 that the ICH opened technical working groups to active participation from experts in non-ICH member regions and countries of the ICH GCG. In addition to the founding members of Japan, the United States, and the EU, the ICH invited five additional regulatory members – Brazil, China, Korea, Singapore, and Taiwan.

The process of incorporating East Asian RCTs into ICH standards raised issues concerning the generalizability of research findings. Researchers and policymakers hoped to establish clinical trial designs and good clinical practices (GCP) that would clarify the influence of ethnic factors on any physiological and behavioral differences in trial test populations in East Asian RCTs. In the end, a technically vague concept of "bridging" was created to make sense of how to extend the applicability of clinical data to a different ethnic population by conducting additional trials with fewer subjects than originally required by local authorities (Kuo 2009, 2012). It is important to note that several ICH guidelines deal with additional differences among subjects (such as age), but the extent of these guidelines varies. For example, the ICH sets no independent guideline regarding inclusion or measurement of gender in clinical trials.

Social and Scientific Challenges in Randomized Controlled Trials

While RCTs have continued to evolve and grow more standardized and globally inclusive, social, economic, political, and internal scientific challenges have continued to complicate both the application of RCTs and the construction of evidence-based medicine (Bothwell et al. 2016; Timmermans and Berg 2003). Additionally, critics have identified the growing impact of commercial interests on the overall ecology of medical evidence. As the pharmaceutical industry has sponsored growing numbers of RCTs since the late 1960s, it has tended to sponsor trials of drugs with substantial potential for use among wealthier populations rather than prioritizing treatments that can transform global public health, such as antibiotics or vaccines for infectious diseases endemic to low-income regions (Bothwell et al. 2016). Pharmaceutical sponsors also have expanded markets by strategically deploying RCTs to establish new drug indications for existing products through trials that claim slightly new therapeutic niches, rather than developing innovative original therapies (Matheson 2017). Researchers conducting industry-sponsored trials have been critiqued for being more susceptible to bias, as comparative analyses have revealed that industry-sponsored trials are more likely to reveal outcomes favoring the product under investigation than publicly funded trials (Bourgeois et al. 2010). Critics have noted that some industry-funded researchers have designed trials in ways that are more likely to reveal treatment effects by selecting narrow patient populations likely to demonstrate favorable results, rather than patients who represent a drug's ultimate target population (Petryna 2009).

Growing interest in assessing treatments in applied clinical settings has also given rise to variations on RCTs. Pragmatic trials, which have been widely discussed and debated, have been proposed more recently as tools to examine medical interventions in the context of their application in clinical practice. Proponents have suggested that pragmatic trials would be most useful during the implementation stage of an intervention or in the post-marketing phase of drug evaluation, once phase 3 trials have been completed (Ford and Norrie 2016). Similarly, as the quantity of therapeutics has expanded over time, researchers also have increasingly conducted randomized comparative effectiveness trials using existing treatments rather than placebos in control arms of trials. The expansion of comparative effectiveness RCTs has responded to a clinical demand for more detailed information not just validating individual therapies but comparing different treatments in current use to guide clinical decision-making (Fiore and Lavori 2016).

New challenges have also emerged in relation to establishing trial endpoints. For example, trial sponsors have pursued surrogate endpoints – intermediate markers anticipated to correlate with clinical outcomes – to achieve statistically significant trial results more quickly. Such trials, however, do not generate comprehensive data on the clinical outcomes experienced by patients. These approaches have had value, such as expediting the evaluation of initial data on the effects of HIV treatments so that more patients could access promising experimental therapies more quickly (Epstein 1996). However, critics have also warned of the shortcomings of the partial data that surrogate endpoints can yield (Bothwell et al. 2016), and there have been important examples of drugs that "improved" the status of a biomarker while leading to worsened clinical outcomes (e.g., torcetrapib raised HDL levels but also increased the risk of mortality and morbidity of patients via unknown mechanisms) (Barter et al. 2007). Some advocates of trial efficiency have also promoted adaptive methods that alter trial design based on interim trial data. The US FDA has examined methodological issues in adaptive designs with their Guidance for Industry on adaptive trials, describing certain methodological challenges in adaptive designs that remain unresolved (US FDA 2018).

While academic critics have identified limitations of RCTs, drug and device industries have used these critiques for their own purposes. In recent years, some industry representatives have embraced criticism of RCTs and evidence-based medicine, seemingly with a goal of undermining major twentieth century attempts to demand clinical trial rigor in the assessment of new therapies. Decriers of regulation have contended that standards for clinical trials are unnecessarily narrow and exacting, increasing research costs and slowing the delivery of new therapies to the market. They make this argument even as other critics argue that regulators such as the FDA have approved some experimental products too rapidly and without sufficient evidence, resulting in poorer patient health outcomes (Kesselheim and Avorn 2017; Ostroff 2015). It is likely that debates over trial design and evidence standards will persist: competing interests continue to have stakes in how medical therapies are regulated and tested. Additionally, academic researchers have competing interests to publish trials with significant results when such publications are criteria for professional advancement (Calabrese and Roberts 2004).

Finally, researchers have continued to face challenges in conducting RCTs of treatments that are less amenable to controlled experimentation. While investigators have long conducted pharmaceutical RCTs comparing active pills and placebos, it has been more challenging to conduct RCTs in certain other areas of medicine, such as surgery. Surgeons, who had long espoused the goal of establishing a rational basis for surgical practice, had recognized the value of control groups in the eighteenth century and had implemented alternate allocation, and then randomization, in the twentieth century. In 1953, for instance, surgeons in New York began a study of surgical and medical management of upper GI bleeding. They began with alternate allocation but switched to randomization for the majority of the study (1955–1963) "to achieve statistically sound conclusions" (Enquist et al., as cited in Jones 2018). By the late 1950s surgeons had randomized patients to tests of many different surgical procedures (Bothwell and Jones 2019). However, RCTs have not become as influential in surgery as they have in pharmaceutical research. Part of this has been a matter of regulation: the FDA does not require RCTs before surgeons start using a new procedure (unless the new procedure relies on a new device for which the FDA deems an RCT appropriate). Surgical epistemology and methodology also pose challenges for RCTs. Since the success of an operation can often seem self-evident, surgeons have been reluctant to randomize patients between radically different modes of therapy (e.g., to a medical vs. surgical treatment for a particular problem; see Jones 2000). There are also few procedures for which surgeons can perform a meaningful sham operation, forcing many surgical trials to be done without blinding. Additionally, variations in practitioner skill can confound trial results: a surgical RCT is not simply a test of the procedure per se, but a test of the procedure as done by a specific group of surgeons whose skills and techniques might or might not reflect those of other surgeons. These challenges have limited the use of RCTs within surgery. When surgical RCTs have been performed historically, it often has not been to validate and introduce a new operation, but rather to test an existing operation which surgeons or nonsurgical physicians have begun to doubt. While RCTs remain an important part of knowledge production in surgery, surgeons have continued to rely extensively on other modes of knowledge production, including case series and registry studies. These problems are not unique to surgery. Challenges have also emerged for RCTs in other medical fields, such as psychotherapy, in which practitioners may have significant degrees of variation in treatment approaches (Bothwell et al. 2016; Jones 2018).

Summary and Conclusion

The foundations of modern RCTs run deep through centuries of thinkers, physicians, scientists, and medical reformers committed to accurately measuring the effects of medical interventions. Clinical trials have taken different forms in different historical social contexts, growing from isolated, small controlled experiments to massive multinational trials. The shifting burden of disease and the interests of trial sponsors have influenced the types of questions investigated in trials – from infectious diseases in the early twentieth century to chronic diseases, particularly those affecting wealthier populations, in contemporary society. Shifts in trial funding and regulatory and ethical policy landscapes have dramatically shaped the historical trajectory of RCTs such that trial design, study location, ethical safeguards for research subjects, investigator accountability, and even the likelihood of favorable trial results have all been influenced by political and economic pressures and contexts. This has not been a linear story of progress. Advances in trial rigor, ethics, and inclusiveness have occurred alongside the emergence of new challenges related to the commercialization of research and pressures to lower regulatory standards for evidence. Many RCTs today have grown so complex and institutionalized that persistent challenges may seem ingrained. However, the history of clinical trials offers numerous examples of how science has been dramatically transformed through the work of individuals committed to rigorous investigations over other competing interests.

Key Facts

1. The historical foundations of RCTs run deep – across time, different societies, and different contexts, investigators have endeavored to create controlled experiments of interventions to improve human health.
2. Social contexts of research – from physical trial settings to funding schemes and regulatory requirements – have significantly impacted the design and scale of trials, the types of questions asked, trial ethics, research subject demographics, and the objectives of trial investigators.
3. The history of RCTs has involved both advances and setbacks: it has not been a linear story of progress. Recent history has revealed persistent challenges for RCTs as well as expanding concerns such as commercial interests in trials that will need to be carefully considered moving forward.

Cross-References

▶ A Perspective on the Process of Designing and Conducting Clinical Trials
▶ Evolution of Clinical Trials Science
▶ Trials in Minority Populations

Permission Segments of this chapter are also published in Bothwell, L., and Podolsky, S. "Controlled Clinical Trials and Evidence-Based Medicine," in Oxford Handbook of American Medical History, ed. J. Schafer, R. Mizelle, and H. Valier. Oxford: Oxford University Press, forthcoming. With kind permission of Oxford University Press, date TBA. All Rights Reserved.

References

Barter PJ et al (2007) Effects of torcetrapib in patients at high risk for coronary events. N Engl J Med 357:2109–2112

Bothwell LE (2014) The emergence of the randomized controlled trial: origins to 1980. Dissertation, Columbia University

Bothwell LE, Jones DS (2019) Innovation and tribulation in the history of randomized controlled trials in surgery. Ann Surg. https://doi.org/10.1097/SLA.0000000000003631

Bothwell LE, Podolsky SH (2016) The emergence of the randomized, controlled trial. N Engl J Med 375:501–504

Bothwell LE, Greene JA, Podolsky SH, Jones DS (2016) Assessing the gold standard – lessons from the history of RCTs. N Engl J Med 374(22):2175–2181

Bourgeois FT, Murthy S, Mandl KD (2010) Outcome reporting among drug trials registered in clinical Trials.gov. Ann Intern Med 153:158–166

Calabrese RL, Roberts B (2004) Self-interest and scholarly publication: the dilemma of researchers, reviewers, and editors. Int J Educ Manag 18:335–341

Carpenter D (2010) Reputation and power. Princeton University Press, Princeton

Chalmers I (2005) Statistical theory was not the reason that randomisation was used in the British Medical Research Council's clinical trial of streptomycin for pulmonary tuberculosis. In: Jorland G et al (eds) Body counts. McGill-Queen's University Press, Montreal, pp 309–334

Chalmers I, Dukan E, Podolsky S, Smith GD (2012) The advent of fair treatment allocation schedules in clinical trials during the 19th and early 20th centuries. J R Soc Med 105(5). See also JLL Bulletin: Commentaries on the history of treatment evaluation. http://www.jameslin dlibrary.org/articles/the-advent-of-fair-treatment-allocation-schedules-in-clinical-trials-during-the-19th-and-early-20th-centuries/. Accessed 17 Mar 2019

Chikenkokusaikakenkyukai [Study group on the globalization of clinical trials] (2013) ICH-GCP Nabgeita: Kokusaitekishitenkaranihonnochiken wo kangaeru. (ICH-GCP navigator: considerations of clinical trials in Japan from an international perspective). Jiho, Tokyo

Cochrane AL (1972) Effectiveness and efficiency: random reflections on the health services. Nuffield Provincial Hospitals Trust, London

Daly J (2005) Evidence-based medicine and the search for a science of clinical care. University of California Press, Berkeley

Epstein S (1996) Impure science: AIDS, activism, and the politics of knowledge. University of California Press, Berkeley

Fiore L, Lavori P (2016) Integrating randomized comparative effectiveness research with patient care. N Engl J Med 374:2152–2158

Ford I, Norrie J (2016) Pragmatic trials. N Engl J Med 375:454–463

Freedman B (1987) Equipoise and the ethics of clinical research. N Engl J Med 317:141–145

Gabriel JM (2014) The testing of Sanocrysin: science, profit, and innovation in clinical trial design, 1926–1931. J Hist Med Allied Sci 69:604–632

Gaudilliere JP, Lowy I (1998) The invisible industrialist: manufactures and the production of scientific knowledge. Macmillan, London

Hill AB (1963) Medical ethics and controlled trials. Br Med J 5337:1043–1049

Jones DS (2000) Visions of a cure: visualization, clinical trials, and controversies in cardiac therapeutics, 1968–1998. Isis 91:504–541

Jones DS (2018) Surgery and clinical trials: the history and controversies of surgical evidence. In: Schlich T (ed) The Palgrave handbook of the history of the surgery. Palgrave Macmillan, London, pp 479–501

Jones DS, Podolsky SH (2015) The history and fate of the gold standard. Lancet 9977:1502–1503

Jones DS, Grady C, Lederer SE (2016) 'Ethics and clinical research' – the 50th anniversary of Beecher's bombshell. N Engl J Med 374:2393–2398

Kaptchuk TJ (1998) Intentional ignorance: a history of blind assessment and placebo controls in medicine. Bull Hist Med 72:389–433

Keating P, Cambrosio A (2012) Cancer on trial. University of Chicago Press, Chicago

Kesselheim AS, Avorn J (2017) New '21st century cures' legislation: speed and ease vs science. J Am Med Assoc 317:581–582

Kuo W-H (2005) Japan and Taiwan in the wake of bio-globalization: drugs, race and standards. Dissertation, MIT

Kuo W-H (2008) Understanding race at the frontier of pharmaceutical regulation: an analysis of the racial difference debate at the ICH. J Law Med Ethics 36:498–505

Kuo W-H (2009) The voice on the bridge: Taiwan's regulatory engagement with global pharmaceuticals. East Asian Science, Technology and Society: an International Journal 3:51–72

Kuo (2012) Transforming states in the era of global pharmaceuticals: visioning clinical research in Japan, Taiwan, and Singapore. In: Rajan KS (ed) Lively capital: biotechnologies, ethics, and governance in global market. Duke University Press, Durham, pp 279–305

Lewontin RC (2008) The socialization of research and the transformation of the academy. In: Hannaway C (ed) Biomedicine in the twentieth century: practices, policies, and politics. IOS Press, Amsterdam, pp 19–25

Lilienfeld L (1982) The fielding H. Garrison lecture: ceteris paribus: the evolution of the clinical trial. Bull Hist Med 56:1–18

Marks HM (1997) The progress of experiment: science and therapeutic reform in the United States, 1900–1990. Cambridge Univ Press, Cambridge

Marks HM (2000) Trust and mistrust in the marketplace: statistics and clinical research, 1945–1960. Hist Sci 38:343–355

Marks HM (2006) 'Until the sun of science … the true Apollo of medicine has risen': collective investigation in Britain and America, 1880–1910. Med Hist 50:147–166

Matheson A (2017) Marketing trials, marketing tricks – how to spot them and how to stop them. Trials 18:105

Meldrum ML (1998) A calculated risk: the Salk polio vaccine field trials of 1954. Br Med J 7167:1233–1236

Milne I (2012) Who was James Lind, and what exactly did he achieve? J R Soc Med 105:503–508. See also JLL Bulletin: Commentaries on the history of treatment evaluation, (2011). http://www.jameslindlibrary.org/articles/who-was-james-lind-and-what-exactly-did-he-achieve/. Accessed 30 Jan 2019

Ostroff SM (2015) 'Responding to changing regulatory needs with care and due diligence' – remarks to the regulatory affairs professional society. United States Food and Drug Administration, Baltimore

Petryna AP (2009) When experiments travel: clinical trials and the global search for human subjects. Princeton University Press, Princeton

Podolsky SH (2006) Pneumonia before antibiotics: therapeutic evolution and evaluation in twentieth-century America. Johns Hopkins University Press, Baltimore

Podolsky SH (2009) Jesse Bullowa, specific treatment for pneumonia, and the development of the controlled clinical trial. J R Soc Med 102:203–207. See also JLL Bulletin: Commentaries on the history of treatment evaluation, (2008). http://www.jameslindlibrary.org/articles/jesse-bullowa-specific-treatment-for-pneumonia-and-the-development-of-the-controlled-clinical-trial/. Accessed 17 Mar 2019

Podolsky SH (2015) The antibiotic era: reform, resistance, and the pursuit of a rational therapeutics. Johns Hopkins University Press, Baltimore

Podolsky SH, Jones DS, Kaptchuk TJ (2016) From trials to trials: blinding, medicine, and honest adjudication. In: Robertson CT, Kesselheim AS (eds) Blinding as a solution to bias: strengthening biomedical science, forensic science, and law. Academic Press, London, pp 45–58

Porter TM (1996) Trust in numbers: the pursuit of objectivity in science and public life. Princeton University Press, Ewing

Ross OB (1951) Use of controls in medical research. J Am Med Assoc 145:72–75

Shapiro AK, Shapiro E (1997) The powerful placebo: from ancient priest to modern physician. Johns Hopkins University Press, Baltimore

Stark L (2011) Behind closed doors: irbs and the making of ethical research. Univ of Chicago Press, Chicago

Tibi S (2006) Al-Razi and Islamic medicine in the 9th century. J R Soc Med 99:206–207. See also James Lind Library Bulletin: Commentaries on the History of Treatment Evaluation, (2005). http://www.jameslindlibrary.org/articles/al-razi-and-islamic-medicine-in-the-9th-century/. Accessed 17 Mar 2019

Timmermann C (2008) Clinical research in post-war Britain: the role of the Medical Research Council. In: Hannaway C (ed) Biomedicine in the twentieth century: practices, policies, and politics. IOS Press, Amsterdam, pp 231–254

Timmermans S, Berg M (2003) The gold standard: the challenges of evidence-based medicine and standardization in health care. Temple University Press, Philadelphia

Tröhler U (2000) To improve the evidence of medicine: the 18th century British origins of a critical approach. Royal College of Physicians of Edinburgh, Edinburgh

United States Food and Drug Administration (1963) Proceedings of the FDA conference on the Kefauver-Harris drug amendments and proposed regulations. United States Department of Health, Education, and Welfare, Washington, DC

United States Food and Drug Administration, Center for Drug Evaluation and Research, Center for Biologics Evaluation and Research (2018) Adaptive design clinical trials of drugs and biologics: guidance for industry (draft guidance). In: United States Department of Health. Education, and Welfare, Rockville

Warner JH (1986) The therapeutic perspective: medical practice, knowledge, and identity in America, 1820–1885. Harvard University Press, Cambridge, MA

Warner JH (1991) Ideals of science and their discontents in late nineteenth-century American medicine. Isis 82:454–478

Evolution of Clinical Trials Science

2

Steven Piantadosi

Contents

Abstract

The art of medicine took two millennia to establish the necessary groundwork for clinical trials which embody the scientific method for making fair comparisons of treatments. This resulted from a synthesis of opposing approaches to the acquisition of knowledge. Establishment of clinical trials in their basic form in the last half of the twentieth century continues to be augmented by advances in disparate fields such as research ethics, computerization, research administration and governance, and statistics.

Keywords

Design · Design evolution

S. Piantadosi (✉)
Department of Surgery, Division of Surgical Oncology, Brigham and Women's Hospital, Harvard Medical School, Boston, MA, USA
e-mail: spiantadosi@bwh.harvard.edu

© Springer Nature Switzerland AG 2022
S. Piantadosi, C. L. Meinert (eds.), *Principles and Practice of Clinical Trials*,
https://doi.org/10.1007/978-3-319-52636-2_198

Introduction

Clinical trials have been with us for about 80 years, using the famous sanocrysin tuberculosis trial as the dawn of the modern era (Amberson et al. 1931). Trials have evolved in various applications and in response to pressures from regulation, ethics, economics, technology, and the changing needs of therapeutic development. Clinical trials are dynamic elements of scientific medicine and have never really been broken, though nowadays everyone seems to know how to fix them.

Neither the science nor the art of trials is static. Perhaps they may eventually be replaced by therapeutic inferences based on transactional records from the point of care, as some people expect. However, most of us who do trials envision only their relentless application. Evolution of clinical trials manifests in components such as organization, technology, statistical methods, medical care, and science (Table 1). Any of these topics is probably worthy of its own evolutionary history.

Every trialist would have their own list of the most important developments that have aided the scope and validity of modern clinical trials. In this discussion I take for granted and omit three mature experiment design principles covered elsewhere in this book: control of random variation using replication, bias control using randomization and masking, and control of extraneous effects using methods such as

Table 1 Evolutionary advancements that have led to improvements in how clinical trials are performed

Area of advancement	Example improvements
Organization	Multicenter management Institutional review boards Data and safety monitoring boards
Ethics and regulation	Ethics standards Evidentiary standards International harmonization
Technology	Computers Analysis software Data systems
Statistical methods	Randomization Survival analysis Missing data methods
Medical care	Imaging Diagnostics Targeted therapeutics
Biological science	Risk and prognosis Pharmacology and drug action Genomic markers
Reporting	Registries Reporting guidelines Meta-analyses
Hybrid	Wearable devices Point of care data Artificial intelligence

placebos, blocking, and stratification. Statisticians have taken these as axioms to be applied consistently since from the beginning of experiment design such as in the early work of Fisher (Fisher 1925).

Maturation of the scientific method was an evolutionary prerequisite for clinical trials. It is equivalent to reconciling dogmatism (rationalism) and empiricism, two opposing philosophies from history. The first part of this chapter discusses why that reconciliation is a bedrock of clinical trials. The second part focuses on some more recent developments that have boosted our ability to conduct clinical trials atop the infrastructure of the scientific method, including ethics, governance models, computerization, multicenter collaborations, and statistical advances. The purpose is to illustrate catalysts for advancement of the science, but not to describe them comprehensively.

Improvements often arrive bundled with counterproductive ideas. Burdensome privacy regulations may be an example, as were required representation in trial cohorts, complex adaptive designs, and centralized institutional review boards (IRB). Scientists tend to view new as better, but even the best intentionally designed improvements carry imperfections. Nearly every such improvement in recent decades makes trials harder and more expensive to perform.

Prior incremental improvements have similarly been bundled, with good ideas emerging in settings or from individuals also holding bad ones. History did not design trials from first principles but gave single methodologic suggestions intermittently. How else can you create something you don't yet understand?

Synthesis of theory (established knowledge) with data is the scientific method. Theory supports the construction of useful biological hypotheses and the paradigm by which they are evaluated. Science relies equally on empirical knowledge derived from data to provide evidence regarding the hypotheses. The ability of data designed for the purpose to disprove hypotheses (falsifiability) is characteristic of the scientific method according to Popper (1959). Clinical trials embody the required interplay between theory, hypotheses, and data.

Cooperation between empirical data and theoretical reasoning synthesizes two trends from history. Rationalism is one trend that itself evolved from dogmatism. Empiricism which disregarded theory in opposition to dogmatism is the other trend. Either approach to knowledge in isolation does not constitute a scientific method. For example, both "empiric" and "dogmatic" continue to be used as pejorative labels. The method of scientific medicine emerges when the contrasting philosophies are joined. Clinical trials could not exist until these two modes of thought learned to collaborate in the experimental method.

The Scientific Method

After Hippocrates, two rival schools of Greek medicine arose, both finding justification in his writings and teachings. One was the Dogmatist (later the rationalist) school, with philosophical perspectives strengthened by the teachings of Plato and Aristotle. Medical doctrines of Diocles, Praxagoras, and Mnesitheus helped to form it (Neuburger 1910). The Dogmatist view of diagnosis and therapeutics was based on pathology and anatomy and sought causes for illness.

The empiric school of medicine arose between 270 and 220 B.C. largely as a reaction to the rigid components of Dogmatist teachings, with underpinnings founded in Skeptic philosophers. Empiric medical doctrines followed the teachings of Philinus of Cos, Serapion of Alexandria, and Glaucias of Nicomedia (Neuburger 1910). Empirics used a "tripod" in their approach to treatment: 1) their own experience (autopsia), 2) knowledge obtained from the experience of others (history), and 3) similarity with other conditions (analogy). A fourth leg was later added to the tripod: 4) inference of previous conditions from present symptoms (epilogism) (Neuburger 1910; Robinson 1931).

Empirics taught that the physician should reject theory, speculation, abstract reasoning, and the search for causes. Physiology and pathology of the time were held in low esteem, and books were written opposing rationalist anatomical doctrines. Thus, empirics were guided almost entirely by experience (King 1982; Kutumbiah 1971). Regarding the search for causes, Celsus (25 B.C.–A.D. 50) stated clearly the empiricist objections:

> Those who are called "empirici" because they have experience, do indeed accept evident causes as necessary; but they contend that inquiry about obscure causes and natural actions is superfluous, because nature is not to be comprehended ... Even in its beginnings, they add, the art of medicine was not deduced from such questionings, but from experience. ... It was afterwards, ... when the remedies had already been discovered, that men began to discuss the reasons for them: the art of medicine was not a discovery following upon reasoning, but after the discovery of the remedy, the reason for it was sought out. (Celsus 1809)

The two components of modern scientific reasoning were separated forcefully in these schools. The two schools of medicine coexisted into the second century when dogmatism (rationalism), embodied by Galen (131–200 A.D.), became dominant. Empiricism nearly died out in the third century, even becoming a disreputable term, and Galen's teachings formed the basis for most western medicine until the sixteenth century. Empiricism was frowned upon in the Middle East as well. For example, Avicenna (980–1037) wrote:

> But truly every science has both a speculative and a practical side. So has medicine. ... When, in regard to medicine, we say that practice proceeds from theory, we do not mean that there is one division of medicine by which we know, and another, distinct therefrom, by which we act. We mean that these two aspects belong together - one deals with the basic principles of knowledge; the other with the mode of operation of these principles. The former is theory; the latter is applied knowledge. (Gruner 1930)

Maimonides wrote in the twelfth century:

> The mere empiricists who do not think scientifically are greatly in error. ... He who puts his life in the hands of a physician skilled in his art but lacking scientific training is not unlike the mariner who puts his trust in good luck, relying on the sea winds which know no science to

steer by. Sometimes they blow in the direction the seafarer wants them to blow, and then his luck shines upon him; another time they may spell his doom. (Muntner 1963)

Rationalist ideas were adopted more broadly in science and the mariner metaphor was a popular one. For example, Leonardo da Vinci (1452–1519) defended the value of theory in scientific thinking by saying:

Those who are enamored of practice without science are like a pilot who goes into a ship without rudder or compass and never has any certainty where he is going. Practice should always be based on a sound knowledge of theory. (da Vinci 1510)

Even so, empiricism was not dead. Theophrastus Bombastus of Hohenheim (Paracelsus) (1493–1541) challenged the existing medical dogma in the early 1500s, literally burning the writings of Galen and Avicenna, and taught that experience with treatments should be the source of knowledge regarding their application (Pagel 1982). The experience of other practitioners was also a worthy source of knowledge. Empiricism was strengthened by thinkers such as Francis Bacon (1561–1626) and J.B. van Helmont (1578–1644). However, the empirics ignored new knowledge or subordinated it to experience, thereby becoming less able to deal with the emerging basic sciences. In contrast, seventeenth-century rationalists such as Rene Descartes (1596–1650), H. Boerhaave (1668–1738), and others adopted new knowledge in anatomy, physiology, and chemistry as a basis for causes of disease.

The dialectic between empiric and rationalist thinking has continued since the seventeenth century. Polemic essays of Thomas Percival (Percival 1767) provide an interesting debate between both positions as an educational device for readers. Percival was the originator of the first code of medical ethics (Editorial 1965; Percival 1803). He appears to be a rationalist who overstated the criticisms of rationalism to make it look better – praising with faint damns. In favor of empiricism, he states:

It is evident that theory is absurd and fallacious, always useless and often in the highest degree pernicious. The annals of medicine afford the most striking proof, that it hath in all ages been the bane and disgrace of the healing art.

In the next essay favoring rationalism, Percival states:

And by thus treading occasionally in unbeaten tracks [the rationalist] enlarges the boundaries of science in general and adds new discoveries to the art of medicine. In a word, the rationalist has every advantage which the empiric can boast, from reading, observation and practice, accompanied with superior knowledge, understanding, and judgment.

By the twentieth century, the scientific method had embraced rationalism and its response to new knowledge in the physical and biological sciences. The development of basic biological science both contributed to and was supported by the rationalist tradition. Clinical medicine remained somewhat more empirical, but increasingly influenced by the scientific method. Abraham Flexner (1866–1959), who was influential in shaping medical education in the USA, recognized the strengths of theory, the usefulness of the scientific method in medicine, and the dangers of purely empiric thinking when he wrote:

> The fact that disease is only in part accurately known does not invalidate the scientific method in practice. In the twilight region probabilities are substituted for certainties. There the physician may indeed only surmise, but, most important of all, he knows that he surmises. His procedure is tentative, observant, heedful, responsive. Meanwhile the logic of the process has not changed. The scientific physician still keeps his advantage over the empiric. He studies the actual situation with keener attention; he is freer of prejudiced prepossession; he is more conscious of liability to error. Whatever the patient may have to endure from a baffling disease, he is not further handicapped by reckless medication. In the end the scientist alone draws the line accurately between the known, the partly known, and the unknown. The empiricist fares forth with an indiscriminate confidence which sharp lines do not disturb. Investigation and practice are thus one in spirit, method, and object. (Flexner 1910)

and

> Modern medicine deals, then, like empiricism, not only with certainties, but also with probabilities, surmises, theories. It differs from empiricism, however, in actually knowing at the moment the logical quality of the material which it handles. ... The empiric and the scientist both theorize, but logically to very different ends. The theories of the empiric set up some unverifiable existence back of and independent of facts ... the scientific theory is in the facts, summing them up economically and suggesting practical measures by whose outcome it stands or falls. (Flexner 1910)

This last quote may seem somewhat puzzling because it states that empirics do, in fact, theorize. However, as the earlier quote from Celsus suggested, the theories of the empiric are not useful devices for acquiring new knowledge.

There is no sharp demarcation when rationalist and empiricist viewpoints became cooperative and balanced. The optimal mixture of these philosophies continues to elude some applications even in clinical trials. R.A. Fisher's work on experimental design (Fisher 1925) might be taken as the beginning of the modern synthesis because it placed statistics on a comparable footing with the maturing biological sciences, providing for the first time the tools needed for the interoperability of theory and data. But the modern form of clinical trials would take another 25 years to evolve.

Biological and inferential sciences have synergized and co-evolved since the middle of the twentieth century. The modern synthesis has yielded great understanding of disease and effective treatments, in parallel with appropriate methods of evaluation. Modern understanding of disease and treatment are flexible enough to accommodate such diverse contexts as molecular biology, chronic disease, psychosocial components of illness, infectious organisms, quality of life, and acupuncture. Modern inferential science, a.k.a. statistics, is applied universally in science. The scientific method can reject theory based on empirical data but can also reject data based on evidence of poor quality, bias, or inaccuracy. An interesting exception to this implied order is the elaborate justification for homeopathy based on empiricism, for example, by Coulter (1973, 1975, 1977). It illustrates the ways in which the residual proponents of purely empirical practices justify them and why biological theory is a problem for such practices.

Some Key Evolutionary Developments

In the remainder of this chapter, we look beyond the historical trends that converged to allow scientific medicine to evolve. Clinical trials have both stimulated and benefitted from key developments in the recent 80 years. These include ethics, governance models, computerization, multicenter collaborations, and statistical advances.

Ethics

Key landmarks in the history of ethics behind biomedical research are well known to clinical trialists because it is a required part of their research training. Historical mistakes have led to great awareness and mechanisms for the protection of research subjects.

With respect to clinical trials specifically, we might take the evolutionary steps in ethics to be Nuremberg, Belmont, and data and safety monitoring boards (DSMB). Some might take a more granular view of ethics landmarks, but this short list has proved to be beneficial to clinical trials. The foundational importance of Nuremberg and Belmont needs no further elaboration here. DSMBs are important because they operationalize some of the responsibilities in institutional review boards (IRB) which otherwise could be overwhelmed without delegating the work of detailed interim oversight.

Ethics principles can be in tension with one another. Resolution of those tensions is part of the evolution of ethics in clinical trials. A good example in recent years has been the debate over content and wording of the Helsinki Declaration regarding the proper use of placebo control groups (Skierka and Michels 2018). Another evolutionary step might be visible in the growing use of "central" IRBs. They are strongly motivated by efficiency but essentially discard the "institutional" local spirit of IRBs as originally chartered.

The modern platform for clinical trials would not exist without public trust founded on ethics principles and review and the risk-benefit protections it affords participants. Ethics is therefore as essential as the underlying biomedical knowledge and clinical trials science.

Governance Models

Multicenter clinical trial collaborations are common today. Their complexity has help improve the management of all trials. They were not as feasible in the early history of clinical trials because they depend on technologies like data systems, rapid communications, and travel that have improved greatly in the last 80 years. Aside from technologies, administrative improvements have also made them feasible. The multicenter model of trial management is not monolithic. Some such collaborations are relatively stable such as the NCI National Clinical Trials Network (NCTN) which has existed in similar form for decades, even following its "reorganization" in the last decade. Other collaborations are constituted de novo with each major research question. That model is used often by the NHLBI and many commercial entities.

Infrastructure costs are high, and a multicenter collaboration must have an extensive portfolio to make the ongoing investment worthwhile. This has been true of cancer clinical trials for many years. Multicenter collaborations overcome the main shortcoming of single-institution trials which is low accrual. They add broad investigator expertise at the same time. The increased costs associated with them are in governance, infrastructure, and management.

The governance model for multicenter projects relies on committees rather than individuals, aside from a Principal Investigator (PI) or Co-PIs. For example, there may be Executive (small) and Steering (larger) Committees. Other efforts scale similarly such as data management, pathology or other laboratory review, publication, and biostatistics. See Meinert (2013) for a concise listing of committee responsibilities. Multicenter collaborations seem to function well even when the various components are geographically separate largely due to advances in computerization.

Computerization

Several waves of computer technology have washed over clinical research in the last 50 years. The first might be described as the mainframe era, during which data systems and powerful and accessible statistical analysis methods began, both of which yielded great benefit to clinical trials. The idea that much could be measured and stored in databases suggested to some in the 1960s and 1970s that designed experiments might be replaced by recorded experience. In fact, data system technology probably did more to advance clinical trials than was appreciated at the time. Even so, the seemingly huge volume and speed of data storage in the mainframe era was trivial by today's standards.

Microcomputers and their associated software comprised the next wave. They created decentralized computing, put unprecedented power in individual hands, and led to the Internet. These technologies allowed breakthroughs in data systems and communication which also greatly facilitated clinical trials. In this period, many commercial sponsors realized the expense of maintaining clinical trial support infrastructure in-house. Those support services could be outsourced more economically to specialist contract research organizations (CROs). This model appears to accomplish the dual aims of maintaining skilled support but paying only for what is needed at the appropriate time.

A third era is occurring presently and might be described as big data or big computation. Increasing speed, storage, computing power, and miniaturization parallels a therapeutic focus on the individual patient. Rapid data capture and transfer of images, video, and genomic data is the rule. Miniaturization is leading to wearable or even ingestible sensors. A major problem now is how to store, summarize, and analyze the huge amount of data available. These developments are changing the course of clinical trials again. Designs can be flexible and their performance tested by simulation. Outcomes can be measured directly rather than reported or inferred. Trials can incorporate individual markers before, during, and after treatment.

Some are expecting a fourth wave of computerization, which might be called true interoperability of data systems. Lack of interoperability by design can be seen in the ubiquitous need for human curation of data sources to meet research needs. As good as they can be, case report forms (CRFs) for clinical trials illustrate the problem. Unstructured data sources must be curated in CRFs to render them computable. Even when data sources are in electronic form, most are not interoperable. This potential wave of computerization will be described below in a brief discussion of the future.

Statistical Advances

Statistics like all other fields of science has made great progress in the last 80 years in both theory and application. Statistics is not a collection of tricks and techniques but is the science of making reliable inferences in the presence of uncertainty. It is our only tool to do so. For that reason, it has found application in every discipline. One might reasonably claim today that there is no science without the integration of statistical methods. The history of statistics has been fleshed out, for example, by Stigler (1980, 1986, 1999), Porter (1986), and Marks (1997).

Statistics is not universally viewed as a branch of mathematics, but probability, upon which statistics is based, is. However, statistics uses the same methods of deductive reasoning and proof as in mathematics. Statistics and mathematics live together in a single academic department in many universities, for example.

Clinical trials and experimental design broadly have stimulated applied statistics and are a major application area. Especially in the domain of data analyses, trials have derived enormous benefit from advances in both statistical theory and methods. The modern wave of "data scientists" may not realize that fundamental tools such as censored data analysis and related nonparametric tests, proportional hazards and similar nonlinear regression methods, pharmacokinetic modeling, bootstrapping, missing data methods, feasible Bayesian methods, fully sequential and group sequential methods, meta-analysis, and dozens of other major advances have come during the era of the modern clinical trial.

Aside from the solid theoretical foundations for these and other methods, computer software and hardware advances have further supported their universal implementation. Procedure-oriented languages evolved in this interval and have moved from mainframes to personal computers while making the newest statistical methods routine components of the language. Importantly all those languages have integrated methods for data *transformations* aside from methods for data *analyses*. Clinical trials could not have their present form without these technological advances. For example, consider a single interim analysis on a large randomized trial as reviewed by the DSMB. The data summaries of treatment effects, multiple outcomes, and formal statistical analyses could not take place in the narrow time windows required without the power of the methods and technologies listed.

A byproduct of both computerization and analysis methods is data integration. This means the ability to assemble disparate sources of data, connect them to facilitate analysis, and show the results of those analyses immediately. Although impressive, clinical trials like many other research applications have minimal need for up to the minute data analysis. Snapshots that are days or weeks old are typically acceptable for research purposes. Live surveys of trial data could be useful in review of data quality or side effects of treatment.

A Likely Future

This collective work is intended to assist the science of clinical trials by defining its scope and content. Much progress necessary in the field remains beyond what scholars can write about. For example, clinical trials still do not have a universal academic home. One must be found. The biostatistics elements of the field have been found in Public Health for 100 years. Biostatisticians have contributed to Public Health so well that most academic institutions function as though that discipline should be present *only* in Public Health. Often the view is reciprocated by biostatisticians inside Public Health who think they must own the discipline everywhere. The result is that there is little biostatistics formally in therapeutic environments despite the huge need there.

Aside from this, biostatistics is not the only component of clinical trials. Training, management, infrastructure, and various clinical and allied sciences are also essential. Where does trial science belong in the academic setting? The answer is not perfectly clear even after 80 years of clinical trials. Options might include departments with various names such as clinical investigation, quantitative science, or medical statistics. In any case, clinical trial science cannot be kept at a distance organizationally and still expect these collaborations to function effectively.

The immediate future of medicine emphasizes economic value. There can be no conversation regarding value unless we also understand efficacy, which is the domain of clinical trials. Organizations that either conduct or consume efficacy evidence to provide high value medical care need internal expertise in clinical trials. Without it, they cannot participate actively in understanding value. It seems likely that this need will be as important in the future as any particular clinical or basic science.

Despite historical progress in computerization, we lack true interoperability of medical records. Electronic health records (EHR) seem to be optimistically misunderstood by the public and politicians alike, who view them as solutions to many problems that realistically have not been solved yet. EHRs are essentially electronic paper created to assist billing, and they have only parchment-like interoperability.

EHRs, like paper, can be sent and read by new caregivers, but this constitutes the lowest form or interoperability. Much of the data contained is unstructured and useless for research without extensive and expensive human curation – hence the need for CRFs. We also know that skilled humans curate EHRs imperfectly, so we can't expect augmented intelligence or natural language processing to fix this problem until EHRs improve. Lack of data model standardization is a major hurdle on that evolutionary path.

Despite the current research-crushing limitations of EHRs, many people have begun to talk about "real-world" data, evidence, or trials which are derived from those sources. This faddish term has a foothold but is bad for several reasons. It implies that 80 years of clinical trials have somehow not reflected practical findings or benefits, which is contrary to the evidence. It also implies that use of EHRs that contain happenstance data, i.e., not designed for purpose, will suffice for therapeutic inferences. This has not been true in the past and remains unproven for current ambitions. In any case, a less catchy but more accurate term is "point of care," indicating data recorded in source documents when and where care is delivered compared to secondary or derived documents like CRFs.

When EHRs evolve to hold essential structured data, data models become standardized, and point of care data become available in adequate volume and quality to address research queries across entire healthcare systems; some questions badly addressed by current clinical trials can be asked. These include what happens in subgroups of the population not represented well in traditional clinical trials, how frequent are rare events not seen in relatively small experimental cohorts, and what outcomes are most likely in lengthy longitudinal disease and complex treatment histories that require multiple changes in therapy. We cannot yet know if we will get accurate answers to these and similar questions using point of care data simply because the inferences will be based on uncontrolled or weakly controlled comparisons.

Final Comments

Clinical trials are quintessential science. They hardwire the scientific method in their design and execution and demand cooperation between theory and data. Trials evolved as science inside science only after rationalism and empiricism began to cooperate and following necessary advances in both statistical theory and biological understanding of disease.

A populist view of science and medicine is that investigative directions are substantially determined by whoever is doing the research. This makes it subject to personal or cultural biases and justifies guidance by political process. While some science is investigator initiated (which does not escape either peer review, sponsor oversight, or accountability), the truth is that science and medicine are obviously guided mostly by economic concerns. Government sponsorship places funding in topic areas that are pursued by scientists. Much research is sponsored by commercial pharmaceutical and device companies, themselves guided nowadays almost solely by marketing considerations. Government allocation of resources is subject to the political process and advocacy and sometimes by personal experiences of lawmakers.

Today, it is not possible to deny the rationalist or scientific nature of medicine or the power of biological theory in understanding disease. We may choose not to use the full power of this method because of constraints such as inefficiency, cost, lack of humanism, or political correctness, but that does not refute the greater usefulness of scientific compared with either dogmatic or empirical thinking. The failure to use well-founded, coherent biological theory can also encourage fraudulent or questionable treatment practices in medicine.

Purely empirical perspectives and their consequences on clinical trials are not without supporters and apologists in the scientific community. History shows us that this is likely to remain true in the future. Claude Bernard was not warm to the application of statistical methods in his day, but likely correct when he said:

> Medicine is destined to escape empiricism little by little, and it will escape in the same way as all the other sciences, by the experimental method. (Bernard 1865)

Key Facts

Clinical trials are an evolving science. Their appearance as a method of scientific medicine depended on a long reconciliation of two competing themes in science – dogmatism and empiricism. The basic tools of designed data production that embody clinical trials have been supplemented in modern times by codification of ethics norms, governance models for complex investigations, multicenter collaborations, advances in computer technology, and improved statistical methods. It is unlikely that therapeutic comparisons provided by clinical trials in their foundational form can be replaced by those based on transactional data.

Cross-References

▶ Leveraging "Big Data" for the Design and Execution of Clinical Trials
▶ Multicenter and Network Trials
▶ Responsibilities and Management of the Clinical Coordinating Center
▶ Social and Scientific History of Randomized Controlled Trials

References

Amberson JB, McMahon BT, Pinner M (1931) A clinical trial of sanocrysin in pulmonary tuberculosis. Am Rev Tuberc 24:401–435
Anon. Editorial (1965) Thomas Percival (1740-1804) codifier of medical ethics. JAMA 194(12): 1319–1320
Bernard C (1865) Introduction a l'Etude de la Medicine Experimentale. J. B. Bailliere et Fils, Paris

Celsus AC (1809) De Medicina. Blackwood and Bryce, Edinburg. Section translated by W. G. Spencer and quoted in Strauss, M. B. (Ed.) (1968). Familiar Medical Quotations. Boston: Little Brown and Company

Coulter HL (1973) Divided legacy. A history of the schism in medical thought. Vol. III, science and ethics in American medicine: 1800–1914. McGrath Publishing Co, Washington, DC

Coulter HL (1975) Divided legacy. A history of the schism in medical thought. Vol. I, the patterns emerge: Hippocrates to Paracelsus. Wehawken Book Co, Washington, DC

Coulter HL (1977) Divided legacy. A history of the schism in medical thought. Vol. II, Progress and regress: J. B. van Helmont to Claude Bernard. Wehawken Book Co, Washington, DC

da Vinci L (c.1510) Manuscript G, Library of the Institut de France (translated by Edward MacCurdy in The Notebooks of Leonardo da Vinci, vol II, Chap XXIX)

Fisher RA (1925) Statistical methods for research workers. Oliver and Boyd, Edinburgh

Flexner A (1910) Medical education in the United States and Canada. Merrymount Press, Boston, p 53

Gruner OC (1930) A treatise on the canon of medicine of Avicenna. Luzac & Co, London

King LS (1982) Medical thinking, a historical preface. Princeton University Press, Princeton

Kluger J (2004) Splendid solution: Jonas Salk and the conquest of polio. G.P. Putnam's Sons, New York. ISBN: 0-399-15216-4

Kutumbiah P (1971) The evolution of scientific medicine. Orient Longman, Ltd, New Delhi

LCSG: Lung Cancer Study Group (1981) Surgical adjuvant intrapleural BCG treatment for stage I non-small cell lung cancer. J Thorac Cardiovasc Surg 82(5):649–657

Marks HM (1997) The progress of experiment: science and therapeutic reform in the United States, 1900–1990. Cambridge University Press, New York

McKneally MF et al (1976) Regional immunotherapy of lung cancer with intrapleural B.C.G. Lancet 1(7956):377–379

Meinert CL (2013) Clinical trials handbook. John Wiley & Sons, Hoboken

Meldrum M (1998) A calculated risk: the Salk polio vaccine field trials of 1954. BMJ 317 (7167):1233–1236

Muntner S (ed) (1963) The medical writings of Moses Maimonides: treatise on asthma. XI, 3. J. B. Lippincott, Philadelphia

Neuburger M (1910) History of medicine, vol 1. Henry Frowde, London

Pagel W (1982) Paracelsus. Karger, Basel

Percival T (1767) Essays medical and experimental. J. Johnson, London

Percival T (1803) Medical ethics; or a code of institutes and precepts adapted to the professional conduct of physicians and surgeons. S. Russell, Manchester

Popper K (1959) The logic of scientific discovery. Hutchinson, London

Porter TM (1986) The rise of statistical thinking, 1820–1900. Princeton University Press, Princeton

Robinson V (1931) The story of medicine. Albert & Charles Boni, New York

Skierka A-S, Michels KB (2018) Ethical principles and placebo-controlled trials – interpretation and implementation of the declaration of Helsinki's placebo paragraph in medical research. BMC Med Ethics 19(1):24

Stigler SM (ed) (1980) American contributions to mathematical statistics in the nineteenth century (2 vols). Arno Press, New York. ISBN 978-0-4051-2590-4

Stigler SM (1986) The history of statistics: the measurement of uncertainty before 1900. Harvard University Press, Cambridge, MA. ISBN 978-0-6744-0341-3

Stigler SM (1999) Statistics on the table: the history of statistical concepts and methods. Harvard University Press, Cambridge, MA. ISBN 978-0-6740-0979-0

Terminology: Conventions and Recommendations

3

Curtis L. Meinert

Contents

C. L. Meinert (✉)
Department of Epidemiology, School of Public Health, Johns Hopkins University, Baltimore, MD, USA
e-mail: cmeiner1@jhu.edu

© Springer Nature Switzerland AG 2022
S. Piantadosi, C. L. Meinert (eds.), *Principles and Practice of Clinical Trials*,
https://doi.org/10.1007/978-3-319-52636-2_200

Abstract

There are dozens of types of trials with specialized vocabularies, but the feature common to all is that they are comparative and focused on differences. If the trial involves just one treatment group, then the focus is on change from enrollment. If the trial is controlled, then the focus is on differences between the treatment groups in outcomes during and at the end of the trial.

Keywords

Language · Usage conventions · Clinical trials · Randomized trials

Introduction

The vocabulary of trials is an admixture of vocabularies from medicine, statistics, epidemiology, and other fields. You need a collection of dictionaries to master the language: medical, statistics (Upton and Cook 2014), epidemiology (Porta 2014), and clinical trials dictionaries (Day 1999; Meinert 2012).

To be sure, terminology varies across trials. To be convinced just read a few publications of results from different investigators. There is nothing that can be done about that variation, but you can standardize vocabulary within your own trial by producing a glossary of accepted terms and sticking to them.

Variation in language during a trial, even in one involving only a few investigators, can lead to confusion in the investigator group. Precision of language is a necessity to avoid confusion on such basic issues as to when a person is counted as enrolled and when a visit is coined as missed and the difference between a person being "off treatment," a dropout, or "lost to followup."

This chapter is about the vocabulary of trials. Definitions, unless otherwise indicated, are from or adapted from *Clinical Trials Dictionary: Terminology and Usage Recommendations* (Meinert 2012).

Clinical Trial

The term "clinical trial" can mean any of the following: 1. The first use of a treatment in human beings. 2. An uncontrolled trial involving treatment of people followed over time. 3. An experiment done involving persons for the purpose of assessing the safety and/or efficacy of a treatment, especially such an experiment involving a clinical event as an outcome measure, done in a clinical setting, and involving persons having a specific disease or health condition. 4. An experiment involving the administration of different study treatments in a parallel treatment design to a defined set of study subjects done to evaluate the efficacy and safety of a treatment in ameliorating or curing a disease or health condition; any such trial, including those involving healthy persons, undertaken to assess safety and/or efficacy of a treatment or health care procedure (Meinert 2012). A publication type in the National Library of Medicine indexing system defined as: *Pre-planned clinical study of the safety, efficacy, or optimum dosage schedule of one or more diagnostic, therapeutic, or prophylactic drugs, devices, or techniques in humans selected according to pre-determined criteria of eligibility and observed for predefined evidence of favorable and unfavorable effects* (National Library of Medicine 1998).

"Clinical" as an adjective means related to the sickbed or to care given in a clinic. The use of the term should be limited to trials involving people with medical conditions and even then usually can be dropped except where necessary to avoid confusion with other kinds of trials, like in vitro trials or trials involving animals.

Trial Versus Study

Trial, when done to test or assess treatments, should be used rather than the less informative term study. Study can mean all kinds of things. Trial conveys the essence of what is being done.

To qualify as a trial there should be a plan – protocol. Trials may be referred to as studies and studies as trials. For example, Ambroise Paré's (Packard 1921) experience on the battlefield in 1537 in regard to use of a digestive medicament for treatment of gunshot victims has been referred to as a clinical trial, but is a misuse of the term because Paré resorted to the medicament when his supply of boiling oil ran out. No protocol.

Ironically, ClinicalTrials.gov (aka, CT.gov), a registration site created specifically for registration of trials, does not use the term, opting instead for "interventional study."

Pilot Study Versus Feasibility Study

A pilot study is one performed as a prelude to a full-scale trial intended to provide training and experience in carrying out the trial.

A feasibility study is one performed for the purpose of determining whether it is possible to perform a full-scale trial.

Name of Trial

The most important words in any publication of results from a trial are the few represented in the title of the manuscript. If it is your trial the words are your choice. Choose wisely. The name you choose will be used hundreds of times. Steer clear of names with special characters or symbols.

Avoid use of unnecessary or redundant terms like "controlled" in "randomized controlled trial"; "randomized" is sufficient to convey "control."

Include the term "trial." Avoid using surrogate terms instead of "trial," like "study" or "project."

Include currency terms like "randomized" and "masked" when appropriate. Include terms to indicate the disease or condition being treated and the treatment being used, for example, as in *Alzheimer's Disease Anti-inflammatory Prevention Trial* (ADAPT Research Group 2009).

If you are looking for publications of results from trials, do not expect to find them by screening titles. A sizeable fraction of results publications do not have "trial" in the title.

Name of the Experimental Variable: Treatment Versus Intervention

The most important variable in trials is the regimen or course of procedures applied to persons to produce an effect. If you have to choose one name, what will it be? Treatment or intervention?

"Treat" as a noun (Merriam Webster; online dictionary) means: 1a: the act or manner or an instance of treating someone or something; b: the techniques or actions customarily applied in a specified situation; 2a: a substance or technique used in treating; b: an experimental condition.

"Intervene" as a verb (Merriam Webster; online dictionary) means: 1: to occur, fall, or come between points of time or events; 2: to enter or appear as an irrelevant or extraneous feature or circumstance; 3a: to come in or between by way of hindrance or modification; b: to interfere with the outcome or course especially of a condition or process (as to prevent harm or improve functioning); 4: to occur or lie between two things; 5: to become a third party to a legal proceeding begun by others for the protection of an alleged interest; b: to interfere usually by force or threat of force in another nation's internal affairs especially to compel or prevent an action.

There is no perfect choice, but "treatment" comes closer to what one wants to communicate than intervention.

The downside with "treatment" is when it refers to nonmedical regimens like counseling schemes to get people to stop smoking, or when the "treatment" involves devices.

The trouble with "intervene" is that technically anything one does to another is a form of intervention, whether or not related to administration of study treatments.

"Intervention" is the term of choice for designating trials on CT.gov. An "interventional study" on the website is defined as "a clinical study in which participants are assigned to receive one or more interventions (or no intervention) so that researchers can evaluate the effects of the interventions on biomedical or health-related outcomes. The assignments are determined by the study protocol. Participants may receive diagnostic, therapeutic, or other types of interventions."

Name for Groups Represented by Experimental Variable: Study Group, Treatment Group, or Arm

Any of the three work, and are used; study group or treatment group preferred though "arm" is often the term of choice in cancer trials.

Persons Studied: Subject, Patient, or Participant

A frequently used label for persons studied is "research subject," "study subject," or simply "subject." The advantage of the labels lies in their generic nature, but the characterization lacks "warmth" as conveyed in a usage note for "subject" as taken from Meinert: *The primary difficulty with the term for persons being studied in the setting of trials has to do with the implication that the persons are research objects. The term carries the connotation of subjugation and, thus, is at odds with the voluntary nature of the participation and requirements of consent. In addition, it carries the connotation of use without benefit; a misleading connotation in many trials and, assuredly, in treatment trials. Even if such a connotation is correct, the term suggests a passive relationship with study investigators when, in fact, the relationship is more akin to a partnership involving active cooperation. Avoid by using more humanistic terms, such as person, patient, or participant* (Meinert 2012).

Patient versus subject? The terms imply different relationships and ethics underlying interactions. "Patient" implies a therapeutic doctor-patient relationship. "Subject" is devoid of that connotation.

Limit "patient" or "study patient" to settings involving persons with an illness or disease and a doctor-patient relationship. Avoid in settings involving well people or when there is a need to avoid connotations of illness or of medical care by using a medically neutral term, such as study participant.

Trial Protocol Versus Manual of Operations

protocol *n* – [MF *prothocole*, fr ML *protocollum*, fr LGk *prōtokollon* first sheet of a papyrus roll bearing date of manufacture, fr Gk *prōt-* prot- + *kollon* to glue together, fr *kolla* glue; akin to MD *helen* to glue] 1. Specifications, rules, and procedures for performing some activity or function. 2. Study protocol. 3. Data collection schedule. 4. Treatment plan. *Usage note*: Often used as a synonym for treatment, as in "on protocol."

    study protocol *n* e – [trials] A written document specifying eligibility requirements, treatments being tested, method of assigning treatment to treatment units, and details of data collection and followup. 5. Treatment protocol. *Usage note*: May refer to unwritten document when used loosely. Often used as a synonym for treatment, as in "on protocol." Assumed to refer to a written document in formal usage; in the context of trials, a written document that is submitted to Institutional Review Board (IRBs) for approval and followed by investigators in conduct of the trial.

    manual of operations (MOO, MoO, MOP, MoP) *n* – 1. A document of instructional material used for performing operations in relation to some defined task or function. 2. Study manual of operations.

    study manual of operations *n* – 1. A document or collection of documents, largely in narrative form, describing the procedures used in a center or set of centers in a study (e.g., study clinics, coordinating center, or reading center) for performing defined functions. 2. Study handbook. *Usage note*: Manual and handbook are sometimes used interchangeably; however, there are differences between the two types of documents. Use manual to characterize a document organized much like a book with a series of chapters and written narrative. Use handbook for a collection of tables, lists, charts, etc., largely devoid of written narrative.

Blocking Versus Stratification and Quotafication

Blocking in relation to treatment assignment is done to ensure that after a specified number of assignments the assignment ratio is satisfied. For example, in a two treatment group design with a 1:1 assignment ratio and blocks of size of 8, assignments are constrained so that after the 8th, 16th, etc., there are the same number of persons assigned to each of the two treatment groups. The purpose of blocking is to ensure balance in the mix of the treatment assignments over enrollment. Time-related shifts in the nature of persons enrolled over the course of a trial can be a confounding variable for treatment comparisons if the mix of persons changes over time and is different by treatment group.

    Blocking should not be confused with stratification. Strata in trials are formed by classifying persons to be enrolled into a trial using some baseline characteristic, for example, gender, and randomizing within strata.

    stratification *n* – 1. Broadly, the act or process of stratifying. 2. An active ongoing process of stratifying as in placing persons in strata as a prelude to randomization. 3. The act or process of classifying treatment units or observations into strata after enrollment for a subgroup analysis. Avoid confusion when both forms of stratification are used in a trial by referring to this form of stratification as post-stratification.

The purpose of stratification is to ensure that treatment assignments are balanced across strata. To be useful, the stratification variable has to be related to the outcome of interest. If it is not, there is no statistical gain from stratification.

Stratification and blocking treatment assignments serve different purposes. Blocking is done to ensure that the assignment ratio for the trial is satisfied at points in time over the course of enrollment; stratification is done to ensure the comparability of the treatment groups with regard to the stratification variable(s).

Likewise stratification and quotafication are different. Stratification merely ensures the mix of people with regard to the stratification variable is the same across treatment groups. The trialist may carry out treatment comparisons by the stratification variable but is not under any obligation to do so.

quotafication *v* – The act or process of imposing a quota requirement on the mix of persons enrolled in a trial. Not to be confused with stratification. The purpose of stratification is to ensure that the different treatment groups in a trial have the same proportionate mix of people with regard to the stratification variable(s). Quotafication is to ensure a study population having a specified mix with regard to the variables used for quotafication.

For example, quotafication for gender would involve enrolling a specified number of males and females and randomizing by gender, that is, with gender also as a stratification variable. The mix of persons enrolled in a trial is determined by the mix of persons seen and ultimately judged eligible for enrollment. Hence, the numbers ultimately represented in the various strata will be variables having values known only after completion of enrollment. The imposition of a sample size requirement for one or more of the strata by imposition of quota requirements will extend the time required for recruitment and should not be imposed unless there are valid scientific or practical reasons for doing so.

Open

Open has various meanings in the context of trials as seen below, including one being a euphemism for unrandomized trials.

open trial *n* – 1. A trial in which the treating physician, some other person in a clinic, or the study participant selects the treatment to be administered. 2. A trial in which treatment assignments are known in advance to clinic personnel or patients, e.g., schemes where the schedule of assignments is posted in the clinic or as in systematic schemes, such as odd-even methods of treatment assignment, where the scheme is known. 3. A trial in which treatments are not masked; nonmasked trial. 4. A trial still enrolling. 5. A trial involving an open sequential design. *Usage note*: Avoid by use of appropriate descriptors to make meaning clear. Use nonmasked in the sense of defn 3. If used in the sense of defns 4 or 5 make certain the term is not taken to denote conditions described in defns 1, 2, or 3.

open label *adj* – [trials] Of or relating to a trial in which study treatments are administered in unmasked fashion. *Usage note*: Avoid; use unmasked.

Controlled

control *n* – 1. A standard of comparison for testing, verifying, or evaluating some observation or result. 2. Something that controls. 3. A person (or larger observation unit) used for comparison, e.g., a control in a case-control study; control patient; control treatment.

controlled *adj* – 1. Restrained; constrained 2. Monitored; watched 3. Any system of observation and data collection designed to provide a basis for comparing one group with another, such as provided in a parallel treatment design with concurrent enrollment to the different study groups represented in the design. 4. Data analysis involving use of control variables. *Usage note*: Often unnecessary as a modifier, especially in relation to design terms that themselves convey the notion of control, as in *randomized* **controlled** *trial* (the modifier **randomized** indicates the nature of the control implied). One assumes that the notion of "control" in the lay sense of usage applies in all research settings. Hence, usage should be limited to those in the sense of defns 1 and 2. However, it is conventional to use the term as a modifier of trial, especially when not preceded or followed by the modifier **randomized**.

controlled clinical trial *n* – MEDLINE defn: *A clinical trial involving one or more test treatments, at least one control treatment, specified outcome measures for evaluating the studied intervention, and a bias-free method for assigning patients to the test treatment. The treatment may be drugs, devices, or procedures studied for diagnostic, therapeutic, or prophylactic effectiveness. Control measures include placebos, active medicine, no-treatment, dosage forms and regimens, historical comparisons, etc. When randomization using mathematical techniques, such as the use of a random numbers table, is employed to assign patients to test or control treatments, the trial is characterized as a randomized controlled trial [publication type]. However, trials employing treatment allocation methods such as coin flips, odd-even numbers, patient social security numbers, days of the week, medical record numbers, or other such pseudo- or quasi-random processes, are simply designated as controlled clinical trials* (National Library of Medicine 1998) (http://www.nlm. nih.gov/archive/20060905/nichsr/ehta/chapter13.html).

Placebo

placebo *adj* – 1. Of or relating to the use or administration of a placebo. 2. Of or relating to something considered to be useless or ineffective. *Usage note*: Limit use to the sense of defn 1. Avoid nonsensical uses such as when the term serves as an adjective for patient or group, as in "placebo patient" or "placebo group"; use placebo-assigned or placebo-treated instead.

placebo *n* – [ME, fr L, I shall please, fr *placēre* to please; the first word of the first antiphon of the service for the dead, I shall please the Lord in the land of the living, fr Roman Catholic vespers] 1. A pharmacologically inactive substance given as a substitute for an active substance, especially when the person taking or receiving it is not informed whether it is an active or inactive substance. 2. Placebo treatment 3. A sugar-coated pill made of lactose or some other pharmacologically inert substance. 4. Any medication considered to be useless, especially one administered in pill form. 5. Nil treatment 6. An ineffective treatment. *Usage note:* Subject to varying use. Avoid in the sense of defns 4, 5, and 6; not to be used interchangeably with sham. The use of a placebo should not be construed to imply the absence of treatment. Virtually all trials involve care and investigators conducting them are obligated to meet standards of care, regardless of treatment assignment and whether masked or not. As a result, a control treatment involving use of a placebo is best thought of as a care regimen with placebo substituting for one element of the care regimen. Labels such as "placebo patient" or "placebo group" create the impression that patients assigned to receive placebos are left untreated. The labels (in addition to being wrong in the literal sense of usage) are misleading when placebo treatment is in addition to other treatments, as usually the case.

placebo control *n* – 1. Placebo-control treatment 2. A treatment involving the use of a placebo.

placebo effect *n* – 1. The effect produced by a placebo; assessed or measured against the effect expected or observed in the absence of any treatment. 2. The effect produced by an inactive control treatment. 3. The effect produced by a control treatment considered to be nil. 4. An effect attributable to a placebo. *rt:* **sham effect** *Usage note*: Limit usage to settings involving the actual use of a placebo. Avoid in the sense of defns 2 and 3 when the control treatment does not involve a placebo.

placebo group *n* – 1. Placebo-assigned group 2. Placebo-treated group 3. A group not receiving any treatment (avoid).

Consent

Usually the modifier "informed" is more an expression of hope than of fact. Its use is best reserved for settings in which there are steps built into the consent process to ensure an informed decision based on evidence of comprehension of what is involved, or for settings in which the decision can be demonstrated to have been informed; otherwise use consent.

Randomization Versus Randomized

Random *adj* – [ME impetuosity, fr MF *randon*, fr OF, fr *randir*, to run, of Gmc origin, akin to OHG *rinnan* to run] [general] 1. Having or appearing to have no specific pattern or objective. 2. Of or designating a process in which the occurrence of previous events is of no value in predicting future events. 3. Haphazard [scientific]. 4. Of or relating to a sequence, observation, assignment, arrangement, etc., that is the result of a chance process with known or knowable probabilities. 5. Of or relating to a process that has the properties of one that is random. 6. Pseudorandom. 7. Of or relating to a single value, observation, assignment, or arrangement that is the result of randomization. *Syn*: **casual, chance, haphazard** *Usage note*: Subject to misuse. Avoid in the absence of a probability base (e.g., as in *random blood sugar*); use haphazard or some other term implying less rigor than random. Misuse in the context of trials arises most commonly in relation to characterizations of treatment assignment schemes as random that are systematic or haphazard. In scientific discourse, reserve the descriptor for uses in the sense of defns 4, 5, 6, and 7.

randomization *n* – 1. An act of assigning or ordering that is the result of a random process such as that represented by a sequence of numbers in a table of random numbers or a sequence of numbers produced by a random number generator, e.g., the assignment of a patient to treatment using a random process. 2. The process of deriving an order or sequence of items, specimens, records, or the like using a random process. *Usage note*: Do not use as a characterization except in settings where there is an explicit or implied mathematical basis for supporting the usage, as discussed in the usage note for random *adj*. Use other terms implying less rigor than implied by randomization, such as haphazardization, quasirandomization, or chance, when that basis is not present or evident.

randomized *n* – [trials] The condition of having been assigned to a treatment via a random process; normally considered to have occurred when the treatment assignment is revealed to any member of the clinic staff, e.g., when an envelope containing the treatment assignment is opened.

Registration Versus Enrollment

registration *n* – 1. Registering; as in entering name and other pertinent information into a register. 2. Enrollment 3. A document certifying the act of registering. 4. The granting of an application or license; in regard to a new drug, the approval of a new drug application by a regulatory agency. 5. The act of registering a trial on CT.gov or other similar registry. *Usage note*: In trials, registration may or may not correspond to enrollment. Usually the act of registration is a necessary but not sufficient condition for enrollment. Hence, registration and enrollment should not be used interchangeably. Registration typically takes place at the first contact with a person during screening; signaled by the act of entering the person's name into a register or log or issue of an identification number for the person. The act of enrollment takes place when the treatment assignment is revealed or treatment is initiated; usually after baseline evaluations have been completed and consent has been obtained.

enrollment *n* – 1. The act of enrolling a person in a research study. 2. The state of having been enrolled. *Usage note*: Ambiguous when used in the absence of detail indicating the point at which enrollment occurs. Generally, in the case of randomized trials, that point when treatment assignment is revealed to clinic personnel. Not to be confused with registration.

Single Center Trial Versus Multicenter Trial

A trial is single center if all activities involved in conducting the trial are housed within the same institution. A trial is multicenter if it has two or more enrollment sites.

single-center trial n – 1. A trial performed at or from a single site: (a) Such a trial, even if performed in association with a coalition of clinics in which each clinic performs its own trial, but in which all trials focus on the same disease or condition (e.g., such a coalition formed to provide preliminary information on a series of different approaches to the treatment of hypertension by control or reduction); (b) A trial not having any clinical centers and a single resource center, e.g., the Physicians' Health Study (Henneken and Eberlein 1985; Physicians' Health Study Research Group Steering Committee 2012). 2. A trial involving a single clinic; with or without satellite clinics or resource centers. 3. A trial involving a single clinic and a center to receive and process data. 4. A trial involving a single clinic and one or more resource centers.

multicenter trial n – 1. A trial involving two or more clinical centers, a common study protocol, and a data center, data coordinating center, or coordinating center to receive, process, and analyze study data. 2. A trial involving at least one clinical center or data collection site and one or more resource centers. 3. A trial involving two or more clinics or data collection sites.

The usual line of demarcation between single and multicenter is determined by whether or not there is more than one treatment or data collection site. Hence, a trial having multiple centers may still be classified as a single-center trial if it has only one treatment or data collection site.

Multicenter Versus Cooperative Versus Collaborative

Multicenter preferred to collaborative or cooperative because cooperation and collaboration is not unique to multicenter trials.

Principal Investigator (PI) Versus Study Chair

In research, "principal investigator" refers to the person having responsibility for conduct of the research; the lead scientist on a research project. "Principal" means first, highest, or foremost in rank, importance, or degree; chief. Hence, uses where reference is to multiple persons in relation to a research project is an oxymoron of sorts. Confusion arises when the term refers to multiple persons in the same study, for example, often as in some multicenter trials. In general, is best avoided in favor of "study chair."

Clinical Investigator Versus Investigator

Investigator is the generic name applied to anyone in a research setting who has a key role in conducting the research or some aspect of the research.

In the context of trials, clinical investigator refers to persons with responsibilities for enrolling and caring for persons enrolled in the trial. Avoid as a designation when used to the exclusion of others having investigator status, for example, as in settings also involving nonclinical investigators as in data coordinating centers.

Steering Committee Versus Executive Committee

steering committee (SC) *n* – In multicenter trials, the committee responsible for conduct of the trial and to which other study committees report. Usually headed by the study chair and consisting of persons designated or elected to represent study centers, disciplines, or activities. *Usage note*: Sometimes executive committee.

executive committee (EC) *n* – A committee within multicenter leadership structures responsible for direction of the day-to-day affairs of the study and accountable to the steering committee; usually consists of the officers of the study and others selected from the steering committee; typically headed by the chair or vice-chair of the steering committee.

Data Monitoring Versus Data Monitoring Committee

data monitoring *v* – 1. Monitoring relating to the process of data collection. 2. Monitoring related to the detection of problems in the execution of a study (performance monitoring) or assessing treatment effects (treatment monitoring).

data monitoring committee (DMC) *n* – A committee with defined responsibilities for data monitoring, e.g., as required in performance or treatment effects monitoring.

treatment effects monitoring *n* – The act of or an instance of reviewing accumulated outcome data by treatment group to determine if the trial should continue unaltered.

Random Versus Haphazard

random *adj* – [ME impetuosity, fr MF *randon*, fr OF, fr *randir*, to run, of Gmc origin, akin to OHG *rinnan* to run] [general] 1. Having or appearing to have no specific pattern or objective. 2. Of or designating a process in which the occurrence of previous events is of no value in predicting future events. 3. Haphazard [scientific]. 4. Of or relating to a sequence, observation, assignment, arrangement, etc., that is the result of a chance process with known or knowable probabilities. 5. Of or relating to a process that has the properties of one that is random. 6. Pseudorandom. 7. Of or relating to a single value, observation, assignment, or arrangement that is the result of randomization. *Syn*: **casual, chance, haphazard** *Usage note*: Subject to misuse. Avoid in the absence of a probability base (e.g., as in *random blood sugar*); use haphazard or some other term implying less rigor than random. Misuse in the context of trials arises most commonly in relation to characterizations of treatment assignment schemes as random that are systematic or haphazard. In scientific discourse, reserve the descriptor for uses in the sense of defns 4, 5, 6, and 7.

pseudorandom *adj* – Being or involving entities that are generated, selected, or ordered by a deterministic process that can be shown to generate orders that satisfy traditional statistical tests for randomness. *Usage note*: Most random number generators are, in fact, pseudorandom number generators, though usually referred to as random number generators. Typically they are built using deterministic computational procedures that rely on a user supplied seed to start the generation process; use of the same seed on different occasions will generate the exact same sequence of numbers.

haphazard *adj* – Occurring without any apparent order or pattern. *Usage note*: Use when characterizing a process that is unordered but not meeting the scientific definition of random, or where there is uncertainty as to whether that definition is satisfied. Do not equate haphazard with random in scientific discourse. Distinct from random, in that there is no mathematical basis for characterizing haphazard processes.

Primary Versus Secondary Outcomes

primary outcome: 1. The event or condition a trial is designed to treat, ameliorate, delay, or prevent. 2. The outcome of interest as specified in the primary objective. 3. The foremost measure of success or failure of a treatment in a trial. 4. The actual occurrence of a primary event in a study participant. 5. Primary endpoint (not recommended). *Usage note*: Not to be used interchangeably with design variable. The modifier, "primary," should be used sparingly, since primariness depends on perspective. Most trials involve observations of various outcomes, each with different implications for well-being or life.

primary outcome measure: 1. That measure specifically designated as primary in the study protocol. 2. That measure, among two or more in a trial, considered to be of primary importance in its design (e.g., the one used for the sample size calculation) or analysis; may be continuous or an event; primary outcome variable. 3. Design variable.

Subject to misuse and confusion. Without access to the study protocol or absent explicit statements as to the primary outcome measure in a manuscript, readers may be hard put to know if the outcome focused onin the analysis is "primary" as represented in definitions above.

Outcome Versus Endpoint

Use outcome instead of endpoint.

An outcome, broadly defined, is something that follows as a consequence of some antecedent action or event. In the context of trials it is an event or measure observed or recorded for a person during or following treatment in a trial. The term may refer to primary or secondary outcome measures.

Endpoint, often used instead of or as a synonym for outcome, but best avoided. Most "endpoints" noted over the course of followup in trials are not indicators of "end" in regard to treatment or followup. Most protocols call for followup over a defined period of time, even in the presence of or following intercurrent events. Therefore, there are no endpoints in the operational sense of usage, except death. Use of the term in protocols and manuals for trials can cause personnel at clinics to stop treatment and followup on the occurrence of an "endpoint" if they mistakenly regard the term as having operational meaning.

Treatment Failure Versus Treatment Cessation

treatment failure *n* – 1. The failure of a treatment, as used in or on a person, to produce a desired effect or result. 2. Such a failure as observed, inferred, or declared by a study physician or other study personnel from measurements, evaluations, or observations on the person in question and resulting in cessation of the treatment or a treatment switch. 3. A person in a trial no longer receiving the assigned treatment; especially cessation of treatment occurring because of concerns regarding the safety or efficacy of the treatment. *Usage note*: The term should be used with caution because of the implied conclusion regarding the treatment and value-laden meaning. Its use should be limited to settings where there is supporting evidence indicating a failure. It should not be used simply as a synonym for treatment cessation.

treatment cessation *n* – 1. Cessation of treatment of a person, especially that due to lack of benefit or intolerable or undesirable side effects associated with treatment. 2. Cessation of a designated treatment regimen in a trial because of lack of benefit, especially such cessation arising from treatment effects monitoring. 3. Treatment termination.

Blind Versus Mask

blind, blinded *adj* – Being unaware or not informed of treatment assignment; being unaware or not informed of course of treatment.

mask, masked *adj* – Of, relating to, or being a procedure in which persons (e.g., patients, treaters, or readers in a trial) are not informed of certain items of information, e.g., the treatment represented by a treatment assignment in a clinical trial. Preferred to blind.

mask *n* – A condition imposed on an individual (or group of individuals) for the purpose of keeping that individual (or group of individuals) from knowing or learning of some condition, fact, or observation, such as treatment assignment, as in single-masked or double-masked trials.

The term "blind," as an adjective descriptor in relation to treatment administration, is more widely used in trials than its counterpart descriptor of "mask" or "masked." The shortcoming of "blind" as a descriptor in relation to treatment administration has do with unfortunate connotations (e.g., as in "blind stupidity") and the fact that the characterization can be confusing to study participants (e.g., in vision trials where loss of vision or blindness is an outcome measure). For these reasons, mask is preferred to blind.

Lost to Followup

Avoid as a generic label. Be specific as to what is lost. Generally used as a synonym for a person who does not show up for followup visits but often such persons can be followed by telephone.

Dropout

Variously defined: 1. One who terminates involvement in an activity by declaration or action; especially one who so terminates because of waning interest or for physical, practical, or philosophical reasons. 2. A person who withdraws from a trial. 3. A person who fails to appear for a followup visit, e.g., a person so classified after having failed to appear for three consecutive followup visits as defined by specified visit time windows. 4. One who refuses or stops taking the assigned treatment. 5. One who stops taking the assigned treatment and whose reasons for doing so is judged not to be related to the assigned treatment.

Subject to varying usage. Most trials require continuing data collection regardless of course of treatment. Hence, a "dropout" in the sense of defn 4 may continue to be an active participant in regard to scheduled data collection. Persons meeting the requirements of defns 4 or 5 are better characterized in relation to treatment adherence. Avoid uses in the sense of defn 5 because of difficulty in making reliable judgments regarding the reason a person stops taking the assigned treatment. The stated reason may not be the real reason. Defn 2 includes those who actively refuse, those who passively refuse, and those who are simply unable to continue followup for physical or practical reasons. Further, the definition allows for the possibility of a person returning for followup. Most long-term trials will have provisions for reinstating persons classified as dropouts if and when they return to a study clinic for required data collection. Avoid in the sense of defn 3 in relation to a single visit or contact in the absence of other reasons for regarding someone as a dropout. Use other language, such as missed visit or missed procedure, to avoid the connotation of dropout. The term should not be confused with lost to followup, noncompliant, withdrawal, or endpoint. A dropout need not be lost to followup if one can determine outcome without seeing or contacting the person (as in some forms of followup for survival) but will be lost to followup if the outcome measure depends on data collected from examinations of the person. Similarly, the act of dropping out need not affect treatment compliance. A person will become noncompliant upon dropping out in settings where doing so results in discontinuation of an active treatment process. However, there may be no effect on treatment compliance in settings where the assigned treatment is administered only once on enrollment and where that treatment is not routinely available outside the trial. Similarly, the term should not be confused with or used as a synonym for withdrawal, since its meaning is different from that for dropout.

Withdrawals

withdrawal n – 1. The act of withdrawing from a trial. 2. The removal of a person from a lifetable analysis at the cessation of followup or at the occurrence of the event of interest; removal due to cessation of followup may occur as a consequence of when the person was enrolled (e.g., calculation of a three-year event rate based on data provided by those who were enrolled at least three years prior to the date of the analysis) or because the person dropped out. 3. Dropout (not a recommended synonym). 4. One who has been removed from treatment; treatment withdrawal. 5. One who is not receiving or taking the assigned treatment (not recommended usage).

The term should not be used as a synonym for dropout or lost to followup. When used in the context of treatment, as in defns 4 and 5, use should be with details indicating the nature of use. Use in the sense of defn 4 involves the act of removing a person from treatment. Use in the sense of defn 5 is neutral with regard to action.

Design Variable Versus Primary Outcome Measure

The design variable is the variable used for determining sample size in planning a trial.

It is usually the same as the primary outcome measure but not always. For example, the design variable could be difference in blood pressure after a specified period of treatment but the outcome of primary interest could be cardiovascular deaths.

Baseline Versus Baseline Period

baseline (Bl, BL) *n* – 1. An observation, set of observations, measurement, or series of measurements made or recorded on a person just prior to or in conjunction with treatment assignment that serves as a basis for gauging change in relation to treatment assignment. 2. An observation, series of observations, measurement, or series of measurements made or recorded at some point after enrollment in relation to some act or event that serves as a basis for gauging change (e.g., a blood pressure measurement made in relation to an increase in dosage of an anti-hypertensive drug to measure the effect of the increase). *Usage note*: Subject to varying uses. Typically, in trials, unless otherwise indicated, reserved for characterizations that are consistent with defn 1. Baseline observations in most trials arise from a series of baseline examinations, separated in time by days or weeks. Hence, the time of observation for one baseline variable, relative to another, may be different.

    baseline period *n* – [general] A period of time that is used to perform procedures needed to assess the suitability and eligibility of a study candidate for enrollment into a study, to collect required baseline data, and to carry out consent processes. [trials] 1. For a study participant, the period defined by the first data collection visit and ending with assignment to treatment. 2. Such a period ending shortly after assignment to treatment. 3. A period of time during the course of treatment or followup of a person, marked by some event, process, or procedure, in which new measurements or observations are made to serve as a base for gauging subsequent change. 4. Enrollment period. *Usage note:* Avoid in the sense of defn 2 or 4 without defining qualifications. Provide qualifying detail for uses in the sense of defn 3. Traditionally, the point defining the end of the baseline period in trials is assignment to or initiation of treatment. The tendency to "stretch" the baseline period, as in defn 2, arises from a desire to reduce missing baseline data. Clearly, the utility of a measure as a baseline measure is diminished if there are possibilities of the observation being influenced by treatment. Hence, the practice is not recommended, even if the time interval following treatment assignment or initiation of treatment is small and even if the likelihood of treatment having had an effect on the variable(s) being observed within that interval is small.

Screened Versus Enrolled

screen, screened, screening, screens *v* – To assess or examine in some systematic way in order to separate persons into groups or to identify a subset eligible for further evaluation or enrollment into some activity, e.g., the process of measuring blood pressures of all persons appearing at a clinic for the purpose of identifying people suitable for enrollment in a study of high blood pressure.

    screening *n* – 1. A search for persons with an identifying marker or characteristic, as determined by results from some test or observation, known or believed to be associated with some disease (or adverse health condition). 2. The process of evaluating study candidates for enrollment into a study. 3. Any of a variety of procedures applied to data to identify outlier or questionable values. 4. A 100% inspection of items, such as in a manufacturing process, in which unacceptable items are rejected.

enrollment n – 1. The act of enrolling a person in a research study. 2. The state of having been enrolled. *Usage note*: Ambiguous when used in the absence of detail indicating the point at which enrollment occurs. Generally, in the case of randomized trials, that point when treatment assignment is revealed to clinic personnel. Not to be confused with registration.

End of Followup Versus End of Trial

Followup for persons enrolled in a trial may end at the same time regardless of when they were enrolled (common closing date design) or may end on a per person basis after a specified period of time after enrollment (anniversary closing date design). End of trial is when all enrollment and data collection activities cease.

Analysis by Assigned Treatment Versus Per Protocol Analysis

Analysis by assigned treatment (aka intention to treat analysis) is an analysis in which persons are counted to the treatment group to which assigned, even if they did not receive any of the assigned treatment. The analysis is the sine qua non of analysis in trials. It may be supplemented by other arrangements but the analysis by assigned treatment is central to whatever conclusions are reached regarding the results.

An alternative analysis is per protocol analysis (PPA) in which persons are arranged by treatment received rather than by assigned treatment. The analysis is considered to provide a more realistic estimate of the actual treatment effect but is subject to selection biases and hence should be presented only as a supplement to analysis by assigned treatment.

Authors of papers are expected to label their analyses so readers know if the results being summarized are per protocol or by treatment assignment.

Bias

bias n – 1. An inclination of temperament, state of mind, or action based on perception, opinion, or impression serving to reduce rational thought or action, or the making of impartial judgments; a specified instance of such an inclination. 2. A tendency toward certain measurements, outcomes, or conclusions over others as a result of a conscious or subconscious mind set, temperament, or the like; a specific expression of such a tendency. 3. Any behavior or performance that is differential across groups in a trial; treatment-related bias. 4. Deviation of the expected value of an estimate of a statistic from its true value. ***Usage note***: Distinguish between uses in which bias (defns 1 or 2) is being proposed in a speculative sense as opposed to an actual instance of bias. Usages in the latter sense should be supported with evidence or arguments to substantiate the claim. Usages in the former sense should be preceded or followed by appropriate modifiers or statements to make clear that the user is speculating. Similarly, since most undifferentiated uses (in the sense of defns 1 or 2) are in the speculative sense, prudent readers will treat all uses as being in that sense, unless accompanied by data, evidence, or arguments to establish bias as a fact. Not to be confused with systematic error. Systematic error can be removed from finished data; bias is more elusive and not easily quantified.

selection bias *n* – 1. A systematic inclination or tendency for elements or units selected for study (persons in trials) to differ from those not selected. 2. Treatment-related selection bias ***Usage note***: The bias defined by defn 1 is unavoidable in most trials because of selective factors introduced as a result of eligibility requirements for enrollment and because of the fact that individuals may decline enrollment. The existence of the bias does not affect the validity of treatment comparisons so long as it is the same across treatment groups, for example, as when treatment assignments are randomized.

treatment-related selection bias *n* – Broadly, bias related to treatment assignment introduced during the selection and enrollment of persons into a trial; often due to knowing treatment assignments in advance of issue and using that information in the selection process. The risk of the bias is greatest in unmasked trials involving systematic assignment schemes (e.g., one in which assignments are based on order or day of arrival of persons at a clinic). It is nil in trials involving simple (unrestricted) randomization, but can arise in relation to blocked randomization if the blocking scheme is known or deduced. For example, one would be able to correctly predict one-half of the assignments before use in an unmasked trial of two study treatments arranged in blocks of size two, if the blocking is known or deduced. The chance of the bias operating, even if the blocking scheme is simple, is minimal in double-masked trials.

Early Stop Versus Nominal Stop

A nominal stop is when all treatment and data collection procedures in the trial cease or are stopped. The usual reason for a nominal stop is when the trial has been completed as planned. Nominal stops can also be the result of loss of funding or because of orders to stop by the funding agency or from a regulatory agency.

Early stops may pertain to all persons enrolled in the trial as in nominal stops or only to a subset. The stop may be due to a clinical hold issued by a regulatory agency or may be due to evidence that a treatment is harmful or ineffective. Typically, early stops are the results of actions taken by investigators based on interim looks at accumulating data over the course of the trial.

Summary

The vocabulary of trials is an admixture of vocabularies principally from medicine, statistics, and epidemiology. Students of trials need collections of dictionaries and glossaries to be competent in the language of trials.

Whether you are a person simply interested in trials or a person designing and conducting a trial, you have to know the language and jargon of trials. You have to be familiar with the difference between "study" and "trial." You have to know the difference between "dropout" and "lost to followup," "open trials" and "open label trials," "control" and "controlled," "endpoint" and "outcome," and "blocking" and "stratification."

References

ADAPT Research Group (2009) Alzheimer's disease anti-inflammatory prevention trial: design, methods, and baseline results. Alzheimers Dement 5:93–104

Day S (1999) Dictionary for clinical trials. Wiley, Chichester, 217pp

Henneken CH, Eberlein K (1985) For the physicians' health study research group: a randomized trial of aspirin and β-carotene among U.S. physicians. Prev Med 14:165–168

Meinert CL (2012) Clinical trials dictionary: terminology and usage recommendations, 2nd edn. Wiley, Hoboken

National Library of Medicine (1998) Medical subject headings – annotated alphabetic list: 1998. National Library of Medicine, Bethesda

Packard FR (1921) Life and times of Ambroise Paré, 1510–1590. Paul B Hoeber, New York

Physicians' Health Study Research Group Steering Committee (2012) Preliminary report: findings from the aspirin component of the ongoing Physicians' health study. New Engl J Med 318:262–264

Porta M (ed) (2014) Dictionary of epidemiology, 5th edn. Oxford University Press, New York, 376pp

Upton G, Cook I (2014) Dictionary of statistics. Oxford University Press, New York, 496pp

Clinical Trials, Ethics, and Human Protections Policies

4

Jonathan Kimmelman

Contents

J. Kimmelman (✉)
Biomedical Ethics Unit, McGill University, Montreal, QC, Canada
e-mail: jonathan.kimmelman@mcgill.ca

© Springer Nature Switzerland AG 2022
S. Piantadosi, C. L. Meinert (eds.), *Principles and Practice of Clinical Trials*,
https://doi.org/10.1007/978-3-319-52636-2_238

Abstract

Clinical trials raise two main sets of ethical challenges. The first concerns protecting human beings when they are used in scientific experiments. The second concerns protecting the welfare of downstream users of medical evidence generated in trials. The present chapter reviews core ethical standards and principles governing the conception, design, conduct, and reporting of clinical trials. This review concludes by suggesting that even the most technical decisions about design and reporting embed numerous moral judgments about how to serve the interests of research subjects and downstream users of medical evidence.

Clinical trials are experiments on human beings. They involve two elements that make them ethically sensitive undertakings. First, the very reagent used in the experiment – the human being – has what philosophers call moral status. That is, human beings are sentient and self-aware, they have preferences and plans, and they have a capacity for suffering. Human beings are thus entitled to having their interests respected and protected when they are themselves the research reagents. Second, clinical trials are aimed at supporting decision-making in health care. Life and death decisions are ultimately based on the evidence we generate from human experiments. Human beings who use that evidence deserve protection from scientific findings that are misleading, incomplete, or biased.

In what follows, I provide a very condensed overview of the ethics of clinical trials. Most writings on the ethics of clinical trials have centered on the protection of human volunteers, treating issues of research integrity as an afterthought, if at all. Two core claims ground this review – claims that perhaps differentiate it from similar overviews of human research ethics. The first is that scientific integrity is a complement to human protections; even the most technical decisions about design and analysis are laden with implicit ethical judgments. The second is that clinical trials present ethical challenges across their full life cycle – not merely in the brief window when a trial is open for enrollment, and where human protection regulations are directed. This review is thus organized according to the life cycle of a clinical trial.

Keywords

Clinical trials · Research ethics · Human protections · Medical evidence · Research oversight

Origins of Research Ethics

The moral and regulatory framework for protecting human subjects has its origins in the aftermath of World War II. The US prosecution of 23 Nazis in the so-called Nazi Doctors' trial led to the first formalized policy on human research ethics, the "Nuremberg Code" (Annas and Grodin 1995). At least in North America, however, the Nuremberg Code went largely unheeded for two decades. Revelations of various research abuses (Beecher 1966), including those surrounding the Tuskegee Syphilis study (an observational study of African American men with middle to late stage syphilis that had run continuously from 1932) led the US Congress to establish the National Commission for the Protection of Research Subjects of Biomedical and Behavioral Research. A key task for this committee was to articulate the basic moral principles of human research. The product of this effort came to be known as the Belmont Report, and regulations established in the USA from this effort include 45 CFR 46 and the Food and Drug Administration's (FDA) equivalent, 21 CFR 50. The first section of the former, which covers the general requirements of human protections, is sometimes called the "Common Rule"; it was revised in 2018 (Menikoff et al. 2017). Various other jurisdictions and bodies have articulated their own policies as well, including the World Health Organization (1982 with several revisions since) (World Health Organization and Council for International Organizations of Medical Sciences 2017), the World Medical Association (1964 with numerous revisions since) (General Assembly of the World Medical Association 2014), and the Canadian Tri-council (1998 with one revision) (Canadian Institutes of Health Research et al. 2018). Though policies around the world vary around the edges, they share a core consensus in expressing principles and policies articulated by the Belmont Report. These principles are respect for persons (implemented by obtaining informed consent or restricting risk for persons lacking capacity); beneficence (implemented by independent establishment of a favorable balance of risk/benefit); and justice (implemented by comparing a trial population to the target population of the knowledge).

The Belmont Principles provide orientation points for thinking about the ethics of a trial. But they are not exhaustive (Kimmelman 2020). Nor do regulations address all duties attending to the conduct of clinical trials. I will return to these gaps periodically.

Conception of Trials

The Belmont Report contains a suggestive and widely overlooked statement: "Radically new procedures of this description should, however, be made the object of formal research at an early stage in order to determine whether they are safe and effective." Nevertheless, there are no regulations or policies that govern the choice of what research questions to address in trials. As far as ethical oversight and drug regulation is concerned, there is no moral distinction between a trial testing a me-too drug for male pattern baldness and a trial testing a promising new treatment for pediatric glioma.

Yet clearly, the resources available for research are finite, and some research questions are more deserving of societal investment than other questions. This is illustrated by the often quoted claim that 90% of the world's resources are committed to addressing health issues that afflict only 10% of the world population (the so-called "10–90% gap") (Flory and Kitcher 2004). It is also illustrated by the historic and unfair exclusion of certain populations from medical research (such as children, women, persons living in economically deprived settings, racial minorities, pregnant women, and elderly populations), or the persistence of medical uncertainty surrounding widely deployed treatments (e.g., the value of PCI for treatment of angina) (Al-Lamee et al. 2018).

Four general considerations might be offered for selecting research hypotheses. First, researchers should direct their attention towards questions that are unresolved. This may seem obvious. However, many trials address questions that have already been adequately resolved. One particularly striking example was the persistence of placebo-controlled trials testing the drug aprotinin, long after its efficacy had been decisively established (Fergusson et al. 2005). Drug companies often run trials that are primarily aimed at promoting a drug rather than testing an unresolved hypothesis (Vedula et al. 2013). Second, researchers should only test hypotheses that are sufficiently mature. For example, researchers generally ought not to initiate phase 1 trials unless there are compelling preclinical studies to motivate them; they should generally not pursue phase 3 studies if there is insufficient grounds to settle on a dose or treatment schedule for testing (again, there are many examples of trials that have been launched absent compelling evidentiary grounds) (Kimmelman and Federico 2017). The best way to ground a claim that a medical hypothesis merits evaluation in clinical trials is with a systematic review (Savulescu et al. 1996; Chalmers and Nylenna 2014; Nasser et al. 2017); some jurisdictions require systematic review before trial conduct (Goldbeck-Wood 1998).

Third, researchers should prioritize clinical questions that are likely to have the greatest impact on health and well-being. To some extent researchers' priorities are constrained by their field, logistical considerations, and funding options. Nevertheless, they can exercise some discretion within these constraints. All else being equal, researchers ought to favor trials involving conditions that cause greater morbidity or mortality (whether because of prevalence or intensity of morbidity) and that afflict unfairly disadvantaged or excluded populations.

Finally, researchers should not initiate trials unless there are reasonable prospects for findings being incorporated into downstream decisions. For example, phase 1 trials should generally meet a more demanding review standard if there is no sponsor to carry encouraging findings forward in a phase 2 trial. Many exploratory trials suggesting the promise of approved drugs in new indications are never advanced into more rigorous clinical trials (Federico et al. 2019). Research that is not embedded within a coordinated research program presents a variety of problems, including a concern about disseminating potentially biased research findings that are incorporated into clinical practice guidelines. The present author has argued that abortive research programs raise questions about the social value of many exploratory trials – especially in the post-approval research context (Carlisle et al. 2018).

Design of Trials

Risk/Benefit

All major policies on research ethics require that risks are favorably balanced against benefits to society in the form of improved knowledge and benefit to subjects (if any). Benefits include direct medical benefits of receiving medical interventions tested in trials (if any) and those expected by addressing a research hypothesis. Inclusion benefit (the benefit patients might receive from extra medical attention they receive when entering trials, regardless of treatment assignment) is generally considered irrelevant for establishing a favorable risk benefit (King 2000).

How, then, are researchers and oversight bodies to operationalize the notion of a favorable risk/benefit balance? The Belmont Report urges an assessment of risk and benefit that is systematic, evidence based, and explicit. One of the most useful approaches is "component analysis" (Weijer and Miller 2004). Clinical trials typically involve a mix of potentially burdensome exposures, including treatment with unproven drugs, venipuncture, imaging or diagnostic procedures, and/or tissue biopsies. Component analysis involves dividing a study into its constituent procedures, and evaluating the risk/benefit for each individual procedure. Importantly, benefits associated with one procedure cannot be used to "purchase" risk for other procedures. For example, the burdens of a painful lumbar puncture cannot be justified by appealing to the therapeutic advantages offered by access to a novel treatment in a trial.

In performing component analysis, procedures can be sorted into two categories. Some procedures, like withholding an established effective treatment, implicate care obligations and are thus termed "therapeutic procedures." Other procedures, like venipunctures to monitor a metabolite, are performed solely to advance a research objective; these are called "demarcated research procedures." Each has a separate process for justifying risk.

Justification of Therapeutic Procedures: Clinical Equipoise

Therapeutic procedures in trials are generally evaluated according to the principle of clinical equipoise. First defined in 1987, clinical equipoise refers to genuine uncertainty within an expert community as to an intervention's clinical value as compared with standard of care (Freedman 1987). A trial that meets these conditions is said to be ethical when, if executed properly, the trial is a necessary step in resolving that expert uncertainty. According to the principle of clinical equipoise, patients should not be assigned to treatments that are known in advance to fall below a standard of care that a patient would receive outside a trial. For example, for Alzheimer's disease, there are currently no proven treatments for reducing progression. Accordingly, assigning a patient to a placebo comparator in a trial testing an Alzheimer's treatment does not deprive that patient of a standard of care that patient would otherwise receive. On the other hand, asking a patient with relapse remitting multiple sclerosis to forgo disease-modifying treatment for a year would fall below standard of care. Placebo-controlled trials of this duration in multiple sclerosis would generally be unethical (Polman et al. 2008).

In one concept, clinical equipoise captures three imperatives for risk/benefit in research. First, it preserves a physician's duty of care when they participate in research. As such, physicians can recruit patients without compromising their fiduciary obligations to patients. Second, the principle of clinical equipoise establishes a standard for acceptable risk in clinical trials by benchmarking risk/benefit in trials to generally accepted standards in medicine. Third, clinical equipoise establishes a standard for scientific value. A trial is only ethical insofar as it is a necessary step towards resolving uncertainty in the expert community. This has subtle implications. For example, it means small, underpowered trials are ethically questionable (unless they are a necessary step towards resolving medical uncertainty, as in the case of phase 2 trials, or designed expressly to be incorporated in future meta-analyses) (Halpern et al. 2002), since "positive" but underpowered trials might be sufficient to encourage further trials, but will generally be insufficient to convince the expert medical community about a treatment's advantage over standard of care.

Though clinical equipoise was first articulated in the context of randomized trials testing new interventions, it can logically be extended to single armed studies that use historical controls as comparators. The concept of clinical equipoise is not without critics (reviewed in London 2007), and its operationalization – like many ethical concepts – can pose challenges (e.g., how much residual uncertainty is necessary for a trial to be ethical). Just the same, no other concept comes close to binding the moral dimensions of trials to their methodology and the obligations of those who conduct them.

Justification of Demarcated Research Procedures

The justification of risks associated with demarcated research procedures proceeds in two steps. In the first, researchers should minimize burdens – for example, by using state-of-the-art techniques for collecting tissue samples. Remaining risks then need to be justified by appealing to the value of the knowledge such procedures enable. If this seems incredibly vague, it is. At best, one can look to the precedent of other studies to ask whether the risks of a research procedure have generally been deemed to have been justified by the incremental gain in knowledge. At worst, this vagueness reveals ongoing unresolved problems for research ethics. As a general rule, demarcated research risks can never exceed minimal risk (or minor increase over minimal risk in the USA) for studies involving minors; for studies in patients that have capacity, they should never involve risk of death or irreversible injury. The sum of all research burdens in component analysis should still be favorably balanced by the value of the trial.

Riskless Research, High Risk Research, Comparative Effectiveness Trials, and Ethics

Both extremes of risk in research pose challenges to the assessment and evaluation of risk in research. Some trials, like early phase trials testing novel strategies, or trials of aggressive treatments in pre-symptomatic patients, present high degrees of risk and uncertainty. Many patients are willing to undertake extraordinary levels of risk, and for patients who have exhausted treatment options, a "standard of care" may be difficult to define for establishing clinical equipoise. Some might argue that, in such circumstances, investigators and ethics review committees should defer to well-informed preferences of research volunteers. However, risk in trials can impact others outside of trials (e.g., third parties), or undermine public confidence (Hope and McMillan 2004). For example, a major debacle or a series of negative trials in a novel research arena can undermine support for parallel research efforts, as occurred with gene therapy in the late 1990s. Though ethics polices and oversight systems do not generally instruct investigators to consider how their trials might affect parallel investigations, some commentators argue that researchers bear duties to steward research programs and refrain from activities that might damage them (London et al. 2010).

At the other extreme are seemingly riskless studies. One category of riskless studies is "seeding trials": trials that involve well-characterized drugs and that are aimed primarily at marketing by habituating doctors to prescribing them (Andersen et al. 2006) or by generating a publication that can function legally as an advertisement through reprint circulation (US Department of Health and Human Services, Food and Drug Administration 2009; Federico et al. 2019) rather than resolving a scientific question. Most human protections policies have little to say about seeding trials, because their risks are so low that little to no scientific value is needed to justify them. Seeding trials are nevertheless an obvious breach of scientific integrity (Sox and Rennie 2008; London et al. 2012). Such studies not only sap scarce human capital for research, but subvert the aims of science (which is aimed at belief change through evidence, not habituation or attentional manipulation) and undermine the credibility of the research enterprise.

Comparative effectiveness and usual care–randomized trials represent a second category of seemingly riskless studies. In these studies, patients are randomly assigned to standards of care in order to determine whether one standard of care is better or noninferior (many such studies do not use any demarcated research procedures). Even when such studies use primary endpoints like mortality or major morbidity, they are often viewed as "riskless" insofar as all patients are receiving the same treatments within trials that they would receive outside of trials (Lantos and Feudtner 2015). Whether "usual care" randomized trials are necessarily minimal risk is hotly debated among research ethicists. The present author would argue that they should not be understood as minimal risk (Kane et al. 2020). First, by using a morbid primary endpoint, researchers are openly declaring they are uncertain as to whether one standard is better than another on a clinically meaningful measure. Second, it is impossible to exclude the possibility that a patient who opts to enter a usual care randomized trial – by having their treatment determined using randomization – is directed toward a treatment trajectory that leaves them worse off against the counterfactual of their not joining the trial. To say that a study fulfills clinical equipoise means that probability of risks and benefit within are very similar to those outside a trial. There may, in fact, be little rational basis for declining trial participation. However, these statements do not entail that the trial is necessarily minimal risk.

Maximizing Efficiencies

Human protections policies are overwhelmingly focused on protecting individual research subjects from undue risk. They are not set up to consider whether a given research question might be addressed with fewer patients, or whether a design is suboptimal. This means that human protections policies have very little to say directly about inefficient research designs, including trials that are overpowered or over-accrue, trials that use uneven randomization ratios, or that divide their alpha excessively over many hypotheses. Yet clearly, if a medical question can be resolved by burdening a smaller number of patients (even though, for each individual patient, there is a favorable risk/benefit balance), that design ought to be preferred (Hey and Kimmelman 2014). Similarly, many studies employ designs that – while riskless per se – cloud the interpretation of results. For example, in one study, 43% of trials in meta-analyses were deemed to show high risk of bias in at least one domain of the risk of bias assessment tool; simple and low-cost design refinements could have halved this figure (Yordanov et al. 2015).

Justice

Fair Subject Selection

The principle of justice, as originally interpreted by the Belmont Report and US regulations, pertains to the relationship between vulnerable populations used in clinical trials and those who benefit from the knowledge acquired in the trials. The principle originated from a concern that disadvantaged research groups, like prisoners, racial minorities, or children, were often enrolled in trials that were aimed at addressing medical uncertainties more relevant for advantaged groups (e. g., racial majorities, adults, etc.). The issue of fair subject selection became a focus of debate in the late 1990s, when questions were raised about the testing of short course AZT for the prevention of perinatal mother to child transmission of HIV. These trials, which were aimed at testing an AZT course that was more suited to the infrastructure and economics of low-income settings, employed a placebo comparator even though a longer (and more expensive and medically demanding) course of AZT had been established as standard of care for high-income countries (Crouch and Arras 1998). Some critics charged the study-violated clinical equipoise, since placebo fell below the high-income standard of care. However, the high-income standard of care was simply inaccessible in low-income countries, where the local standard of care was nontreatment.

Following this episode, international policies like the Declaration of Helsinki and others were revised to articulate two core expectations for research funded by high-income sponsors and conducted in vulnerable groups. The first is that trials must make provisions for post-trial access for patients/participants in a trial in the event a treatment shows benefit. The second is "responsiveness," articulated in the Declaration of Helsinki (to pick one definition) as "research [that] is responsive to the health needs or priorities of this group and [that] cannot be carried out in a non-vulnerable group this group should stand to benefit from the knowledge, practices or interventions that result from the research." In some cases, as in trials testing economical approaches to treating tropical disease, responsiveness is easy to establish. In other cases, the connection of trials to health needs of disadvantaged populations is more attenuated.

The high costs and regulatory demands of conducting trials have motivated many drug companies to pursue trials in low- and middle-income countries (Glickman et al. 2009). For instance, many pivotal cancer drug trials include recruitment sites in former Eastern Bloc countries. Cancer treatments are among the most expensive drugs in the modern pharmacopeia. While health care systems in countries like Romania and the Ukraine confront cancer, the extent to which they are likely to absorb the costs of new cancer treatments is unclear. Of note, one of the most influential regulatory documents for clinical trial research ethics, the International Conference on Harmonization "Good Clinical Practice" policy (International Council for Harmonisation 1996) – omits language pertaining to such justice concerns; this omission is inconsistent with nearly every other influential and contemporary policy on human protections (Kimmelman et al. 2009).

Inclusion

A second major salient for expansion of the justice principle in the 1990s was inclusion. By the 1990s, it had become increasingly clear that certain populations had been excluded – often systematically – from research, unfairly depriving these populations of medical evidence for managing their conditions. These populations have variously included gay men, African Americans, women, children, pregnant women, and the elderly (Palmowski et al. 2018).

Major policy reforms in the USA at funding agencies and with drug regulation have encouraged greater inclusion of (and analysis of subgroups for) children (US Department of Health and Human Services, Food and Drug Administration 2005), women (Elahi et al. 2016), and racial minorities (US Department of Health and Human Services, Food and Drug Administration 2016). Though ethical review of trial protocols does not typically focus on inclusion and representativeness, it is now widely recognized that, absent a compelling scientific or policy rationale, clinical trial investigators should strive to maximize the representativeness of the populations they recruit into trials – particularly in later phase trials that are aimed at directly informing regulatory approvals and/or health care. Even with these policy reforms, there are suggestions that certain populations continue to be underrepresented in clinical research relative to incidence of disease in these populations (Dickmann and Schutzman 2017; Ghare et al. 2019). Studies that do enroll diverse populations often do not report stratified analyses, potentially frustrating the aim of broader inclusion.

Trial Inception

Respect for Persons

Only after a trial has been deemed to fulfill the above expectations is informed consent relevant. All major policies require that investigators offer prospective research subjects the opportunity to consider a study's risks, burdens, and benefits against their preferences, values, and goals. This consent, expressed at the outset of screening and enrollment, must be ongoing for the duration of a clinical trial.

Elements of Valid Informed Consent

Valid informed consent is said to consist of three core elements (Faden and Beauchamp 1986). The first is capacity. Prospective research participants must have the cognitive and emotional resources to render informed judgments about trial participation. Generally, capacity is a clinical judgment. In cases where there are concerns, there are tools for assessing capacity to participate in research. Some populations, like children, trauma victims, or persons with dementia, lack competence to provide informed consent. Under such circumstances, there are other provisions for respecting persons (see below).

The second element of valid informed consent is understanding. Prospective research subjects must receive, comprehend, and appreciate information that is material to their decision to enroll in a trial. Information includes (but is not limited to): risk/benefit, study procedures, study purpose, and alternatives to participation. There is a very large literature showing that patients often report inability to recall basic information about study features. In particular, many patients struggle to accurately understand the probability of benefit (therapeutic overestimation) (Horng and Grady 2003) or the way research participation may constrain ability to pursue individualized care (therapeutic misconception) (Appelbaum et al. 1987).

The third element of a valid informed consent is voluntariness. Prospective research participants should be free of controlling influences, such as coercion (i.e., threatening to make an individual worse off, or threatening to withhold something that is owed to the individual) or undue manipulation (i.e., alterations to choice architecture, disclosure processes, or interactions) that encourage compliance. Some forms of manipulation are considered ethical – at least for certain routine research settings. Healthy volunteer phase 1 studies often use financial payment to manipulate an individual's enrollment in a trial. Key to judging whether a manipulation is "undue" is whether it involves an offer that is disrespectful (Grant and Sugarman 2004) (i.e., offering to pay an individual to override a moral commitment) or whether an offer is irresistible. Compensation, that is, covering expenses associated with lost wages, parking, or travel, is different from inducement and does not involve manipulation.

Research Without Informed Consent

There are several circumstances where human research can be ethically and legally conducted without valid informed consent of research subjects. One is in studies involving persons lacking decisional competence. Generally, three protections are established for such populations. First, demarcated research risk is limited to minimal risk or minor increase over minimal risk (though policies vary). Second, surrogate consent is sought from parents or guardians (in the case of children) or from a designated agent (e.g., an individual designated as such in an advanced directive, or a family member) for incapacitated adults. Third, where applicable, assent (i.e., agreement and cooperation) is sought from the research subject.

A second circumstance where consent can be waived, at least in some jurisdictions, is emergency research (e.g., testing trauma or resuscitation trials). As above, demarcated research procedures cannot exceed minimal risk. Because surrogate consent cannot typically be obtained in emergency research, there are provisions for public disclosure and community consultation before such studies are launched (Halperin et al. 2007).

Many proposals have circulated about expedited or waived informed consent, particularly in the context of usual care trials. One such example is Zelen's consent, which pre-randomizes patients and bypasses informed consent for those assigned to treatments that are identical to those they would receive had they not enrolled in a trial. This particular design is generally subject to strong ethical criticisms, since patients who are randomly assigned to standard treatments are denied the opportunity to consent to research participation (Hawkins 2004). However, other similar trial designs have been proposed that, according to some, correct these ethical deficiencies while preserving expedience. The reader is directed elsewhere for discussions (Flory et al. 2016).

Informed Consent Documents

One of the main vehicles for informed consent is the informed consent document (ICD). ICDs typically contain a description of key disclosure elements of a study. ICDs are widely criticized for their readability, their length, and their ineffectiveness in supporting understanding among research participants. However, ICDs can be better understood as a supplement for face-to-face discussions, which are much more effective at achieving understanding (Flory and Emanuel 2004). They also provide Institutional Review Boards (IRB, described in the next section) a proxy of what will be covered in these discussions. Effort spent fussing over wording, if redirected towards an appraisal of risk and benefit, would probably be a better investment for members of IRBs.

Independent Review

As Henry Beecher noted in his 1966 exposé (Beecher 1966), physicians harbor divided loyalties when they conduct clinical research. Judgments about risk and benefit, informed consent, and fair subject selection are refereed prospectively by submitting trial protocols to independent review bodies (in the USA, these committees are called Institutional Review Boards or IRBs; in Canada they are called "Research Ethics Boards" or REBs). Various policies stipulate the composition of REBs, as well as the range of issues they should (or should not) consider. Different models of REB review have emerged in the past decade or so, including for profit REB review, centralized review mechanisms, and specialized review mechanisms for fields like gene therapy or cancer trials (Levine et al. 2004).

Before trial launch, REB approval must be obtained. All design elements and planned analyses for the trial should be pre-specified in a trial protocol. The protocol should have been reviewed for scientific merit. And main design details, hypotheses, and planned analyses should be registered prospectively in a public database like clinicicaltrials.gov.

Conduct

Trials and Ethics Across Time

Trials occur over time. New information emerges from within a trial as it unfolds, or from concurrent research or adverse events documented outside of trials. This information can alter a study's risk/benefit balance, necessitating an alteration of study design, reconsenting, and sometimes halting a trial. Similarly, slow recruitment can compromise a study's risk/benefit balance, since under-accrual can stymie the ability of a trial to achieve the quantum of social value that was projected during ethical review, and the options available outside the trial can change. Accordingly, risk/benefit must always be monitored as a study proceeds. In studies involving higher levels of risk, this duty typically devolves to investigators and data safety monitoring boards (DMSBs). DSMBs confront myriad policy, ethical, and statistical challenges; the reader is directed elsewhere for further discussions of trial monitoring (DeMets et al. 2005).

Reporting

Publication and Results Deposition

Once a trial is complete, the fulfillment of the risk/benefit established at trial outset requires that results be disseminated to relevant knowledge users. Until recently, there were few expectations and regulations on trial reporting. Numerous studies have shown that many clinical trials are never published. For example, the present author's own work showed that only 37% of pre-license trials of drugs that stalled in clinical development were published within 5 years of trial closure (Hakala et al. 2015). Many policies, like Declaration of Helsinki or Canada's Tricouncil Policy Statement articulate a requirement of deposition of results for all clinical research. The US FDA also requires deposition of clinical trial results in clinicaltrials.gov within 12 months of completion of primary endpoint collection (US Department of Health and Human Services 2016). However, many clinical trials are exempt from this requirement, including phase 1 trials as well as trials testing nonregulated products (e.g., surgeries, psychotherapies (Azar et al. 2019), or any research not pursued as part of an IND). Some funders, institutions, and journals have policies intended to address these gaps.

Methods and Outcome Reporting

The main way findings in trials are disseminated is through publication. Trials should also provide a frank and transparent description of methods and results. This entails at least three considerations. First, methods should be described in sufficient detail to support valid inferences. Methods in the report should be consistent with the study protocol. Second, results should be reported in full, and consistent with planned analyses. For example, all planned subgroup analyses should be reported; any new subgroup analyses should be labeled as post hoc analyses. Third, study reports should explain limitations and what new results mean in the context of existing evidence. There is a wealth of literature showing these three aspirations are not always fulfilled in trials. Regarding the first, systematic reviews show that many trials do not adequately describe methods such as how allocation was concealed or how randomization sequences were generated (Turner et al. 2012), or have reported primary outcomes that are inconsistent with those stated in trial protocols (Mathieu et al. 2009). Regarding complete reporting, safety outcomes are often not well reported in trials (Phillips et al. 2019). Lack of balance in reports is suggested by the frequent use of "spin" in trial reports (Boutron et al. 2014), or by the selective presentation of positive subgroup analyses in study abstracts (Kasenda et al. 2014).

The Afterlife of Trials

Researchers and sponsors continue to have ethical obligations to research participants and evidence consumers. For instance, many commentators argue that there is an obligation to share trial results with study participants (Partridge and Winer 2002; Dixon-Woods et al. 2006). Response to researcher queries, sharing unpublished analyses, or making data available can interact with the value and burden associated with research (Bauchner et al. 2016). One area where these obligations are contended is access to individual patient data. Recently, several medical journals have proposed (and some endorsed) an expectation that researchers who publish in their venues make provisions for sharing individual patient data (Loder and Groves 2015). Most patient participants favor sharing individual patient data provided safeguards are in place (Mello et al. 2018). Model safeguards for patient privacy and research integrity are described elsewhere (Mello et al. 2013).

Synthesis

The above review is, by necessity, cursory and leaves many dimensions of clinical trial ethics unaddressed. These include questions about protecting third parties like caregivers in research (Kimmelman 2005), the ethics of incidental findings (Wolf et al. 2008), and ancillary care obligations (Richardson and Belsky 2004). New trial methodologies like adaptive trial designs (Bothwell and Kesselheim 2017) or cluster-randomized trials (Weijer et al. 2011) pose challenges for implementing the ethical standards described above.

It is tempting to view human protections and research ethics as a set of considerations that are only visited once a clinical trial has been designed and submitted for ethical review. However, decisions about what hypotheses to test, how to test them, how the trial is conducted, and how to report results are saturated with ethical judgments. Most of these judgments occur absent clear regulatory guidance, or outside the gaze of research ethics boards. In that way, every scientist participating in the conception, design, reporting, and uptake of clinical research is practicing research ethics.

Cross-References

▶ ClinicalTrials.gov
▶ Clinical Trials in Children
▶ Consent Forms and Procedures
▶ International Trials
▶ Reporting Biases

References

Al-Lamee R, Thompson D, Dehbi H-M et al (2018) Percutaneous coronary intervention in stable angina (ORBITA): a double-blind, randomised controlled trial. Lancet 391:31–40. https://doi.org/10.1016/S0140-6736(17)32714-9

Andersen M, Kragstrup J, Søndergaard J (2006) How conducting a clinical trial affects physicians' guideline adherence and drug preferences. JAMA 295:2759–2764. https://doi.org/10.1001/jama.295.23.2759

Annas GJ, Grodin MA (eds) (1995) The Nazi doctors and the Nuremberg Code: human rights in human experimentation, 1st edn. Oxford University Press, New York

Appelbaum PS, Roth LH, Lidz CW et al (1987) False hopes and best data: consent to research and the therapeutic misconception. Hast Cent Rep 17:20–24

Azar M, Riehm KE, Saadat N et al (2019) Evaluation of journal registration policies and prospective registration of randomized clinical trials of nonregulated health care interventions. JAMA Intern Med. https://doi.org/10.1001/jamainternmed.2018.8009

Bauchner H, Golub RM, Fontanarosa PB (2016) Data sharing: an ethical and scientific imperative. JAMA 315:1238–1240. https://doi.org/10.1001/jama.2016.2420

Beecher HK (1966) Ethics and clinical research. N Engl J Med 274:1354–1360. https://doi.org/10.1056/NEJM196606162742405

Bothwell LE, Kesselheim AS (2017) Thereal-world ethics of adaptive-design clinical trials. Hast Cent Rep 47:27–37. https://doi.org/10.1002/hast.783

Boutron I, Altman DG, Hopewell S et al (2014) Impact of spin in the abstracts of articles reporting results of randomized controlled trials in the field of cancer: the SPIIN randomized controlled trial. J Clin Oncol 32:4120–4126. https://doi.org/10.1200/JCO.2014.56.7503

Canadian Institutes of Health Research, Natural Sciences and Engineering Research Council of Canada, Social Sciences and Humanities Research Council of Canada, Secretariat on Responsible Conduct of Research (Canada) (2018) Tri-Council policy statement: ethical conduct for research involving humans

Carlisle B, Federico CA, Kimmelman J (2018) Trials that say "maybe": the disconnect between exploratory and confirmatory testing after drug approval. BMJ 360:k959. https://doi.org/10.1136/bmj.k959

Chalmers I, Nylenna M (2014) A new network to promote evidence-based research. Lancet 384:1903–1904. https://doi.org/10.1016/S0140-6736(14)62252-2

Crouch RA, Arras JD (1998) AZT trials and tribulations. Hast Cent Rep 28:26–34. https://doi.org/10.2307/3528266

DeMets DL, Furberg CD, Friedman LM (eds) (2005) Data monitoring in clinical trials: a case studies approach, 2006 edition. Springer, New York

Dickmann LJ, Schutzman JL (2017) Racial and ethnic composition of cancer clinical drug trials: how diverse are we? Oncologist. https://doi.org/10.1634/theoncologist.2017-0237

Dixon-Woods M, Jackson C, Windridge KC, Kenyon S (2006) Receiving a summary of the results of a trial: qualitative study of participants' views. BMJ 332:206–210. https://doi.org/10.1136/bmj.38675.677963.3A

Elahi M, Eshera N, Bambata N et al (2016) The Food and Drug Administration Office of Women's Health: impact of science on regulatory policy: an update. J Women's Health 25:222–234. https://doi.org/10.1089/jwh.2015.5671

Faden RR, Beauchamp TL (1986) A history and theory of informed consent. Oxford University Press, New York

Federico CA, Wang T, Doussau A et al (2019) Assessment of pregabalin postapproval trials and the suggestion of efficacy for new indications: a systematic review. JAMA Intern Med 179:90–97. https://doi.org/10.1001/jamainternmed.2018.5705

Fergusson D, Glass KC, Hutton B, Shapiro S (2005) Randomized controlled trials of aprotinin in cardiac surgery: could clinical equipoise have stopped the bleeding? Clin Trials 2:218–232. https://doi.org/10.1191/1740774505cn085oa

Flory J, Emanuel E (2004) Interventions to improve research participants' understanding in informed consent for research: a systematic review. JAMA 292:1593–1601. https://doi.org/10.1001/jama.292.13.1593

Flory JH, Kitcher P (2004) Global health and the scientific research agenda. Philos Public Aff 32:36–65. https://doi.org/10.1111/j.1467-6486.2004.00004.x

Flory JH, Mushlin AI, Goodman ZI (2016) Proposals to conduct randomized controlled trials without informed consent: a narrative review. J Gen Intern Med 31:1511–1518. https://doi.org/10.1007/s11606-016-3780-5

Freedman B (1987) Equipoise and the ethics of clinical research. N Engl J Med 317:141–145. https://doi.org/10.1056/NEJM198707163170304

General Assembly of the World Medical Association (2014) World Medical Association Declaration of Helsinki: ethical principles for medical research involving human subjects. J Am Coll Dent 81:14–18

Ghare MI, Chandrasekhar J, Mehran R et al (2019) Sexdisparities in cardiovascular device evaluations: strategies for recruitment and retention of female patients in clinical device trials. JACC Cardiovasc Interv 12:301–308. https://doi.org/10.1016/j.jcin.2018.10.048

Glickman SW, McHutchison JG, Peterson ED et al (2009) Ethical and scientific implications of the globalization of clinical research. N Engl J Med 360:816–823. https://doi.org/10.1056/NEJMsb0803929

Goldbeck-Wood S (1998) Denmark takes a lead on research ethics. BMJ 316:1185. https://doi.org/10.1136/bmj.316.7139.1185j

Grant RW, Sugarman J (2004) Ethics in human subjects research: do incentives matter? J Med Philos 29:717–738. https://doi.org/10.1080/03605310490883046

Hakala A, Kimmelman J, Carlisle B et al (2015) Accessibility of trial reports for drugs stalling in development: a systematic assessment of registered trials. BMJ 350:h1116. https://doi.org/10.1136/bmj.h1116

Halperin H, Paradis N, Mosesso V et al (2007) Recommendations for implementation of community consultation and public disclosure under the Food and Drug Administration's "exception from informed consent requirements for emergency research": a special report from the American Heart Association Emergency Cardiovascular Care Committee and Council on Cardiopulmonary, Perioperative and Critical Care: endorsed by the American College of Emergency Physicians and the Society for Academic Emergency Medicine. Circulation 116:1855–1863. https://doi.org/10.1161/CIRCULATIONAHA.107.186661

Halpern SD, Karlawish JHT, Berlin JA (2002) The continuing unethical conduct of underpowered clinical trials. JAMA 288:358–362

Hawkins JS (2004) The ethics of Zelen consent. J Thromb Haemost 2:882–883. https://doi.org/10.1111/j.1538-7836.2004.00782.x

Hey SP, Kimmelman J (2014) The questionable use of unequal allocation in confirmatory trials. Neurology 82:77–79. https://doi.org/10.1212/01.wnl.0000438226.10353.1c

Hope T, McMillan J (2004) Challenge studies of human volunteers: ethical issues. J Med Ethics 30:110–116. https://doi.org/10.1136/jme.2003.004440

Horng S, Grady C (2003) Misunderstanding in clinical research: distinguishing therapeutic misconception, therapeutic misestimation, and therapeutic optimism. IRB 25:11–16

International Council for Harmonisation (1996) Guideline for good clinical practice. https://database.ich.org/sites/default/files/E6_R2_Addendum.pdf

Kane PB, Kim SYH, Kimmelman J (2020) What research ethics (often) gets wrong about minimal risk. Am J Bioeth 20:42–44. https://doi.org/10.1080/15265161.2019.1687789

Kasenda B, Schandelmaier S, Sun X et al (2014) Subgroup analyses in randomised controlled trials: cohort study on trial protocols and journal publications. BMJ 349:g4539. https://doi.org/10.1136/bmj.g4539

Kimmelman J (2005) Medical research, risk, and bystanders. IRB Ethics Hum Res 27:1

Kimmelman J (2020) What is human research for? Reflections on the omission of scientific integrity from the Belmont Report (accepted). Perspect Biol Med 62(2):251–261

Kimmelman J, Federico C (2017) Consider drug efficacy before first-in-human trials. Nature 542:25–27. https://doi.org/10.1038/542025a

Kimmelman J, Weijer C, Meslin EM (2009) Helsinki discords: FDA, ethics, and international drug trials. Lancet 373:13–14. https://doi.org/10.1016/S0140-6736(08)61936-4

King NMP (2000) Defining and describing benefit appropriately in clinical trials. J Law Med Ethics 28:332–343. https://doi.org/10.1111/j.1748-720X.2000.tb00685.x

Lantos JD, Feudtner C (2015) SUPPORT and the ethics of study implementation: lessons for comparative effectiveness research from the trial of oxygen therapy for premature babies. Hast Cent Rep 45:30–40. https://doi.org/10.1002/hast.407

Levine C, Faden R, Grady C et al (2004) "Special scrutiny": a targeted form of research protocol review. Ann Intern Med 140:220–223

Loder E, Groves T (2015) The BMJ requires data sharing on request for all trials. BMJ 350:h2373. https://doi.org/10.1136/bmj.h2373

London AJ (2007) Clinical equipoise: foundational requirement or fundamental error? In: The Oxford handbook of bioethics. Oxford University Press, Oxford, pp 571–596

London AJ, Kimmelman J, Emborg ME (2010) Beyond access vs. protection in trials of innovative therapies. Science 328:829–830. https://doi.org/10.1126/science.1189369

London AJ, Kimmelman J, Carlisle B (2012) Rethinking research ethics: the case of postmarketing trials. Science 336:544–545. https://doi.org/10.1126/science.1216086

Mathieu S, Boutron I, Moher D et al (2009) Comparison of registered and published primary outcomes in randomized controlled trials. JAMA 302:977–984. https://doi.org/10.1001/jama.2009.1242

Mello MM, Francer JK, Wilenzick M et al (2013) Preparing for responsible sharing of clinical trial data. N Engl J Med 369:1651–1658. https://doi.org/10.1056/NEJMhle1309073

Mello MM, Lieou V, Goodman SN (2018) Clinical trial participants' views of the risks and benefits of data sharing. N Engl J Med. https://doi.org/10.1056/NEJMsa1713258

Menikoff J, Kaneshiro J, Pritchard I (2017) The common rule, updated. N Engl J Med 376:613–615. https://doi.org/10.1056/NEJMp1700736

Nasser M, Clarke M, Chalmers I et al (2017) What are funders doing to minimise waste in research? Lancet 389:1006–1007. https://doi.org/10.1016/S0140-6736(17)30657-8

Palmowski A, Buttgereit T, Palmowski Y et al (2018) Applicability of trials in rheumatoid arthritis and osteoarthritis: a systematic review and meta-analysis of trial populations showing adequate proportion of women, but underrepresentation of elderly people. Semin Arthritis Rheum. https://doi.org/10.1016/j.semarthrit.2018.10.017

Partridge AH, Winer EP (2002) Informing clinical trial participants about study results. JAMA 288:363–365. https://doi.org/10.1001/jama.288.3.363

Phillips R, Hazell L, Sauzet O, Cornelius V (2019) Analysis and reporting of adverse events in randomised controlled trials: a review. BMJ Open 9:e024537. https://doi.org/10.1136/bmjopen-2018-024537

Polman CH, Reingold SC, Barkhof F et al (2008) Ethics of placebo-controlled clinical trials in multiple sclerosis: a reassessment. Neurology 70:1134–1140. https://doi.org/10.1212/01.wnl.0000306410.84794.4d

Richardson HS, Belsky L (2004) The ancillary-care responsibilities of medical researchers. An ethical framework for thinking about the clinical care that researchers owe their subjects. Hast Cent Rep 34:25–33

Savulescu J, Chalmers I, Blunt J (1996) Are research ethics committees behaving unethically? Some suggestions for improving performance and accountability. BMJ 313:1390–1393. https://doi.org/10.1136/bmj.313.7069.1390

Sox HC, Rennie D (2008) Seeding trials: just say "no". Ann Intern Med 149:279–280

Turner L, Shamseer L, Altman DG et al (2012) Consolidated standards of reporting trials (CONSORT) and the completeness of reporting of randomised controlled trials (RCTs) published in medical journals. Cochrane Database Syst Rev 11:MR000030. https://doi.org/10.1002/14651858.MR000030.pub2

U.S. Department of Health and Human Services (2016) 42 CFR 11: clinical trials registration and results information submission

U.S. Department of Health and Human Services, Food and Drug Administration (2005) Guidance for industry: how to comply with the Pediatric Research Equity Act

U.S. Department of Health and Human Services, Food and Drug Administration(2009) Good reprint practices for the distribution of medical journal articles and medical or scientific reference publications on unapproved new uses of approved drugs and approved or cleared medical devices

U.S. Department of Health and Human Services, Food and Drug Administration(2016) Collection of race and ethnicity data in clinical trials

Vedula SS, Li T, Dickersin K (2013) Differences in reporting of analyses in internal company documents versus published trial reports: comparisons in industry-sponsored trials in off-label uses of gabapentin. PLoS Med 10:e1001378. https://doi.org/10.1371/journal.pmed.1001378

Weijer C, Miller PB (2004) When are research risks reasonable in relation to anticipated benefits? Nat Med 10:570. https://doi.org/10.1038/nm0604-570

Weijer C, Grimshaw JM, Taljaard M et al (2011) Ethical issues posed by cluster randomized trials in health research. Trials 12:100. https://doi.org/10.1186/1745-6215-12-100

Wolf SM, Paradise J, Caga-anan C (2008) The law of incidental findings in human subjects research: establishing researchers' duties. J Law Med Ethics 36(361–383):214. https://doi.org/10.1111/j.1748-720X.2008.00281.x

World Health Organization, Council for International Organizations of Medical Sciences (2017) International ethical guidelines for health-related research involving humans. CIOMS, Geneva

Yordanov Y, Dechartres A, Porcher R et al (2015) Avoidable waste of research related to inadequate methods in clinical trials. BMJ 350:h809. https://doi.org/10.1136/bmj.h809

History of the Society for Clinical Trials

5

O. Dale Williams and Barbara S. Hawkins

Contents

Abstract

This chapter provides a synopsis of the events leading to the creation of the Society for Clinical Trials (SCT). The Society was officially incorporated in September 1978 and celebrated its 40th anniversary during its annual meeting in New Orleans May 19–22, 2019.

O. D. Williams (✉)
Department of Biostatistics, University of North Carolina, Chapel Hill, NC, USA

Department of Medicine, University of Alabama at Birmingham, Birmingham, AL, USA
e-mail: odalewilliams@yahoo.com

B. S. Hawkins
Johns Hopkins School of Medicine and Bloomberg School of Public Health, The Johns Hopkins University, Baltimore, MD, USA
e-mail: bhawkins@jhmi.edu

© Springer Nature Switzerland AG 2022
S. Piantadosi, C. L. Meinert (eds.), *Principles and Practice of Clinical Trials*,
https://doi.org/10.1007/978-3-319-52636-2_208

Keywords

Clinical trials · Greenberg report · Coordinating center · CCMP · Models Project · National Conference · Directors

Introduction

The Society for Clinical Trials, Inc. (SCT) is a professional society for advocates, designers, and practitioners of clinical trials, regardless of medical specialty or area of expertise. SCT was incorporated in September 1978. It was created with the purpose:

- To promote the development and exchange of information for design and conduct of clinical trials and research using similar methods
- To provide a forum for discussion of philosophical, ethical, legal, and procedural issues involved in the design, organization, operations, and analysis of clinical trials and other epidemiological studies that use similar methods (Society for Clinical Trials Board of Directors 1980).

Background: 1967–1972

In the early 1970s, there was an expanding and evolving awareness that clinical trials were going to play a vital and key role in the development and implementation of improved strategies for addressing important public health and medical issues. At that time, only a few large multicenter trials had been undertaken, including the University Group Diabetes Program (UGDP) and the Coronary Drug Project (CDP), both sponsored by the National Institutes of Health (NIH). Experience in these projects highlighted the theoretical, organizational, and operational challenges such studies presented. It was clear that clinical trials were a valuable tool for evaluating and comparing interventions; however, there was significant concern among sponsors and practitioners as to their cost, management, and duration before they reached a conclusion regarding the effectiveness and safety of interventions under evaluation. Donald S. Fredrickson (1924–2002; Director, National Heart Institute 1966–1974; NIH Director 1975–1981) summarized these issues eloquently in an address to the New York Academy of Science on January 23, 1968. In this address, for which the full text is available2, he described field trials as indispensable ordeals that are necessary for avoiding perpetual uncertainty.

In 1967, the National Heart Institute (later the National Heart, Lung, and Blood Institute [NHLBI]) created the Heart Special Project Committee (chaired by Bernard G. Greenberg, Chair of Biostatistics, University of North Carolina) to review the approach to cooperative studies. The resulting report, known as the Greenberg Report, was presented to the National Advisory Heart Council later in the same year. The Greenberg Report (Heart Special Project Committee 1988) highlighted three essential components:

- Organization of local units under good leadership
- Establishment of a coordinating center
- Critical "interrogation" of the data

It also provided guidelines for organizational structure and operations, many of which continue to be followed to this day.

Many of the technology elements now taken for granted were not available in the early 1970s. Communication by telephone and postal mail was more difficult, fax capability was not fully available, and desktop computers were still under development. Word processing and other essential software applications, including those for data management, also were not available. Further, telephone conferencing was in its early phases and was expensive and less than fully reliable. It required an operator to contact participants and add them to the call. Video conferencing was beyond the imagination of most clinical trialists.

In spite of these and other constraints, it was clear that the volume of large-scale multicenter trials was likely to grow and that they would require techniques and operations not yet fully developed. During the early 1970s, the National Heart Institute initiated three large-scale multicenter activities that included large clinical trials: the Lipids Research Clinics (LRC) Program with its Coronary Primary Prevention Trial, the Hypertension Detection and Follow-up Program (HDFP), and the Multiple Risk Factor Intervention Trial (MRFIT). These were large, multicenter long-term studies designed to address mechanisms of and interventions for critical aspects of heart disease, the leading cause of death among men in the United States (USA) at that time.

Steps in the Creation of the Society for Clinical Trials

So the stage was set for the creation of an organization of designers and others engaged in multicenter clinical trials. Key steps in this process were:

1. Annual meetings of personnel from coordinating centers for trials already underway that began in 1973
2. Meeting of interested individuals with the NIH Clinical Trials Committee, 1976
3. National Conference on Clinical Trials Methodology, October 1977
4. SCT incorporation, September 1978
5. Publication of first issue of *Controlled Clinical Trials,* May 1980

It may be surprising that the first step listed is meetings of coordinating center personnel. However, as noted above, the Greenberg Report indicated that coordinating centers were essential components of cooperative studies, such as large-scale multicenter clinical trials. The annual meetings were facilitated by NHLBI under the leadership of Robert I. Levy. Levy understood that coordinating center capabilities and the pool of relevant expertise needed to be expanded to meet current and future needs for successful conduct of large studies. These meetings began in 1973 and continued until 1981; they initiated a sequence of events that ultimately led to the creation of the SCT.

Meetings of Coordinating Center Personnel

The initial 1.5-day meeting of coordinating center personnel was held in May 1973 in Columbia, Maryland. More than 60 people participated, including 9 from NIH; participants represented 11 institutions. This initial meeting was mostly a "show and tell" by investigators from coordinating centers for major NHLBI-sponsored multi-center studies:

- Lipid Research Clinics Program
- Hypertension Detection and Follow-Up Program
- Multiple Risk Factor Intervention Trial
- Hypertension, Thrombolysis, and Exercise
- Coronary Drug Project

Organization of and participation in the initial meeting was facilitated by NHLBI primarily through existing funding awards to individual investigators.

The full sequence of meetings of coordinating center personnel, meeting locations, and host institutions are listed by year in Table 1. The host institution typically was the location of one or more of the NHLBI-supported coordinating centers. Beginning in 1976, these meetings were sponsored by NHLBI through the Coordinating Center Models Project (Curtis L. Meinert, principal investigator), described below. The last two meetings were held in conjunction with the first and second annual scientific meetings of the Society for Clinical Trials.

The breadth and depth of these meetings evolved over time. For example, by the time of the fourth meeting in Chapel Hill, the 166 attendees represented 40 multicenter studies. Presentations focused on data quality assurance, computer

Table 1 Locations and host organizations for meetings of personnel from clinical trial coordinating centers, 1973–1981

Year	Meeting location	Host organization
1973	Columbia, MD	University of Maryland
1974	–	–
1975	Plymouth, MN	University of Minnesota
1976	Houston, TX	University of Texas
1977	Chapel Hill, NC	University of North Carolina
1978	Washington, DC	George Washington University
1979	Boston, MA	
1980	Philadelphia, PA	Society for Clinical Trials
1981	San Francisco, CA	Society for Clinical Trials

–, no meeting held

operations and cost, and survival analysis. Also, the Coordinating Center Models Project was introduced. The guest speaker was Levy, who addressed "Decision Making in Large-Scale Clinical Trials." Organizers of these meetings already had adopted the format of typical scientific society meetings.

Coordinating Center Models Project

Two important activities occurred in 1976. One was NHLBI funding of the Coordinating Center Models Project (CCMP [1976–1979]). The CCMP purpose was to study existing coordinating centers for large, multicenter trials with the aim of establishing guidelines and standards for organization and operations of coordinating centers for future multicenter trials. The seven CCMP reports are available from the National Technical Information Service (Coordinating Center Models Project Research Group. Coordinating Center Models Project 1979a, b, c, d, e, f, 1980).

Also during 1976, Williams, Meinert, and others met with Robert S. Gordon, Jr., who was special assistant to the NIH Director (Frederickson) and other key leaders at NIH. Later that year, a group consisting of Fred Ederer (National Eye Institute) and Meinert, Williams and Harold P. Roth (National Institute of Arthritis, Metabolism, and Digestive Disease) met with the NIH Clinical Trials Committee. This group proposed that a professional society that addressed the general issues of clinical trials be created and asked for the Committee's support. The Committee members expressed interest in the concept but indicated that evidence for widespread participatory support was lacking. Instead, the Committee proposed holding a conference to assess the level of support for such a society. As a result, a Planning Committee was formed under the leadership of Roth.

Although thus far we have described activities in the USA sponsored primarily by the NHLBI, other sponsors and practitioners of clinical trials were interested in creating a forum for sharing experiences, methods, and related developments. The National Cancer Institute (NCI) created the Clinical Trials Cooperative Group Program in 1955; the National Cancer Act of 1971 enhanced the role of these cooperative groups and their coordinating centers. In 1962, the U.S. Veterans Administration (VA; now the U.S. Department of Veterans Affairs) established four regional research support centers for the VA Cooperative Studies Program (VA CSP) under the leadership of Lawrence Shaw (https://www.vascp.research.va.gov/CSP/history.asp). In 1967 and 1970, findings from a major trial of antihypertensive agents conducted by a VA Cooperative Studies Group were published (Veterans Administration Cooperative Study Group on Antihypertensive Agents 1967, 1970). In 1972, two of the regional research support centers were designated to house CSP coordinating centers to support "multicenter clinical trials that evaluated novel therapies or new uses of standard treatments" (Streptomycin in Tuberculosis Trials Committee 1948). Two more CSP coordinating centers were established during the next 6 years. In the United Kingdom (UK), the Medical Research Council had sponsored randomized trials, following the landmark trial of streptomycin for tuberculosis (Streptomycin in Tuberculosis Trials Committee 1948). Thus, the group of sponsors and individuals potentially interested in a professional society for clinical trialists extended well beyond NHLBI and its awardees.

National Conference on Clinical Trials Methodology

The 1977 National Conference on Clinical Trials Methodology was held in Building 1 on the NIH campus on October 3 and 4, 1977. Somewhat to the surprise of almost everyone involved in its planning, the conference attracted more than 700 participants from around the USA who represented much of NIH and other current and potential sponsors of clinical trials. Attendees were welcomed by Gordon and Fredrickson; the program included presentations within broad topics:

- When and how to stop a clinical trial?
- Who will be effective as a clinical trials investigator, and what are adequate incentives?
- Patient recruitment: problems and solutions.
- Quality assurance of clinical data.
- Ethical considerations in clinical trials.

One of the more important sessions was on communications, which addressed the question "Should mechanisms be established for sharing among clinical trial investigators experience in handling problems in design, execution and analysis?" The discussion leaders were Roth and Genell Knatterud, with Louis Lasagna, Meinert, and Barbara Hawkins. Harold Schoolman and Fred Mosteller also contributed. The conference and this session on communications played a key role in the creation of the SCT. The conference proceedings were published 2 years later (Roth and Gordon 1979).

Soon after this conference, in September, 1978, the Society for Clinical Trials was incorporated. The members of the initial board of directors are listed in Table 2. One

Table 2 Members of the initial board of directors of the Society for Clinical Trials

Thomas C. Chalmers, MD, *Chair,* Mt. Sinai School of Medicine
Harold O. Conn, MD, Yale University School of Medicine and West Haven VA Hospital
Fred Ederer, MA, National Eye Institute, National Institutes of Health
Robert S. Gordon, Jr., MD, National Institutes of Health
Curtis L. Meinert, PhD, The Johns Hopkins University
Christian R. Klimt, MD, DrPH, University of Maryland and Maryland Medical Research Institute
Paul Meier, PhD, University of Chicago
Charles G. Moertel, MD, Mayo Clinic
Thaddeus E. Prout, MD, The Johns Hopkins University and Greater Baltimore Medical Institute
Harold P. Roth, MD, National Institute of Diabetes and Digestive Diseases, NIH
Maurice J. Staquet, MD, Representative of the International Society for Clinical Biostatistics
O. Dale Williams, PhD, University of North Carolina

of the first acts of the Board was to develop plans for the first meeting of the Society. A Program Committee (Williams, Chair) was created; as noted above, this meeting was planned and undertaken in conjunction with the seventh annual meeting of coordinating center personnel. The result was a four-day meeting May 5–8, 1980, in Philadelphia. Sponsors included NHLBI, NEI, National Institute for Neurologic Conditions, Deafness, and Stoke (NINDS), National Institute for Addiction and Infectious Diseases (NIAID), and Maryland Medical Research Institute. This important meeting included three key presentations (Combined Annual Scientific Sessions Society for Clinical Trials 1980):

- Fredrickson, NIH Director: "Sorting out the doctor's bag"
- Seymour Perry, Director National Center for Health Care Technology: "Introduction to the National Center for Health Care Technology"
- Charles G. Moertel, Chair, Comprehensive Cancer Center, Mayo Clinic: "How to succeed in clinical trials without really trying"

The second annual meeting, also with Williams as Program Committee Chair, was held in conjunction with the eighth and final annual meeting of coordinating center personnel.

Journals of the Society for Clinical Trials

In conjunction with the incorporation of the Society, negotiations began with a publisher to initiate a journal, *Controlled Clinical Trials,* with Meinert to serve as Editor and Williams as Associate Editor. The editorial arrangement continued for about 10 years until Williams stepped down from his role. The journal had been adopted as the official journal of the Society by the time the first issue was published in 1980. Janet Wittes, (1995–1998), and James Neaton, (1999–2003), each served as a later editor of *Controlled Clinical Trials.*

Controlled Clinical Trials was unique when it originated because of its publication of articles on a variety of topics that represented the broad and varied interests and expertise of the SCT membership. These spanned clinical trial design, conduct, logistics, ethics, regulation, policy, analysis, and methodology. In particular, it was prescient in being one of very few or perhaps the only journal at that time to publish "design papers," i.e., papers devoted solely to presenting the design and key protocol elements of planned clinical trials. The idea that protocols are both scholarly outputs and should be publicly described was enshrined in the later formation of clinicaltrials.gov, and the idea has also been adopted by a wide variety of fields today under the rubric of "Registered Reports."

In 2004, the Society decided to part ways with Elsevier, the publisher of the Society's journal. Because the journal's name was owned by Elsevier (albeit subsequently changed by them to *Contemporary Clinical Trials*), the Society in effect launched a new journal, albeit with the same editorial board. This new journal was named *Clinical Trials: the Journal of the Society for Clinical Trials* and is published by Sage. Steven N. Goodman was the originating editor of the new journal from 2004 to 2013 and succeeded by Colin Begg in 2013.

International Participation

The Society has been enhanced by membership and meeting attendees from outside the USA, essentially from its outset. In fact, Maurice J. Staquet was a member of the initial board of directors as a representative of the International Society for Clinical Biostatistics. Also, meetings have been held in other countries. The first was the 7th meeting, held in Montreal, Canada, May 1986. The 11th meeting was held in Toronto, Canada, May 1990; the 12th was the first joint meeting with the International Society for Clinical Biostatistics, held in Brussels, Belgium, July 1991; the 18th was the second meeting of the Society and the International Society for Clinical Biostatistics, held in Boston, July 1997; the 21st was held in Toronto, Canada, April, 2000; the 24th was the third joint meeting with the International Society for Clinical Biostatistics, held in London, England, July 2003; the 28th was held in Montreal, Canada, May, 2007; the 32nd in Vancouver, Canada, May, 2011; the 37th was held in Montreal, Canada, May 2016; and the 38th was held in Liverpool, England, May 2017.

Summary and Conclusion

By 1981, the Society for Clinical Trials was fully functional; *Controlled Clinical Trials* was in publication. Beginning in 1980, scientific meetings of the Society have been held annually. Programs of annual meetings and abstracts of contributed presentations, along with other information, are online at https://www.sctweb.org; many have been published in the official SCT journals. Although clinical procedures and information technology have evolved since 1981, many of the practical issues persist; for example, the methods for promoting and monitoring data quality have evolved but the need for data of high quality remains. As in other areas of clinical trials methodology, the practices to achieve a desired result may change over time, but the principles are permanent. Thus, the goals of the SCT remain pertinent to today's clinical trialists.

Many different individuals contributed importantly to the creation and early operation of the SCT. Of those mentioned above, three are especially important. Fredrickson saw the need for an entity such as the SCT and supported it from the highest levels of NIH. Gordon was tireless in meeting with interested advocates for a professional society for clinical trialists, eliciting and securing support across NIH, and helping to lead the overall creation effort. Levy saw a compelling need for enhanced coordinating center capability and made sure the meetings of coordinating center personnel that led directly to the creation of the Society were supported and well organized. Many other individuals deserve significant credit as well, but these three are especially deserving of recognition for their important and timely contributions.

References

Abstracts. Combined Annual Scientific Sessions Society for Clinical Trials and seventh annual symposium for coordinating clinical trials. May 6–8, 1980, Marriott Inn, Philadelphia, PA (1980) Control Clin Trials 1:165–178

Coordinating Center Models Project Research Group. Coordinating Center Models Project (1979a, March 1) A study of coordinating centers in multicenter clinical trials. Design and methods, vols 1 and 2. NTIS Accession No. PB82-143730 and PB82-143744. National Technical Information Services, Springfield

Coordinating Center Models Project Research Group. Coordinating Center Models Project (1979b, March 1) A study of coordinating centers in multicenter clinical trials. RFPs for coordinating centers: a content evaluation. NTIS Accession No. PB82143702. National Technical Information Services, Springfield

Coordinating Center Models Project Research Group. Coordinating Center Models Project (1979c, August 1) A study of coordinating centers in multicenter clinical trials. Terminology. NTIS Accession No. PB82-143728. National Technical Information Services, Springfield. Bibliographic resource for clinical trials. April 1, 1980. NTIS Accession No. PB87-??????

Coordinating Center Models Project Research Group. Coordinating Center Models Project (1979d, September 1) A study of coordinating centers in multicenter clinical trials. Phases of a multicenter clinical trials. NTIS Accession No. PB82-143751. National Technical Information Services, Springfield

Coordinating Center Models Project Research Group. Coordinating Center Models Project (1979e, September 1) A study of coordinating centers in multicenter clinical trials. Enhancement of methodological research in the field of clinical trials. NTIS Accession No. PB82-143710. National Technical Information Services, Springfield

Coordinating Center Models Project Research Group. Coordinating Center Models Project (1979f, June 1) A study of coordinating centers in multicenter clinical trials. CCMP manuscripts presented at the annual symposia on coordinating clinical trials. NTIS Accession No. PB82-143694. National Technical Information Services, Springfield

Coordinating Center Models Project Research Group. Coordinating Center Models Project (1980, September 1) A study of coordinating centers in multicenter clinical trials. Coordinating centers and the contract process. NTIS Accession No. PB87-139101? National Technical Information Services, Springfield

Frederickson DS (1968) The field trial: some thoughts on the indispensable ordeal. Bull N Y Acad Med 44(2):985–993

Heart Special Project Committee (1988) Organization, review, and administration of cooperative studies (Greenberg report): a report from the Heart Special Project Committee to the National Advisory Heart Council. Control Clin Trials 9:137–148. [Includes a list of members of the Heart Special Project Committee]

https://www.vascp.research.va.gov/CSP/history.asp. Accessed 12 Aug 2019

Roth HP, Gordon RS (1979) Proceedings of the national conference on clinical trials methodology. Clin Pharmacol Ther 25(5, pt 2):629–765

Society for Clinical Trials Board of Directors (1980) By-laws. Control Clin Trials 1(1):83–89

Streptomycin in Tuberculosis Trials Committee (1948) Streptomycin treatment of pulmonary tuberculosis. Br Med J 2:769–782

Veterans Administration Cooperative Study Group on Antihypertensive Agents (1967) Effects of treatment on morbidity in hypertension. Results in patients with diastolic blood pressures averaging 115 through 129 mm Hg. JAMA 202(11):116–122

Veterans Administration Cooperative Study Group on Antihypertensive Agents (1970) Effects of treatment on morbidity in hypertension. II. Results in patients with diastolic blood pressures averaging 90 through 114 mm Hg. JAMA 213(7):1143–1152

Part II

Conduct and Management

Investigator Responsibilities

6

Bruce J. Giantonio

Contents

B. J. Giantonio (✉)
The ECOG-ACRIN Cancer Research Group, Philadelphia, PA, USA

Massachusetts General Hospital, Boston, MA, USA

Department of Medical Oncology, University of Pretoria, Pretoria, South Africa
e-mail: bgiantonio@ecog-acrin.org

© Springer Nature Switzerland AG 2022
S. Piantadosi, C. L. Meinert (eds.), *Principles and Practice of Clinical Trials*,
https://doi.org/10.1007/978-3-319-52636-2_29

Abstract

The research atrocities committed during World War II using human subjects prompted the development of a body of regulations, beginning with the Nuremberg Code, to ensure that human subjects' research is safely conducted and prioritizes the rights of the individual over the conduct of the research. The resultant regulations guiding human subjects' research affect protocol design, the selection of participants, safety reporting and oversight, and the dissemination of research results. The investigator conducting research on human subjects must be familiar with those regulations to meet his/her responsibility to protect the rights and welfare of research participants.

Keywords

Belmont Report · The Common Rule · Delegation of tasks · Drug accountability · Good clinical practice · Informed consent process · Institutional review board (IRB) · Investigator · Noncompliance · Scientific misconduct

Introduction

Clinical research is the foundation for evidence-based, high-quality medical care. The individuals who participate in clinical research are central to advancing our knowledge of disease, yet inherent in the conduct of clinical research is the risk of harm to the research participant. Since the development of the Nuremberg Code in 1947, regulations and guidelines for performing clinical research that balance the common good of scientific advancement with protecting the rights and welfare of individuals provide the framework for the ethical conduct of clinical research with human subjects. Building on the Nuremburg Code, the Belmont Report delineates the boundary between practice and research and describes three basic principles relevant to the ethics of research involving human subjects: the principles of respect of persons, beneficence, and justice. These principles provide the foundations for the "Common Rule" and "good clinical practice" (GCP). (Of note, the "Common Rule" is used to describe subpart A of Title 45, part 46 (45 CFR 46) of the Code of Federal Regulations. The CFR represents the codification of the general and permanent rules of the departments and agencies of the US Federal Government.)

Regulations and policies governing clinical research and defining the responsibilities of the investigator will be found at the federal, state, and local level and can vary by region of the world. Additional responsibilities may be required by funding agencies, sponsors, and research institutions. In section "References," we list the regulations and guidance documents with the greatest impact on the conduct of clinical research and from which the responsibilities of the investigator are derived.

Definitions

Research

Research is defined in 45 CFR 46 as a systematic investigation, including research development, testing, and evaluation, designed to develop or contribute to generalizable knowledge.

Investigators

The definitions of investigator used in the existing guidelines and policies vary but in general describe any individual responsible for the conduct of research involving human subjects. The conduct of clinical research can be limited to one research site or performed across hundreds of sites, and the term investigator (or principal investigator) can apply to the person responsible either for the study as a whole, or for an individual site. For purposes of clarity, and unless otherwise stated, we will use the term investigator to encompass the investigator of single-site research, the lead investigator of multi-site research, and site-specific investigators of multi-site research.

Overall Responsibilities of Investigators

Research that requires the participation of human subjects includes prospective clinical trials of drugs, devices, or other interventions; translational biologic and imaging analyses; participant-based surveys and questionnaires; and retrospective data analyses. Regardless of the type of investigation being conducted, a clinical investigator's primary responsibility is to protect the rights and welfare of the participants (Bear et al. 2011).

In general this requires that the clinical research is scientifically justifiable and uses research methods and a trial design appropriate to the question being studied and that there must be safeguards for the participants proportional to the level of risk of the research.

We will review the specific responsibilities of the investigator according to the two broad, albeit overlapping, categories of research study design and conduct and safeguard to protect research participants.

Research Study Design and Conduct

Design

The investigator of a single-site clinical research study, or the lead investigator of a multi-site study, has direct responsibility for the design of the proposed research.

Table 1 Seven requirements for the ethical conduct of clinical research

1. Value	Enhancements of health or knowledge must be derived from the research
2. Scientific validity	The research must the methodologically rigorous
3. Fair subject selection	Scientific objectives, not vulnerability or privilege, and the potential for and distribution of risks and benefits should determine communities selected as study sites and the inclusion criteria for individual subjects
4. Favorable risk-benefit ratio	Within the context of standard clinical practice and the research protocol, risks must be minimized, and potential benefits enhanced and the potential benefits to individuals and the knowledge gained for society must outweigh the risks
5. Independent review	Unaffiliated individuals must review the research and approve, amend, or terminate it
6. Informed consent	Individuals should be informed about the research and provide their voluntary consent
7. Respect for enrolled subjects	Subjects should have their privacy protected, the opportunity to withdraw, and their well-being monitored

Four of the seven requirements for the ethical conduct of clinical research (Emanuel et al. 2000) relate to the design of the research: value, scientific validity, fair subject selection, and a favorable risk-benefit ratio (Table 1).

To justify exposing participants to potential harm, the proposed research must provide generalizable knowledge that contributes to the common good. There must be uncertainty among the medical community, or "clinical equipoise," for the question being asked by the research, and the methodology for obtaining that knowledge must be appropriate to the question and rigorously applied. Risks to participants must be minimized, and subject selection must be done such that both the risks and benefits of the research are fairly distributed with subjects excluded only for valid safety or scientific reasons.

Conduct

Qualifications, Training, and Delegation of Tasks

The investigator of a single-site study, the lead investigator for a multi-site study, and individual site-specific investigators are responsible for conducting or supervising the research.

All investigators involved in the research must have the appropriate level of education, training, and experience to conduct the research. This includes maintenance of records of all training required by their institutions and research sponsors, updated as necessary and relevant over time. In addition, the investigator must have sufficient time and resources to properly conduct and supervise the research for which they are responsible.

The rationale for the study and the requirements for its safe and appropriate conduct must be fully understood by the investigator and the research conducted in compliance with the specifics of the study. Investigators must have no conflicts of interest, financial, or otherwise, that could influence their judgment for the inclusion of subjects in the research or the interpretation of the findings.

The Clinical Research Team

The complexity of conducting clinical research has rendered it nearly impossible for an investigator to meet his or her responsibilities to the research without the assistance of others. It is common for certain types of clinical research to be supported by a team of individuals who assist the investigator including co-investigators, clinical research associates, and research pharmacists. In these instances the investigator will serve as the leader of the team with responsibility for its supervision.

The delegation of tasks related to the conduct of the research by the investigator to other qualified individuals is accepted practice. Most institutions that conduct clinical research have programs designed to support their research activities that include offices staffed with those individuals who assist the investigator. The extent to which research-related tasks are delegated, and to whom, is affected by and must comply with federal, state, and local regulations.

It is the responsibility of the investigator that all members of the research team to whom tasks are delegated must have appropriate education, training, and experience in both the conduct of clinical research in general and for the specific study. The supervision of the staff performing the delegated tasks is also the responsibility of the investigator, regardless of the employment arrangements of the staff. In addition, the members of the research team must also be free of conflicts of interest.

Accountability of Investigational Agents

In clinical research that involves investigational agents, the investigator is responsible for drug accountability. This includes oversight of the proper handling and storage of the agent, its correct administration, and the return or destruction of unused agent. The chain of custody of the agent must be clearly documented from the time of the arrival of the investigational agent until its return or destruction. It is appropriate to delegate these tasks to an individual such as a pharmacist who has been trained on the handling, storage, and use of investigational agents.

Data Collection, Research Record Maintenance, and Retention

Data is the lingua franca of clinical research. The accuracy of the data is essential to the sound and safe conduct of the research, and all reported data must be verifiable in the source documents and/or electronic record.

Investigators are ultimately responsible for the accuracy of research data, its storage, and the necessary confidentiality protections according to the specifics of the protocol and its consent form. For large multi-site studies, the storage of research data is centralized and managed by a sponsor or an institution in accordance with their policies. "Shadow charts" maintained at the research site are subject to the same regulations.

All records and communications related to the research are to be securely maintained by the investigator, or his or her representatives. This includes all versions of the protocol and research plan, consent documents, and institutional review board (IRB)/ethics committee correspondence. The research records must be made available upon request by regulatory agencies and research sponsors.

The duration of retention of research data and records may vary by country and local requirements and the specifics of the research. In general, the duration of retention should be in compliance with the regulation requiring the longest duration of record retention.

Reporting of Research Findings

The results of the research, regardless of outcome, are to be reported in a timely manner. To not publish the results of clinical research violates the commitment made to the participant that their involvement in the research will contribute to generalizable knowledge.

Safeguards to Protect Research Participants

Participants in clinical research can be individuals with, or at risk for, a particular disease, or they can be entirely well. The acceptable level of risk that the participant in a research study is subject to must consider the potential benefit to society, and the design of the research study must include steps to protect the participants from untoward harm. Risks to participants can include immediate and long-term physical and emotional harm, financial damage, and privacy violations.

Some of the risk associated with participation in clinical research is mitigated by appropriate study design and research methods, as described above.

Adverse Event Reporting

The recording and monitoring of adverse events encountered during research is essential to protecting the safety of research participants. The investigator must have processes in place that allow for the timely review of adverse events. Any serious or unanticipated adverse events must be promptly reported according to the specifics of the study to the IRB of record for the research project, to any regulatory agency as appropriate, and to the study sponsor.

The investigator is responsible for ensuring that reasonable medical care is provided to the research participants for issues related to the study participation and for the facilitation of care for other health issues that might arise during the study.

Safety Oversight

In addition to an IRB, the oversight of participant safety for a specific research project may utilize a Data and Safety Monitoring Committee (DSMC). Such committees are comprised of individuals with experience in the conduct of clinical research and expertise in the particular disease being studied, the majority of whom are unaffiliated with the specific research project and are free from other conflicts of interest.

Both IRBs and DSMCs are provided with safety data during the conduct of the study. Any severe or unanticipated adverse event is to be reported in a timely manner and according to requirements included in the protocol; all others are submitted according to a preplanned review schedule. Data and Safety Monitoring Committees review not only adverse effects but also outcomes data at preplanned intervals to ensure that the continuation of the research is justified. The reports from Data and Safety Monitoring Committees are usually submitted to the IRB of record for the specific research project.

IRB Requirements

Unless exempt from review, investigators are responsible for interactions with the IRB, including initial IRB approval, approval for any modifications to the research, safety reporting, and, as required, continuing review of the research.

In order for the IRB to effectively evaluate and monitor a clinical research project, investigators must provide the IRB of record with sufficient information to make their determinations regarding the initiation of the clinical research and its ongoing conduct. This includes new safety and outcomes information, deviations to study specified or IRB requirements (section "Protocol Noncompliance and Research Misconduct" below), as well as unanticipated problems involving risks to subjects or others.

Additionally, the investigator is responsible for informing the IRB of record of any significant new finding that emerges during the conduct of the research that might affect a participant's willingness to continue to participate in the research. Based on the significance of the new findings, the investigator may be responsible for providing the new findings to the registered participants, and modifications to the study to account for the new findings may require a suspension in accrual.

It is important to note that the inclusion of vulnerable populations (such as children, students, prisoners, and pregnant women) in clinical research may require additional IRB-approved safeguards for their participation, and the investigator is responsible for implementing those safeguards.

Informed Consent Process

The informed consent process and the consent form are required to ensure that a potential participant in a clinical research project has enough information about the specific project, and about clinical research in general, to make an informed and autonomous decision about their participation.

For clinical research that requires the participant's informed consent, the investigator is responsible for ensuring that consent is obtained and documented as approved by the IRB and according to federal, state, and local requirements. In addition, each participant is to be provided a copy of the informed consent document when written consent is required.

Investigators are required to allow for monitoring and auditing of the research by the IRB of record, sponsors, and any applicable regulatory agencies.

Protocol Noncompliance and Research Misconduct

The investigator is responsible for reporting to the IRB any instances of protocol noncompliance and misconduct. Reporting to the sponsor and other regulatory agencies may be required as well. In addition, the suspension or termination of an IRB approval may also require reporting to the sponsor and to the appropriate federal, state, and local regulatory agencies.

Protocol Noncompliance

As discussed, the protection of the rights and welfare of research participants requires an appropriate trial design. The investigator is responsible for compliance with all protocol-specified requirements during the conduct of the research. This is to ensure both the safety of the participants and the scientific integrity of the research. However, deviations and/or violations (the terms are used interchangeably by some) to protocol-specified criteria can occur and in some instances may be justified. In general protocol deviations are either intentional, or discovered, after they occur.

An intentional protocol deviation represents a change in the research that requires prior IRB review and approval before the change is allowed. In some instances, however, deviations from the protocol for safety reasons are allowed in advance of IRB review and approval.

Research protocol deviations that are discovered after they occur may need to be reported to the IRB. The IRB will determine if the violations represent serious noncompliance or continuing noncompliance. Additional reporting to the sponsor and to regulatory agencies may be required.

- Serious noncompliance: any deviation from protocol-specified requirements that may affect the rights and welfare of participants or adversely affects the scientific integrity of a study.
- Continuing Noncompliance: a pattern of noncompliance that may affect the rights and welfare of participants or adversely affects the scientific integrity of a study.

Research Misconduct

Research misconduct is generally defined by regulatory agencies as fabrication, falsification, or plagiarism in proposing, performing, or reviewing research, or in reporting research results (From: https://ori.hhs.gov/definition-misconduct). In addition, misconduct is not limited to the researcher but includes sponsors, institutions, and the journals publishing the research.

Scientific misconduct violates the investigator's commitment to the ethical conduct of research and exposes research participants to unjustifiable risk. Corrective actions that result from misconduct can include the retraction of the published findings, a loss of research privileges and funding, monetary fines and criminal charges, and a public distrust of the clinical research enterprise. The investigator has a responsibility to report any findings of misconduct, intentional or unintentional, by the research team to the sponsor, to the IRB of record, and to any federal, state, and local regulatory authorities.

Summary and Conclusion

The responsibilities of the clinical research investigator can cover the lifespan of the study and are intended to protect rights and welfare of the research participants and the integrity of the research itself. And while much of the work of clinical research is delegated to others, the overall responsibility remains with the investigator. Noncompliance with the requirements of the research protocol can compromise both participant safety and study integrity.

Key Facts

- The clinical investigator's primary responsibility is to protect the rights and welfare of the participants.
- Research is a systematic investigation, including research development, testing, and evaluation, designed to develop or contribute to generalizable knowledge.
- The Belmont Report identifies three principles for the ethical conduct of research involving human subjects: respect of persons, beneficence, and justice.
- Risk of harm to research participants is mitigated by appropriate study design and research methods.
- All investigators involved in clinical research must have the appropriate level of education, training, and experience to conduct the research.
- The investigator is responsible for the accuracy of research data, its storage, and the necessary confidentiality.
- Noncompliance with all protocol-specified requirements during the conduct of the research can compromise participant safety and the scientific integrity of the research.
- Intentional protocol deviation requires IRB review and approval before the change is allowed. In some instances deviations from the protocol for safety reasons are allowed in advance of IRB review and approval.
- Scientific misconduct violates the investigator's commitment to the ethical conduct of research and exposes research participants to unjustifiable risk.

Regulations and Policies

Regulations and Policies upon which the investigator responsibilities are derived:

a. The Belmont Report: US Department of Health and Human Services, Office for Human Subjects Research: Belmont Report. Ethical Principles and Guidelines for the Protection of Human Subjects of Research.

http://www.hhs.gov/ohrp/humansubjects/guidance/belmont.html

b. US Code of Federal Regulations

eCFR – Code of Federal Regulations

The two relevant sections of the Code of Federal Regulations that apply to the conduct of clinical research are Title 21 CFR Food and Drugs and 45 CFR Public Welfare.

i. Title 21 CFR: Food and Drugs

https://gov.ecfr.io/cgi-bin/text-idx?SID=027d2d7bd97666fc9f896c580d5039dc&mc=true&tpl=/ecfrbrowse/Title21/21tab_02.tpl

This section establishes many of the regulations concerning the investigation of new agents and devices and forms the basis of the policies of the Food and Drug Administration. Relevant sections of 21 CFR are:

21 CFR 312.50: General Responsibilities of Investigators

21 CFR 812.100: Responsibilities of Investigators: Biologics

21 CFR 812.110: Responsibilities of Investigators: Devices

21 CFR 11: Electronic records/Electronic signature

21 CFR 50: Protections of Human Subject

21 CFR 54: Financial Disclosure by Clinical Investigators

21 CFR 56: Institutional Review Boards

ii. Title 45 CFR: Public Welfare

Section 45 CFR 46: "Regulation for the Protection of Human Subjects in Research"

https://gov.ecfr.io/cgi-bin/text-idx?SID=6ddf773215b32fc68af87b6599529417&mc=true&node=pt45.1.46&rgn=div5

45 CFR 46 applies to all research involving human subjects that is conducted or funded by US Department of Health and Human Services (DHHS) and has been widely adopted as guidance for clinical research outside of that funded by DHHS.

Subpart A: The Common Rule

Subpart B: Additional protections for pregnant women, human fetuses and neonates

Subpart C: Additional protections for prisoners

Subpart D: Additional protections for children

c. Good Clinical Practice Guidelines (GCP ICH-E6R2)

The International Council for Harmonisation of Technical Requirements for Pharmaceuticals for Human Use (ICH) was established in 1990 with the stated mission to achieve greater harmonization worldwide to ensure that safe, effective, and high-quality medicines are developed and registered in the most resource-efficient manner.

GCP ICH-E6R2 is one of the products created by this organization to define "good clinical practices" for clinical research. These guidelines are commonly used guide clinical research around the world. Of note, the use of the term "good clinical practice" in this context is distinct from that applied to day-to-day patient care.

https://www.ich.org/products/guidelines/efficacy/efficacy-single/article/integrated-addendum-good-clinical-practice.html

d. CIOMS International Ethical Guidelines for Biomedical Research

The Council for International Organizations of Medical Sciences (CIOMS) is an international nongovernmental organization in an official relationship with World Health Organization (WHO). The guidelines focus primarily on rules and principles to protect humans in research and to reliably safeguard the rights and welfare of humans.

https://cioms.ch/shop/product/international-ethical-guidelines-for-health-related-research-involving-humans/

e. Additional Guidance Documents

Attachment C: https://www.hhs.gov/ohrp/sachrp-committee/recommendations/2013-january-10-letter-attachment-c/index.html

FDA Guidance for Industry on Investigator Responsibilities: https://www.fda.gov/downloads/Drugs/.../Guidances/UCM187772.pdf

Cross-References

▶ Data and Safety Monitoring and Reporting
▶ Financial Conflicts of Interest in Clinical Trials
▶ Fraud in Clinical Trials
▶ Good Clinical Practice
▶ Institutional Review Boards and Ethics Committees
▶ Qualifications of the Research Staff
▶ Trial Organization and Governance

References

Baer AR, Devine S, Beardmore CD, Catalano R (2011) Clinical investigator responsibilities. J Oncol Pract 7:124–128. https://doi.org/10.1200/JOP.2010.000216

Emanuel EJ, Wendler D, Grady C (2000) What makes clinical research ethical? JAMA 283:2701–2711. https://doi.org/10.1001/jama.283.20.2701

Centers Participating in Multicenter Trials

7

Roberta W. Scherer and Barbara S. Hawkins

Contents

Abstract

Successful conduct of multicenter trials requires many different types of activities, implemented by different types of centers. Resource centers are those involved in planning the trial protocol, overseeing trial conduct, and analyzing and interpreting trial data. They include clinical and data coordinating centers, reading centers, central laboratories, and others. Clinical centers prepare for the trial at their setting and

R. W. Scherer (✉)
Department of Epidemiology, Johns Hopkins Bloomberg School of Public Health, Baltimore, MD, USA
e-mail: rschere1@jhu.edu

B. S. Hawkins
Johns Hopkins School of Medicine and Bloomberg School of Public Health, The Johns Hopkins University, Baltimore, MD, USA
e-mail: bhawkins@jhmi.edu

© Springer Nature Switzerland AG 2022
S. Piantadosi, C. L. Meinert (eds.), *Principles and Practice of Clinical Trials*,
https://doi.org/10.1007/978-3-319-52636-2_30

accrue, treat, and follow up study participants. Each center has specific responsibilities, which are tied to the trial phase and wax and wan over the course of the trial. Activities during the planning phase are mostly the purview of the clinical and data coordinating centers, which are responsible for obtaining funding and designing a trial that will answer the specific research question being asked. The initial design phase and the protocol development and implementation phase see both resource centers and clinical centers making preparations for the trial to be conducted. The main responsibilities of clinical centers during the participant recruitment, treatment, and follow-up phases are to recruit, randomize, treat, and follow study participants and collect and transmit study data to the data coordinating center. The resource centers manage drug or device distribution, receive and manage data, and monitor trial progress. Clinical centers complete closeout visits during the participant closeout phase, while resource centers complete final data management activities, data analysis, and interpretation. The termination phase finds investigators from all centers involved in manuscript writing activities. Collaboration among all centers during all phases is essential for the successful completion of any multicenter trial.

Keywords

Resource center · Clinical center · Coordinating center · Reading center · Central laboratory · Multicenter trial · Trial phase

Introduction

In this chapter, we discuss the types of centers that form the organizational units of a multicenter trial. As implied by the term multicenter, different types of centers are typically required to conduct a multicentered trial, each with specific responsibilities but which together perform all required functions. Resource centers are those with expertise and experience in performing specific tasks and include groups such as coordinating centers, data management centers, central laboratories, reading centers, and quality control centers among others. Distinct from the resource centers are clinical centers, whose main function is the accrual, treatment, and follow-up of study participants, thus forming an integral part of any multicenter trial.

Roles and Functions of Resource Centers

Although all aspects of a single-center trial may be performed within a single institution, responsibilities may be assigned to individual departments or divisions of the institution that provide special expertise. In a multicenter trial, some responsibilities may be assigned to a facility or institution that houses people with special expertise and facilities that serve the entire trial, i.e., resource centers, sometimes referred to as central units or support centers. The types of resource centers selected for an individual trial vary with the design and goals of the trial. Resource centers may be established to provide expertise to multiple clinical trials, and possibly other types of research studies, or may be organized to serve a specific trial or group of trials.

Coordinating Centers

All multicenter trials have at least one center with overall responsibility for the scientific conduct of the trial. Two types of coordinating centers are common: clinical coordinating centers and data or statistical coordinating centers. In multinational trials, there may be multiple regional or national coordinating centers (Brennan 1983; Alamercery et al. 1986; Franzosi et al. 1996; Kyriakides et al. 2004; Larson et al. 2016).

Clinical Coordinating Centers

Clinical coordinating centers sometimes are known as the trial chair's office, principal investigator's office, or treatment coordinating center, depending on the types of responsibilities assigned to the center, sponsor, and medical setting of the trial. Responsibilities in some trials have included:

- Identification of clinical and resource centers to collaborate in the conduct of the trial
- Obtaining and maintaining funding for the trial
- Disbursement of funds to participating clinical centers and resource centers
- Training of clinical investigators to standardize diagnostic or treatment procedures
- Responding to queries from clinical investigators regarding protocol interpretation
- Scheduling and organizing meetings of the trial investigators and personnel
- Developing and disseminating information about the trial to aid participant recruitment
- Marketing the trial to the medical community

In other trials, some of these responsibilities may be assigned to another resource center, such as the data or statistical coordinating center. Typically, the clinical coordinating center does not have responsibility for data collection, storage, or analysis, except possibly information regarding clinical center performance. Those responsibilities are usually assigned to a data coordinating center. Regardless of the distribution of responsibilities, typically there is close collaboration between personnel in the clinical coordinating center and those in the data coordinating center.

Data Coordinating Centers

Data (or statistical) coordinating centers often are known as coordinating centers without a modifier, particularly when some of the responsibilities described above for clinical coordinating centers are assigned to the (data) coordinating center. The senior statistician for the trial typically is located at the data coordinating center and may be the principal investigator (or a co-investigator) for the funding award to this center. In some cases, an epidemiologist or a person with other related expertise may be the principal investigator.

Typically, the expected principal investigator and/or the senior trial statistician participates in the design of the trial and preparation of the trial protocol (Williford et al. 1995).

Coordinating centers often serve as the trial communications center and information source for investigators, trial leadership, other trial personnel, and sponsor. Personnel at these centers provide expertise regarding research design and methods and, often, experience gained from participation in other clinical trials. They oversee the treatment allocation (randomization) process and serve as the scientific conscience of the investigative group. This trial resource center has primary responsibility for assembling and maintaining an accurate, complete, and secure trial database and for analysis of data accumulated for the trial.

Typical responsibilities of data coordinating centers include:

- Select and implement the information technology methods that will be used for the trial (McBride and Singer 1995).
- Design and implement the methods for collecting and recording the data required to address the goals of the trial (Hosking et al. 1995).
- Design and implement the randomization schema and the methods for assigning trial participants to treatment arms and communicating the assignment to participants and trial personnel as required.
- Develop and monitor methods for masking trial personnel and participants to treatment assignment as required to preserve the integrity of the trial.
- Develop methods for storing, managing, securing, and reporting accumulating trial data reported by clinical centers, other resource centers, and committees assigned responsibility for coding events or other aspects of participant follow-up.
- Provide for regular communication with personnel at clinical centers and other resource centers regarding protocol issues and data anomalies.
- Develop methods for assessing and reporting data quality, including data provided by participants, clinical center personnel, and personnel at other resource centers (Gassman et al. 1995).
- Develop methods for reporting accumulated data for groups assigned to monitor the progress of the trial, data quality, and comparative safety and effectiveness of trial treatments (McBride and Singer 1995).
- Cooperate with external monitors of the coordinating center (Canner et al. 1987).
- Participate in preparation of manuscripts to report trial methods and outcomes. In particular, the trial statisticians typically are responsible for performing all data analyses included in reports, including selecting and describing appropriate methods of statistical analysis and verifying all data reported and their interpretation.

- Retain all documentation regarding data analyses included in manuscripts and reports for future reference as needed.
- Participate in development of procedures for closing trial participation and debriefing of participants (McBride and Singer 1995; Dinnett et al. 2004).
- Archive the database when the trial is completed so that the data are available for future exploratory analyses (Hawkins et al. 1988).
- Store minutes of committee meetings and reports.

To meet these responsibilities, staff of the data coordinating center must include personnel with expertise in several areas. There is no formula that applies to every trial. Besides statistical and information technology expertise at various levels, personnel typically include clerical and other types of personnel. It is essential that coordinating center personnel be able to interact effectively with trial investigators and personnel at other trial centers. When some of the trial data are collected by coordinating center personnel, for example, through telephone interviews for patient-reported outcomes or central long-term follow-up of participants for outcomes (Peduzzi et al. 1987), the personnel may include telephone interviewers. Regardless of the expertise or roles of individual coordinating center personnel, all must be trained in the trial protocol and procedures.

The manuals of operations/procedures prepared for individual trials are useful resources for identifying the many responsibilities assigned to data coordinating centers, the ways in which personnel and investigators at those centers have met their responsibilities, and the organizational structure of data coordinating centers.

In clinical trial networks, a single coordinating center may serve all trials, or subgroups of personnel may be designated to participate in individual trials (Blumenstein et al. 1995). A data coordinating center also may be created to participate in a single multicenter trial. The organization of the coordinating center depends on the trial setting and, often, the trial sponsor and funding source. In the United Kingdom, clinical trials units (another name for coordinating centers) currently undergo registration to assure that they meet requirements regarding (1) expertise, continuity, and stability; (2) quality assurance; (3) information systems; and (4) statistical input (McFadden et al. 2015). The importance of development and documentation of standard operating procedures (SOPs) for these units is emphasized in the UK registration process (McFadden et al. 2015) and by others (Krockenberger et al. 2008).

Because coordinating center responsibilities evolve during the course of a trial, it is useful to consider changes in responsibilities by trial phase. Phases of a trial, adapted from the Coordinating Center Models Project [CCMP], are defined in Table 1. Common coordinating center responsibilities by trial phase are summarized in Table 2.

Other Resource Centers

Other resource centers required for an individual trial depend on the goals of the trial and the need for standardization of trial procedures. Resource centers may be created

Table 1 Phases of a multicenter clinical trial. (Adapted from Coordinating Center Models Project Report No. VI)

Planning and pilot phase: Ends with submission of funding application(s) to sponsor
Initial design phase: Ends with funding for the trial
Protocol development and implementation phase: Ends with initiation of participant recruitment
Participant enrollment phase: Ends with completion of participant recruitment
Treatment and follow-up phase: Ends with initiation of participant closeout
Participant closeout phase: Ends with completion of participant closeout
Termination phase: Ends with termination of funding for the trial
Post-funding phase: Ends with completion of all trial activities and publications
Comment
Phases of an individual trial are not always clearly defined regarding beginning and ending dates or events. Activities of a phase may overlap with those of another; hence the end of each phase is defined above by an "event." Activities of the trial centers vary by trial phase; in fact, the coordinating center investigators must be constantly planning for the next phase

to serve an individual trial or serve multiple trials that have similar needs. Some of the responsibilities assigned to resource centers have been:

• Establish pre-randomization eligibility or confirm post-randomization eligibility of trial participants based on review of images or biologic specimens from trial participants, possibly together with selected clinical data.
• Interpret images from participants made at baseline and/or follow-up examinations.
• Prepare and distribute trial medications, and possibly other supplies, with appropriate masking of trial personnel and participants.
• Monitor accuracy of assays made at local laboratories.
• Monitor/confirm clinical center adherence to treatment protocol.
• Collect and analyze participant diaries, regarding, for example, nutrient intake, adherence to study medication, or exercise program.
• Collect and store biospecimens for analysis for the current trial or future research.

As an example, resource centers that participated in the Collaborative Ocular Melanoma Study (COMS) and their responsibilities are described in Table 3. The COMS was a multicenter study with two randomized trials of radiotherapy versus enucleation (removal of the eye) for choroidal melanoma in adults. Of the resource centers listed in Table 3, three relocated with the center investigators during the 20 years that trial activities were underway, an important lesson for investigators who design trials with long accrual or follow-up periods expected.

Central laboratories have a long history in US multicenter trials, extending back to the University Group Diabetes Program and the Coronary Drug Project (Hainline et al. 1983) and possibly earlier in oncology trials for standard analysis of biochemical specimens. An extensive literature exists regarding central laboratories, particularly from the perspective of the pharmaceutical industry (Habig et al. 1983;

Table 2 Common responsibilities of [data] coordinating centers and clinical centers by trial phase. (Adapted from the Coordinating Center Models Project and other sources)

[Data] coordinating centers	Clinical centers
Planning and pilot phase	
Participate in literature review/meta-analyses to assess and document need for contemplated trial	
Participate in design and analysis of pilot studies to assess feasibility of trial design and methods	Conduct pilot studies
Meet with investigators expected to direct other resource centers	
Visit one or more clinical centers expected to participate in trial	Engage in discussions regarding possible participation in trial
Initial design phase	
Estimate required sample size	
Outline the data collection schedule	
Outline quality assurance and monitoring procedures	
Outline data analysis plans	
Outline data intake and editing procedures	
Prepare funding proposal for the [data] coordinating center	Review proposed clinical center budget
Participate in preparation of qualifications of clinical centers and the selection process	
Work with the proposing study chair to coordinate the overall funding application package	
Coordinate development of a draft manual of procedures for the trial	Provide input on manual of procedures if asked
Protocol development and implementation phase	
Register or assure registration of trial in a clinical trials registry	Determine feasibility of integrating trial into clinic setting
Develop patient treatment allocation (randomization) procedures	Constitute study team and select primary clinical coordinator
Develop computer software and related procedures for receiving, processing, editing, and analyzing study data	Complete Good Clinical Practice and ethics training
Develop and test study data forms and methods used for completion and submission by clinical center personnel	
Oversee development of interfaces for data transmission between individual resource centers and clinical centers	Organize infrastructure including telephone, computer and Internet, courier services
Coordinate drug or device distribution	Procure equipment, including refrigerators or freezers, lockable cabinets, and any special equipment

(continued)

Table 2 (continued)

[Data] coordinating centers	Clinical centers
Train clinical center personnel in the data collection and transmission process	Attend training meeting
Implement training certification in the trial protocol at clinical centers	Complete certification requirements
Distribute study forms and related study material for use in next phases of the trial	
Designate one or more coordinating center investigators to serve on each trial committee	Institute interdepartmental communication pathways, including pharmacy, radiology, laboratory, etc.
Modify and refine manual of procedures and distribute to all trial centers	Organize filing system and binders, including those for essential documents
Develop and document internal procedures for coordinating center operations and responsibilities	Organize space, including interview or exam rooms, storage areas for confidential materials, and drugs or devices
Act as a repository for official records of the trial: minutes of meetings, committee reports, etc.	
When agreed with sponsor, reimburse clinical centers and other resource centers and others based on the funding award	Complete budgeting and contractual negotiations
Participate in creating the application for local and/or study-wide institutional review boards/ethics committees	Incorporate trial protocol and informed consent statement template into local ethics board template and submit for approval
Develop and implement dedicated website with trial information suitable for access by multiple stakeholders	
Participant recruitment phase	
Develop templates for recruitment materials	Develop recruitment materials or use templates developed by coordinating center; submit to local ethics review board
	Implement recruitment activities
Administer treatment assignments. Periodically check (1) baseline comparability of treatment arms and (2) characteristics of participants versus target population and eligibility criteria	Screen potential study participants; complete eligibility testing on potential study participants
Implement editing procedures to detect data deficiencies	Complete all baseline data collection forms to determine eligibility of potential study participant
Develop monitoring procedures and prepare data reports to summarize performance of participating clinical centers with patient recruitment	Obtain formal informed consent from study participant and complete randomization process
Develop monitoring and reporting procedures to detect evidence of adverse or beneficial effects of trial treatments	

(continued)

Table 2 (continued)

[Data] coordinating centers	Clinical centers
Respond to requests for reports and data analyses from within the trial organization	
Implement and lead quality assurance and monitoring program	
Schedule and participate in site visits to clinical centers and other resource centers	Participate in site visits, and respond to queries by site visitors
Prepare progress reports for trial sponsor	
Prepare, or collaborate in preparing, any requests for continued or supplemental funding by the sponsor	
Prepare a manuscript to describe the trial design	
Participant treatment and follow-up phase	
Monitor drug or device distribution	Administer treatment as assigned by randomization, including accountability activities for study medications or devices
Monitor treatment adherence	Complete required documents, or provide materials related to treatment adherence
Prepare periodic reports of the data concerning adverse and beneficial effects of trial treatments	
Monitor and report adverse events to sponsors as required	Identify and report all serious adverse events as required by trial and federal agencies and local ethics committees
Prepare periodic reports of the performance of all trial centers	Identify and resolve all protocol deviations
	Schedule all study visits, including any logistical issues (e.g., travel for participant(s), scheduling radiology or surgery, etc.)
Evaluate data handling procedures and modify as necessary	Complete all study follow-up visits and associated data collection forms, and transmit data to data coordinating center
Analyze baseline and related data for publication, as appropriate	Respond to data queries from coordinating center
Prepare materials for investigator meetings	Attend all investigator group meetings
Prepare summary of trial results for individual participants for use in closeout discussion and final data collection	
Develop and test data forms for patient closeout phase	
Initiate/lead searches for participants lost to follow-up by clinical centers	
Work with trial leadership and investigators to develop a publication plan	
Coordinate participant closeout process	

(continued)

Table 2 (continued)

[Data] coordinating centers	Clinical centers
	Complete annual progress reports for ethics review boards
Participant closeout phase	
Collect participant closeout data	Complete closeout study visit
Coordinate and monitor progress with participant closeout	
Monitor adherence to closeout procedures	
Develop plans for final checks on completeness and accuracy of trial database	Complete all remaining data queries from coordinating center
Develop and test analysis programs for any additional data summaries or analyses	
Develop plan for final disposition of final trial database and accumulated materials	
Participate in reorganization of trial for final phases, including disengagement of clinical centers	Complete all center closeout activities, including final reports
Continue to participate in preparation of manuscripts to disseminate trial findings and methods	
Coordinate and monitor progress with trial manuscripts	Participate in manuscript writing, as required
Termination phase	
Perform final quality checks of trial database	
Implement plans for documentation and disposition of final database and other trial records	
Advise clinical center personnel regarding disposition of local trial records	Archive or dispose of all study documents as required by sponsor
Continue activities regarding preparation and publication of manuscripts	Participate as co-author on study publications, if requested
Monitor collection and disposal of unused study medications and supplies	Complete accountability of study medications or devices and all study materials
Undertake final efforts to determine or confirm the vital status of all trial participants	
Provide writing teams with data analyses and summaries needed to complete manuscripts	Present study findings at a conference, as requested
Circulate manuscripts for review by trial investigators prior to submission for publication	Review final manuscripts

Cooper et al. 1986; Rosier and Demoen 1990; Davey 1994; Davis 1994; Dijkman and Queron 1994; Harris 1994; Wilkinson 1994; Lee and Hill 2004; Sheintul et al. 2004; Strylewicz and Doctor 2010). The integration of local and central roles in an international multicenter trial has been described by Nesbitt et al. (2006).

Table 3 Example of resource centers and selected responsibilities in the Collaborative Ocular Melanoma Study

Study chairman's office
Organize planning meetings of prospective center investigators
Identify potential clinical centers and resource centers
Interact with sponsor to assess feasibility of support
Prepare core study funding applications in collaboration with coordinating center investigators
Design and develop informational materials for prospective study participants
Design and disseminate materials to inform community oncologists and ophthalmologists about the trials
Schedule meetings of investigators and committees; develop meeting agendas in collaboration with coordinating center investigators and committee chairs
Monitor adherence of investigators to study policy for presentation and publication of study data
Participate in preparation of manuscripts to disseminate trial findings
Advise the coordinating center investigators regarding issues outside their areas of expertise
Coordinating center
Coordinate preparation and submission of funding applications to sponsor
Coordinate study communications
Enroll and randomize eligible participants
Maintain the *COMS Manual of Procedures*
Develop methods for and coordinate data collection
Maintain the COMS database
Monitor data quality at other centers and internally
Analyze and report accumulating data to appropriate groups
Maintain study documents
Coordinate preparation of manuscripts to report trial findings
Archive the final database and documentation after study completion
Ophthalmic echography reading center
Train clinical center echographers in study methods
Confirm diagnosis of choroidal melanoma based on photographs from baseline echographic examination
Monitor quality of echography
Measure tumor height to monitor changes after brachytherapy
Assess topographic features of tumors
Photograph reading center
Train clinical center photographers in study methods
Monitor quality of photography
Confirm diagnosis of choroidal melanoma based on characteristics observed on photographs and fluorescein angiograms of tumor
Describe changes in boundaries of tumor base
Describe retinopathy following brachytherapy
Pathology center
Describe tumor characteristics based on external and microscopic examinations of enucleated eyes

(continued)

Table 3 (continued)

Provide technical processing of enucleated eyes sent from clinical centers
Coordinate activities of the Pathology Review Committee
Radiological physics center
Participate in development of radiotherapy protocols with radiation oncologist study co-chair
Assess accuracy of clinical center calculation of radiation dose, and notify clinical center in case of disagreement
Disseminate instructive findings to clinical center personnel
Sponsor: National Eye Institute
Monitor overall study progress
Observe adherence to study goals

Image analysis and interpretation centers were used in early multicenter for standard interpretation of echocardiographic tracings from participants (Prineas and Blackburn 1983; Rautaharju et al. 1986). Over time, manual review and coding largely has been replaced with automated methods (Goodman 1993). Resource centers with similar roles for other types of images have become common as new imaging methods have been developed and implemented clinically to monitor the effects of treatment. They have been widely used in oncology (Chauvie et al. 2014; Gopal et al. 2016) and ophthalmology trials (Siegel and Milton 1989; Danis 2009; Price et al. 2015; Toth et al. 2015; Domalpally et al. 2016; Rosenfeld et al. 2018) but also in trials in other medical settings (Desiderio et al. 2006; Ahmad et al. 2016).

Central pharmacies/procurement and distribution centers also have a long history in multicenter clinical trials. They have been established to aid with masking of treatment assignments in pharmaceutical trials and with distribution of supplies to clinical centers and participants (Fye et al. 2003; Martin et al. 2004; Peterson et al. 2004; Rogers et al. 2016).

Adjudication centers or committees have been created for many trials to confirm or code outcomes reported by clinical center personnel or trial participants (Moy et al. 2001; Pogue et al. 2009; Marcus et al. 2012; Barry et al. 2013). The need for central adjudication of outcomes such as death has been debated (Granger et al. 2008; Meinert et al. 2008).

Other types of resource centers have been less common but have played important roles in multicenter clinical trials to date (Glicksman et al. 1985; Kempson 1985; Sievert et al. 1989; Carrick et al. 2005; Henning 2012; Shroyer et al. 2019). A registry of resource centers with various types of expertise and experience with participation in multicenter clinical trials would be a useful resource for designers of future trials. Similarly, a registration system similar to that used in the United Kingdom for clinical trials units could be modified to be applicable to other types of resource centers.

Regardless of the role of a resource center, interactions with the (clinical and data) coordinating centers and clinical center personnel are required to assure that transmission of information and materials from clinical centers to the resource center is timely and accurate and that the information transmitted to the trial database is linked to the correct trial participant and examination.

Resource centers may be funded independently of other trial centers or may receive funding from the clinical or data coordinating center budgets. The expertise and number of personnel at these centers depend on the type of collaboration provided. As noted by Farrell (1998), expertise acquired at resource centers is a valuable resource and should be recognized.

Typical responsibilities of resource centers, other than coordinating centers, include:

- Maintain secure and accurate local records of trial participant identifiers.
- Log receipt of materials, track progress with processing, and store materials securely.
- Establish the format and frequency of data to be transmitted to the trial database.
- Respond promptly in trials where eligibility of candidate participants depends on reading or interpretation of baseline materials or specimens.
- Notify clinical center personnel of deficiencies in transmission/shipment or quality of specimens/materials.
- Provide periodic monitoring of internal data quality.
- Collaborate with external monitors of data quality.
- Provide progress reports to trial sponsor and committees at agreed intervals.
- Adhere to local institutional regulations and policies.
- Establish and monitor clinical trial budget for the center.
- Document internal procedures relative to the trial.
- Collaborate with site visitors on behalf of the trial.
- Prepare manuscripts to describe central methods used for the trial.

Clinical Centers

Clinical centers are a unique "resource" center. Without a committed and fully functioning clinical center, a multicenter trial is doomed to failure. Clinical centers or sites are the engines that generate the data needed to answer the research question posed by the trial. The historical model for a clinical center has been a single academic center, but other workable models have emerged with the inclusion of clinical practice sites (Submacular Surgery Trials Research Group 2004; Dording et al. 2012), nontraditional sites such as nursing homes (Kiel et al. 2007), and international centers (Perkovic et al. 2012). In some cases, with the organization of the clinical trial networks, a network of dedicated clinical sites may contribute to multiple related trials (Beck 2002; Sun and Jampol 2019). Even though clinical centers may be located at any one of these types of sites, all are responsible for administrative functions, patient interactions, data management functions, and interactions with coordinating and other resource centers. Similarly, personnel within a clinical center can vary depending on the complexity of the trial being conducted, but all clinical centers have a principal investigator who is usually the clinician actively involved in the trial and a clinical coordinator, who handles day-to-day functions. Overall, clinical centers communicate with and are responsive to the clinical coordinating or data coordinating center and often with other resource centers. In addition to administrative functions, clinical center responsibilities always include recruitment and accrual of study participants, including determination of eligibility, elicitation of an informed consent, administration of treatment, and completion of follow-up visits. Secure and confidential data collection is ongoing during these processes.

Clinical center responsibilities during each phase of the trial are summarized in Table 2 and described in the following sections.

The Implementation Phase

The first responsibility of the clinical center is to learn about the incipient trial. As the principal investigator, the clinical center director must have a thorough understanding of the research question, the trial design, the operations, and the possible impact on the clinic if the decision is to be part of the investigative group. The primary clinical coordinator optimally is selected at this phase of the trial, and the clinical director and coordinator together perform many of the tasks necessary to integrate the trial into the clinic setting.

Following clinical center selection, the clinical center enters into negotiations for contractual or funding arrangements. Because operational failures are often based on insufficient allocation of resources (Melnyk et al. 2018), it is important to ensure sufficient funding for all phases of the trial, including both start-up and final visit data collection. Certainly, given the time commitment required by a trial, either time protected from clinical responsibilities or appropriate reimbursement for research time is helpful, if not necessary, for the principal investigator (Herrick et al. 2012). Different models for clinical center funding exist from fixed funding based on personnel effort and anticipated costs to capitation with reimbursement based on completion of all data entry for enrollment and study visits by participants. A combination with some fixed up-front costs and further reimbursement based on completed visits also has been used successfully (Jellen et al. 2008).

Organizing the Site

To participate fully in a multicenter trial, the site must be organized to ensure adequate space, telecommunications, and computer systems. Rooms for physical examinations or private participant interviews may be necessary depending on the specific trial. Lockable cabinets are also necessary to store study participant binders and other confidential patient information. Special equipment or materials may be required (e.g., specific charts or instrumentation). In some cases, trial-specific equipment, such as laptop computers, may be supplied as part of the trial. If biospecimens are to be obtained, then laboratory equipment, such as a centrifuge, and refrigerators or freezers to store samples are required. The principal investigator must ascertain whether the required equipment is available and make provisions for maintenance and upkeep of the equipment for the duration of the trial.

Given the collaborative nature of a multicenter trial, it is necessary to have clear communication pathways between the involved parties, so adequate computer and Internet service is essential. Integration of the site with other facilities or departments may also be required, such as radiology or the chemistry laboratories. If biospecimens are required to be sent to a central laboratory, required supplies and courier services need to be set up. Administration of a study drug mandates either an appropriate cabinet or safe locked for storage of study drug or involvement of the local pharmacy.

Assembling the Study Team

Hand in hand with organizing the site is assembling the study team. Depending on trial needs, staff in addition to the principal investigator and coordinator may include specialty physicians, imaging technicians, laboratory personnel, psychometricians, regulatory monitors, or other technical staff. In choosing trial staff, the principal investigator should build a coalition of persons capable of sustained group effort to maintain continuous communication among staff members (Chung and Song 2010). Notwithstanding the size or attributes of the staff at a clinical site, the principal investigator is ultimately responsible for the performance and integrity of the site. On the other hand, all members of the clinical center team should have a commitment to the trial and have a voice in the local decision-making (Fiss et al. 2010).

Attributes of the Principal Investigator

The principal investigator should be an experienced clinical researcher with an understanding of the structure and conduct of randomized trials, have completed Good Clinical Practice training, be open to new ideas, and have impeccable integrity. Any potential conflicts of interest must be disclosed both at the beginning and also throughout the trial. The principal investigator should be a leader and have the ability to delegate tasks and engender a spirit of teamwork and collaboration among the clinical center staff.

Attributes of the Clinical Coordinator

The importance of a skilled coordinator cannot be overstated. This person is crucial to the proper functioning of a clinical site. Many trials require clinic coordinators to have specific credentials and/or certification (e.g., nursing degree). Responsibilities reported by most oncology trial clinical coordinators included patient registration and randomization, recruitment, follow-up, case report form completion, serious adverse event reporting, managing study files, and preparing for, and attending, audits (Rico-Villademoros et al. 2004). Empathy, an essential attribute for a coordinator (Jellen et al. 2008), provides an incentive for study participants to remain in the trial and complete all follow-up visits. A coordinator is flexible, works independently, and has superlative organizational skills.

As Jellen stated (Jellen et al. 2008):

> Responsibility for protocol adherence ultimately rests with the principal investigator, but ensuring that it is achieved falls primarily to the clinic coordinator.

There may be a single coordinator at a clinical center or multiple coordinators with each performing a specific task or serving as backup when necessary.

The coordinator or a separate regulatory monitor also coordinates all compliance issues. A "regulatory monitor" is responsible for financial and contractual arrangements and all interactions with ethics review board and federal drug agencies. A monitor also may review the protocol for feasibility and develop and monitor the clinical center budget together with the principal investigator. Other responsibilities include all communications and interactions with the local ethics board and appropriate and timely reporting of adverse events.

Interactions with the Team

Once funding is secured, and the team assembled, the principal investigator typically meets with the staff to orient them to the trial and individual responsibilities delegated to each staff member. These meetings, coordinated by the study coordinator, optimally continue on a regular basis, either as a group or singly, depending on the required input.

Ethical Approval

Before participating in the trial, local ethics board or a commercial review board approval is required to conduct the trial at each institution. Often the coordinator or regulatory monitor drafts the required materials for ethics review by using templates of the study protocol and consent forms provided by the data or clinical coordinating center. Continuing interactions with the ethics committee include obtaining approval for any amendments to the protocol, approval for ancillary studies, notification of any serious adverse events that occur, and submission of annual progress reports. If there is a data monitoring committee for the trial as a whole, clinical centers also submit the report of this committee following each meeting.

Organization Binders/Files

Prior to trial initiation, the coordinator or regulatory monitor typically sets up all the requisite binders and trial files, whether paper-based or electronic, and organizes all correspondence. Binders include those for essential documents as mandated by Good Clinical Practice, a current manual of procedures or handbook, required logbooks, ethics board correspondence, a scheduling book, and study participant binders, among others. The coordinator maintains currency of these documents and files as the trial progresses.

Certification and Training

Trial-specific training invariably is required for the principal investigator, coordinator, and all other involved staff. Training typically takes place at a "kickoff" full investigative group meeting over 1 or 2 days at a convenient location. There often are breakout sessions where responsibilities specific to the coordinator and possibly other clinic personnel are covered. Topics typically covered during training for coordinators include research integrity, trial protocol, governance, timeline, and trial-specific processes for randomization, treatment administration, data management, and adverse event reporting. Associated with training is documentation of basic knowledge about the trial and role-specific understanding and knowledge through the process of certification to participate in the trial. Usually there are requirements for certification that must be met to allow data collection or treatment administration within the trial. The purpose of certification is to demonstrate knowledge of the trial and competency in the role the staff member will hold. Requirements may include reading the manual of procedures, demonstrating understanding of the trial objectives, and design and skill in administration of tests or questionnaires. Certification may also require submission of "dummy" data collection forms or data collected using trial materials (e.g., an audiotape for counseling). For surgical procedures, documentation of experience or submission of videotapes may be required. With staff replacements, training and certification continue during the trial, especially for longer trials (Mobley et al. 2004). While the trial is ongoing, staff may be trained by an existing certified staff member or a member of the clinical coordinating center or data coordinating center who visits the clinical center for this purpose. Other options include special training meetings, webinars with didactic lectures and/or videotapes, or slides sets or videotapes from previous training meetings.

Participant Enrollment Phase

Recruitment

Following ethics review board approval, accrual of study participants, or recruitment, proceeds. Recruitment materials, such as educational brochures or poster templates, are used to facilitate identification of potential study participants. These materials are either prepared using templates provided by study resource centers or may be developed at the clinic and specifically aimed at the local population (Mullin et al. 1984). Other recruitment activities include disseminating information through grand rounds or local presentations or directly using letters or personal meetings with colleagues or other persons who have access to the potential patient population.

Screening and Randomization

Screening of potential participants is the first step in determining eligibility for the trial and when the informed consent process begins. Assignment of an identification number to each candidate often happens at screening to facilitate confidentiality. Following a positive screening, clinical center staff further assess eligibility and continue the informed consent process by explaining the trial to the potential participant in greater detail. The coordinator and principal investigator review collected data to verify eligibility prior to enrollment in the trial. A binder or file is prepared for every person who undergoes screening and eligibility testing, while information for those failing eligibility testing may be filed separately.

Following confirmation of eligibility, a designated staff member proceeds with obtaining final informed consent from the study participant to enroll in the trial. The staff member who obtains informed consent makes sure that the potential participant understands the risks and benefits and his or her responsibilities within the trial. Formal informed consent is documented by the participant signing the informed consent statement; a copy is given to the participant, and a copy is kept for the clinic and is stored in a binder or file designated for that purpose. Randomization and treatment assignment typically occurs only after informed consent has been obtained and documented. Randomization is often achieved via an online system, although in small or single-center studies, sealed opaque-coded envelopes may be issued to provide the assigned treatment. Documentation related to randomization is stored in the participant binder or file.

Treatment and Follow-Up Phase

The next step is to implement the assigned treatment. If a drug or pharmaceutical is assigned, the drug must be obtained from the pharmacy or from the storage cabinet where study drug is held, carefully checked to ensure that the assigned code matches that on the bottle or other drug container, and given to the participant with instructions. Similarly, if the assignment involves a device, then the device must be retrieved or ordered and may require matching codes. If the assignment is a specific surgical procedure, the surgery and operating room must be scheduled within the required time window for treatment. A counseling or other behavioral intervention requires scheduling within the designated time frame. For all assignments, it is imperative that the intervention given to the study participant matches that assigned at randomization.

Scheduling and Communications

For the most part, the clinic coordinator becomes the face of the trial for the study participant. The coordinator schedules all study visits and ensures that all required procedures and data collection take place during the study visit. Preparations may include ensuring examination or interview space is available and all imaging, physical, or psychological examinations that are required for that visit are scheduled. If study drug is to be distributed, then the drug must be obtained from the pharmacy or storage area to give to the study participant. The clinic coordinator either arranges travel or investigates transportation options when required for overnight visits or for participants unable to drive themselves to the clinic. At the study visit, the coordinator makes sure that the contact information for the study participant is up to date and arranges for meals for long visits. Between visits, especially with long intervals between visits, the coordinator may contact the study participant to make sure everything is going well. The study coordinator serves as a patient advocate and educator and can provide referrals to social services or other needed resources (Larkin et al. 2012). Throughout trial interactions, the coordinator builds a relationship with each study participant, establishing a rapport as they work together on the trial as a team.

Adverse Events

Adverse events that occur during a trial, particularly serious adverse events, must be handled correctly and in a timely manner. Appropriate medical care for the study participant overrides the trial protocol, especially for serious adverse events or events that may be related to a trial intervention. The assigned treatment may need to be discontinued and appropriate documentation prepared. All regulatory bodies, including trial sponsors, local ethics board, and pertinent regulatory agencies, must be notified within the time frame designated by the trial protocol.

Data Collection

Data are the backbone of clinical research, mandating proper data collection and management. Data may be collected using paper forms, directly onto electronic media, or indirectly through review of medical charts, taped interviews, or other methods. Data sources include participant self-report, scheduled interviews or examinations, or imaging or laboratory findings. Collection of external data also may be required, e.g., death certificates for determination of cause of death, hospital records, or operative notes from surgical procedures. Data are collected at various points during a participant's sojourn in the trial and possibly in multiple ways. At screening and eligibility assessment, eligibility criteria are verified, and baseline data used to assess change over follow-up may be collected. Treatment administration requires data related to treatment adherence or compliance and associated treatment-related adverse events. Outcome data and adverse events are collected during follow-up. Clinical center staff must ensure faithful and accurate data collection. Data forms should be checked for completeness and accuracy prior to transmission to the data coordinating center. Transmission of data may be implemented using various modes (e.g., paper forms, online, submission of electronic files) but should be completed expeditiously and accurately while maintaining confidentiality. In addition to collecting participant-related data, the clinic also manages other study-related data, such as drug accountability or biospecimen collection and shipment. There may also be specific data forms dealing with study-related events, such as protocol deviations or adherence to treatment.

Data Management

Although the database may have checks to provide for accurate entry and double-data entry be employed, there still may be missing, out of range, or inconsistent data items. Errors may occur within a single form, across forms, or across visits. Typically, the data coordinating center routinely reviews the data and queries the clinical center about perceived errors. Clinic staff then review each query and, if an error had occurred, correct the paper forms or electronic record and transmit the corrected item to the data coordinating center. These data management activities typically take more time at the beginning of a trial or during slow recruitment when more errors occur (Taekman et al. 2010). The amount of effort for all data management activities requires a substantial time commitment by the coordinator (Goldsborough et al. 1998).

Site Visits

Site visits are a quality assurance measure that typically includes a review of the clinic setting, implementation of the trial protocol, and routine audits of the data. Having a site visit scheduled often provides an incentive for a clinical center to make sure all documents are current and well-organized. During the site visit, the site visitors typically will observe administration of a clinical procedure, determine that adequate space and required facilities are available to conduct the trial, review that essential documents (paper or electronic) are current and that signed informed consent documents are available for each study participant, and conduct a data audit. During an audit, data in the database are compared with those recorded on paper forms or in other ways. Discrepancies are treated as data errors and require review and correction. Common problems encountered during site visits are inadequate consent documentation, problems with drug accountability, and protocol nonadherence (Turner et al. 1987).

Study Meetings

Goals of full investigative group meetings vary, but generally are designed to build collaboration between investigators and coordinators. Topics covered may include trial progress; problem-solving, especially during the recruitment phase; and issues related to implementing the protocol in the clinic setting. Protocol amendments may be discussed and reviewed, as well as performance reports and accumulating baseline data. Continuing education also may be provided, by either engaging outside speakers or having a trial investigator provide updates on the scientific literature in the trial topic area.

Participant Closeout Phase

Final Follow-Up Visit

Relationships that the study participant may have forged with the coordinator over the past year or more are changed at the last study visit. The principal investigator should ensure that there are no untoward events associated with termination of treatment. He or she should also provide for ongoing medical care for the study participant and provide information from trial participation to facilitate future care.

Post-Funding Phase

Dissemination of Study Results

The recognition received for completing a well-conducted trial comes with dissemination of the trial result; the clinical center principal investigators typically are key to this process. Their role may entail presenting trial results at a conference, being on a Writing Committee for a journal publication, or presenting results locally.

Summary and Conclusion

Different types of centers form the nodes in the organizational structure of a multicenter trial. Resource centers perform designated functions as required within specific trials; they include coordinating centers, reading centers, central laboratories, and others. Clinical center responsibilities encompass functions related to accrual, treatment, and follow-up of study participants. Specific responsibilities of both types of centers change depending on the phase of the trial. Collaboration among all resource centers and clinical centers is essential as they aim toward the common goal of successfully completing a multicenter trial.

Key Facts

- Centers participating in multi-center clinical trials may include clinical or data coordinating centers and clinical centers, along with others as required by trial design.
- Specific responsibilities of centers change across trial phases.
- Clinical and data coordinating centers provide scientific oversight of the trial, and oversee data management and analyses.
- Clinical centers are responsible for accrual, treatment, and follow-up of study participants.

Cross-References

▶ Administration of Study Treatments and Participant Follow-Up
▶ Consent Forms and Procedures
▶ Data Capture, Data Management, and Quality Control; Single Versus Multicenter Trials
▶ Design and Development of the Study Data System
▶ Funding Models and Proposals
▶ Implementing the Trial Protocol
▶ Investigator Responsibilities
▶ Multicenter and Network Trials
▶ Paper Writing
▶ Participant Recruitment, Screening, and Enrollment
▶ Procurement and Distribution of Study Medicines
▶ Qualifications of the Research Staff
▶ Responsibilities and Management of the Clinical Coordinating Center
▶ Selection of Study Centers and Investigators
▶ Training the Investigatorship
▶ Trial Organization and Governance

References

Ahmad HA, Gottlieb K, Hussain F (2016) The 2 + 1 paradigm: an efficient algorithm for central reading of Mayo endoscopic subscores in global multicenter phase 3 ulcerative colitis clinical trials. Gastroenterol Rep (Oxf) 4(1):35–38

Alamercery Y, Wilkins P, Karrison T (1986) Functional equality of coordinating centers in a multicenter clinical trial. Experience of the International Mexiletine and Placebo Antiarrhythmic Coronary Trial (IMPACT). Control Clin Trials 7(1):38–52

Barry MJ, Andriole GL, Culkin DJ, Fox SH, Jones KM, Carlyle MH, Wilt TJ (2013) Ascertaining cause of death among men in the prostate cancer intervention versus observation trial. Clin Trials 10(6):907–914

Beck RW (2002) Clinical research in pediatric ophthalmology: the Pediatric Eye Disease Investigator Group. Curr Opin Ophthalmol 13(5):337–340

Blumenstein BA, James KE, Lind BK, Mitchell HE (1995) Functions and organization of coordinating centers for multicenter studies. Control Clin Trials 16(2 Suppl):4s–29s

Brennan EC (1983) The Coronary Drug Project. Role and methods of the Drug Procurement and Distribution Center. Control Clin Trials 4(4):409–417

Canner PL, Gatewood LC, White C, Lachin JM, Schoenfield LJ (1987) External monitoring of a data coordinating center: experience of the National Cooperative Gallstone Study. Control Clin Trials 8(1):1–11

Carrick B, Tennyson M, Lund B (2005) Managing a blood repository for use by multiple ancillary studies in the Women's Health Initiative. Clin Trials 2(Suppl 1):S73

Chauvie S, Biggi A, Stancu A, Cerello P, Cavallo A, Fallanca F, Ficola U, Gregianin M, Guerra UP, Chiaravalloti A, Schillaci O, Gallamini A (2014) WIDEN: a tool for medical image management in multicenter clinical trials. Clin Trials 11(3):355–361

Chung KC, Song JW (2010) A guide to organizing a multicenter clinical trial. Plast Reconstr Surg 126(2):515–523

Cooper GR, Haff AC, Widdowson GM, Bartsch GE, DuChene AG, Hulley SB (1986) Quality control in the MRFIT local screening and clinic laboratory. Control Clin Trials 7(3 Suppl):158s–165s

Danis RP (2009) The clinical site-reading center partnership in clinical trials. Am J Ophthalmol 148 (6):815–817

Davey J (1994) Managing clinical laboratory data flow. Drug Inf J 28:397–402

Davis JM (1994) Current reporting methods for laboratory data at Zeneca Pharmaceuticals. Drug Inf J 28:403–406

Desiderio LM, Jaramillo SA, Felton D, Andrews LA, Espeland MA, Tan JC, Bryan NR, Perry J, Liu DF (2006) A multi-institutional imaging network: application to Women's Health Initiative Memory Study. Clin Trials 3(2):193–194

Dijkman JHM, Queron J (1994) Feasibility of Europe-wide specimen shipments. Drug Inf J 28:385–389

Dinnett EM, Mungall MM, Kent JA, Ronald ES, Gaw A (2004) Closing out a large clinical trial: lessons from the prospective study of pravastatin in the elderly at risk (PROSPER). Clin Trials 1 (6):545–552

Domalpally A, Danis R, Agron E, Blodi B, Clemons T, Chew E (2016) Evaluation of geographic atrophy from color photographs and fundus autofluorescence images: Age-Related Eye Disease Study 2 report number 11. Ophthalmology 123(11):2401–2407

Dording CM, Dalton ED, Pencina MJ, Fava M, Mischoulon D (2012) Comparison of academic and nonacademic sites in multi-center clinical trials. J Clin Psychopharmacol 32(1):65–68

Farrell B (1998) Efficient management of randomised controlled trials: nature or nurture. BMJ 317 (7167):1236–1239

Fiss AL, McCoy SW, Bartlett DJ, Chiarello LA, Palisano RJ, Stoskopf B, Jeffries L, Yocum A, Wood A (2010) Sharing of lessons learned from multisite research. Pediatr Phys Ther 22(4): 408–416

Franzosi MG, Bonfanti I, Garginale AP, Nicolis E, Santoro E, N. Investigators (1996) The role of a regional data coordinating centre (RDCC) in a multi-national large phase-II trial. Control Clin Trials 17(Suppl 2S):104S–105S

Fye CL, Gagne WH, Raisch DW, Jones MS, Sather MR, Buchanan SL, Chacon FR, Garg R, Yusuf S, Williford WO (2003) The role of the pharmacy coordinating center in the DIG trial. Control Clin Trials 24(6 Suppl):289s–297s

Gassman JJ, Owen WW, Kuntz TE, Martin JP, Amoroso WP (1995) Data quality assurance, monitoring, and reporting. Control Clin Trials 16(2 Suppl):104s–136s

Glicksman AS, Reinstein LE, Laurie F (1985) Quality assurance of radiotherapy in clinical trials. Cancer Treat Rep 69(10):1199–1205

Goldsborough IL, Church RY, Newhouse MM, Hawkins BS (1998) How clinic coordinators spend their time. Appl Clin Trials 7(1):33–40

Goodman DB (1993) Standardized and centralized electrocardiographic data for clinical trials. Appl Clin Trials 2(6):34, 36, 40–41

Gopal AK, Pro B, Connors JM, Younes A, Engert A, Shustov AR, Chi X, Larsen EK, Kennedy DA, Sievers EL (2016) Response assessment in lymphoma: concordance between independent central review and local evaluation in a clinical trial setting. Clin Trials 13(5):545–554

Granger CB, Vogel V, Cummings SR, Held P, Fiedorek F, Lawrence M, Neal B, Reidies H, Santarelli L, Schroyer R, Stockbridge NL, Feng Z (2008) Do we need to adjudicate major clinical events? Clin Trials 5(1):56–60

Habig RL, Thomas P, Lippel K, Anderson D, Lachin J (1983) Central laboratory quality control in the National Cooperative Gallstone Study. Control Clin Trials 4(2):101–123

Hainline A Jr, Miller DT, Mather A (1983) The Coronary Drug Project. Role and methods of the Central Laboratory. Control Clin Trials 4(4):377–387

Harris RAJ (1994) Clinical research aspects of sampling, storage, and shipment of blood samples. Drug Inf J 28:377–379

Hawkins BS, Gannon C, Hosking JD, James KE, Markowitz JA, Mowery RL (1988) Report from a workshop: archives for data and documents from completed clinical trials. Control Clin Trials 9(1):19–22

Henning AK (2012) Starting a genetic repository. Clin Trials 9(4):523

Herrick LM, Locke GR 3rd, Zinsmeister AR, Talley NJ (2012) Challenges and lessons learned in conducting comparative-effectiveness trials. Am J Gastroenterol 107(5):644–649

Hosking JD, Newhouse MM, Bagniewska A, Hawkins BS (1995) Data collection and transcription. Control Clin Trials 16(2 Suppl):66s–103s

Jellen PA, Brogan FL, Kuzma AM, Meldrum C, Meli YM, Grabianowski CL (2008) NETT coordinators: researchers, caregivers, or both? Proc Am Thorac Soc 5(4):412–415

Kempson RL (1985) Pathology quality control in the cooperative clinical cancer trial programs. Cancer Treat Rep 69(10):1207–1210

Kiel DP, Magaziner J, Zimmerman S, Ball L, Barton BA, Brown KM, Stone JP, Dewkett D, Birge SJ (2007) Efficacy of a hip protector to prevent hip fracture in nursing home residents: the HIP PRO randomized controlled trial. JAMA 298(4):413–422

Krockenberger K, Luntz SP, Knaup P (2008) Usage and usability of standard operating procedures (SOPs) among the coordination centers for clinical trials (KKS). Methods Inf Med 47(6):505–510

Kyriakides TC, Babiker A, Singer J, Piaseczny M, Russo J (2004) Study conduct, monitoring and data management in a trinational trial: the OPTIMA model. Clin Trials 1(3):277–281

Larkin ME, Lorenzi GM, Bayless M, Cleary PA, Barnie A, Golden E, Hitt S, Genuth S (2012) Evolution of the study coordinator role: the 28-year experience in Diabetes Control and Complications Trial/Epidemiology of Diabetes Interventions and Complications (DCCT/EDIC). Clin Trials 9(4):418–425

Larson GS, Carey C, Grarup J, Hudson F, Sachi K, Vjecha MJ, Gordin F (2016) Lessons learned: infrastructure development and financial management for large, publicly funded, international trials. Clin Trials 13(2):127–136

Lee JY, Hill A (2004) A multicenter lab sample tracking system. Clin Trials 2:252–253

Marcus P, Gareen IF, Doria-Rose P, Rosnbaum J, Clingan K, Brewer B, Mille AB (2012) Did death certificates and a mortality review committee agree on lung cancer cause of death in The National Lung Screening Trial? Clin Trials 9(4):464–465

Martin DE, Pan J-W, Marticn JP, Beringer KC (2004) Pharmacy management for randomized pharmacotherapy trials: the MATRIX web data management system. Clin Trials 1(2):248

McBride R, Singer SW (1995) Interim reports, participant closeout, and study archives. Control Clin Trials 16(2 Suppl):137s–167s

McFadden E, Bashir S, Canham S, Darbyshire J, Davidson P, Day S, Emery S, Pater J, Rudkin S, Stead M, Brown J (2015) The impact of registration of clinical trials units: the UK experience. Clin Trials 12(2):166–173

Meinert CL, Martin BK, McCaffrey LD, Breitner JC (2008) Do we need to adjudicate major clinical events? Clin Trials 5(5):557; author reply 558

Melnyk H, Rosenfeld P, Glassman KS (2018) Participating in a multisite study exploring operational failures encountered by frontline nurses: lessons learned. J Nurs Adm 48(4):203–208

Mobley RY, Moy CS, Reynolds SM, Diener-West M, Newhouse MM, Kerman JS, Hawkins BS (2004) Time trends in personnel certification and turnover in the Collaborative Ocular Melanoma Study. Clin Trials 1(4):377–386

Moy CS, Albert DM, Diener-West M, McCaffrey LD, Scully RE, Willson JK (2001) Cause-specific mortality coding. Methods in the collaborative ocular melanoma study coms report no. 14. Control Clin Trials 22(3):248–262

Mullin SM, Warwick S, Akers M, Beecher P, Helminger K, Moses B, Rigby PA, Taplin NE, Werner W, Wettach R (1984) An acute intervention trial: the research nurse coordinator's role. Control Clin Trials 5(2):141–156

Nesbitt GS, Smye M, Sheridan B, Lappin TR, Trimble ER (2006) Integration of local and central laboratory functions in a worldwide multicentre study: experience from the Hyperglycemia and Adverse Pregnancy Outcome (HAPO) Study. Clin Trials 3(4):397–407

Peduzzi P, Hatch HT, Johnson G, Charboneau A, Pritchett J, Detre K (1987) Coordinating center follow-up in the Veterans Administration Cooperative Study of Coronary Artery Bypass Surgery. Control Clin Trials 8(3):190–201

Perkovic V, Patil V, Wei L, Lv J, Petersen M, Patel A (2012) Global randomized trials: the promise of India and China. J Bone Joint Surg Am 94(Suppl 1E):92–96

Peterson M, Byrom B, Dowlman N, McEntegart D (2004) Optimizing clinical trial supply requirements: simulation of computer-controlled supply chain management. Clin Trials 1(4):399–412

Pogue J, Walter SD, Yusuf S (2009) Evaluating the benefit of event adjudication of cardiovascular outcomes in large simple RCTs. Clin Trials 6(3):239–251

Price MO, Knight OJ, Benetz BA, Debanne SM, Verdier DD, Rosenwasser GO, Rosenwasser M, Price FW Jr, Lass JH (2015) Randomized, prospective, single-masked clinical trial of endothelial keratoplasty performance with 2 donor cornea 4 degrees C storage solutions and associated chambers. Cornea 34(3):253–256

Prineas RJ, Blackburn H (1983) The Coronary Drug Project. Role and methods of the ECG Reading Center. Control Clin Trials 4(4):389–407

Rautaharju PM, Broste SK, Prineas RJ, Eifler WJ, Crow RS, Furberg CD (1986) Quality control procedures for the resting electrocardiogram in the Multiple Risk Factor Intervention Trial. Control Clin Trials 7(3 Suppl):46s–65s

Rico-Villademoros F, Hernando T, Sanz JL, Lopez-Alonso A, Salamanca O, Camps C, Rosell R (2004) The role of the clinical research coordinator – data manager – in oncology clinical trials. BMC Med Res Methodol 4:6

Rogers A, Flynn RW, McDonnell P, Mackenzie IS, MacDonald TM (2016) A novel drug management system in the Febuxostat versus Allopurinol Streamlined Trial: a description of a pharmacy system designed to supply medications directly to patients within a prospective multicenter randomised clinical trial. Clin Trials 13(6):665–670

Rosenfeld PJ, Dugel PU, Holz FG, Heier JS, Pearlman JA, Novack RL, Csaky KG, Koester JM, Gregory JK, Kubota R (2018) Emixustat hydrochloride for geographic atrophy secondary to age-related macular degeneration: a randomized clinical trial. Ophthalmology 125(10): 1556–1567

Rosier J, Demoen P (1990) Labeling of clinical trial samples: an overview of some regulatory requirements. Drug Inf J 24:583–590

Sheintul M, Lun R, Cron-Fabio D, Krishtul R, Xue H, Lin K-H (2004) The challenges of designing a clinical research laboratory database. Clin Trials 1(2):219–220

Shroyer ALW, Quin JA, Wagner TH, Carr BM, Collins JF, Almassi GH, Bishawi M, Grover FL, Hattler B (2019) Off-pump versus on-pump impact: diabetic patient 5-year coronary artery bypass clinical outcomes. Ann Thorac Surg 107(1):92–98

Siegel D, Milton RC (1989) Grading of images in a clinical trial. Stat Med 8(12):1433–1438

Sievert YA, Schakel SF, Buzzard IM (1989) Maintenance of a nutrient database for clinical trials. Control Clin Trials 10(4):416–425

Strylewicz G, Doctor J (2010) Evaluation of an automated method to assist with error detection in the ACCORD central laboratory. Clin Trials 7(4):380–389

Submacular Surgery Trials Research Group (2004) Clinical trial performance of community- vs university-based practice in the Submacular Surgery Trials: SST report no. 2. Arch Ophthalmol 122:857–863

Sun JK, Jampol LM (2019) The Diabetic Retinopathy Clinical Research Network (DRCR.net) and its contributions to the treatment of diabetic retinopathy. Ophthalmic Res 62:225–230

Taekman JM, Stafford-Smith M, Velazquez EJ, Wright MC, Phillips-Bute BG, Pfeffer MA, Sellers MA, Pieper KS, Newman MF, Van de Werf F, Diaz R, Leimberger J, Califf RM (2010) Departures from the protocol during conduct of a clinical trial: a pattern from the data record consistent with a learning curve. Qual Saf Health Care 19(5):405–410

Toth CA, Decroos FC, Ying GS, Stinnett SS, Heydary CS, Burns R, Maguire M, Martin D, Jaffe GJ (2015) Identification of fluid on optical coherence tomography by treating ophthalmologists versus a reading center in the comparison of age-related macular degeneration treatments trials. Retina 35(7):1303–1314

Turner G, Lisook AB, Delman DP (1987) FDA's conduct, review, and evaluation of inspections of clinical investigators. Drug Inf J 21(2):117–125

Wilkinson M (1994) Carrier requirements for laboratory samples. Drug Inf J 28:381–384

Williford WO, Krol WF, Bingham SF, Collins JF, Weiss DG (1995) The multicenter clinical trials coordinating center statistician: more than a consultant. Am Stat 49(2):221–225

Qualifications of the Research Staff

8

Catherine A. Meldrum

Contents

Abstract

Through the use of clinical trials, the global research community have paved the way for new medical interventions and ground breaking new therapies for patients. In the past 60 years we have embraced rigorous scientific standards for assessing and improving our therapeutic knowledge and practice. These scientific standards dictate that a research workforce possessing knowledge, skills, and abilities is crucial to the success of a study. The many challenging (and ever changing) rules and regulations inherent in the clinical research arena also require diligent trained staff be available to conduct the study. While it is well known that the Principal Investigator is ultimately responsible for the conduct of the study, it is generally a team of individuals who conduct the daily operations of the study. This chapter discusses qualifications and training of other research staff members and why these are important for achieving success in clinical trials.

C. A. Meldrum (✉)
University of Michigan, Ann Arbor, MI, USA
e-mail: cathymel@umich.edu; cathymel@med.umich.edu

© Springer Nature Switzerland AG 2022
S. Piantadosi, C. L. Meinert (eds.), *Principles and Practice of Clinical Trials*,
https://doi.org/10.1007/978-3-319-52636-2_283

Keywords

Clinical research staff · Qualifications · Education · Clinical research coordinator

Introduction

Development and subsequent licensing of new pharmaceutical agents and devices are highly regulated processes. Clinical trials protocols have become more complex. Regulations and guidelines for managing clinical research trials have also increased (Infectious Disease Society of America 2009; NIH 2012). This then translates into the need for adequately trained research staff who conduct research to be knowledgeable in research ethics and scientific education and have sufficient training and education in the areas where they work. For high quality large scale clinical trials to be completed, the research staff involved should have the skills and knowledge to truly advance science. Study quality and integrity can be severely compromised if a very inexperienced individual is managing the research study without assistance from a more experienced individual. Meeting the needs of a research study means that each staff member has the responsibility to understand and apply the ethical tenets, principals, and regulatory requirements of Good Clinical Practice (GCP). That being said the research community understands the benefits and challenges of finding that seasoned professional to hire.

Commonly in research, industry dictates an individual have 2 years of professional experience upon hire but how does one get that experience if no one hires them. Furthermore, one could consider that although research studies require accuracy and diligence in performing them, maybe it is possible to hire novice staff with a blend of senior staff for oversight. Given the national shortage of clinical research staff for these positions, it is possible to consider staff having complete core competencies and not be so stringent on experience (ACRP 2015). Organizations could develop training programs that include internal and external education that meet the high expectations required in clinical research. Certainly this is a profession still under development and we need to evaluate previous history and future needs in the clinical research arena to best formalize and guide advancement of clinical research staff. Only then can it be assured the protection and well-being of the research participants are fulfilled and that research activities are conducted according to regulatory guidelines.

History of Clinical Research Staff

The Principal Investigator (PI) of a research study is the primary individual responsible for the overall research study though we are keenly aware it takes a village to actually complete a successful research study. It is not unusual for many required study tasks be delegated from the PI to members of the research team but who are the members of the research team and more importantly how have they been trained. Do the study members possess the experience and skill needed to assure compliance with guidelines and regulations set forth by regulatory agencies and/or institutions?

Unlike many professions the professional research staff role is really in its infancy in terms of development. While the nursing profession, widely recognized and licensed, flourished in 1860 when the first school of nursing was opened in Europe, the creation of research staff roles really began less than 40 years ago. Due to the early stage development of this career pathway, there has been less consensus on standardized job descriptions for this profession. There is no state licensure required for this type of work nor is the expectation that baseline experience is the same between institutions. The actual roles and titles of the research staff conducting a clinical trial are also widely varied. Titles may include: Clinical Research Coordinator, Study Nurse, Clinical Research Nurse, Research Nurse Coordinator, Clinical Research Assistant, Study Coordinator, and many more.

In nursing, the use of research nurses in oncology trials was common though their roles within the research project were not well defined. Many nurses worked with oncology patients clinically, though lacked clear direction or training to work with patients in a research capacity. An oncology research nurse may have complementary functions and roles with oncology chemotherapy nurses, but there are unique characteristics required of the research nurse that are not applicable to the oncology chemotherapy nurse (Ocker and Pawlik Plank 2000). In 1982, the Oncology Nursing Society sought to standardize job descriptions for oncology nurses who were involved in research studies (Hubbard 1982). Subsequently, as clinical trials grew in both numbers and complexity, there was a further push to define the scope of practice in the role of the research nurse. In 2007, the Clinical Center Nursing at the National Institute of Health launched an effort to help define Clinical Research Nursing (CRN). Later, in 2009 the first professional organization, the International Association of Clinical Research Nurses (IACRN) for research nurses was founded. This organization is not specific to oncology nurses but supports the professional development of nurses that specialize in any research domain thus, regardless of the title for this occupation or the research domain, nurses engaged in clinical trials develop, coordinate, and implement research and administrative strategies vital to the successful management of research studies.

Though it was common to use nurses in the research enterprise in oncology, there are many other areas outside of oncology that do not rely solely on a Clinical Research Nurse/Research Nurse Coordinator. Many staff hired to complete a research project are not trained as nurses. In fact, it is common to hire varied ancillary personnel to get the research study/project done. Without industry job description standards much of the initial workforce sort of "fell into the role." As noted early on it was quite common for an Investigator to utilize a nurse to assist in research. The nurse would begin to take on other responsibilities within research until it literally grew into some type of research role. Eventually other staff that may have worked in allied health or even in a clerical position began to take on additional duties, again eventually inheriting the role of study coordinator. Within the past decades there has been a tremendous growth in clinical research and with this, the need for more individuals conducting clinical research grew. No longer could just on-the-job training be the answer nor could pulling additional staff in at random times to assist in a research study be deemed sufficient as that individual may lack the proper training. A job entity/title for this profession was clearly needed. This led to several job titles and descriptions for research professionals as noted above but probably most common are Study Coordinator or Clinical Research Coordinator (CRC). Today many of the titles are interchangeable though for the purposes of this chapter we will refer to the Research Professional as a Clinical Research Coordinator (CRC).

A CRC does work under the direction of the Principal Investigator (PI); however, the background of the CRC can be quite diverse. Traditionally, a high percentage of CRCs did possess a nursing background (Davis et al. 2002; Spilsbury et al. 2008), and given the nursing curriculum and their experience with patients, this could be considered a well-suited career move for a nurse. Transitioning from the bedside nursing position to a CRC position while not difficult does require additional training, but the registered nurse (RN) already possesses some of the major key attributes required in the CRC role. Certainly understanding medical terminology, documentation skills, and good people skills help facilitate the transition. If an individual has a medical background other than nursing such as pharmacy, respiratory therapy, or another allied health field, they also understand medical terminology and are likely skilled in working with patients. More recently, individuals with these types of medical backgrounds are clearly more abundant in the research community as they pursue advanced training to work in the field of research. Individuals who would like to work as a CRC and have a nonmedical background may require even more additional training to sufficiently work in the clinical research arena but this can be achieved.

Although it is evident that it takes many personnel needed to effectively and efficiently carry out clinical research, the regulations require the Principal Investigator (PI) ensure that all the study staff are adequately trained and maintain up-to-date knowledge about the study (FDA 2000). Frequently, Co-Investigators (CO-I) are available to support the principal investigator in the management and leadership of the research project but the actual day to day operations of the study are carried out with ancillary personnel other than a PI or CO-I. In most studies the PI (or a delegate) hire personnel to assist in carrying out the study yet what really needs to be considered is: do the individuals hired have the appropriate training and skills necessary to fulfill the high demands of a clinical research study. This can be challenging as many times it may not even be the PI doing the actual hiring of the candidate. The individual doing the hiring needs to be fully aware of what the needs are for the study and be able to assess whether the potential candidate can meet those needs.

Staff Qualifications

As with any job position you have to find the person who best suits your needs. There are certainly times when an entry level candidate can assist in performing the activities needed for the research study but usually a highly experienced staff member is needed to oversee the study especially if it is a complex study. The overall question facing the researcher (or PI) is what type of individual do I need to complete the study successfully? Some broad topics that should be considered when hiring staff are:

- Educational background (medical/science)
- Research experience
- Patient care experience (people oriented)
- Experience with databases and collection of data
- Communication skills
- Organization skills
- Detail oriented
- Flexibility

Hiring can also be complicated since the length of time a research study is ongoing is quite varied; thus, the person you hire for that particular research study may not be the same type of individual you need for the next research study. A PI must consider the long term needs of their research enterprise and gauge what the staff composition should look like to fulfill their goals.

For most health care professions, entry level requirements include a focused didactic curriculum usually from an academic institution followed by some hands on experience. This has not been the case with entry level staff in clinical research. An individual cannot pursue this degree as a new student at an academic institution as no academic institution has entry level programs in this type of discipline.

There is also no license mandate to practice in clinical research as required in other medical disciplines though research staff may obtain professional certification credentials within the field. Frequently in clinical research entry level people perform such tasks as data entry, data management, and basic patient care tasks such as taking a blood pressure, measuring height and weight, or performing a manual count for returned medications. As one achieves more experience, they may gradually move up the clinical ladder with added responsibilities and commonly take on the title of Clinical Research Coordinator (or some facsimile of this).

CRCs work in a variety of settings such as private and public institutions, device pharmaceutical and biotechnology companies, private practice, Clinical Research Organizations (CRO), Site Management Organizations (SMO), and varied independent organizations involved in clinical research. Being a CRC is a multifaceted role with many responsibilities. They are really at the center of the research enterprise with multiple roles. Previous work has demonstrated that one research coordinator may be responsible for between 78 and 128 different activities (Papke 1996). With the growth in clinical research studies, there are still many more activities in the future that may be required of the research coordinator. The additional complexities of research ethics that have evolved over time and regulatory and economic pressures that continue to mount create the need for a skilled individual in this role (NIH 2006). Though the duties of clinical research staff vary from each institution, they likely include some or all of the following:

- Recruitment and enrollment of participants
- Protocol development
- Protocol implementation
- Assurance of participant safety
- Development of informed consent documents
- Development of case report forms
- Development of research budgets
- IRB submission
- Maintenance of drug accountability
- Accurate data collection
- Accurate data entry
- Data monitoring/Data analysis of people
- Staff education

While the above list is not an exhaustive list of duties, it illuminates the need for clinical research staff to have expert clinical skills and well-developed thinking skills. To achieve the best possible outcomes for research participants and the overall research process, they must be well versed in the regulatory, ethical and scientific domains of clinical research. Thus, it is crucial that PI assure the study employ at least one highly skilled individual to conduct a clinical trial. This leads us to discuss "How does staff obtain training?"

Training

In traditional University settings, there are no adequate curriculums in any disciplines that prepare a student to graduate with a bachelor's degree and work in clinical research though in the United States there are many clinical research administration programs that provide either a post graduate certificate or a master's degree. Online courses and online curriculums are also available but these can be costly. Conference symposiums are offered around the country though these types of courses usually provide a specialized topic (such as informed consent documentation, clinical trial initiation, FDA forms and procedures, regulatory documents and binder maintenance, source documents, study initiation and close-out visits, compliance and retention, drug compliance/storage/documentation, IRB submissions and HIPAA, adverse events and safety monitoring, quality assurance audits and monitor visits and preparing for FDA audits). Though the above may seem fairly thorough, these topics are not done in enough detail to provide adequate comprehensive training for a novice staff member so generally attending a one-day conference symposium is not considered sufficient training for entry level staff. These types of conference symposiums are mean to be adjunct materials for a research coordinator. On-the-job training and mentoring from more experienced staff are also training methods for that are used by many employers.

Training for a particular research study is generally done by the Sponsor. Once training is complete the individual signs a Delegation of Authority Log (DOA). This log serves to ensure that the research staff member performing study-related tasks/ procedures has been appropriately trained and authorized by the investigator to perform such tasks. Although a delegation log is not federally mandated, it may be a Sponsor requirement and must be completed and maintained throughout the trial. ICG/GCP guidance (E6 4.1.5) requires an investigator maintain a list of qualified staff to whom the investigator has designated study-related activities.

In 2012, a Clinical & Translational Science Awards Program (CTSA) taskforce found insufficient training, and lack of support among CRC's employed at Clinical Translational Science Institutes (CTSI) (Speicher et al. 2012). They also observed a low job satisfaction within this field. Recognizing the evolving demands of the clinical research enterprise across the nation, the Task Force's study reiterated the need for support and educational development while recognizing that there are insufficient numbers of adequately trained and educated staff for these roles.

One year after the CTSA study Clinical Research was formally accepted as a profession by Commission on Accreditation of Allied Health Education Programs (CAAHEP) though at the time of this writing the occupational description, job description, employment characteristics, and educational programs available for the role are still not available on the CAAHEP website (CAAHEP 1994).

Increasing clinical research studies and newer technologies create a demand for an evenr newer skillset in the research workforce, and this is where professional competencies come into play. In 2014, the Joint Task Force (JTF) for Clinical Trial Competency published a landmark piece on defining the standards for professionalism in the research industry (Sonstein et al. 2014). This universal Core Competency Framework has undergone three revisions with the most recent publication in October 2018 (Sonstein et al. 2018). It now incorporates three levels (Fundamental, Skilled, and Advanced), whereas more standard roles, assessments, and knowledge can be assessed within the eight domains. The domains include: Scientific Concepts and Research Design, Ethical and Participant Safety Considerations, Investigational Products Development and Regulation, Clinical Study Operations, Study and Site Management, Data Management and Informatics, Leadership and Professionalism, and Communication and Teamwork. A diagram of the framework is provided below (Fig. 1):

Credentialing Organizations in Clinical Research

To date there are two organizations that credential research staff. They are the Association of Clinical Research Professionals (ACRP) and The Society of Clinical Research Associates (SOCRA). Both of these organizations are international in scope. SOCRA currently has chapters in six international countries (Belgium, Brazil, Canada, Nigeria, Poland, Saudi Arabia) and certification testing can be done at a PSI testing center throughout the world. ACRP is located in more than 70 countries with about 600 testing centers available internationally.

Credentialing is achieved by way of an examination through both organizations. Interestingly though is that both organizations require at least 2 years of documented

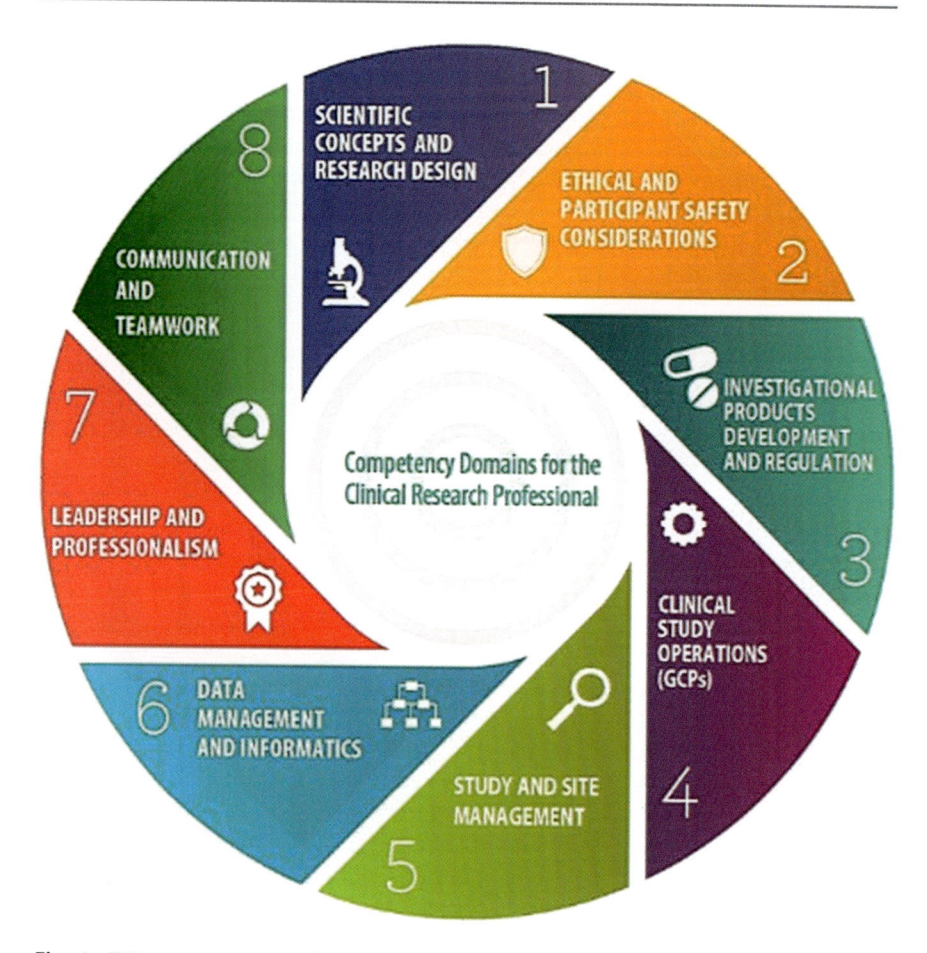

Fig. 1 JTF core competency domains. (JTF, Joint Task Force for Clinical Trial Competency, Sonstein and Jones 2018)

clinical research experience to take the examination (Association of Clinical Research Professionals 2018; Society of Clinical Research Associates 2018). The oldest organization is the Association of Clinical Research Professionals (ACRP). Founded in 1976 they have over 32,000 certified clinical researchers. This organization has several certification programs available for those employed in the clinical research workforce. These include: Certified Clinical Research Associate (CCRA), Certified Clinical Research Coordinator (CCRC), Certified Principal Investigator (CPI), and Professional certification (ACRP-CP). A CRA works on behalf of the sponsor and is not involved in obtaining research data, changing or manipulating data. Their duties largely revolved around independent monitoring of the data; thus, they are technically not part of the day to day operations in a clinical research study. A CRC is the individual largely tasked with day to day operations of participating in the study under the direction of the PI. Those seeking ACRP-CP certification are involved in planning, conducting, and overseeing the overall study.

To maintain certification a CCRC must submit an application and pay a recertification fee. The applicant must demonstrate competency by retaking the certification exam every 2 years or have accumulated 24 contact hours in continuing education activities. At least 12 of the continuing education activities must be research related. The remaining educational credit activities are obtained through Continuing Involvement or Continuing Education activities of the applicants' choice. This designates continued understanding of new knowledge relevant to clinical research study conduct.

SOCRA was incorporated in 1991 with a strong focus on providing education and credentialing for oncology coordinators. Through its growth it has emerged into a leading research organization providing education opportunities for clinical research staff in all therapeutic areas supporting government, industry, and academic institutions. Similar to ACRP the background of the research staff is varied and may include nursing, pharmacy, biology, teaching, medical technology, business administration, and other areas. Eligibility for taking the certification exam requires the applicant be working with Good Clinical Practice (GCP) guidelines with protocols that have been approved by either an Institutional Review Board (IRB), Institutional Ethics Committee (IEC), or a Research Ethics Board (REB). Additionally, the applicant must quality under one of three categories with a combination of work and/or educational experience. Upon successfully completion of the examination, the individual may use the title of Certified Clinical Research Professional (CCRP). This designation represents the individual has understanding, knowledge, and conduct application of clinical research that involves human subjects according to International Conference on Harmonization Guideline for Good Clinical Practice (E6) (ICH/GCP), ICH Clinical Safety Data Management: Definitions and Standards for Expedited Reporting (E2A), the United States Code of Federal Regulations (CFR) and the ethical principles of the Nuremberg Code, the Belmont Report. Duties may include: data collection, preparation of reports, protocol development, development or monitoring of case report forms, development of informed consent documents, protection of subject and subjects' rights, and reporting of adverse events throughout the study.

Certification is maintained by completion of 45 continuing education credits within a 3-year time period or retaking the examination. A minimum of 22 of the credits must be related to Clinical Research polices, regulations, etc. The remaining continuing education credits are generally related to ones' therapeutic area. Similar to ACRP an application and a fee for recertification is required.

Competency guidelines for Clinical Research Coordinators were recently developed by the ACRP (ACRP 2015). These guidelines were developed with input from over forty industries ranging from pharmaceutical, academic medical institutions, Medical Research Corporations, and a variety of Foundations. The guidelines are intended to serve many purposes such as standardize CRC performance, develop competency-based job descriptions, enhance CRC retention, increase CRC recruitment, and professional development and improve clinical trial quality.

Both ACRP and SOCRA are overwhelming accepted by industry standards as professional organizations assisting in establishing professional identities for Clinical Research Staff.

Summary

While there is still no standard education level for a position in clinical research, it is often associated with a bachelor's degree and some type of clinical trial research experience. Increased technology has essentially pushed the clinical research enterprise to expect that clinical research staff have a higher skillset than in previous decades. Certainly the importance of having a trained workforce in clinical research ultimately impacts the integrity of clinical research. The research field has come a long way in education and job description roles for research staff but there is still have a long road ahead. The field is evolving towards somewhat more standardized job descriptions even with the historical lack of clear consistent definitions for research staff titles and their responsibilities. This evolution should allow transparency that standardizes job classifications and education expectations while providing new growth opportunity for advancement in the clinical research profession. This will ultimately allow the profession to mature increasing workforce development and increased job satisfaction within the profession. If the universal competencies, certifications, and accepted job descriptions are not adopted, it may end up in the hands a government who would license this professional group.

Key Facts

1. Historically education and training of clinical research staff is highly variable.
2. Responsibilities and duties of the clinical research staff have increased due to increasing regulatory demands.
3. SOCRA and ACRP are international organizations that have assisted in the creation of guidance for more standardized job descriptions within the field of research.

Cross-References

▶ Documentation: Essential Documents and Standard Operating Procedures
▶ Implementing the Trial Protocol
▶ Investigator Responsibilities
▶ Selection of Study Centers and investigators

References

ACRP (2015) A New Approach to Developing the CRA Workforce. Retrieved January 30, 2019 from https://www.acrpnet.org/resources/new-approach-developing-cra-workforce/
Association of Clinical Research Professionals (2018) CRC Certification. Available at: https://www.acrpnet.org/certifications/crc-certification/

CAAHEP (1994) Consortium of academic programs in clinical research. https://www.caahep.org/
    Students/Program-Info/Clinical-Research-Professional.aspx. Retrieved January 31, 2019
Davis AM, Hull SC, Grady C, Wilfond BS, Henderson GE (2002) The invisible hand in clinical
    research: the study coordinator's critical role in human subjects protection. J Law Med Ethics
    30:411–419
Hubbard SM (1982) Cancer treatment research: the role of the nurse in clinical trials of cancer
    therapy. Nurs Clin N Am 17(4):763–781
Infectious Diseases Society of America (2009) Grinding to a halt: the effects of the increasing
    regulatory burden on research and quality improvement efforts. Clin Infect Dis 49:328–335
National Institutes of Health (2006) Regulations and ethical guidelines. Retrieved January 17, 2019
    from https://grants.nih.gov/policy/humansubjects.htm
NIH Policies and Procedures for Promoting Scientific Integrity (2012) Retrieved January 31, 2019
    from https://www.nih.gov/sites/default/files/about-nih/nih-director/testimonies/nih-policies-pro
    cedures-promoting-scientific-integrity-2012
Ocker BM, Pawlik Plank D (2000) The research nurse role in a clinic-based oncology research
    setting. Cancer Nurs 23(4):286–292
Papke A (1996) The ACW national job analysis of the clinical research coordinator. Monitor 46:45–
    53
Society of Clinical Research Associates (2018) Certification program overview. Available at:
    https://www.socra.org/certification/certification-programoverview/introduction/
Sonstein SA, Jones CT (2018) Joint task force for clinical trial competency and clinical research
    professional   workforce   development.   Fronti   Pharmacol.   https://doi.org/10.3389/
    fphar.2018.01148
Sonstein SA, Seltzer J, Li R, Jones CT, Silva H, Daemen E (2014) Moving from compliance to
    competency: a harmonized core competency framework for the clinical research professional.
    Clin Res 28(3):17–12
Sonstein SA, Namenek Brouwer RJ, Gluck W, Kolb HR, Aldinger C, Bierer BE, Jones CT (2018)
    Leveling the joint task force core competencies for clinical research professionals. Ther Innov
    Regul Sci 216847901879929
Speicher LA, Fromell G, Avery S, Brassil D, Carlson L, Stevens E, Toms M (2012) The critical
    need for academic health centers to assess the training, support, and career development
    requirements of clinical research coordinators: recommendations from the clinical and transla-
    tional science award research coordinator taskforce. Clin Transl Sci 5:470–475
Spilsbury K, Petherick E, Cullum N, Nelson A, Nixon J, Mason S (2008) The role and potential
    contribution of clinical research nurses to clinical trials. J Clin Nurs 17(4):549–557
United States Food and Drug Administration (2000) Retrieved February 5, 2019, from http://www.
    fda.gov

Multicenter and Network Trials

9

Sheriza Baksh

Contents

Abstract

Multicenter clinical trial designs offer a unique opportunity to leverage the diversity of patient populations in multiple geographic locations, share the burden of resource acquisition, and collaborate in the development of research questions and approaches. In a time of increasing globalization and rapid technological advancement, investigators are better able to conduct such projects seamlessly, benefiting investigators, sponsors, and patient populations. Regulatory agencies have embraced this shift towards the use of multicenter clinical trials in product development and have issued statements and guidance documents promoting their utility and offering best practices. Some governmental health agencies have even formed clinical trial networks to facilitate the use of multicenter clinical trials to answer a broad range of clinical questions related to a disease or disease area. This chapter will cover design considerations, data coordination,

S. Baksh (✉)
Johns Hopkins Bloomberg School of Public Health, Baltimore, MD, USA
e-mail: sbaksh4@jhu.edu

regulatory requirements, and study monitoring of multicenter clinical trials as well as how they can be conducted with a clinical trial network.

Keywords

Multicenter clinical trials · Clinical trial networks · Trial consortiums · Cooperative group clinical trials

Introduction

The conduct of clinical trials sometimes requires multiple clinical sites in order to complete studies in a timely manner and maximize the external generalizability of trial results. Increased globalization and inherent improvements in global coordination of data and research activities have made this study design the preferred option when large study populations, generalizable study results, and fast turnaround are the primary goals. Multicenter clinical trials allow for the streamlining of trial resources, collaborative consensus for research decisions, greater precision in study results, increased generalizability and external validity, and a wider range of population characteristics. Multicenter clinical trials conducted in various regions of the world may also bring clinical care options that would otherwise not be available to study participants in lower- and middle-income countries. There are special considerations for multicenter clinical trials that must be incorporated into protocols, statistical analysis plans, and data monitoring plans. Additionally, data collection, data management, and treatment guidance must be coordinated across study sites to comply with local standards.

Multicenter clinical trial designs have been in use for several decades, necessitating additional guidance on trial conduct from national and multinational regulatory and funding agencies. Many places such as Brazil, China, The European Union, and the United States use consensus documents, such as those produced in the International Conference for Harmonisation (ICH) as the basis for their own guidance on the conduct of clinical trials. For instance, the South African Good Clinical Practice Guidelines draws from source documents developed by ICH, the Council for International Organisations of Medical Sciences, World Medical Association, and the UNAIDS, but heavily emphasizes the importance of incorporating the local South African context into the design of multicenter clinical trials conducted in South Africa (Department of Health 2006). In the United States, since the passage of Kefauver-Harrison Amendments in 1962, multicenter clinical trials conducted in foreign countries have been used for regulatory submissions. However, the United States Food and Drug Administration (United States Food and Drug Administration 2006a, b, 2013) and the United States National Institutes of Health (NIH) (National Institutes of Health 2017) have only recently developed guidelines for trialists who are either submitting multicenter clinical trial data for regulatory approval or being funded for a multicenter clinical trial through the federal government. Each of the Institutes of the NIH have also developed specific guidelines for multicenter clinical trial grants under their purview. These guidelines address the nuances of trial conduct, coordination, data analysis, and ethical considerations across many trial designs conducted in a multicenter setting. These guidelines are also heavily based on those developed by ICH. Other countries implementing and tailoring ICH guidelines include Brazil, Singapore, Canada, Korea, and others.

The ICH of Technical Requirements for Pharmaceuticals for Human Use E17 Guideline for multi-regional clinical trials outline principles for the conduct of multicenter clinical trials for submission to multiple regulatory agencies (The International Conference on Harmonisation of Technical Requirements for Registration of Pharmaceuticals for Human Use 2017). The document discusses important considerations in study design, such as regional variability on the measured treatment effect, choice of study population, dosing and comparators, allowable concomitant medications, and statistical analysis planning. Additionally, E17 highlights the benefit of incorporating multi-regional clinical trials into the global product development plan to decrease the need for replication in various regions for each submission. Study investigators should consider the regulatory requirements of different regions, outcome definitions, treatment allocation strategies, and subpopulations of interest when designing multicenter clinical trials across different regions. This may require consultation with multiple regulatory agencies in the design of the trial. Safety reporting should also conform to the local requirements for all study sites. By coordinating study activities to meet the regulatory requirements in different regions, sponsors can efficiently leverage study results for timely reviews of investigational products.

The ICH has created additional guidance on the potential impact of ethnic differences across study sites that should be considered when conducting multicenter clinical trials in different countries (The International Conference on Harmonisation of Technical Requirements for Registration of Pharmaceuticals for Human Use 1998). The E5 Guideline discusses intrinsic and extrinsic factors that have the potential to modify the association between treatment and safety, efficacy, and dosing. Characterization of treatment effect may differ based on factors such as genetic polymorphism, receptor sensitivity, socioeconomic factors, or study endpoints. The clinical data package should have sufficient documentation of pharmacokinetics, pharmacodynamics, safety, and efficacy in the study population for each region in which the trial will be submitted for regulatory consideration. In the absence of that, additional bridging data that assesses the sensitivity of the treatment effect to specific ethnic factors unique to the target population in a particular region can help regulators extrapolate from study results accordingly. While the ICH E5 Guideline was developed for multicenter clinical trials in an international context, it can be applied to any multicenter clinical trial with heterogeneity in study populations across clinical sites.

Multicenter clinical trials can also be conducted via clinical trial networks. This mechanism allows for collaborative research and the alignment of research priorities among a core group of investigators. Networks are typically organized around a specific disease area and consist of investigators with common research initiatives. Clinical trial networks can serve to advance innovation in research methodologies for a particular clinical area, accelerate translational research, facilitate a measured approach to researching multiple questions surrounding a poorly understood disease or condition, and leverage existing patient populations for larger clinical trials in rare diseases.

This chapter highlights the nuances of conducting a multicenter clinical trial, in contrast to a single center trial, and highlight aspects of doing so within a clinical trial network.

Multicenter Clinical Trials

Formation

This chapter will delve into the conduct of multicenter clinical trials within the United States, with selected comparisons to contexts in other countries. The examples presented here are typical of an NIH-funded, investigator-initiated, multicenter clinical trial. As there are other models for multicenter clinical trials such as industry trials for regulatory approval, this chapter will highlight other notable design aspects when applicable. For the purposes of this chapter, the principal investigator (PI) is the lead clinical scientist who has received funds from government or private entities for the conduct of a multicenter clinical trial. The funder is the provider of financial support for the clinical trial. The sponsor is the responsible party for the clinical trial and may or may not be the same party as the funder.

Multicenter clinical trials are clinical trials conducted under a single protocol that utilize multiple clinical sites in different geographical locations to recruit participants for a clinical trial answering a specific clinical question. The clinical site principal investigators typically contribute to the study leadership and collaborate in the development and refinement of the study question and design. Communication among the sites and between the sites and the study PI is often coordinated by a data coordinating center and often directed by the PI.

Multicenter clinical trials understandably require a considerable deal of coordination, both administratively and functionally. The decision for which clinical sites to include in a clinical trial can be determined during the study planning phase and finalized after the start of the trial. During this time, the PI may invite clinical sites to apply to join the multicenter clinical trial. PIs can choose to invite individual clinical trial sites within their professional networks, existing clinical trial networks, or sites identified through clinical trial site directories or trial registries. During the application process, potential clinical sites are asked to list their proposed study team, clinical site resources, confirmation of ability to conduct clinical research activities, and their ability to coordinate ethical approvals across sites. These applications can be accompanied by a site assessment visit, where site monitors can visit the potential clinical site to inspect the facilities and capabilities of the applicant site. These visits can be useful in the design phase of the study, when the site monitors consider which research activities may or may not be feasible for each clinical site and what tasks might better be completed centrally. This is also an opportunity for the site monitors to ascertain the types of patients a clinic typically receives, what proportion would meet study eligibility criteria, and discuss appropriate recruitment goals with the potential clinical site investigator. Site monitors may also use the site visit as an opportunity to conduct a risk assessment of the site's ability to complete study recruitment and quality goals.

Once the PI and the clinical site decide to pursue collaboration on the clinical trial, they enter into a contract that outlines the rights, roles, and responsibilities of each party. The contract may also address payment schedules to the sites, any resource transfers to or sharing with the individual sites, data storage and security liability, and event reporting responsibilities. If there are specimen collections in the clinical trial, the contract might also specify who holds ownership for those specimens and material transfer agreement details.

Earlier collaboration and consensus between the clinical sites and the PI in the development of the study and investment by the clinical sites in the clinical trial are two benefits to engaging and onboarding potential sites earlier in the planning phase. The Wrist and Radius Injury Surgical Trial (WRIST) group highlighted three techniques they employed in consensus building during their trial planning phase: focus group discussion, nominal group technique, and the Delphi method (Chung et al. 2010; Van De Ven and Delbecq 1974). Each of these methods require different levels of structure in reaching consensus. The PI for the clinical trial must assess whether the group of clinical site investigators have existing relationships with each other and whether or not some voices might carry more weight than others. For example, in a focus group discussion on increasing study recruitment, dominant voices may decrease democratic decision-making through the discussion, and less vocal investigators may have fewer opportunities to voice their ideas, resulting in a net loss to innovation in problem-solving. Pre-existing relationships may lend themselves to an established group dynamic that may or may not accommodate the addition of new voices. The nominal group technique is better suited for this type of situation in that it requires participation from all members (Van de Ven and Delbecq 1972). In the study recruitment example, by offering everyone an opportunity to share their ideas, innovation around recruitment strategies can be readily shared and amplified through voting by others in the group. It can be difficult to implement however, since it involves face-to-face meetings in order to prioritize and vote on decisions. Additionally, PIs should consider whether each investigator has an equal opportunity to voice his/her opinion in the course of designing and implementing the clinical trial. This includes ensuring that each investigator has his/her research interests considered for incorporation into the study objectives and is given an equal chance at authorship for manuscripts resulting from the trial. If the investigator group consists of researchers with varying levels of experience and seniority, the ideas of those more junior may be lost in the conversation. In this scenario, the Delphi method might be a more appropriate means of reaching consensus, as this method uses anonymity to minimize the effect of dominant voices (Dalkey 1969). Using the recruitment strategy example, this technique might further allow for the amplification of novel strategies, regardless of who presents the idea.

Trial Leadership

In contrast to a single-site clinical trial where study leadership primarily consists of the PIs and a lead coordinator, sponsors may ask PIs to establish a steering committee for larger multicenter clinical trials ("Trial Governance," 2015). As the name suggests, the steering committee steers the direction of the day-to-day activities and priorities of clinical and data coordinating centers (Daykin et al. 2016). The steering committee typically consists of the PI, the head of the data coordinating center, senior investigators from each clinical site, study statistician, and independent researchers who advise the PI throughout the study. This is one of many possible configurations of a steering committee; however, their key responsibility is to vote on major study decisions regarding design and analysis issues, study procedures, data sharing, allocation of study resources, and priorities for meeting competing demands of the study, should they arise. Of note, members of the steering committee may not all be voting members. The committee monitors the progress of the study, considers outside research that could affect the interpretation of the trial results and the appropriateness of the study design and analysis, and communicates study progress to interested parties. The steering committee is usually blinded and privy to the recommendations of the data safety monitoring board/committee in order to effectively direct study activities.

In situations where major study decisions must be made on a schedule that makes it difficult to convene the full steering committee, a smaller executive committee may meet to resolve routine issues that arise. The executive committee may consist of a handful of investigators, such as the study chair (usually the study PI), vice chair, director of the data coordinating center, and key study personnel to communicate and implement the decisions made. This smaller group of study leadership are tasked with resolving day-to-day issues in study conduct, prepare policies and proposals for steering committee review, address higher level administrative issues, develop plans to correct deficiencies in study conduct, review publications and presentations of study findings for steering committee approval, and review any proposed ancillary studies before approval by the steering committee. The executive committee may meet more frequently than the steering committee to address such issues in a timely manner and prepare for larger group review during the steering committee meetings. They may also work directly with other study team members to execute their assigned tasks.

There are several managerial and administrative duties that are often delegated in a multicenter clinical trial. Study leadership may decide to set up a chairman's office to undertake some of these tasks, consisting of the PI, study account manager, administrative coordinator, and potentially a clinical coordinating center. They carry the responsibility of distributing funds to the various clinics, labs, specimen repositories, and data coordinating center. They may also manage the contracts with each of these entities. The chairman's office may meet with the data coordinating center in executive committee meetings to coordinate start-up activities, data collection procedures, and other study logistics. Scheduling steering committee, executive committee, and data safety monitoring board/committee meetings for the study are additional responsibilities of the chairman's office. If the chairman's office also handles clinical coordinating activities, they may arrange for training and research group meetings to ensure that all study personnel are kept abreast of changes to study procedures and policies, as well as to address any issues in the day-to-day activities of the study. The chairman's office may also be in charge of communicating study-wide changes to procedure, new recruitment initiatives, and concerns about study progress.

There may be situations where some or all of these clinical coordinating duties are delegated to the data coordinating center, depending on available resources, and pre-determined study roles and responsibilities. Data coordinating centers also play an integral role in disseminating information about data collection procedures, data standardization, study monitoring, and data audits. The data coordinating center may be heavily involved in collecting details about study adverse events and protocol deviations for dissemination to sites for local reporting in addition to central reporting to the single investigational review board (sIRB). They may also conduct site visits to assess site performance and conduct quality checks. Reports from these visits are usually shared with the steering committee. These reports can serve to highlight unique approaches to study hurdles as well as identify areas for improvement. By sharing these reports with the entire steering committee, local site PIs can solicit feedback for improvement and share their successes with the group during the discussions of the reports. Finally, the data coordinating center monitors and facilitates timely data entry for the purpose of required reporting to the data safety monitoring board/committee, sIRB, study leadership, and study sponsor.

Design Considerations

There are a few design considerations unique to multicenter clinical trials. First, when a study statistician develops the randomization scheme for a multicenter clinical trial, he/she typically stratifies the randomization by clinical site. This reduces potential bias due to measured and unmeasured differences across clinical sites. In the case of stratifying by clinical site, the investigators control for the potential interaction between clinical site and primary outcome measures (Senn 1998; Zelen 1974). Stratification by clinical site maximizes the probability of balanced numbers of participants receiving each treatment arm in the study. Without this balance, there is potential for bias if one clinical site experiences different outcomes on average than other clinical sites. One can imagine a situation where clinical sites might have catchment areas with different socioeconomic statuses, patient demographics, and clinical characteristics. All of these could potentially affect baseline risk for the primary outcome in the study population at each site.

The second point of consideration is the target number of randomizations for each site. After a site has agreed to participate, the data coordinating center typically establishes recruitment goals for each site participating in the study to ensure that the overall recruitment goal for the study is met. These site-specific recruitment goals should consider what the clinical capacity is at each site, length of study visits and contacts, full-time equivalents dedicated to the study at each site, recruitment goals of other sites in the study, the timeline for completion of study recruitment, and the flexibility around adding additional sites to the study. Different recruitment goals across sites should not bias results or result in less precision, especially if randomization is stratified by clinical site (Senn 1998). Recruitment goals at each site should be roughly similar with allowances for faster and slower recruitment at sites; these goals should not be uniform and driven by extremes.

Third, multicenter clinical trial designs can benefit from built in flexibility for adding sites at any point during the trial. In order to facilitate this process, PIs should seriously consider the burden both on the data coordinating center and the prospective sites of the site start-up procedures. While multicenter trials inherently increase power, the benefits of adding a site as a collaborator should outweigh the administrative and logistical hurdles of doing so. Having a start-up package of forms for clinical sites to complete, a mini handbook of start-up activities, and a start-up training can ease this burden and allow for transparency.

Coordination of Study Activities and Logistics Between Sites

Sites involved in a multicenter clinical trial should all have the resources or capacity to acquire the resources necessary for the execution of all study procedures. This includes key personnel, study materials, and regulatory infrastructure (if applicable). PIs should bear in mind these potential limitations at each site as they design the study. In extreme cases, this may mean that study budgets may have to account for infrastructure support to ensure that each site has the minimum required resources to conduct study activities.

Through the course of a multicenter clinical trial, the data coordinating center works to ensure uniformity in study procedures, data collection, and adverse event and protocol deviation reporting across sites. To accomplish this, they coordinate a number of study logistics in an orchestrated manner. This begins when a site is chosen to join the clinical trial and has agreed to participate. For example, in the United States, all clinical sites are asked to join an sIRB designated for the multicenter clinical trial. As of 2016, all National Institutes of Health (NIH) sponsored multicenter clinical trials are required to use an sIRB of record for their ethical review (National Institutes of Health 2016). This move was intended to streamline the review of studies, promote consistency of reviews, and alleviate some of the burdens to investigators (Ervin et al. 2016). There are situations when a site may be unable to join an sIRB (i.e., foreign jurisdiction or highly restrictive local regulations). If a site agrees to rely on the sIRB for the study, they must complete a reliance agreement documenting this arrangement between the sIRB of record and their site. The letter of indemnification corresponding to this reliance outlines the scope of reliance, claims, and governing laws. Australian regulatory agencies have endorsed a similar approach through the National Mutual Acceptance (NMA) system. Through this agreement, health departments across Australian states and territories agree to recognize the ethical reviews conducted in member states for multicenter trials.

Similarly, the government of Ontario, Canada has supported Clinical Trials Ontario to streamline the ethical review of study protocols across the province. While a single ethical review may not be possible for protocols for all multicenter clinical trials, streamlining these activities when possible has been endorsed by sponsors and regulatory agencies.

After a site has received ethical approval from either the study's sIRB or their local institutional review board, then the data coordinating center can work with the clinic staff to prepare for initiating the study at their site. The data coordinating center may hold a training session for all certified clinic staff to orient them with the study protocol and data entry system. In preparation for this training session, clinic staff may be asked to review the protocol as well as any handbook (i.e., manual of procedures or standard operating procedures). This smaller training session during the onboarding process is an opportune time for clinic staff to clarify any technical issues with the protocol or identify any difficulties with data entry. By conducting this training with every site, the data coordinating center reinforces uniformity in study activities across sites. The coordinators introduce the data collection instruments at this time and indoctrinate clinic staff into the formatting requirements of the data as well as any nuances to the data system. Data collection instruments are standardized across the entire study and do not differ between clinical sites; however, sites are allowed to maintain their own local records of study participants. As the study proceeds, the data and/or clinical coordinating center may hold regular teleconferences or webinars with clinic staff to communicate important study changes, assess and triage any challenges, and solicit feedback from sites. This is also an opportunity for sites to learn from the experience of the other sites.

Given the potential for a large number of clinical sites, data coordinating centers may utilize risk-based approaches to remote and on-site data monitoring. This is a multipronged strategy for monitoring that prioritizes the most important aspects of patient safety, study conduct, and data reporting (Organization for Economic Co-operation and Development 2013; United States Food and Drug Administration 2013). Key features of risk-based monitoring include statistical approach to central monitoring, electronic access to source documents, timely identification of systemic issues, and greater efficiency during on-site monitoring. This risk-based monitoring plan is usually developed after a risk assessment of critical data and procedures to be monitored throughout the trial both remotely and on-site. In contrast to regular visits to all clinical sites with 100% data audits, this approach to monitoring allows study sponsors to effectively use resources to centralize data quality checks and use site visits as an opportunity to further investigate any data anomalies, observe clinic and study activities, and gather feedback about ease of data procedures and the data system. This may mean that monitors conduct source data verification on selected data items, a random sample of data forms, or a hybrid approach of source data verification of 100% of key data collection instruments and a sample of the remaining forms. This is another opportunity for study monitors to reinforce uniformity across sites in the conduct of study procedures. These on-site monitoring visits are seen as particularly useful at the beginning of a trial, with supplementary centralized monitoring through the duration of the trial. If clinics are found to be "higher risk" with regards to errors, then additional on-site monitoring visits and re-training can be arranged in a targeted manner.

Clinical Trial Networks

Multicenter clinical trials can be conducted within clinical trial networks, also referred to as trial consortiums or cooperative group clinical trials. Clinical trial networks can be organized around a common clinical or disease area, can span multiple countries, and can be publicly or privately funded. Table 1 lists several clinical trial networks around the world, their sponsors, and mission. They range in specificity of their missions, and in some cases, their goals have evolved since their establishment. Some may focus on research areas on therapeutic testing for neglected diseases or diseases that have high mortality with few to no treatment options. Many of the institutes within the United States National Institutes of Health sponsor clinical trial networks to accelerate research in priority areas.

Table 1 Clinical Trial Network Examples

Name	Sponsor	Overview
Alzheimer's Clinical Trials Consortium	National Institute on Aging	Comprised of 35 sites in 24 states Mission to provide infrastructure, centralized resources, and shared expertise for the accelerated development of Alzheimer's disease and related disorders
Platform for European Preparedness for Re(emerging) Epidemics (PREPARE)	European Commission	Hundreds of sites across Europe and Western AustraliaMission to establish a framework for harmonized clinical research on infectious disease, prepared for rapid response, and real-time evidence
Ozwaldo Cruz Foundation (FIOCRUZ) Clinical Research Network	Ozwaldo Cruz Foundation	Network of clinical research groups, steering committee, executive secretary, and communities of practice across Brasil Mission to strengthen the role of clinical research at FIOCRUZ, overcome technological hurdles, and establish national clinical research program
Korea National Enterprise for Clinical Trials (KoNECT) Collaboration Center	Government of Korea	Multiple clinical research sites across Korea Mission to foster a community of clinical research and networking for product development
East African Consortium for Clinical Research (EACCR2)	European Union	Multiple research nodes across East Africa supported by a network of European and African country governments Mission to conduct rigorous clinical trials on poverty-related diseases and neglected diseases

Clinical trial networks in Europe may build on the existing relationships between governments in the European Union (EU) and apply for European Research Infrastructure Consortium (ERIC) designation. This allows for clinical trial networks to be legally recognized across all EU member states, to fast-track the development of an international organization, and to be exempt from Value Added Tax (VAT) and excise duty. Countries outside of Europe are also allowed to join ERICs. Clinical trial networks interested in this designation must provide evidence that they have the infrastructure necessary to carry out the intended research, that the research is a value-add to the European Research Area (ERA), and the venture is a joint European

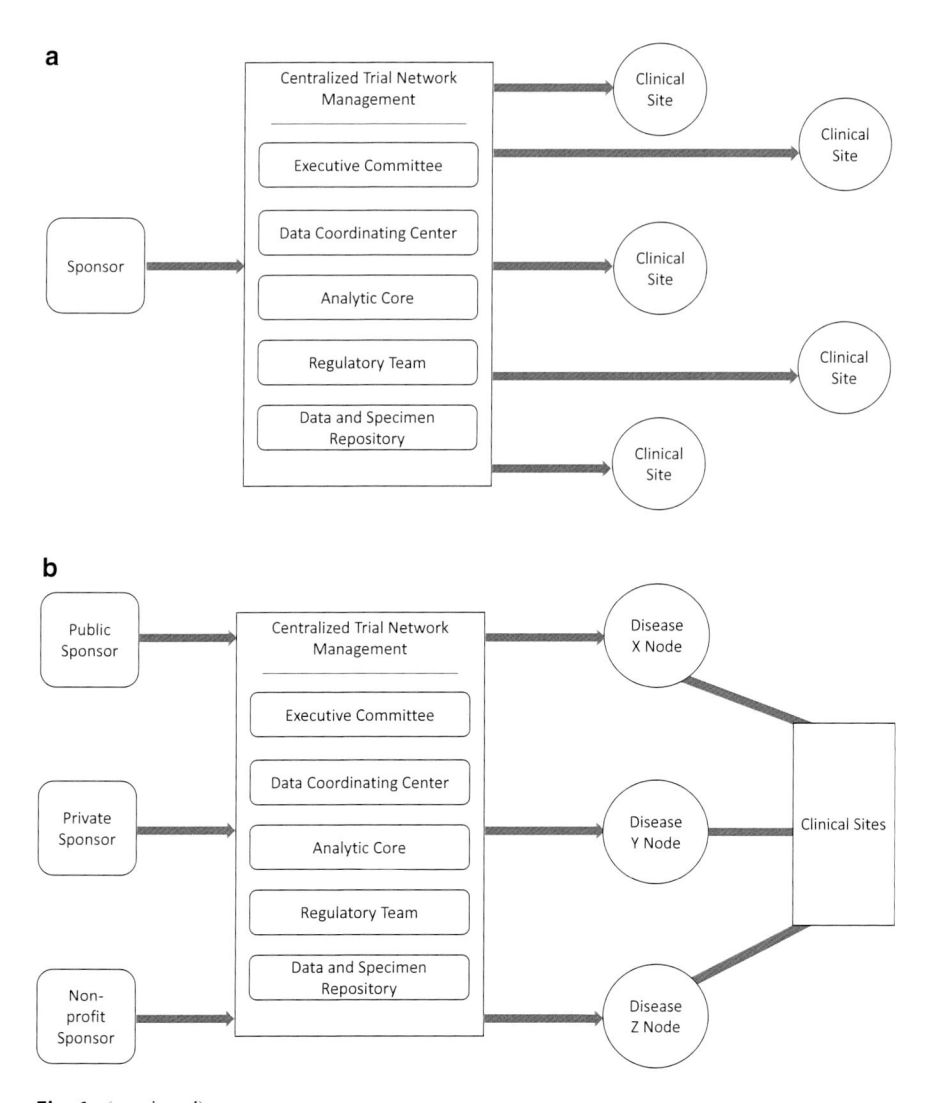

Fig. 1 (continued)

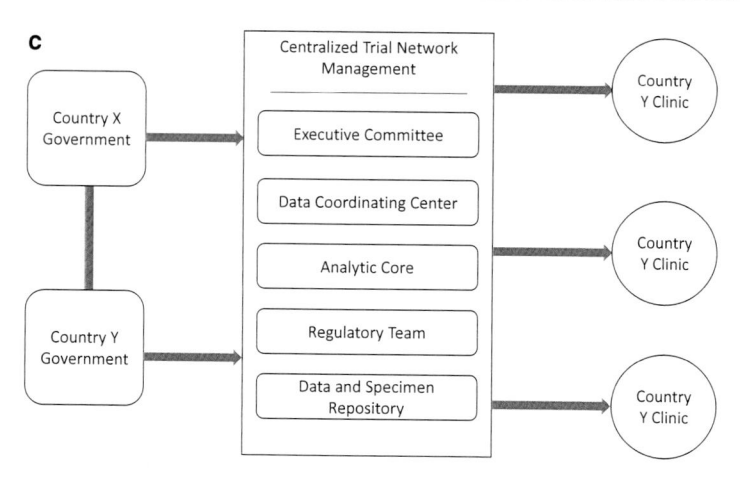

Fig. 1 Clinical Trial Network Structure Examples. (**a**) Clinical trial network with one sponsor who works directly with the centralized trial network management to direct and coordinate research at multiple clinics. (**b**) Clinical trial network with multiple public and private sponsors who work directly with the centralized trial network management to direct and coordinate research nodes, focusing on different diseases, that then coordinate research at multiple clinal sites. (**c**) Clinical trial network with public sponsors from different governments who work directly with the centralized trial network management to direct and coordinate research at multiple clinics in one country; typically, seen with one northern country sponsoring government and one southern country sponsoring government, with research conducted in the southern country

initiative intended to disseminate research results to benefit the entire ERA (European Commission 2009).

There are a variety of ways in which a clinical trial network can be organized. Figure 1 depicts common structures. Despite their differences in design, there are several unique elements common to most clinical trial networks. Due to their inherent complexity, clinical trial networks tend to have centralized operations management. This may consist of some executive body that directs the mission and research programs for the network. They may include a representative from the funding organization to inform the direction of the research agenda. This group may task one or more working groups to coordinate between clinical investigators to execute such initiatives. Clinical trial networks may also include a dedicated, centralized, regulatory arm that handles the regulatory reporting responsibilities of all studies conducted within the network. Data coordination can also be done centrally for a number of studies within the network. Along with data coordination, a clinical trial network may have a dedicated analytic core to perform all study analyses. This group may also be charged with developing novel trial designs that are best suited to answer questions related to the clinical area of interest for the network. Because the network pulls participants from the same patient pool, investigators can recruit for multiple studies within the network at once, leading to better enrollment for all network trials, particularly those that require highly specific patient populations (Liu et al. 2013; McCrae et al. 2012). This often means that patient data that feeds into a data repository can serve to inform several trials with minimal associated administrative overhead (Massett et al. 2019). Finally, clinical trial networks have a formal system for building consensus around research priorities, resource allocation, and network leadership (Organization for Economic Co-operation and Development 2013). Developing the protocol for reaching consensus is essential when clinical trial networks are large and multinational with differing regulatory oversight and clinical standards.

Clinical trial networks offer many benefits to various stakeholders. They provide an opportunity for investigators with similar research interests to exchange ideas, develop novel trial methodologies for their clinical area, share resources, and leverage a large pool of potential participants to push their field forward (Bentley et al. 2019; Davidson et al. 2006). In cases where there is national buy-in from local governments, this becomes an important public-private partnership to accelerate national research agendas in an efficient manner. Initiating trials within an existing infrastructure of research groups with existing relationships between each other and with the sponsor, organizational competence, and administrative support contribute to this efficiency. The inherent structure of clinical trial networks lends itself to comparative effectiveness research that can inform government reimbursement decisions and potential guideline changes. Smaller clinical sites wishing to develop relationships with certain sponsors can benefit from joining clinical trial networks as well. Sub-studies are also easier to execute for clinical sites with limited resources by leveraging existing infrastructure. Lastly, all clinical sites, regardless of capacity, can benefit from the increased exchange of ideas through the frequent meetings.

Despite these benefits, clinical trial networks can carry limitations worth considering. There is a common perception that enrollment is the standard metric of success within a network. As such, payment structures may be based on the number of participants enrolled at each site, with little consideration of overhead costs. This could be a deterrent for investigators from academic institutions with high overhead costs or for study investigators with study protocols requiring high resource utilization, as investigators are dependent on their institution's cooperation and support of the endeavor. Clinical trial networks can also fall victim to inadequate staffing, with consequences more substantial than would be in a single clinical research group (Baer et al. 2010). Additionally, participation in a clinical trial network may mean involvement in multiple clinical trials; however, not all of these may lead to significant credit or publications for every investigator (Bentley et al. 2019). The decision for investigators to participate in a clinical trial network should weigh the benefits and limitations of their home institution, existing patient pool, and potential for professional growth in their group and contribution to science.

Summary and Conclusions

Clinical trial networks provide an efficient platform for investigators to conduct a large number of multicenter clinical trials, simultaneously, in niche research areas. They also allow for trial innovation in ways that are specifically catered to the needs of a clinical area. While this is a highly structured manner to conduct many multicenter clinical trials, they can be done on a single trial basis with a different group of investigators each time. Multicenter clinical trial designs are a welcoming platform for smaller clinical centers wishing to engage in clinical trials for which the patient population is hard to recruit and for which trial conduct is resource intense. This approach then allows for engagement of investigators and patient pools that would otherwise be excluded from such research. Multicenter clinical trials allow for an efficient, timely approach to conduct a clinical trial with a representative patient population. They are utilized by both private and public entities for evidence used in product development and informing guidelines and reimbursement decisions.

Key Facts

1. Multicenter clinical trials are a resource conservative approach to engage investigators in large clinical trials, particularly those for which patients are rare or hard to recruit.
2. As clinical research moves towards electronic records and virtual assessments, multicenter clinical trials are becoming more feasible in resource poor locations, as data coordination, study monitoring, and regulatory submissions are managed centrally.
3. Government agencies can accelerate priority research by establishing clinical trial networks around these areas to engage investigators in multiple, simultaneous clinical trials for disease therapeutics and interventions.
4. While multicenter clinical trials offer an efficient way to conduct clinical trials, they do have considerable levels of oversight from trial leadership and require site investigators to cede some autonomy.

Cross-References

▶ Data Capture, Data Management, and Quality Control; Single Versus Multicenter Trials
▶ Institutional Review Boards and Ethics Committees
▶ Responsibilities and Management of the Clinical Coordinating Center
▶ Selection of Study Centers and Investigators
▶ Trial Organization and Governance

References

Baer AR, Kelly CA, Bruinooge SS, Runowicz CD, Blayney DW (2010) Challenges to National Cancer Institute-Supported Cooperative Group clinical trial participation: an ASCO survey of cooperative group sites. J Oncol Pract 6(3):114–117. https://doi.org/10.1200/jop.200028
Bentley C, Cressman S, van der Hoek K, Arts K, Dancey J, Peacock S (2019) Conducting clinical trials – costs, impacts, and the value of clinical trials networks: a scoping review. Clin Trials 16(2):183–193. https://doi.org/10.1177/1740774518820060

Chung KC, Song JW, Group, WS (2010) A guide to organizing a multicenter clinical trial. Plast Reconstr Surg 126(2):515–523. https://doi.org/10.1097/PRS.0b013e3181df64fa

Dalkey NC (1969) The Delphi method: an experimental study of group opinion. Santa Monica, CA: RAND Corporation, 1969. https://www.rand.org/pubs/research_memoranda/RM5888.html

Davidson RM, McNeer JF, Logan L, Higginbotham MB, Anderson J, Blackshear J, . . . Wagner GS (2006) A cooperative network of trained sites for the conduct of a complex clinical trial: a new concept in multicenter clinical research. Am Heart J 151(2):451–456. https://doi.org/10.1016/j.ahj.2005.04.013

Daykin A, Selman LE, Cramer H, McCann S, Shorter GW, Sydes MR, . . . Shaw A (2016) What are the roles and valued attributes of a Trial Steering Committee? Ethnographic study of eight clinical trials facing challenges. Trials 17(1):307. https://doi.org/10.1186/s13063-016-1425-y

Department of Health (2006) Guidelines for good practice in the conduct of clinical trials with human participants in South Africa. https://www.dst.gov.za/rdtax/index.php/guiding-documents/south-africangood-clinical-practice-guidelines/file

Ervin AM, Taylor HA, Ehrhardt S (2016) NIH policy on single-IRB review – a new era in multicenter studies. N Engl J Med 375(24):2315–2317. https://doi.org/10.1056/NEJMp1608766

European Commission (2009) Report from the Commission to the European Parliament and the council on the application of Council Regulation (EC) No 723/2009 of 25 June 2009 on the community legal framework for a European Research Infrastructure Consortium (ERIC). (COM (2014) 460 final). European Commission, Brussels. Retrieved from https://ec.europa.eu/info/sites/info/files/eric_report-2014.pdf

Liu G, Chen G, Sinoway LI, Berg A (2013) Assessing the impact of the NIH CTSA program on institutionally sponsored clinical trials. Clin Transl Sci 6(3):196–200. https://doi.org/10.1111/cts.12029

Massett HA, Mishkin G, Moscow JA, Gravell A, Steketee M, Kruhm M, . . . Ivy SP (2019) Transforming the early drug development paradigm at the National Cancer Institute: the formation of NCI's Experimental Therapeutics Clinical Trials Network (ETCTN). Clin Cancer Res 25(23):6925–6931. https://doi.org/10.1158/1078-0432.Ccr-19-1754

McCrae N, Douglas L, Banerjee S (2012) Contribution of research networks to a clinical trial of antidepressants in people with dementia. J Ment Health 21(5):439–447. https://doi.org/10.3109/09638237.2012.664298

National Institutes of Health (2016) Final NIH policy on the use of a single institutional review board for multi-site research. Bethesda. Retrieved from http://grants.nih.gov/grants/guide/notice-files/NOT-OD-16-094.html

National Institutes of Health (2017) Guidance on implementation of the NIH policy on the use of a single institutional review board for multi-site research. Bethesda. Retrieved from https://grants.nih.gov/grants/guide/notice-files/NOT-OD-18-004.html

Organization for Economic Co-operation and Development (2013) OECD recommendation on the governance of clinical trials. Retrieved from http://www.oecd.org/sti/inno/oecdrecommendationonthegovernanceofclinicaltrials.htm

Senn S (1998) Some controversies in planning and analysing multi-centre trials. Stat Med 17(15–16):1753–1765. https://doi.org/10.1002/(sici)1097-0258(19980815/30)17:15/16<1753::aid-sim977>3.0.co;2-x; discussion 1799–1800

The International Conference on Harmonisation of Technical Requirements for Registration of Pharmaceuticals for Human Use (1998) ICH E5(R1) ethnic factors in the acceptability of foreign clinical data. cited European Medicines Agency. Available from: https://www.ema.europa.eu/en/documents/scientific-guideline/iche-5-r1-ethnic-factors-acceptability-foreign-clinical-data-step-5_en.pdf

The International Conference on Harmonisation of Technical Requirements for Registration of Pharmaceuticals for Human Use (2017) ICH E17 general principles for planning and design of multi-regional clinical trials. Available from: The International Conference on Harmonisation of Technical Requirements for Registration of Pharmaceuticals for Human Use. ICH E17 General Principles for Planning and Design of Multi-Regional Clinical Trials. 2017

Trial Governance (2015) Field trials of health interventions: a toolbox, 3rd edn. In: Smith P, Morrow R, Ross D (Eds). OUP Oxford, Oxford, UK

United States Food and Drug Administration (2006a) Guidance for clinical trial sponsors – establishment and operation of clinical trial Data Monitoring Committees. Rockville. Retrieved from https://www.fda.gov/media/75398/download

United States Food and Drug Administration (2006b) Guidance for industry – using a centralized IRB review process in multicenter clinical trials. Retrieved from https://www.fda.gov/regulatory-information/search-fda-guidance-documents/using-centralized-irb-review-process-multicenter-clinical-trials

United States Food and Drug Administration (2013) Guidance for industry – oversight of clinical investigations – a risk-based approach to monitoring. Silver Spring. Retrieved from https://www.fda.gov/media/116754/download

Van de Ven AH, Delbecq AL (1972) The nominal group as a research instrument for exploratory health studies. Am J Public Health 62(3):337–342. https://doi.org/10.2105/ajph.62.3.337

Van De Ven AH, Delbecq AL (1974) The effectiveness of nominal, Delphi, and interacting group decision making processes. Acad Manag J 17(4):605–621. https://doi.org/10.2307/255641

Zelen M (1974) The randomization and stratification of patients to clinical trials. J Chronic Dis 27(7–8):365–375. https://doi.org/10.1016/0021-9681(74)90015-0

Principles of Protocol Development

10

Bingshu E. Chen, Alison Urton, Anna Sadura, and
Wendy R. Parulekar

Contents

Abstract

Randomized clinical trials are essential to the advancement of clinical care by providing an unbiased estimate of the efficacy of new therapies compared to current standards of care. The protocol document plays a key role during the life cycle of a trial and guides all aspects of trial organization and conduct, data collection, analysis, and publication of results.

Several guidance documents are available to assist with protocol generation. The SPIRIT (Standard Protocol Items: Recommendations for Interventional Trials) Statement comprises a checklist of essential items for inclusion in a

B. E. Chen · A. Urton · A. Sadura · W. R. Parulekar (✉)
Canadian Cancer Trials Group, Queen's University, Kingston, ON, Canada
e-mail: bechen@ctg.queensu.ca; aurton@ctg.queensu.ca; asadura@ctg.queensu.ca;
wparulekar@ctg.queensu.ca

© Springer Nature Switzerland AG 2022
S. Piantadosi, C. L. Meinert (eds.), *Principles and Practice of Clinical Trials*,
https://doi.org/10.1007/978-3-319-52636-2_32

protocol document. Other essential references include those generated by the International Conference on Harmonization and the Declaration of Helsinki which inform the design and conduct of trials that meet the highest scientific, ethical, and safety standards.

Keywords

SPIRIT Statement · International Conference on Harmonization · Declaration of Helsinki

Introduction

The protocol serves as the reference document for the conduct, analysis, and reporting of a clinical trial which must satisfy the requirements of all stakeholders involved in clinical trial research including trial participants, ethics committees, regulatory and legal authorities, funders, sponsors, public advocates, as well as the medical and scientific communities that are the direct consumers of the research findings.

An inadequate or erroneous protocol has significant consequences. A deficient protocol may result in delayed or denied regulatory or ethical approval, risks to the safety of study subjects, investigator frustration and poor accrual, inconsistent implementation across investigators, as well as increased workload burden and financial costs due to unnecessary amendments. Ultimately, the trial results may not be interpretable or publishable.

The purpose of this chapter is to outline the general principles of protocol development with an emphasis on use of standard definitions and criteria for protocol content where applicable. Essential reading for this chapter is the SPIRIT 2013 Statement (Chan et al. 2013a) and accompanying Elaborations and Explanations paper (Chan et al. 2013b). The SPIRIT Initiative was launched in 2007 to address a critical gap in evidence-based guidance documents for protocol generation. Using systematic reviews, a formal Delphi consensus process, and face-to-face meetings of key stakeholders, a 33-item checklist relating to protocol content was generated and subsequently field tested prior to publication. Although the SPIRIT checklist was primarily developed as a guidance document for randomized clinical trials, the principles and application extend to all clinical trials, regardless of design. The reader is also directed to the SPIRT PRO extension which builds on the methodology of the SPIRIT Statement and provides recommendations for protocol development when a patient-reported outcome is a key primary or secondary outcome (Calvert et al. 2018).

Key principles that underpin the content of high-quality clinical trial protocols relate to the originality and relevance of the primary research hypothesis contained therein, use of design elements to adequately test the hypothesis, and inclusion of appropriate measures to protect the rights and safety of trial participants. Guidance documents generated by the International Conference on Harmonization (ICH) are useful references and address multiple topics of interest such as the E6 *Good Clinical Practice* (GCP) and E8 General Considerations for Clinical Trials (https://www.ich.org/products/guidelines/efficacy/efficacy-single/article/integrated-addendum-good-clinical-practice.html). Another important reference document is the Declaration of Helsinki which was developed by the World Medical Association and represents a set of principles that guides the ethical conduct of research involving humans (https://www.wma.net/policies-post/wma-declaration-of-helsinki-ethical-principles-for-medical-research-involving-human-subjects).

What follows is a brief summary of key protocol content topics annotated with the associated SPIRIT checklist items. Additional comments to assist with comprehension or use of SPIRIT protocol items are included as appropriate.

Administrative Information: SPIRIT Checklist Items 1–5d

The administrative information relates to protocol title, unique trial registry number, amendment history, and contact information for trial conduct from scientific, operational, and regulatory perspectives. The title should indicate the trial phase, interventions under evaluation and disease settings/trial population (Fig. 1)

The Declaration of Helsinki (revised 2008) mandates the registration of all clinical trial in a publicly accessible database before recruitment of the first subject.

Trial registration in a primary register of the WHO International Clinical Trials Registry Platform (ICTRP) or in ClinicalTrials.gov has been endorsed by the International Committee of Medical Journal Editors (http://www.icmje.org/recommendations) since both registries meet the criteria of access to the public at no charge, oversight by a not for profit organization, inclusion of a mechanism to ensure

Fig. 1 Sample protocol title page

Protocol Version Date

Research Organization

Protocol Title (number/code)

Trial Registration Number

Study Chair:

Steering Committee:

Biostatistician:

Collaborating Research Organizations:

Regulatory Sponsor:

Support Providers: Grant Agencies:

Pharmaceutical Companies:

validity of registry information, and searchability by electronic means. Effective April 18, 2017, trial registration for applicable clinical trials became mandatory under the US Federal Food, Drug, and Cosmetic Act (FD&C Act). Registration promotes informed decision-making by reducing publication bias, ensures researchers and potential study participants are aware of trial opportunities, avoids duplication of trials, and can identify gaps in clinical research. Registries may also require submission of basic study results.

A protocol is a dynamic document that is responsive to new information that emerges during the life cycle of a trial from external or internal sources. Amendment history is recorded in the protocol document using date and version control; a master list of changes to the protocol must be maintained in the trial master file. The content of the amendment will guide the rapidity with which the protocol is modified and circulated to investigators. Amendments based on safety considerations are the highest priority and are processed rapidly; administrative changes or clarifications can be issued when there are sufficient cumulative changes in a trial to justify the workload associated with approval of the amendment by regulators and ethics committees. Designation of key roles and responsibilities to specific individuals involved in trial design and conduct and their contact information are an essential resource for trial participants and the research community and are provided in the protocol document.

Background and Rationale and Objectives: SPIRIT Checklist Items 6–7

The justification for a research study is the single most important component of any clinical results of trial that will not contribute meaningfully to the advancement of healthcare and research represents a waste of resources and is unethical, regardless of adherence to checklists and standards for research involving human subjects.

The background section should summarize the current literature about the research topic and the hypothesis that will be addressed by the clinical trial. A review of ongoing trials addressing the same or similar research questions will demonstrate non-duplication of research efforts. Finally, explicit statements regarding the anticipated impact of the trial results – either positive or negative – provide a powerful justification for trial conduct. This section should be updated as required to reflect important advances in knowledge as they relate to the research question, especially if they result in changes to trial design or conduct.

The objectives of the trial enable the research hypothesis to be tested and are listed in order of importance as primary and secondary objectives. The primary objective links directly to the statistical design of the trial which allow the results to be interpreted within a pre-specified set of statistical parameters (see Section Statistical Methods). Secondary objectives are selected to provide additional information to support interpretation of the primary analysis data and typically focus on additional measures of efficacy, safety, and tolerability associated with a given intervention. Tertiary objectives are exploratory in nature and may address preliminary research questions related to disease biology or response to treatment.

Trial Design: SPIRIT Checklist Item 8

The trial design is driven by the research hypothesis under evaluation. For example, new therapeutic strategies with the potential for greater disease control compared to standard of care may be tested in a parallel group superiority trial; a non-inferiority trial may be suitable to test a therapy associated with less toxicity or greater ease of delivery for which a small loss of efficacy may be acceptable. In addition to a description of the trial framework, the protocol must clearly indicate the randomization allocation ratio. Deviation from the usual 1:1 allocation may be justified by the desire for a more in-depth characterization of treatment-associated safety and tolerability and may increase participant willingness to be enrolled in a specific trial if there is a greater chance of receiving a new treatment compared to standard of care. Crossover in treatment administration is another important aspect of trial design and is used frequently in studies of chronic diseases which are relatively stable, and therapeutic interventions result in amelioration but not cures of the condition, e.g., pain syndromes or asthma. Patients are randomly allocated to predefined sequence of treatments administered over time periods, and the outcome of interest is measured at the end of each treatment time period unit.

A design of increasing interest and use is the pilot study. This type of trial is to is conducted using the same randomization scheme and interventions but on a smaller scale. The goal of the pilot study is to gather information regarding trial conduct such as ability to randomize patients, administer the therapeutic interventions, or measure the outcomes measure(s) of interest but not to estimate relative treatment efficacy between the interventions (Lancaster et al. 2004; Whitehead et al. 2014).

Participants, Interventions, and Outcomes: SPIRIT Checklist Items 9–17b

Participants

The population selected for trial participation must meet specific criteria to ensure safety and enable the primary and secondary objectives to be met.

For trials testing drug interventions, adequate organ function is based on the known pharmacokinetic and pharmacodynamic properties of the drug. Surgical or radiotherapy trials may require additional tests of fitness for the required intervention including lung function tests, adequacy of coagulation, and ability to tolerate an anesthetic.

A patient is enrolled on a trial based on the assumption that he/she will contribute meaningful information to the outcome measure(s) with a small loss of data due to trial dropouts or withdrawals. The eligibility criteria should ensure that enrolled patients can contribute data to enable the trial objectives to be met. For example, a trial examining the impact of a therapeutic intervention on pain response must enroll symptomatic patients with a specific pain threshold; trials evaluating the ability of interventions to control or shrink disease must have a quantifiable disease burden, e.g., radiological evidence of cancer in a trial evaluating anticancer activity of different therapies. Given the significant resource required for the conduct of a randomized trial, a natural tendency is to include as many outcome measures as possible to maximize the yield of the data generated by the trial. This approach is not recommended since it increases the burden of study conduct and participation and the risk of noncompliance with data submission and may negatively impact accrual if enrollment is contingent on ability to provide data on multiple outcome measures. The overall false-positive rate could be inflated when multiple numbers of hypotheses are being tested and proper adjustment for multiple tests is required.

Patient-reported outcomes (PROs) are frequently included in trials of therapeutic interventions to provide a patient perspective on their health status during the course of a trial. Specific eligibility criteria related to participation in PRO data collection, e.g., language ability, comprehension of questionnaires, and access to electronic devices for direct patient to database submissions, should be adequately described in the eligibility criteria. Similarly, criteria related to other research objectives such as submission of biological tissue for analyses related to disease prognosis or predictors of response to therapeutic interventions or health utility questionnaires for economic analyses are included in the eligibility criteria as appropriate. The mandatory versus optional nature of the criteria for tissue submission and patient-reported outcome must be stipulated.

A long-standing criticism of clinical trials is that the results may have limited real-world applicability due to the highly selected patient population enrolled. Linked to this concern is the issue of screen failures, i.e., patients who are appropriate candidates to participate in the trial but cannot be enrolled due to inability to meet the stringent eligibility criteria. In response to this concern, efforts are underway by research and advocacy organizations to broaden criteria to allow greater participation in clinical trials by removing barriers such as the presence of comorbidities, organ dysfunction, prior history of malignancies, or minimum age (Gore et al. 2017; Kim et al. 2017; Lichtman et al. 2017).

Interventions

The treatment strategies under evaluation must be clearly described in the protocol, to allow participating centers to safely administer the intervention and the medical community to reproducibly administer the intervention should it be adopted or used on a wider basis. A basic trial schema included early in the protocol document provides a visual illustration of the interventions (Fig. 2).

For drug trials, dose calculation and guidelines regarding administration and dose modification are provided. A tabular format is a convenient method to illustrate the dose modification requirements mandated by specific laboratory values and/or adverse events. In addition, guidance regarding dose modifications should a patient experience multiple adverse events with conflicting recommendations regarding dose adjustments is essential information for the protocol. Nondrug interventions

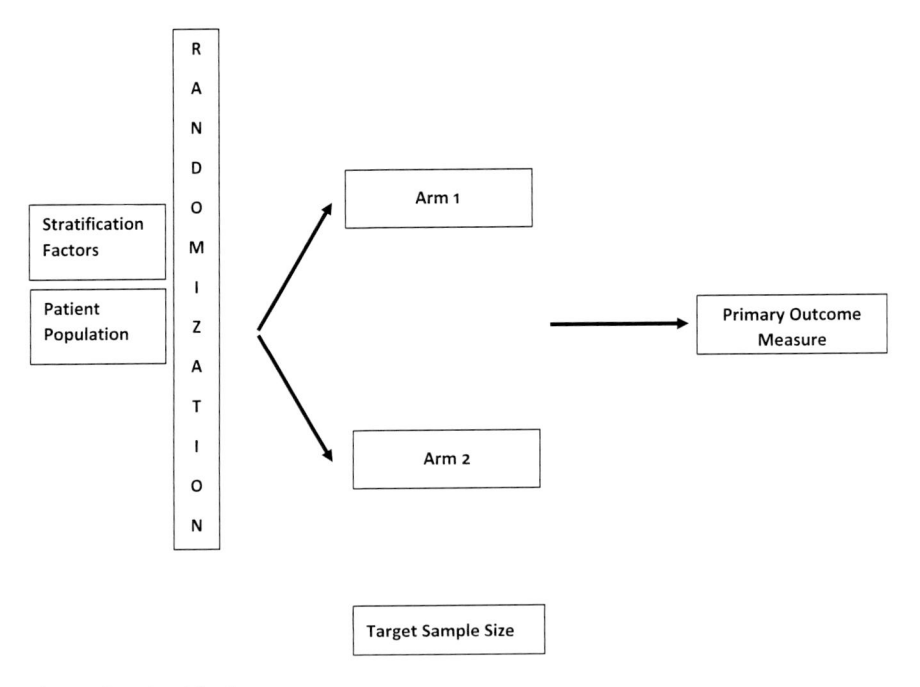

Fig. 2 Sample trial schema

such as surgery, radiotherapy, or use of other devices require additional protocol guidance related to credentialing requirements of those administering the intervention and the setting of administration.

The protocol should also include details regarding strategies to maintain compliance with trial interventions and how these will be measured. Inclusion of this information will optimize exposure of the participants to the interventions of interest and interpretation of efficacy estimates and inform the uptake of the intervention by the clinical community if the intervention is beneficial. Caution is advised when choosing the instrument(s) to measure compliance. For example, oral dosing of a drug may be monitored by patient diaries and/or pill counts at the end of a predefined treatment period. Maintaining a medication diary may be burdensome and inaccurate for patients who are treated over long periods of time. In addition, using both diary entries and pill returns to measure compliance may be problematic if these measures provide conflicting information about drug exposure.

Concurrent therapies or care administered on a trial may impact the adverse event experience and compliance with the intervention of interest and may have the potential to alter the disease outcome, leading to biased estimates of efficacy for a given intervention. To minimize this problem, permissible and non-permissible therapies should be clearly listed in a protocol combined with guidance regarding dose adjustments or discontinuation in the case of administration of a prohibited therapy.

Outcomes

The outcome measures selected in a clinical trial are of paramount importance – they form the basis for data collection, statistical analysis, and results reporting. An appropriate outcome measure must have a biologically plausible and clinically relevant link to the intervention(s) under evaluation and be objectively and reliably measured and reported using appropriate nomenclature.

Standardization of outcome measures has been identified by the research community as a goal to improve the general interpretability of the results of individual trials and to enhance the integration and analysis of results from multiple trials. The COMET (Core Outcome Measures in Effectiveness Trials) initiative is an example of a collaborative effort to define a minimum core set of outcomes to be measured and reported in clinical trials (http://www.comet-initiative.org). In addition to providing guidance regarding disease-specific outcome measures, the COMET initiative represents a rich resource of relevant methodologies for interested researchers.

Composite outcome measures are often used to evaluate the efficacy of therapeutic interventions and deserve specific mention. As with single-item outcome measures, the individual components of a composite measure must be clearly defined and evaluable. In addition, the hierarchy of importance of the individual components of a composite outcome measure must be prospectively identified to assist with data collection and reporting. For example, if disease worsening can be defined by radiological investigations or measurement of a blood-based marker, guidance for reporting must be included in the protocol should both outcome events occur simultaneously.

Perhaps the most important and challenging criterion to satisfy when selecting an outcome measure relates to clinical benefit or meaningfulness. If the ultimate goal of a therapeutic intervention is to live longer or better, the outcome measure must be correlated to clinical benefit. Overall survival is considered the gold standard outcome measure for trials testing therapeutic interventions for life-threatening diseases but may be challenging to measure and interpret if death occurs years after enrollment in a trial or if multiple efficacious therapies are administered after the intervention of interest has failed to control the disease. Use of an intermediate, clinically meaningful outcome measure may be justified in circumstances when overall survival measurement is not feasible, especially when the alternative outcome measure is a validated surrogate for overall survival, e.g., metastasis-free survival in early prostate cancer (Xie et al. 2017).

Participant Timeline, Sample Size Recruitment (Items 13–15)

The schedule of investigations and interventions is included in all protocols to enable meaningful participation of patients and researchers. Baseline and post-randomization evaluations should be displayed in easy to understand format such as tables or schematic diagrams. Timing of evaluations is linked to safety and efficacy oversight. The former is dictated by the schedule of treatment administration and safety profile of the treatment intervention; the latter must be symmetric between arms to avoid biased assessment of treatment efficacy. Classification of investigations by disease and treatment trajectory is a logical way to convey the information to trial participants, i.e., prior to randomization, treatment phase, and follow-up phase after the treatment has been completed or discontinued. Only essential investigations should be included in a protocol to minimize the burden of participation on patients and healthcare facilities. An important principle guiding protocol development relates to alignment of study assessments to usual care. Tests or interactions within the healthcare systems that deviate from current practice will increase the risk of noncompliance of participants with protocol-mandated assessments and may lead to incomplete data collection and an impact on enrollment. To minimize this risk, the protocol schedule of assessments and follow-up should be shared with prospective participants for review prior to trial initiation.

Sample Size

The sample size justification is directly linked to the trial hypothesis and primary objective. The statistical and clinical assumptions that inform the sample size calculation must be clearly stated. The relevant information includes identification of the primary outcome measure, expected primary outcome in the control group, and the targeted difference in the primary outcome measure between treatment groups, primary statistical test, type I and II errors rates, and measures of precision. In general, a minimal clinically important difference (MCID) shall be used in sample size calculation. Sample size adjustments for missing data and/or interim analyses should be detailed. Additional important details to include in this section relate to the planned duration of accrual and follow-up required to compile sufficient data to enable the primary analysis.

Recruitment

The success of a trial is directly related to its ability to meet the pre-specified accrual target. Given the tremendous effort and resource required to conduct a randomized trial, every effort must be made to ensure the enrollment of consenting patients in a timely manner. Details of recruitment plans are included in the protocol and will vary with the patient population and interventions of interest, participating research networks, and duration of accrual. Oversight measures to ensure adequacy of accrual are described in this section.

Assignment of Interventions (for Controlled Trials): Spirit Checklist Items 16–17b

The single most powerful design aspect of a controlled clinical trial is the process of randomization or random assignment of enrolled subjects/patients to protocol treatments. The purpose of randomization is to reduce the impact of bias of known and unknown factors on treatment comparisons as a means of isolating the treatment effect on patient outcome. Multiple methods of randomization exist. Blocked randomization ensures balance of treatment assignment within a pre-specified number of enrollments. For example, with a block size of eight and a 1:1 randomization, four patients will have been randomized to each treatment after completion of a block (Altman and Bland 1999). To reduce selection bias, random block size is recommended in the randomized trial, and block size should be concealed from the trial investigators. Another technique of randomization is known as stratified randomization. This method balances treatment allocations within pre-specified strata defined by factors which may impact disease outcomes independent of treatment assignment (Zelen 1974; Kernan et al. 1999). Minimization is another method frequently used in clinical trial conduct that adaptively assigns patients to treatments based on the last treatment assignment of the trial taking into account pre-specified stratification factors. This technique represents a rigorous method to achieve balance of treatment assignment for predefined patient factors as well as for the enrollment number for each treatment group (Pocock and Richard 1975). All stratification factors at randomization (except for center unit) shall be taken into account in the statistical analysis.

The protocol document must clearly outline the procedures for trial entry/enrollment. This includes the requirements for activation of a participating center. Specific requirements such as investigator or center credentialing for treatment delivery must be outlined including reference to appropriate appendices for additional guidance.

A step by step description of the enrolment process should also be provided. This includes instructions regarding the enrollment system in use, means of access, and hours of operation as well as the data fields required to complete the enrollment. Details on how a successful enrollment and treatment allocation will be communicated to the participating center are also outlined in the protocol document.

Data Collection/Management and Analysis: SPIRIT Checklist Items 18a–20c

Data Collection

Data collection must align with the protocol specifications and thus not exceed what has been approved by regulators, ethics boards, and consenting patients. Several principles guide data collection during trial conduct: protection of identity and confidentiality of trial participant data, adequacy of data to meet the primary and secondary objectives of the trial, use of standard criteria to collect and report data, and non-duplication of data collection unless justified and pre-specified in the protocol document. The protocol must specify the data points of interest, methods of collection, and frequency of reporting. Standard dictionaries for data collection and reporting should be used where available, e.g., TNM (tumor, lymph node, metastases) system for solid tumor cancer staging in oncology trials. Use of validated questionnaires or other instruments to enable accurate measurement of outcome measures will ensure consistency of reporting and enhance the quality and interpretation of the statistical analyses, e.g., EORTC QLQ-C30 questionnaire for global quality of life evaluation in cancer patients (Aaronson et al. 1993) (Table 1).

Table 1 Sample patient evaluation flow sheet

Required investigations	Pre-study prior to registration/ randomization	During protocol treatment	After protocol treatment
History and physical exam			
xx	Within x days		
Hematology			
xx			
Coagulation			
xx			
Biochemistry			
xx			
Radiology			
xx			
Other investigations			
xx			
Correlative studies			
xx			
Adverse events			
xx			
Quality of life			
xx			
Health economics			

Data Management

To demonstrate adherence to guidelines and regulations for database compilation, storage, and access, the protocol or associated documents must detail the infrastructure and oversight procedures for data management. This includes information regarding how trial conduct will be monitored at participating sites to enable data verification, ethics compliance, and review of pharmacy documentation for drug trials.

Guidance documents for retention of essential documents at participating sites should be cited as appropriate. For example, ICH GCP 4.9.5 guidance refers to the number of years that essential documents must be retained at an investigative site; GCP 4.9.7 outlines investigative site obligations to allow direct access to trial-related documents by an oversight bodies such as a regulatory authority, research ethics board, or monitors/auditors (https://ichgcp.net/4-investigator/).

The integrity of a database is related to the quality of data contained therein. To ensure the submission of high-quality data by trial participants, including accurate, complete, and timely submission, data collection forms should include clear instructions and unambiguous data entry fields. Submitted data should be consistent with source records. Data management guidebooks are useful tools to address topics such as data entry and editing; methods to record unknown data; how to add comments and how to respond to queries. Specific trial-related procedures can also be detailed in protocol appendices or guides, e.g., collection and submission procedures for biological samples.

Statistical Analysis

The statistical analysis section must be described in sufficient detail to allow replication of the analysis and interpretation of the trial results by the scientific and clinical community. Inclusion of an experienced statistical member/team in the protocol writing, trial conduct, and analysis phases is essential to meet these goals. The parameters of interest include the outcome measure to be compared; the population whose data will be included, e.g., all randomized versus eligible; and the statistical methods used to analyze the data. Details regarding the use of censoring and methods to deal with missing data should also be included. When stratification was used at randomization, the statistical test for primary hypothesis shall account for the stratification factors (e.g., stratified Cochran-Mantel-Haenszel test for response rate and stratified log-rank test for time to event outcome). For example, a clinical trial comparing the impact of a new therapy compared to standard of care on overall survival may utilize a time to event analysis. Appropriate statistical methods to analyze the survival experience of all randomized patients grouped by assigned treatment include graphical display using the Kaplan-Meier method and comparison using an appropriate log-rank test (Rosner 1990) with additional exploratory comparisons adjusted for prognostic covariates (Cox 1972).

Subgroup analyses are of great interest to the clinical community to understand the treatment effect of a given intervention on different populations defined by specific covariates such as those related to disease burden, exposure to prior treatment, or patient characteristics. Given the exploratory nature of subgroup analyses, these should be prospectively justified and defined in the protocol with the appropriate statistical tests to determine if there is an interaction between treatment and subgroup.

Analyses of secondary outcome measures should inform interpretation of the primary analysis and, ultimately, the research hypothesis. Sufficient details regarding these analyses to justify their inclusion in the protocol and the associated data collection plans are required. Using quality of life as an example, the specific questionnaire/domains of interest, definition of meaningful change in score(s), time point of data collection for analysis, and methods to control the type I error due to multiplicity of testing should be outlined in the statistical section (Calvert et al. 2018).

Monitoring: SPIRIT Checklist Items 21–23

Monitoring activities of a trial relate to real-time oversight of accumulating data related to safety and efficacy as well as trial conduct in participating centers.

Data Monitoring

Oversight of data is integral to the regulatory, safety, and ethical obligations for any trial. It is expected that all phase III randomized trials will be monitored in a real time and ongoing basis by an independent Data and Safety Monitoring Committee/Board (DSMC/DSMB). According to ICH GCP, the oversight committee responsibilities include assessment of trial progress, review of safety and critical efficacy data, and providing recommendations on trial continuation, modification, and/or termination as appropriate.

The protocol should refer to the existence of this oversight body and the reporting obligations of the trial sponsor to the DSMC/DSMB relating to the progress of the clinical trial, safety, and critical efficacy analyses. Specific terms of reference or charters for the DSMC/DSMB may be contained in non-protocol documents that are available on demand.

Efficacy

Interim analyses of the primary outcome measure allow for early termination of a clinical trial if extreme differences between the treatment arms are seen. Given the potential for misleading results and interpretations due to multiple analyses of accumulating data (Geller and Pocock 1987), all prospectively planned interim analyses must be described in detail in the statistical section. The description will include the timing or triggers for the interim analyses, the nominal critical p-values for rejecting the null and alternative hypotheses that may lead to early disclosure of results or termination of the trial, and required statistical adjustment to preserve the overall type I error of the trial.

Harm

Safety monitoring is continuous during trial conduct and is multifaceted. It includes adverse event reporting, laboratory, and organ-specific surveillance testing such as EKCs as well as physical examinations of enrolled trial participants. An adverse event is defined by the ICH E2A guideline as *any untoward medical occurrence in a patient or clinical investigation subject administered a pharmaceutical product and which does not necessarily have to have a causal relationship with this treatment* (www.ich.org). Key components of this definition relate to the temporal association of the untoward sign, symptom, or disease with the pharmaceutical product, regardless of causality. The ICH 2sA guideline further defines the term *serious adverse event* as any medical experience that result in death, is life-threatening, requires inpatient hospitalization or prolongation of existing hospitalization, results in persistent or significant disability/incapacity, or is a congenital anomaly/birth defect. For protocol development, these definitions of adverse event and serious adverse events apply to any medical procedure, not just pharmaceutical products.

To enable safety oversight in a given trial, the lexicon for adverse event classification and submission timelines by research personnel must be referred to in the protocol and provided in a companion document or appendix. One example of such a lexicon is the Common Terminology Criteria for Adverse Events (CTC AE) developed by the US National Cancer Institute and widely utilized in oncology and non-oncology clinical trials (www.ctep.cancer.gov/protocoldevelopment). These criteria provide standard wording and severity ratings for adverse events, grouped by organ or system class. An essential component of safety reporting relates to requirements for expedited or time-sensitive adverse event reporting by participants and sponsor obligations for reporting adverse event data to other organizations involved in trial conduct, such as national and international regulatory authorities, pharmaceutical partners, and participating centers.

On a practical note, the safety elements embedded in any protocol should reflect the developmental stage of a therapeutic agent and the research objectives of the trial. For example, the adverse event reporting requirements for a drug that is approved and used within indication in a trial may be streamlined to focus on higher-grade events with expedited reporting mandated only for serious events that are unexpected and related. If a stated research objective is to characterize late or organ-specific side effects of a therapeutic intervention, the protocol should outline the specific requirements for collection and reporting of adverse events of interest.

Quality Assurance (Monitoring/Auditing)

The quality management and quality assurance process is essential to the successful conduct of clinical trials to ensure human subject protection and the integrity of trial results. Systems should be in place to manage quality in all aspects of the trial through all stages. The quality assurance process should be defined in the trial protocol and be supported by standard operating procedures and plans. Details of the plan must comply with applicable regulations and guidelines, health authority expectations, and sponsor standard operating procedures. This includes details regarding visit frequency, scope of review, and extent of compliance and source data assessment. Risk factors to consider in development of the plan include but are not limited to population, phase of trial, safety profile of agent, trial objectives and complexity, accrual, performance history, and regulatory filing intent.

Quality assurance may include monitoring, either central or on-site, and auditing activities. Per GCP these activities may be risk adapted. GCP 1.38 defines monitoring as "the act of overseeing the progress of a clinical trial, and of ensuring that it is conducted, recorded, and reported in accordance with the protocol, standard operating procedures, Good Clinical Practice, and the applicable regulatory requirements (s)," whereas GCP 1.6 defines audit as "a systematic and independent examination of trial related activities and documents to determine whether the evaluated trial activities were conducted, and the data were recorded, analyzed, and accurately reported according to the protocol, sponsor's standard operating procedures, Good Clinical Practice, and the applicable regulatory requirements." Quality assurance activities may include reviews at participating sites and vendors, internally with respect to sponsor procedures. The objectives are to verify patient safety, to verify the accuracy and validity of reported data, and to assess the compliance with regulations/guidelines and standard operating procedures. In general, components of review related to informed consent, protocol compliance and source data verification, ethics and essential documents part of the trial master file which includes standard operating procedures and training, and handling of investigational medicinal product as applicable.

Ethics and Dissemination: SPIRIT Checklist Items 24–31c

Ethics

An ethical trial is one that addresses an important research question while protecting the safety, rights, and confidentiality of trial participants. The protocol must include sufficient detail to reflect adherence to regulatory and guidance documents pertaining to these principles. This includes adherence to the Declaration of Helsinki and other reference documents such as the Tri-Council guidelines (*Tri-Council Policy Statement: Ethical Conduct for Research Involving Humans, December 2014*. Retrieved from http://www.pre.ethics.gc.ca/pdf/eng/tcps2-2014/TCPS_2_ FINAL_Web.pdf) regarding research in vulnerable populations as defined by the ability to make independent decisions or susceptibility to coercion. The protocol should contain specific wording regarding enrollment of vulnerable individuals.

ICH GCP Section 4.8 provides guidance on the informed consent process. This includes the requirement for an ethics committee-approved, signed informed consent document prior to enrollment in the trial, the need to identify the most responsible parties in a trial from compliance and liability perspectives, the use of a translator to obtain informed consent, the methods to consent a participant who cannot read, and the obligation to disclosure new information to a trial participant during trial conduct. Guidance regarding pregnancy reporting and follow-up is also required if applicable to the trial population.

ICH GCP 4.8 also provides guidance regarding the explanations of the trial to be included in the consent document. The explanations cover topics related to the experimental nature of the research and the research question; the treatments under evaluation and likelihood of assignment; trial-mandated interventions and categorization of which are experimental versus nonexperimental; the risks and benefits of trial participation including exposure of unborn embryos, fetuses, or nursing infants to protocol therapies; the existence of alternative treatment options; the trial sample size; and anticipated duration.

Topics relating to legal and ethical oversight of the trial must also be addressed in the consent document including the roles of regulatory and ethics bodies in trial conduct, the voluntary nature of trial participation, the rights of an enrolled participant including the ability to withdraw consent to participate or submit data to the sponsor, compensation for injuries should they occur, and the protection of confidentiality, which trial-related organizations will have direct access to original patient data and how data will be stored. Specific contact information for all trial-related questions or in the case of emergency is also provided.

Optional consents are utilized if there is a nonmandatory aspect of trial conduct in which enrolled patients can participate. An example of an optional consent is one that allows banking of tissue samples for future biomarker analyses related to disease prognosis or predictors of response to the treatment strategies under investigation in a trial.

Practically speaking, a consent must be written in clear, nontechnical language aimed for the general readership rather than a research savvy/legally trained participant. Content-specific sections should be clearly identified using appropriate headings and inclusive of the critical information required for an *informed* decision regarding trial participation to be made. In reality, the process of ensuring that the consent is informed extends beyond a written signature of a consent and the protocol document. Adequate time and resources must be available prior to and after the actual signature is obtained to respond to questions and provide information regarding the clinical trial. The actual consent document is retained as a permanent part of the healthcare record and is a useful resource for continued dialogue during the entire trajectory of the trial including the analysis, publication, and dissemination process (Resnick 2009; www.fda.gov/patients/clinical-trials-what-patients-need-know/informed-consent-clinical-trials).

Dissemination

Dissemination of results of a trial is usually done via presentations at scientific meetings and/or a peer-reviewed research manuscript published in a scientific journal. The International Committee of Medical Journal Editors (ICMJE) has established four general criteria for authorship in a medical journal that must be met for all named individuals on a submitted manuscript (http://www.icmje.org/):

- Substantial contributions to the conception or design of the work or the acquisition, analysis, or interpretation of data for the work
- Drafting the work or revising it critically for important intellectual content
- Final approval of the version to be published
- Agreement to be accountable for all aspects of the work in ensuring that questions related to the accuracy or integrity of any part of the work are appropriately investigated and resolved

The protocol should make reference to authorship guidelines as well as related, specific policies of the trial sponsor. The mechanism of assigning and ensuring accountability of author roles rests with the trial leadership and sponsor rather than the journal editor/editorial staff.

An important part of the dissemination process includes direct communication of results of the trial and resulting publication to participants, including the enrolled patient or subject as well as the research staff involved in trial conduct. The process of communication should be described in the protocol as well as the informed consent document. Trials registered in a clinical trials registry may be subject to results reporting requirements at a specified time point.

Data sharing is considered an integral part of the clinical trial process as a means of optimizing a culture of transparency while enhancing scientific knowledge and inquiry as well as resource utilization (http://www.iom.edu/activities/research/sharingclinicaltrialdata.aspx. 2015). Plans and policies for making publicly available the protocol, statistical analysis report, and/or individual patient data should be outlined in the protocol if known at the time of study conduct. Associated timelines for dissemination of this information and administrative requirements for access should also be described.

Conclusion

The protocol is the pivotal guidance document for a clinical trial that communicates the essential details of the research plan to trial participants and organizations involved in research oversight. A well-written protocol has internal consistency and logical and clear designation of specific protocol sections and is written using unambiguous wording. Guidance documents for protocol development and content are useful resources for all stakeholders involved in clinical trial research.

References

Aaronson NK, Ahmedzai S, Bergman B, Bullinger M, Cull A, Duez NJ, Filiberti A, Flechtner H, Fleishman SB, de Haes JC, Klee M, Osoba D, Razavi D, Rofe PB, Schraub S, Sneeuw K, Sullivan M, Takeda F (1993) The European Organization for Research and Treatment of Cancer QLQ-C30; a quality-of-life instrument for use in international clinical trials in oncology. J Natl Cancer Inst 85:365–376

Altman DG, Bland JM (1999) How to randomise. BMJ 319:703–704

Calvert M, Kyte D, Mercieca-Bebber R, Slade A, Chan AW, King MT, The SPIRIT-PRO Group, Hunn A, Bottomley A, Regnault A, Chan AW, Ells C, O'Connor D, Revicki D, Patrick D, Altman D, Basch E, Velikova G, Price G, Draper H, Blazeby J, Scott J, Coast J, Norquist J, Brown J, Haywood K, Johnson LL, Campbell L, Frank L, von Hildebrand M, Brundage M, Palmer M, Kluetz P, Stephens R, Golub RM, Mitchell S, Groves T (2018) Guidelines for inclusion of patient-reported outcomes in clinical trial protocols: the SPIRIT-PRO extension. JAMA 319(5):483–494

Chan AW, Tetzlaff JM, Altman DG (2013a) SPIRIT 2013 statement: defining standard protocol items for clinical trials. Ann Intern Med 158:200–207

Chan AW, Tetzlaff JM, Gotzsche PC (2013b) SPIRIT 2013 explanation and elaboration: guidance for protocols of clinical trials. BMJ 346:e7586. https://doi.org/10.1136/bmj.e7586

Cox DR (1972) Regression models and life tables (with discussion). J R Statist Soc Ser B34:187–220

Geller NL, Pocock SJ (1987) Biometrics 43(1):213–223

Gore L, Ivy SP, Balis FM, Rubin E, Thornton K, Donoghue M, Roberts S, Bruinooge S, Ersek J, Goodman N, Schenkel C, Reaman G (2017) Modernizing clinical trial eligibility: recommendations of the American Society of Clinical Oncology–friends of Cancer research minimum age working group. J Clin Oncol 35:3781–3787

Kernan WN, Viscoli CM, Makuch RW, Brass LM, Horwitz RI (1999) Stratified randomization for clinical trials. J Clin Epidemiol 52(1):19–26

Kim ES, Bruinooge SS, Roberts S, Ison G, Lin NU, Gore L, Uldrick TS, Lictman SM, Roach N, Beavre JA, Sridhara R, Hesketh PJ, Denicoff AM, Garrett-Mayer E, Rubin E, Multani P, Prowell TM, Schenkel C, Kozak M, Allen J, Sigal E, Schilsky RL (2017) Broadening eligibility criteria to make clinical trials more representative: American society of clinical oncology and friends of cancer research joint research statement. J Clin Oncol 35:3737–3744

Lancaster GA, Dodd S, Williamson PR (2004) Design and analysis of pilot studies: recommendations for good practice. J Eval Clin Pract 10:307–312

Lichtman SM, Harvey RD, Smit MAD, Rahman A, Thompson MA, Roach N, Schenkel C, Bruinooge SS, Cortazar P, Walker D, Fehrenbacher L (2017) Modernizing clinical trial eligibility criteria: recommendations of the American Society of Clinical Oncology–friends of Cancer research organ dysfunction, prior or concurrent malignancy, and comorbidities working group. J Clin Oncol 35:3753–3759

Pocock SJ, Richard S (1975) Sequential treatment assignment with balancing for prognostic factors in the controlled clinical trial. Biometrics Int Biometric Soc 31(1):103–115

Resnick DB (2009) Do Informed Consent Documents Matter?. Contemp Clin Trials 30(2):114–115

Rosner B (1990) Fundamentals of biostatistics, 3rd edn. PWS-Kent, Boston

Whitehead AL, Sully BG, Campbell MJ (2014) Pilot and feasibility studies: is there a difference from each other and from a randomised controlled trial? Contemp Clin Trials 38(1):130–133

Xie W, Regan MM, Buyse M, Halabi S, Kantoff PW, Sartor O, Soule H, Clarke NW, Collette L, Dignam JJ, Fizazi K, Paruleker WP, Sandler HM, Sydes MR, Tombal B, Williams SG, Sweeney CJ (2017) J Clin Oncol 35(27):3097–3104

Zelen M (1974) J Chronic Dis 27:365–375

Procurement and Distribution of Study Medicines

11

Eric Hardter, Julia Collins, Dikla Shmueli-Blumberg, and Gillian Armstrong

Contents

E. Hardter · J. Collins · D. Shmueli-Blumberg
The Emmes Company, LLC, Rockville, MD, USA
e-mail: ehardter@emmes.com; jcollins@emmes.com; dblumberg@emmes.com

G. Armstrong (✉)
GSK, Slaoui Center for Vaccines Research, Rockville, MD, USA
e-mail: gillian.x.armstrong@gsk.com

© Springer Nature Switzerland AG 2022
S. Piantadosi, C. L. Meinert (eds.), *Principles and Practice of Clinical Trials*,
https://doi.org/10.1007/978-3-319-52636-2_34

Abstract

When compared to clinical trials involving a new (unapproved for human use) drug or biologic, utilizing an approved, commercially available medication in a clinical trial can introduce a new set of variables surrounding procurement and distribution, all of which are fundamental to successful trial implementation. Numerous procurement factors must be considered, including the identification of a suitable vendor, manufacturing of a matching placebo, and expiration dating, all of which can become more intricate when the study increases in complexity by involving factors like active comparators, drug tapering regimens, and research sites in more than one country. Distribution is a similarly complex operation, which involves adherence to regulatory requirements and consideration of aspects such as blinded study designs or utilization of additional safeguards with the use of controlled substances. This chapter will review the basic factors to be taken into consideration during the planning and operational stages of a clinical trial involving a marketed medication and provide examples of how to manage these factors, all of which are aimed at ensuring compliance with both applicable local and international laws and with guidance documents aimed at protecting the rights, safety, and well-being of trial participants.

Keywords

Investigational product (IP) · Placebo · Current Good Manufacturing Practices (cGMPs) · Blinded/blinding · Manipulation · Procurement · Controlled substance · Vendor · Accountability · Distribution

Introduction

The International Council for Harmonisation of Technical Requirements for the Registration of Pharmaceuticals for Human Use (ICH) Good Clinical Practice (GCP) guidelines (▶ Chap. 35, "Good Clinical Practice") defines investigational product (IP) as a pharmaceutical form of an active ingredient being tested or used as a reference in a clinical trial or the corresponding placebo (ICH E6, 2016). As the pharmaceutical form (tablet, liquid, sterile injectable, etc.,) and type (active, active comparator, or placebo) of IP or study medication required in a clinical trial are driven by the study goals and protocol design, the procurement and distribution of IP should be considered early during protocol development and be a key part of early study planning activities. A lack of planning and anticipation of the impact of study design on IP procurement and distribution may lead to insurmountable roadblocks during study implementation, including excessive costs, extended time-lines, compliance problems, and logistical issues at both the Sponsor and site level.

Although clinical trials are primarily conducted to examine the safety and efficacy of a new active ingredient, studies are also often conducted using an IP with an ingredient that is approved by a competent authority (CA), such as the US Food and

Drug Administration (FDA), for use in a specific indication (combination of a disease and patient population). These latter types of clinical trials are often performed to assess the safety and efficacy of an approved drug or biologic outside of its initial indication or to gain further information about an approved use, such as when given via a new route of administration, at a higher dose, or in combination with another therapy. As it can be purchased "off the shelf," using an approved IP in a clinical trial may seem simpler than using an unapproved IP at first glance; however, these trials come with their own set of challenges and potential pitfalls surrounding procurement and distribution, which must be carefully considered during study planning.

Although an IP may be available commercially via prescription from a pharmacy, a Sponsor supporting a clinical trial involving IP may still need to file an Investigational New Drug (IND) application (or regional equivalent) to the FDA or local CA, depending on the indication to be studied and the goal of the clinical trial. For example, in the USA, while some criteria to be exempt from filing an IND as per 21 Code of Federal Regulations (CFR) 312.2 are straightforward (e.g., not intending to use the data collected to support a new indication or change in advertising for the IP), it can be challenging to present an argument that a clinical trial does not "significantly increase the risk (or decrease the acceptability of the risk) associated with the use of the drug product" (21 CFR 312.2(b)(iii)). Some typical examples of IND trials using marketed medication are shown in Fig. 1. If ever in doubt about whether an IND or equivalent is required, Sponsors should seek guidance from the CA with oversight over the clinical trial (e.g., the FDA can provide this guidance by way of a pre-IND meeting and a written request for IND exemption or via formal and/or informal communications).

Regardless of the requirement to file an application with the local CA prior to trial initiation, adherence to ICH GCP guidelines and all applicable in-country regulatory requirements (e.g., federal and state laws in the USA) is paramount to protect the rights and well-being of human subjects taking part in the clinical trial and to ensure the integrity of the data collected. This includes adherence to applicable Current Good Manufacturing Practices (cGMPs, 21 CFR 210 and 211 in the USA, and ICH Q7, 2000) during the manufacture of blinded medication (such as manipulation of commercially sourced medication for blinding purposes, manufacture of a matching placebo, etc.), repackaging or relabeling IP, and appropriate tracking of inventories at and shipments from the distributor/central pharmacy and clinical site. This chapter

---

- An increase in the daily dose or dosing duration of a medication
- Utilization of a new combination of therapies that could increase the risks of use than either single therapy alone.
- A new participant population outside of the approved indication, e.g. children, pregnant women.
- An indication not currently approved.

Fig. 1 Examples of clinical trials using marketed medication usually requiring an IND or regional equivalent will outline the main components and points to consider for IP procurement (including sourcing, manipulation of dosage forms, and compounding) and distribution (tracking, restocking, and destruction) throughout the life of a clinical trial.

Procurement of Investigational Product

Investigational Product Procurement Planning

The extent to which a study drug must be manipulated for the clinical trial will dictate selection of not only an initial source of the commercially available drug but also the requirement for all other IP-related vendors or suppliers. Thus, it is critically important for the Sponsor to decide upon all IP-related protocol aspects during the planning phase, prior to selecting a supplier, and to make minimal changes to the protocol that can impact IP during study conduct. For small open-label clinical studies where IP is administered once, IP procurement may be as simple as the on-site physician ordering the medication from an appropriate commercial vendor or pharmacy and dispensing to participants, tracking lot numbers as per institutional practices. However, IP procurement requirements can quickly become more complicated for later phase trials (phase 2 and 3), which can last longer, require blinded medication, and/or have many participating sites (national and international). This complexity can be compounded further by IP-driven storage requirements (controlled, refrigerated, or frozen medication).

Once the initial protocol design is finalized, the identification of a suitable commercially approved drug or biologic is the first step in procurement planning. This should be a dosage form (tablet, capsule, liquid, etc.), strength, and formulation (oral, injectable, topical, etc.) suitable for use in the study, given the proposed schedule and route of administration, with factors such as color, taste, shape, etc., as well as the availability of immediate-release or extended-release formulations, taken into consideration (if appropriate). Pricing of each of the available options for the study should then be performed to allow an initial check against the study budget. If the proposed clinical trial is being conducted by an academic institution or public health agency, it can be worthwhile to approach the pharmaceutical company manufacturing the drug to ask about any programs through which the IP needed to conduct the trial may be obtained for free or at a lower cost. In such situations, the company donating the drug may dictate the packaging/labeling for their IP and the process that must be utilized to supply medication to the study sites. A detailed agreement should be in place regarding the provision of IP; the requirement, if any, for clinical sites to return unused medication to the manufacturer; the ability of the trial Sponsor to cross-reference the manufacturer's investigational or marketing application as required; and any specific safety reporting related to product quality that the manufacturer requires for their post-marketing obligations.

Use of a Generic Drug

In many countries around the world, innovative drugs are protected from generic intrusion by a patent or a period of marketing exclusivity. In the USA, the former is a legal protection obtained through and afforded by the US Patent and Trademark Office, while the latter is provided to a manufacturer by FDA. Both have an ability to prohibit competitors from seeking approval of a drug or biologic therapeutically equivalent to the innovator drug, which often increases drug availability and can push prices down. International regulatory authorities, such as Health Canada and the European Medicines Agency (EMA), have similar data exclusivity protections. Having only a single source of IP can not only make IP prohibitively expensive but may also delay or halt the study if there is a market shortage of the drug.

If neither a patent nor marketing exclusivity applies, purchasing options may increase to potentially include generic versions of an IP. Prior to marketing authorization, generic drugs must be considered therapeutically equivalent to the innovator drug. The FDA considers drugs pharmaceutical equivalents if they contain the same active ingredients, are of the same dosage form and route of administration, are formulated to contain the same amount of active ingredient, and meet the same compendial or other applicable standards (i.e., strength, quality, purity, and identity). Generic drugs will differ in characteristics such as shape, scoring config-uration, release mechanisms (for immediate- or extended-release formulations), packaging, excipients (including colors, flavors, preservatives), expiration dating, and, within certain limits, labeling, all important factors to take into consideration when selecting a generic version of an approved drug to use as an IP. In the USA, therapeutically equivalent generic drugs will receive an "A" rating in the FDA *Approved Drug Products with Therapeutic Equivalence Evaluations* book (also known as the *Orange Book*).

Considerations for IP Procurement/Manipulation in Blinded Trials

Blinded studies will require additional consideration as the drug or comparator will be manipulated prior to being used in the trial, e.g., covered with another color to obscure identifying markers (i.e., inking or debossing) to allow the manufacture of a matching placebo (▶ Chaps. 43, "Masking of Trial Investigators" and ▶ 44, "Masking Study Participants"). A blinded study design is used to reduce bias and involves the study participants being unaware of which treatment assignment or study group they are randomized to (single-blind) or all parties (the Sponsor, investigator, and participant) being unaware of a participant's treatment assignment (double-blind). For placebo-controlled studies, a commercially sourced IP must be disguised, and a matching placebo must be manufactured, if not already available from the commercial IP manufacturer as part of their study support. In comparison, open-label medication trials do not disguise the IP, as both the participants and investigators are aware of the assigned treatment. IP can be obtained and managed in a more straightforward fashion, both during drug procurement and throughout the implementation of open-label clinical trials.

Generic medications, each of which vary in shape, color, and/or debossing/imprinting (for tablets), can provide additional challenges or potential benefits for blinding in a clinical trial, as certain shapes/sizes may be easier to insert into a capsule, to replicate in a placebo, or to disguise for blinded use; e.g., a tablet that has a letter or logo printed in ink on the surface can be easier to disguise by overspraying than a tablet with a similar marking which is debossed, since the latter contains a gap that must be filled.

Once a marketed product has been selected, securing a reliable IP source for the entire duration of the study is the most important next step. Key parameters to consider are the lead time for procuring the IP, quantity available, the time needed to manipulate (i.e., spray coat, repackage, etc.,), and the expiration date of the IP available. Lead time and available quantity could be subject to change pending a potential shortage of drug. The time needed to get the IP ready to ship to sites is dependent on the degree of manipulation, whereas expiration date of the IP is directly tied to its stability profile, with drug wholesale companies usually providing their "oldest" stock for shipment over stock which can remain on their shelves longer. While the use of generic medication may reduce initial costs, availability over an extended period may still become an issue for longer trials, necessitating IP restocking. Further, generic drugs can be removed from the market without warning, affecting the entire supply chain for a clinical trial. Thus, it is important to consider the longevity of generic manufacturing (i.e., the likelihood of continuation of IP manufacture for the duration of the trial) prior to selecting a manufacturer.

In a blinded trial, the purchased IP (and active comparator, if one is available) must be manipulated (and the matching placebo manufactured) prior to study start. For example, an IP in tablet form may be obscured via discoloration (e.g., overspraying) to cover identifying markers/debossing and to allow the manufacture of a matching placebo. An injectable medication, however, may only require relabeling if the color can be matched with a placebo. The extent to which purchased IP is manipulated for the clinical trial will dictate the selection of an appropriate supplier or vendor for this manipulation, set the timeline from procurement to shipping to the clinical site, and also set expectations for IP-related data to be collected during the study. For example, manipulation of a study drug may require release and ongoing stability testing to ensure its continued identity, purity, and potency.

Impact of IP-Related Factors: Controlled Substances

If the IP is a controlled substance, there are additional steps and/or regulations surrounding the preparation, testing, shipment, storage, dispensation, and return for destruction of the drug that the Sponsor must consider during protocol design. This includes the requirement for registration of parties handling the IP (site, central pharmacy, manufacturing facility, etc.) with applicable local authorities, such as the Drug Enforcement Administration (DEA) in the USA.

Identification of Qualified Vendors

By purchasing a commercially available drug or biologic, the identity, potency, purity, sterility, and stability of purchased IP can be assured, as continued cGMP compliance is a condition of marketing authorization. Any IND, or similar filing to a CA or Institutional Review Board (IRB), should therefore reference the marketing application for the commercial product to be purchased for the trial. The manipulation of the purchased product (active IP and active comparator, where applicable) to make it suitable for use in the clinical trial must also be described in these filings, including manufacture of a matching placebo, where applicable. It is the Sponsor's responsibility (Sponsor Requirements) to ensure that this manipulation is conducted according to the applicable regulations and any potential impact on the product attributes (identity, potency, purity, sterility, and stability) is identified and managed appropriately. Planning activities involve the identification of tasks required to support IP quality followed by the identification of reliable and qualified vendors who can conduct their assigned tasks according to the applicable regulations, i.e., cGMPs, according to the timelines dictated by the study and within the budget assigned.

Depending on vendor expertise and logistics (e.g., IP storage and transport), study-related IP activities involving multiple steps (e.g., overcoating tablets, manufacturing matching placebo, packaging/labeling of both release and stability testing) can be carried out at a single facility or multiple facilities. A facility with the broadest ability to do all required work is likely to be a licensed cGMP manufacturer registered with a CA, such as FDA, with experience in the required activities, with all applicable tasks occurring in a cGMP-compliant manner. However, full-service facilities can be busy and therefore difficult to schedule, pushing up costs and extending the timelines.

For IP that is produced on a very small scale, a pharmacist-led facility, such as a 503A compounding pharmacy in the USA, may be an option. Classically, both in routine clinical care and for clinical trials, production of IP in one of these facilities is done on a per-patient, per-prescription basis and is performed by a pharmacist to tailor a medication to a specific use, e.g., to produce a topical formulation of an active ingredient usually given orally. The constraint of requiring individual prescriptions for each participant effectively precludes the utilization of these facilities in larger clinical trials. For slightly larger studies, a licensed outsourcing facility (termed a 503B outsourcing facility in the USA) would be a better option. Since these facilities must adhere to cGMPs, assurance is provided to study Sponsors regarding the identity, purity, and potency of the study IP. Common activities at such facilities may include procedures such as re-encapsulation of drug capsules and overcoating of drug tablets to obscure their appearance, as well as production of matched placebo.

The more a commercial drug product is manipulated, the greater the likelihood that these activities will have an impact on the quality attributes of the IP used in the trial. These trials therefore require management of this risk, including release testing and subsequent monitoring during the study.

Packaging Considerations

The IP should be packaged to prevent contamination and unacceptable deterioration during transport and storage (ICH E6 5.13.3). The packaging configuration should also take into consideration how the IP will be provided to the study participants. Blister packages or IP kits are often useful for IP which needs to be tapered up and down, ensuring the correct dose is taken; however, larger packs may be wasteful if a participant drops out or a kit is lost.

For both open-label and blinded studies, IP repackaging and relabeling activities are very likely required. In the USA, FDA describes repackaging as the act of taking a finished drug product from the container in which it was distributed by the original manufacturer and placing it into a different container *without further manipulation of the drug* (FDA Guidance for Industry: Repackaging of Certain Human Drug Products by Pharmacies and Outsourcing Facilities 2017). This activity can be performed by a vendor/supplier or by a licensed study pharmacist. Alteration of exterior packaging, such as a secondary box for medication contained in a blister pack, would not be considered a repackaging activity. This type of repackaging is a process associated with a very low risk of impact on the IP, as long as storage instructions are followed during the repackaging activities. However, repackaging activities during which tablets are transferred into a different bottle can impact the stability profile; similarly, repackaging a sterile liquid into smaller single-use vials can impact sterility. Therefore, the identification of the requirement for specialized vendors (e.g., for sterile repackaging or handling medication which is refrigerated/frozen) and for stability testing, including testing performed, time points, storage conductions, and acceptance criteria, should be defined prior to IP manipulation.

Manufacturing and Packaging Considerations for Blinded Trials

If, for the purposes of blinding, a commercial drug product is inserted into a capsule, sprayed to change color, etc., the impact of these changes should be taken into consideration and testing performed to ensure that the quality attributes of the IP are maintained and that patient safety and study integrity are also maintained. For example, depending on the dissolution rate of the tablet, placing it into an opaque gelatin capsule for blinding purposes may change the rate of drug release and therefore impact the onset of drug action, which can be important if a drug has a narrow therapeutic window, so performing re-encapsulation (emptying current capsules and transferring content to a new capsule) may be a preferable option. An IP that is sensitive to light should be repackaged under appropriate conditions, utilizing amber/opaque bottles or suitable blister packages. While placebo has no expectation of potency, it typically still needs to undergo testing for characteristics such as sterility, appearance, and odor during stability studies. Neither drug nor placebo should be released for use in the study until it meets all applicable release testing requirements, with testing usually performed according to local Pharmacopeia monographs (standards for identity, quality, purity, strength, packaging, and labeling).

Certain commercially available drug products may contain active ingredients with defining characteristics (e.g., odor, color, taste). For placebo-controlled studies, Sponsors should ensure that a manufacturing vendor can mimic these characteristics in the matched placebo as much as possible. As a resource, FDA maintains databases of allowable inactive ingredients, excipients, and substances generally recognized as safe (GRAS) for the development of a placebo, which manufacturers can utilize to ensure the placebo mirrors the study drug in all facets, excepting potency.

Each time a commercial drug product is manipulated, e.g., emptied from a bottle or sprayed to change its color, there is a possibility that some supply may be diverted from the clinical trial due to loss during these procedures (including equipment and user errors, tablet breakage, etc.). Additional supply may also be needed for process development and in-process testing. Lastly, when required, additional supply of the final IP may need to be diverted and placed into stability testing for the duration of the clinical study. To account for these activities, the total amount of IP needed should be increased by at least 10–20% during the Sponsor's estimations.

Overall, given the breadth of possible IP manipulation activities that may take place for a given clinical trial, the selection of the right vendors is critical, as they are going to be key partners throughout the clinical trial. Indeed, if a facility is determined to be non-compliant after initial selection, there may be loss of study drug and a delay in timelines while things are corrected. Expectations on the quality of the IP and the timelines associated with key steps during IP manipulation must be clear to both sides at project start. In the worst case, study start may be delayed, while alternative vendors are identified and qualified. In 2015, for example, an FDA inspection of the Pharmaceutical Development Section of the NIH Clinical Center triggered the inactivation and premature closure of multiple NIH intramural studies, with others delayed pending the identification of alternate vendors. This example serves to highlight the overarching significance of the selection of the right vendor.

Managing the risk of such an adverse outcome requires a proactive approach, such as checking public inspection databases, such as the FDA web site, for records for previous examples of non-compliance (e.g., Warning Letters and Forms FDA 483) for a specific manufacturing facility and also ensuring the vendor is able to conduct the tasks as assigned, usually via the vendor qualification process, performed as per the Sponsor's standard operating procedures (SOPs). Depending on the scope of activities, an on-site audit can be part of this process, performed by representatives with expertise in regulatory affairs, quality assurance, and cGMP compliance. Timing of the audit should ideally be early during the planning stage if the vendor is not already qualified, so that it allows time for appropriate follow-up and corrections to procedures/practices and reauditing if necessary.

International Clinical Trials

As discussed in the "Investigational Product Procurement Planning" section, multisite trials with international locations have the potential to add elements of complexity (▶ Chap. 19, "International Trials"). The primary consideration for such studies surrounds the regulatory status of the commercial product chosen (and the active ingredient) in each country (e.g., approved for marketing, approved but no longer available, etc.), as this influences the ability to import IP and the requirement for a clinical trial application locally. For example, a multinational study utilizing IP which is FDA-approved may only require IRB oversight in the USA, without an IND application, provided the study meets all criteria in 21 CFR 312.2. However, if the same drug does not have marketing approval in Canada, it will require full reporting to Health Canada under a Clinical Trial Application (CTA), an assessment by the study Research Ethics Board, and an environmental assessment by Environment Canada. Such regulatory approvals, or lack thereof, influence drug sourcing options. In the scenario described above, IP would need to be exported from the US manufacturer and imported into Canada. This requires prior approval of the CTA and appropriate labeling of the exported drug, along with sign-off from an importing agent in Canada (who must be a Canadian resident); otherwise, the IP will be seized at the border by the Canadian Border Services Agency that works in conjunction with Health Canada.

Similarly, IP manufacturing requirements may differ between countries. While ICH member states typically overlap in this regard, small differences may result in additional levels of compliance. For example, an IP manufactured in the USA and intended for import to a European Union member state (e.g., Germany and France), for a clinical trial, will require release by a qualified person (QP). The QP is responsible for verifying that the IP meets a certain degree of cGMP compliance for import into the country and thus will likely require access to IP batch records to determine cGMP adherence. In some instances, the QP may wish to assess the batch manufacture in person, depending on the risk of the activities undertaken during the manufacturing process. It should be noted that, while the above scenario remains plausible, mutual recognition agreements often exist between CAs (typically between ICH members). These agreements effectively state that the competent regulatory authority from an importing country will defer to a cGMP inspection of the competent regulatory authority from the exporting country (or from another ICH country, if such an inspection has been performed), without necessitating additional inspection. Therefore, choice of a commercially available drug manufactured by a company that has already obtained marketing authorizations for it in the countries to be used in the clinical trial may lead to a quicker study start-up, as the local CAs will be familiar with the IP and only the manipulation for the clinical trial will need to be described.

Distribution of Investigational Product

The tracking of IP inventory available at the distributor/central pharmacy and distribution to each clinical site is not only important for compliance with ICH E6 GCPs but also to ensure that IP is available for each participant. Tracking can be achieved several ways, such as by utilizing a system provided by the central IP distributor or vendor. Regardless of the distribution method, basic measures of drug management and accountability must be followed. Particular IP characteristics and study design parameters, such as the use of controlled substances or whether the study is blinded, can also influence the process.

Documents to Support Release of IP to Qualified Sites

As per ICH E6 GCP, many documents must be generated and be on file prior to study start, which is often considered the initial shipment of IP to a clinical site. These documents include those relating to the release of IP by the manufacturer, for example, a Certificate of Analysis, which ensures that the IP fulfills the quality attributes set for it. A subset of documents is also collected from the site and includes documents related to the investigator's ability to conduct the trial (documentation of relevant qualifications and training), the favorable review of the study protocol and other documents by the IRB or International Ethics Committee (IEC), (▶ Chap. 36, "Institutional Review Boards and Ethics Committees") and an agreement to follow the study protocol, including the requirements for the reporting of adverse events. These documents should be reviewed for their accuracy and suitability to support study conduct prior to authorizing IP shipment and will often include ensuring that the site has the appropriate documents and training for handling IP, including IP disposition logs. If the IP is a controlled medication, the applicable local registrations for the site to receive and prescribe controlled substances, such as DEA registration in the USA, are particularly important and will have to be provided to the central distributing facility to ensure they comply with the facility's SOPs.

In a clinical trial with a small number of sites, it may be feasible to collect and manage these regulatory documents using a paper system; however, in a larger-scale, multicenter clinical trial, the collection and management of regulatory documents throughout the life of the study is more challenging and complex. When multiple sites are involved, the use of an electronic trial master file (eTMF) and a linked clinical trial management system (CTMS) can help facilitate this task and assist the Sponsor in maintaining compliance with applicable regulations (Zhao et al. 2010). For example, some systems can automatically trigger alerts and notifications for upcoming expiration dates of documents filed in the system, as well as generate reports that can be used to quickly identify any missing documents. Only once all required documents have been collected and the required national and local approvals are in place can the Sponsor or designee supply an investigator or institution with IP. Setting clear expectations early in study start-up for the number and quality of documents to be collected from the site prior to IP shipment is key to on-time study start. Also, routine frequent monitoring of site documents, including IP logs, at the site will ensure that the documents are maintained and are inspection ready at the end of the study.

Use of Controlled Substances in Clinical Trials

The World Health Organization (WHO) provides guidance on the scheduling of substances that can be of potential harm due to their psychoactive and/or dependence-producing properties, as well as providing technical expertise to the United Nations (UN) on drugs of abuse under the United Nations Single Convention on Narcotic Drugs (1961) and the United Nations Convention on Psychotropic Substances (1971). These two treaties, along with the United Nations Convention against the Illicit Traffic in Narcotic Drugs and Psychotropic Substances (1988), provide the legal basis for the international prevention of drug abuse (WHO 2018). The UN system categorizes narcotics and psychotropic substances into four classifications, based on their harmfulness, which includes the risk of abuse and other health dangers. Many countries and regions have their own classification systems for controlled substances. In one article that investigated classification systems across 23 countries (including countries in North America, Western Europe, the Middle East, and Asia), it was found that the range of controlled substance schedules varied from 2 to 15 different schedules of drug (Dragic et al. 2015); therefore, local regulations should be carefully reviewed to assess the local requirements for clinical trials utilizing IP which could be considered a controlled medication.

In the USA, the DEA classifies drugs, substances, and certain chemicals used to make drugs into five categories or schedules depending upon the drug's acceptable medical use and abuse or dependency potential (21 CFR 1308.11–1308.15). Schedule I drugs have a high potential for abuse and the potential to create severe psychological and/or physical dependence (e.g., heroin), while Schedule V drugs represent the least potential for abuse (e.g., cough preparations containing not more than 200 mg of codeine per 100 ml or per 100 g, such as Robitussin AC (US DEA 2018) (Fig. 2)). In the USA, all clinical trials involving controlled substances are regulated under the federal Controlled Substances Act (CSA). In addition, many states have local regulations regarding the use of controlled substances in clinical trials, and often these local regulations can be more restrictive than federal guidelines. For example, California Law requires that any clinical investigation involving either Schedule I or Schedule II medication as the main study drug be reviewed and approved by the Research Advisory Panel of California in the Attorney General's office (State of California Department of Justice 2018).

In the USA, there are eight key control measures that directly impact all clinical trials with controlled substances (Fig. 3). These include the scheduling of the drug (I through V), registration and licensing of investigators, importation and exportation controls, setting quotas for Schedule 1 and 2 substances, and on-site security measures designed to restrict access to controlled substances. Additional control measures involve strict and rigorous record keeping requirements for all controlled substances, reporting requirements for theft or loss of these substances, and DEA inspections (Woodworth 2011). Investigators outside the USA should review local laws and look for a similar level of control.

DEA Schedule	Description	Example Substance(s)
I	No currently accepted medical use in the US, a lack of accepted safety for use under medical supervision, and a high potential for abuse.	heroin, lysergic acid diethylamide (LSD), marijuana (cannabis)
II/IIN	High potential for abuse which may lead to severe psychological or physical dependence.	hydromorphone, oxycodone (Schedule II); amphetamine (Adderall®) (Schedule IIN (stimulants))
III/IIIN	Have a potential for abuse less than substances in Schedules I or II and abuse may lead to moderate or low physical dependence or high psychological dependence.	Tylenol with Codeine®; buprenorphine; ketamine
IV	Have a low potential for abuse relative to substances in Schedule III.	alprazolam (Xanax®); diazepam (Valium®)
V	Have a low potential for abuse relative to substances listed in Schedule IV and consist primarily of preparations containing limited quantities of certain narcotics.	Cough preparations containing not more than 200 milligrams of codeine per 100 milliliters or per 100 grams (Robitussin AC®)

Source: US DEA Diversion Control Division 2018.

Fig. 2 List of US DEA categories or "schedules." Drugs are categorized into schedules based on their acceptable medical use and abuse or dependency potential (United States Department of Justice Drug Enforcement Administration, Diversion Control Division 2018)

IP Inventory Management for Complex Study Designs

Inventory management is driven primarily by study design, the specific drugs used (special handing requirements, e.g., controlled substances, frozen/refrigerated), the number of clinical sites, and the countries involved. For example, as mentioned, IP for an open-label study conducted at a single site can be prescribed locally and dispensed as needed to the participants following institutional procedures. Conversely, more intricate study designs, particularly those involving blinded IP, increase the complexity of the drug supply process. To accommodate these complexities, electronic systems have evolved to include more streamlined, auditable, and user-friendly drug assignment and distribution processes. Systems such as a CTMS, IRT (interactive response technologies), and/or electronic data capture (EDC) systems (▶ Chap. 13, "Design and Development of the Study Data System") are used alone or in conjunction with each other, interfacing and automatically updating to assign IP to a participant, track site inventory, and request resupplies. The key benefits to these systems are the ability to monitor the IP in real time, the immediate allocation of IP (bottle, kit, or single dose) available at the site to a participant according to an overall randomization scheme, tracking of expiration of IP, and the possibility for automatic replenishment of IP once a predetermined

Control Measure	Key Information
1. Scheduling of the drug or substance	See Table 2. The parties involved in determination of drug classification or scheduling are the US Department of Health and Human Services or HHS (including FDA and NIDA) and DEA (Title 21, CSA, 811(b)).
2. Federal registration and state licensing of clinical investigators to prescribe, dispense, administer and conduct research with controlled substances	**Registration:** A federal DEA *practitioner registration* is required for an investigator to handle controlled substances in any manner. A DEA "Practitioner" registration is valid for three years and a separate registration is required for each principal place of business or professional practice at one general physical location where controlled substances are manufactured, distributed, imported, exported, or dispensed by a person (21 CRF §1301.12(a)). DEA Registrations for *receipt of medication* at a clinical research site are required when using scheduled drugs as investigational products, subject to DEA regulations. There are several types of DEA Registrations (designations) that can be used for receipt of medication (e.g., Pharmacy, Hospital/Clinic, etc.). An individual DEA Registration (e.g., Practitioner, Researcher) may be used for shipping and receipt of study medication as long as the address of record is the site address or the local pharmacy where the drug is to be shipped and received. **Licensing:** At the state level, licensing is generally accomplished via a license that covers clinical practice and research; however, requirements may vary by state.
3. Importation and exportation controls	In general, the nation exporting controlled substances must obtain a written permit or other form of permission in advance for each transnational shipment from the country to which the substance is being shipped (Article 31, Single Convention on Narcotic Drugs, 1961 and Article 12, Convention on Psychotropic Substances, 1971).
4. Setting quotas for Schedule I and Schedule II substances	The Controlled Substances Act requires the DEA to determine the maximum amount of Schedule I and Schedule II controlled substances that may be manufactured in the U.S. every calendar year (Title 22, United States Code, Section 826).
5. Security measures that must be put in place at the clinical site to restrict access to controlled substances	Investigators are required to store controlled substances in a "securely locked, substantially constructed cabinet" (21 CFR 1301.75) and to segregate (e.g., separate box, separate shelf) by clinical study (if > 1) and by DEA registration number. "Double lock" security, such as a locked cabinet inside a locked room, is recommended as a best practice. Furthermore, Schedule I substances can't be stored with Schedules II-V and all controlled substances must be separated from non-controlled medications.
6. Comprehensive, stringent recordkeeping requirements for all controlled substances	Once a controlled substance is received on site, the PI is required to maintain a detailed inventory (i.e., physical count) of all controlled substances on hand at that site. Inventory must be taken at least once every two years; however, it is recommended that investigators complete this much more frequently (such as every time medication is dispensed or returned, or biweekly/monthly) (21 CFR 1304.11). The records must include the name and address of the person to whom the medication was dispensed, the date of dispensing, the number of units or volume dispensed, and the written or typewritten name or initials of the individual who dispensed or administered the substance (21 CFR 1304.22 (c)).
7. Reporting requirements	Although there are several reporting requirements that those involved in the drug supply chain must meet, Investigators are only required to report "any theft or significant loss of a controlled substance" to the DEA (Title 21, Code of Federal Registrations, Section 1301.76 (b)).
8. DEA inspections	The DEA typically only performs routine investigations of clinical sites when a Schedule I controlled substance is being used in a trial.

Fig. 3 Key control measures impacting clinical trials with controlled substances (adapted from Woodworth 2011)

threshold is reached. In blinded studies, the EDC can bypass the requirement for any direct staff involvement in resupply. One component of these systems is careful planning in setup of not only the system but also the IP itself, as the Sponsor must ensure that any system-specific information, such as a bottle or kit identifying number and corresponding barcode for electronic systems, is included to allow the IP to be tracked. Overall, these systems can help minimize last-minute supply requests, oversupply at a single site, and waste at clinical sites.

Site Name	Supply Name	Current Inventory	Threshold	Expiration Date
Research Site A		9-Aug-18		
	XR-NTX Medication Kit	10	5	8/31/2018
	Suboxone 4mg strips	750	400	12/31/2019
	Suboxone 8mg strips	300	350	11/30/2019
Research Site B		9-Aug-18		
	XR-NTX Medication Kit	8	5	8/31/2018
	Suboxone 4mg strips	615	400	12/31/2019
	Suboxone 8mg strips	425	350	11/30/2019
Research Site C		9-Aug-18		
	XR-NTX Medication Kit	4	5	5/31/2019
	Suboxone 4mg strips	375	400	12/31/2019
	Suboxone 8mg strips	428	350	11/30/2019

Fig. 4 Example Inventory Form for IP/study medication. IP levels at or below threshold or past their expiration date appear in red

IP Accountability

One method for utilizing electronic IP management systems is to ask research staff to report IP inventory periodically (e.g., weekly) directly in the EDC system. These data are subsequently pulled into specifically programmed reports, which can be reviewed to identify reorder needs based on predetermined thresholds and usage at each site. Color-coding of these reports is useful for quick visual identification of supplies that are nearing expiration or are below the desired threshold. Of note, to maximize efficiency, inventory forms may also include study supplies other than the IP (e.g., blood draw equipment) (not reflected in figure) (Fig. 4). Shipments should be carefully timed, and the appropriate amount of IP (taking site storage capacity and projected enrollment rate/target into account) should be distributed with each shipment to minimize the amount of IP and other supplies left unused at the site while ensuring there are sufficient supplies on site for active study participants. The latter can often be predicted based on participant enrollment rates at the site and the IP distribution schedule delineated in the study protocol. The ideal ratio and time will reduce shipping costs and waste.

Drug accountability is more than simply counting pills; it goes hand in hand with inventory management and refers to the record keeping associated with the receipt, storage, and dispensation of an investigational product. When done correctly, it should provide a complete and accurate accounting of drug handling from initial receipt on site to final disposition (e.g., utilization in the study, return, or destruction). While the study Sponsor is responsible for procurement of study medication (Sponsor Requirements) (including the processes delineated at the start of this chapter), once at the sites, it is the responsibility of the principal investigator (PI) to maintain adequate records of the product's handling and dispensation (ICH GCP 4.6.1) (► Chap. 6, "Investigator Responsibilities"). In accordance with ICH GCP, the PI can choose to delegate responsibility of IP accountability to an "appropriate pharmacist or another appropriate individual" of whom they have oversight (ICH GCP 4.6.2). It should be ensured that this delegation and the qualifications of the individual are documented appropriately.

By nature, working with human research subjects introduces participant-level error with regard to study drug accountability, particularly when IP is "sent home" with the participant. For example, participants might forget doses, misplace or lose some or all of the study IP, share IP with others, or sell it illegally. To account for these situations, clinical trial protocols often require participants to return any unused IP at designated intervals throughout the study (e.g., weekly, monthly) before providing them with more. Once IP is returned, qualified study staff complete an inventory (e.g., number of remaining capsules/tablets) to evaluate medication compliance and perform IP accountability (the latter is particularly important when the IP is a controlled substance). To address the expected level of participant error in IP management during a clinical trial, there are certain strategies that study Sponsors can employ to attempt to increase medication adherence and enhance subsequent drug accountability. These methods may range from basic paper-and-pencil record keeping, such as providing participants with a small calendar to mark the dates and times that they took their medication, to leveraging technology-based options. One such option involves real-time medication adherence monitoring by using a "smart" pill bottle, which may perform tasks such as indicating or recording whether the patient took their medication on schedule (e.g., through a glowing light or via a counting tool built into the bottle cap), measuring the time that elapses between doses using a stopwatch function, or even sending automatic medication reminders to patients via text message on their smart phone (Choudhry et al. 2017)). Another technology-based option is providing patients with a QR (quick response) code to access easy-to-understand pharmacist counseling videos, which guide patients through how to take the medication, any potential side effects, etc. (Yeung et al. 2003). Although all materials provided to a patient during a clinical trial can require IRB review, an IRB may request additional oversight of compliance and require that a participant take daily videos of themselves taking the study medication and securely share these with the study team for compliance measurement purposes. Potential study participants will be informed of such a mechanism during the informed consent process (► Chap. 21, "Consent Forms and Procedures").

Enhancing medication adherence is not only beneficial for study data reliability, but it also plays a role in overall IP accountability. As such, it is the responsibility of the study Sponsor to become familiar with the available options for participant IP adherence and select a method (or methods) that is appropriate for the population being studied and makes sense within the larger context of the clinical trial. The PI must also ensure proper security and storage of the investigational drug while on site (ICH GCP 4.6). Even when research pharmacists or vendors are involved, the PI retains this responsibility (► Chap. 6, "Investigator Responsibilities"). Finally, drug dispensation at the site must be documented in a clear and comprehensive way. Often Sponsors will provide tools such as drug inventory and tracking logs to assist the site staff, including pharmacists, in study-specific requirements for tracking drug receipt and dispensation (e.g., see Fig. 5). However, if no tools are offered by the Sponsor, the site should follow local institutional practices.

Shipping and Receipt of IP

In some clinical trials, IP is shipped to research sites directly from a manufacturer, while other studies utilize the services of a central pharmacy, which receives study drug from a manufacturer and distributes it to the study sites. Any such distributor must be in full compliance with applicable regulations (e.g., International Air Transport Association (IATA) or, in the USA, regulations set by the FDA, DEA, and the US Environmental Protection Agency (EPA)) and possess the required licenses and permits required by federal, state, and local authorities for the safe operation of a Drug Distribution Center. The distributor would need to have the capability to store IP per cGMPs and labeled storage conditions and also maintain packaging and shipping supplies (e.g., wet and dry ice, frozen cold packs, liquid nitrogen, qualified Styrofoam shipping containers) needed for the uninterrupted supply of study medication.

Proper storage during drug distribution (i.e., shipment) is critical to preserve the quality of the investigational product. In their totality, good storage and distribution practices should facilitate IP movement through a supply chain involving multiple parties (i.e., supplier, manufacturer, pharmacy, and sites) that are controlled, measured, and analyzed for continuous improvement and maintain the integrity of the IP (USP <1079>). Both during distribution and when stored on site, the IP(s) should be stored as specified by the Sponsor in the label and in accordance with applicable regulatory requirement(s) (ICH GCP 4.6.4), as well as the study protocol, investigational brochure, or marketed medication information sheet (e.g., package insert, or summary of product characteristics). To meet these specifications, Sponsors should utilize both qualified, validated shipping materials and environment-tracking devices that "alarm" when out of the specified range, such as temperature monitors (e.g., TempTales) and humidity sensors. The Sponsor should determine the storage requirements including the acceptable storage temperatures, storage conditions (e.g., protection from light), storage times, reconstitution fluids and procedures, and devices for product infusion, if any. The Sponsor should inform all involved parties (e.g., monitors, investigators, pharmacists, storage managers) of these determinations via the study protocol, instructional manual, or direct study-specific training (ICH GCP 5.13.2).

In accordance with institutional practices and GCP requirements, the PI (or designee, such as a qualified pharmacist) at the clinical site should maintain records of the product's delivery to the site (e.g., the packing slip denoting what was included in the shipment and any required shipment confirmation documentation, such as a confirmation form that must be emailed or faxed back to the supplier).

Site Medication Inventory Log (4mg sublingual film)

Site Name: _____

Page ____ of ____

RECEIVED INTO INVENTORY			REMOVED FROM INVENTORY					DISPOSITION			
Date Received (mm/dd/yyyy)	Quantity (#4mg films)	Received by (initials)	Date Dispensed (mm/dd/yyyy)	Dispensed by (initials)	Amount Dispensed (#films)	Lot #	Assigned to (ppt ID - 4 digits)	Disposition (dispensed, returned, expired)	Confirmed by (initials/date)	Comments	Inventory Balance (4mg films)
			███████████								

Fig. 5 Example study drug inventory and tracking log for a clinical trial

These records should include dates, quantities, batch/serial numbers, expiration dates, and the unique code numbers assigned to the investigational product(s) and trial subjects, if applicable (ICH GCP 4.6.3). When study drug is received at the clinical site, it is critical to inspect the shipment thoroughly and as quickly after receipt as possible. The packing slip should be compared to both the order form and the contents of the shipment to confirm that there are no discrepancies, and the items themselves should be checked to confirm that they are intact. If a temperature and/or moisture sensor is included in the shipment, ensure that it has not "alarmed" or been activated; if so, the temperature and/or moisture levels may have surpassed the acceptable threshold during shipment, potentially compromising IP integrity. Some studies (often at the request of the manufacturer/distributor) may require that the packing slip be signed, dated, and returned to the shipper to acknowledge receipt of the shipment, while other studies may utilize an online portal or supply chain management software to digitize this process. If it appears that the shipment is incomplete or was damaged in transit, the Sponsor or designee should be contacted immediately. Often, it is helpful to prepare comprehensive inventory logs for the sites in advance, to ensure all key information is captured (see Fig. 5). Furthermore, if the site does not already have a local SOP for the receipt of drug, it is recommended that they create one prior to study start. Requiring documentation within an SOP and study staff training on this SOP ensures that the process has been thought out and that site staff is ready to properly receive and document the receipt of drug.

Quality Assurance

The Sponsor is responsible for ensuring that adequate quality assurance procedures are followed throughout the drug procurement and distribution process ("Sponsor Requirements"). Specific to IP receipt and accountability, ICH GCP guidelines indicate that "the Sponsor should ensure that written procedures include instructions that the investigator/institution should follow for the handling and storage of investigational product(s) for the trial and documentation thereof" (ICH GCP 5.14.3). Detailed procedures (e.g., in the study protocol or pharmacy manual) should address the proper receipt, handling, storage, dispensing, and final disposition of the investigational product. Once IP is on site, the PI is required to follow all applicable laws and regulations regarding IP administration and distribution to participants, such as adhering to the dosing guidelines in the investigator's brochure or package insert and keeping detailed records of the IP (e.g., lot number, amount) that is distributed to each study participant. Those tasked with observing the research sites in person to ensure that the study procedures are being properly followed, often termed clinical trial monitors, should also periodically ensure that procedures related to IP, such as adequate IP storage, temperature monitoring during shipment, and appropriate documentation for receiving and dispensing drug throughout the trial, are in place and are being followed.

Summary and Conclusion

IP procurement and distribution can be a complex process, and the level of complexity depends on variables such as study design, scope, the specific IP being utilized (e.g., controlled substances), and the number of sites and countries involved. Whatever the level of complexity, the process requires advanced planning, attention to detail, and compliance with local and regional regulations. The process of IP procurement and distribution is carried out by an assortment of organizations and individuals (all of whom need careful oversight and management by the study Sponsor or appropriate designee) who may be involved in the manufacturing, testing, packaging, labeling, documentation and accountability, shipping, and storage of study drug. Clear communication and efficient coordination of the groups and procedures involved are crucial, as are well-defined and unambiguous instructions to the clinical sites. Deviation from appropriate drug accountability measures and the various federal, state, and local regulations may potentially alter participant safety as well as safety and efficacy study outcome measures. Thoughtful planning in the pre-implementation stage of a clinical trial can mitigate these possible risks and help ensure consistent and dependable standards are used throughout the lifecycle of the clinical trial.

Key Facts

- Factors to consider during IP procurement include identification of a suitable vendor, manipulation of IP and manufacturing of matching placebo, and expiration dating, all of which increase in complexity in studies with active comparators, drug tapering regimens, and/or multiple research sites.
- To avoid insurmountable roadblocks during study implementation, it is important to consider procurement and distribution (in the context of the overall study design) early in the protocol development process as part of the study planning activities.
- The local competent authority can provide guidance as to whether an IND application (or regional equivalent) is required for a trial with a currently marketed IP.
- To protect the safety of human research participants, clinical trials using IP must adhere to cGMPs when manufacturing blinded medication, repackaging or relabeling IP, shipping IP to sites, and storing IP on site or at the central distributor or pharmacy.
- Basic measures of drug accountability and management need to be followed when IP is distributed to clinical sites, and various tools (such as clinical trial management systems) are available to streamline these processes.
- IP characteristics and study design parameters (such as studies involving controlled substances or blinded trials) influence the drug distribution process and should be carefully considered when planning and implementing a clinical trial.

References

Choudhry N, Krumme A, Ercole P et al (2017) Effect of reminder devices on medication adherence: the REMIND randomized clinical trial. JAMA Intern Med 177(5):624–631

Dragic L, Lee E, Wertheimer A, et al. (2015) Classifications of controlled substances: insights from 23 countries. Inov Pharm 6(2):Article 201

State of California Department of Justice (2018) Research advisory panel. https://oag.ca.gov/research. Accessed 06 Sep 2018

United Nations (1961) Single convention on narcotic drugs. https://www.unodc.org/pdf/convention_1961_en.pdf. Accessed 04 Oct 2018

United Nations (1971) Convention on psychotropic substances. https://www.unodc.org/pdf/convention_1971_en.pdf. Accessed 04 Oct 2018

United Nations (1988) Convention against illicit traffic in narcotic drugs and psychotropic substances. https://www.unodc.org/pdf/convention_1988_en.pdf. Accessed 04 Oct 2018

United States Department of Justice Drug Enforcement Administration, Diversion Control Division (2018) Control substance schedules. https://www.deadiversion.usdoj.gov/schedules/. Accessed 04 Oct 2018

United States Drug Enforcement Administration (2018) Drug scheduling. https://www.dea.gov/drug-scheduling. Accessed 04 Oct 2018

US Department of Health and Human Services Food and Drug Administration Center for Drug Evaluation and Research (2017) Guidance for industry: re-packaging of certain human drug products by pharmacies and outsourcing facilities. https://www.fda.gov/downloads/Drugs/Guidances/UCM434174.pdf. Accessed 19 Oct 2018

Woodworth T (2011) How will DEA affect your clinical study? J Clin Res Best Pract 7(12):1–9

World Health Organization (WHO) (2018) Substances under international control. http://www.who.int/medicines/areas/quality_safety/sub_Int_control/en/. Accessed 06 Sep 2018

Yeung D, Alvarez K, Quinones M et al (2003) Low-health literacy flashcards & mobile video reinforcement to improve medication adherence in patients on oral diabetes, heart failure, and hypertension medications. J Am Pharm Assoc 57(1):30–27

Zhao W, Durkalski V, Pauls K et al (2010) An electronic regulatory document management system for a clinical trial network. Contemp Clin Trials 31:27–33

Selection of Study Centers and Investigators

12

Dikla Shmueli-Blumberg, Maria Figueroa, and Carolyn Burke

Contents

Abstract

Site and investigator selection has traditionally been the result of a comprehensive process by which a study sponsor and/or designated representative, often a contract research organization (CRO), evaluates prospective investigative teams and associated clinical sites for clinical trial participation. A list of criteria is often

D. Shmueli-Blumberg (✉) · M. Figueroa · C. Burke
The Emmes Company, LLC, Rockville, MD, USA
e-mail: dblumberg@emmes.com; mfigueroa@emmes.com; cburke@emmes.com

© Springer Nature Switzerland AG 2022
S. Piantadosi, C. L. Meinert (eds.), *Principles and Practice of Clinical Trials*,
https://doi.org/10.1007/978-3-319-52636-2_35

compiled and used by the sponsor to grade site and investigator suitability for study participation.

In implementing a study, sponsors and site teams become partners in achieving study goals. For longer-term or complex studies, this partnership can become extensive. Sponsors and site teams must mutually invest in respective stakeholder perspectives and approaches to answer research questions. Site teams interested in the research question, with sufficient and qualified staff, and with access to the desired participant population, are key to conducting sound research. Sponsors that appreciate site perspectives, consider site operations and logistics in protocol design, support efforts to mitigate site challenges, communicate updates on broader perspectives of study activities, and offer fair compensation for site resources are key factors in implementing a successful study. Conversely, disconnected relationships between investigative teams and study sponsors can disrupt the timetable for research, contributing to compromised morale, cost overruns, and increased variability in administrating the protocol resulting in reduced ability to detect treatment differences, and may result in an unsuccessful trial.

A site and investigator selection process should be designed to ensure that both sponsors and site teams thoroughly evaluate whether the protocol design, resources, sponsor/team relationships, general timelines, and site facilities are compatible in achieving the goals of the study.

Keywords

Site · Investigator · Sponsors · Investigator selection plan · Site selection · Recruitment · Investigator qualification · Investigative team · Qualification visit

Introduction

Site and investigator selection is not a one-size-fits-all activity. It's not unusual for a site to be labeled a "good site" or a "bad site" in research, yet the criteria for such conclusions are ill-defined. What qualities do those designations represent, and how are those qualities best assessed? More importantly perhaps is the philosophy that there is no universally "good" or "bad" site, but rather the partnership or "fit" between the site team and the sponsor in executing a specific protocol at a specific site can be better, or worse, given the site resources and protocol requirements. A site team that successfully contributed to achieve study goals in one study may not necessarily have the same success in a subsequent, similar study. A sponsor that may have been a positive partner to a study team on a previously successful study may not be a positive partner under a subsequent study.

Site teams and sponsors with established relationships from prior partnerships can use their experiences to evaluate potential future partnerships. These relationships often are not devoid of subjective considerations, but objective measures should be incorporated into evaluations to the extent possible.

This chapter is entitled ▶ "Selection of Study Centers and Investigators", with inherent connotations of the traditional hierarchical approach that sponsors enlist centers (referred to as sites throughout this chapter) and investigators to contribute to research. Readers are encouraged to consider the sponsor and study teams as partners in identifying relationships that are conducive to achieving the goals of research.

Site and Investigator Selection Plan

As a study protocol evolves, sponsors consider the site facilities and teams that may best complement the goals of the study. The protocol context can have a significant impact on site characteristics and serve to narrow the field of potential sites quickly. A documented site and investigator selection plan can be useful in defining the site and investigator characteristics that are expected to complement the study requirements.

Investing time developing a site and investigator selection plan encourages the sponsor to review the protocol with perspective for anticipated needs and challenges associated with subject recruitment, site and subject compensation, quantity and location of sites (e.g., single country or international, rural or urban), site type (e.g., academic, commercial, private practice), study visit schedules, operations and logistics, staffing experience and credentials, equipment, and applicable regulations. Given the scope of potential factors to evaluate, a comprehensive plan assists sponsors and site teams to objectively evaluate sponsor and site compatibility more efficiently and possibly mitigate potential for subjective factors that can introduce bias in selection. For example, an objective and transparent plan can limit potential for hurt feelings based on pre-existing relationships. Plans should include documented timepoints intended to evaluate the effect of the plan, once applied, to identify any potential areas in the site and investigator selection approach requiring modification.

Once a site and investigator selection plan has been developed, sponsor and site teams should have common understanding and insight into potential study requirements before considering partnering in a research project. At minimum, a detailed protocol synopsis, if not an initial draft of the protocol, should be available for site teams to evaluate feasibility and potentially offer perspectives and experience that could support further, more robust, protocol development. With access to detailed information about a prospective study, site teams may be able to enhance the integrity of a site application by offering objective and specific examples of resources and past performance. In turn, this may create opportunities for more candid review and discussion among both site and sponsor teams for evaluating suitability for a study. Considerations that could be mutually applied to both the sponsor and site team could include quantitative categories associated with level of engagement, response time, adherence to timelines, and resolutions to action items/ troubleshooting initiatives. At the site level, considerations may include protocol and regulatory compliance, subject recruitment and retention, number of queries generated in and the time to query resolution, and data completion. Even the best possible site teams will "fail" if the protocol requirements are not suitable for their site and the budget is inadequate to support their efforts.

Site Selection

The scope of potential qualities and characteristics to consider in evaluating site compatibility for any research project is vast. Desired characteristics are specific to the proposed project and defined in the selection plan. More general concepts are described below (Fig. 1).

Facility Resources

Key considerations in assessing the suitability of sites for a research study include evaluation of the research space, which may include exam room features, secure and appropriate areas to store study drug or devices, specialized equipment needs, availability of and access to a pharmacy, and laboratory and imaging capabilities.

Important factors to evaluate include the availability of adequate infrastructure, staff availability (e.g., hours/days of week), staff depth (e.g., coverage for key staff on leave, attrition management), and staff credentials and expertise such as clinicians representing a disease specialty. Alternatively, if there is a possibility of supporting capacity-building activities such as staff training at a site, then there could be more flexibility regarding this criterion. The facility itself would be ideally located in close proximity, or easily accessible via public transportation, to the subject population of interest. Other important facility-related considerations include accounting for institutional standards of care, attitudes and participation of the various departments in the facility, the ability to support data management operations, Internet connectivity, immediate and long-term record storage capabilities, and other study-specific operational concerns.

Site and Process Flow

With study subjects as key partners in research, sites and sponsors should invest time and resources to streamline the subject experience during study visits. Consideration

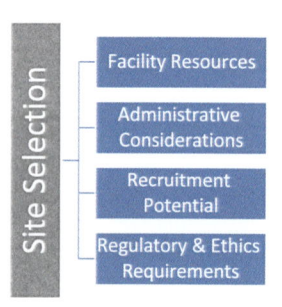

Fig. 1 Site selection considerations

for who, what, when, where, and how study requirements will be completed will help site teams evaluate their processes and either identify areas for modifications to accommodate the subject experience or may determine they will not be able to satisfy the study requirements.

In addition to the subject experience, the same considerations should be applied to improve overall efficiency at the site. For example, if a protocol requires laboratory sample analysis within 2 h of a subject's arrival in an Emergency Room, the site team will need to identify means to collect that sample shortly after consent, get the sample to the lab quickly, and place a stat order for analysis. The sample collection and analysis are already challenging, but if the laboratory happens to be on the other side of an academic campus, or site policies require specific site personnel to transport the sample that may not be immediately available, then there is increased risk of compromising protocol requirements in ensuring sample analysis within 2 h.

Sites that have a central laboratory facility and equipment resources consistent with protocol requirements (e.g., specific Tesla MRI machine) and can follow study-wide standards of operations (SOPs) and/or guidelines may be more timely in preparing for site initiation than sites that do not have such resources.

Administrative Considerations

Study costs may differ between research sites for a variety of reasons, including the presence or absence of a national healthcare system in each country, regional standards of care, or routine patient care costs that a form of Medicare or private insurance carriers in that area will cover. Individual study budgets may not be known during the site selection process, but investigating key budget-related questions (e.g., institutional overhead fees) might be informative even in the most preliminary phase of the process.

Policies and legal requirements of both the sponsor and the site should be explored. Time requirements for negotiating budgets and contract terms should be considered. Sites with extensive legal contract and budget reviews may be less favorable depending on study timelines. Additionally, there may be requirements (e.g., protection from liability) either from the sponsor or at the site that cannot be accommodated, instantly ruling out study participation. Alternatively, requirements that can be accommodated but require negotiation may prolong time needed between site selection and site initiation, ultimately impacting the overall project budget and timelines. Such factors will also impact timelines for implementing protocol and contract amendments after the study is initiated.

Recruitment Potential

Research questions cannot be answered without study subjects who are engaged in the trial and eager to support activities to answer the research question. The more collaborative the sponsor and site team are in encouraging and supporting subject recruitment and retention, the better.

Many trials in the past have failed to reach their enrollment goal within the anticipated timeframe or ever. A primary factor to consider in site selection is whether the site team has access to a target population with the condition of interest and who are willing to participate in a trial. Recruitment potential is a necessary, but insufficient, stand-alone criterion for selection. Sites may have a history of reaching their recruitment goals, but a careful selection process must also assess whether subjects were good research subjects, once enrolled, by reviewing compliance and retention rates.

The investigator should be able to demonstrate that they have adequate recruitment potential for obtaining the required number of subjects for that study. This could be based on retrospective data, such as showing the number of patients who have come in for a similar treatment at that facility over the past 12 months.

Ideally, site and sponsor teams will have experience in compiling and executing a recruitment and retention plan centered around the subject experience. Even without such experience, it's never too late to try a new approach. Considerations for such a plan include streamlined study activity workflow, potential compensation, subject access to transportation, availability of childcare, snack/meal options during visits, flexible scheduling hours, personnel dispositions, general hospitality, and even facility aesthetics that will better support recruitment and retention initiatives.

Regulatory and Ethics Requirements

The globalization of clinical research makes attention to regulatory requirements particularly important. Considering relevant regulatory authorities, affiliation with central or distributed or local Institutional Review Boards (IRBs) or Independent Ethics Committees (IECs), and issues related to drug procurement and distribution may be important when assessing the fit of a site to a specific study. Regulatory requirements between countries should be compared to identify potential regulations that may only be required in select countries but need to be applied in all countries to ensure compliance. Depending on the study, more granular questions regarding assurances, certifications, and accreditations (such as local clinical laboratory licensing) may be relevant as well.

Timelines to ensure compliance with regional regulatory requirements and corresponding review can be significant in the overall project timeline. In some countries, country-level regulatory review can take at least 90 days.

Investigator Selection

Investigators hold a key role in clinical trials, and the success or failure of a trial may hinge in part on finding a suitable individual to fill this important position. It is important for sponsors and prospective investigators to have a mutual understanding of the roles and responsibilities of a site investigator and the investigative team in ensuring study subject privacy and safety and protocol and regulatory compliance during a research project. Without appreciation for protocol and regulatory requirements prior to implementing a study, investigative teams can experience unfortunate consequences. Most consequential, the rights and welfare of study subjects, the true champions for research, can be compromised. Such consequences can ultimately contribute to imposed study termination, resulting in an inability to answer the research question, and lost money, time, and resources. For various reasons, some sponsors may predetermine a PI or several PIs to participate in a trial. There is an inherent risk in finalizing the selection of these individuals to the critical role of investigator without proper attention to their specific qualifications based on objective measures. The section below offers a review of investigator responsibilities and training requirements.

Investigator Responsibilities

The International Council for Harmonization (ICH) defines an investigator as the individual responsible for the conduct of the clinical trial at a study site (ICH, GCP 1.34). If there is a larger team of people conducting the study at any site, then the investigator is considered the responsible leader of that team and may be called the principal investigator (PI). In multicenter trials, each clinical site has its own PI who provides oversight and leads the research site staff at that site in implementing the study. A successful PI has the time to engage in the study and demonstrates a commitment to the research team, to study subjects, and to the integrity of the trial itself. The PI's actions set the tone for the research staff by implying the importance of the trial and setting work expectation standards. The responsibilities of the investigator are varied and related to the different phases throughout the study life cycle. Investigator responsibilities generally include the following:

- Knowledge of the study protocol, ensuring other research staff are informed about the protocol, and conducting their roles in accordance with the processes and procedures outlined in the current version of that document.
- Maintaining proper oversight of the study drug, device, or investigational product including documenting product receipt, handling, administration, storage, and destruction or return. An investigator has a responsibility to inform potential study subjects when drugs or devices are being used for investigational purposes.
- Reporting safety events throughout the implementation of a clinical trial (21 CFR 312.64). Investigators should document adverse events (AEs) which are untoward medical occurrences associated with the use of a drug in humans that occur during the study and, sometime, even for period after the study closure. They must carefully follow the protocol and Federal guidelines for the appropriate procedures (cite OHRP, FDA) for reporting AEs and serious adverse events (SAEs) as needed.

To illustrate the scope of investigator responsibilities, below is an example of responsibilities an investigator would be asked to accept for a study under an investigational new drug (IND) application with the Food and Drug Administration (FDA) in the United States (Fig. 2).

9. COMMITMENTS

I agree to conduct the study(ies) in accordance with the relevant, current protocol(s) and will only make changes in a protocol after notifying the sponsor, except when necessary to protect the safety, rights, or welfare of subjects.

I agree to personally conduct or supervise the described investigation(s).

I agree to inform any patients, or any persons used as controls, that the drugs are being used for investigational purposes and I will ensure that the requirements relating to obtaining informed consent in 21 CFR Part 50 and institutional review board (IRB) review and approval in 21 CFR Part 56 are met.

I agree to report to the sponsor adverse experiences that occur in the course of the investigation(s) in accordance with 21 CFR 312.64. I have read and understand the information in the investigator's brochure, including the potential risks and side effects of the drug.

I agree to ensure that all associates, colleagues, and employees assisting in the conduct of the study(ies) are informed about their obligations in meeting the above commitments.

I agree to maintain adequate and accurate records in accordance with 21 CFR 312.62 and to make those records available for inspection in accordance with 21 CFR 312.68.

I will ensure that an IRB that complies with the requirements of 21 CFR Part 56 will be responsible for the initial and continuing review and approval of the clinical investigation. I also agree to promptly report to the IRB all changes in the research activity and all unanticipated problems involving risks to human subjects or others. Additionally, I will not make any changes in the research without IRB approval, except where necessary to eliminate apparent immediate hazards to human subjects.

I agree to comply with all other requirements regarding the obligations of clinical investigators and all other pertinent requirements in 21 CFR Part 312.

Fig. 2 Excerpt from FDA Form 1572, Section 9: Investigator Commitments

This form represents a commitment by the PI to personally conduct or supervise the trial, which involves appropriate delegation of activities to other investigators and qualified research staff, allocating time to adequately interact and supervise those staff members periodically, and oversight of any third parties involved at their site, if any. Other documentation, such as a protocol signature page, or a signed protocol document may also serve as a commitment that the PI and sub-investigators will follow the procedures and requirements outlined in the protocol.

The consequences of not adhering to these obligations can be serious. Investigators could be barred from participating in future research, lose professional licensure, and face legal action. Warning Letters from the FDA (which are posted on the FDA website) commonly involve an investigator's failure to appropriately follow the protocol, informed consent violations, and not maintaining adequate records (Anderson et al. 2011). Anderson et al. also state that determining whether a PI has personally conducted or supervised the trial has been emphasized during FDA clinical investigator inspections as well. Enforcement strategies include regulatory warning letters, disqualifications, restrictions and debarments, criminal prosecutions, prison, and/or fines if warranted based on the circumstances of the violations.

Investigator Qualification

The US Code of Federal Regulations specifies that clinical trial investigators should be qualified by training and experience as "appropriate experts to investigate the drug" (21 CFR 312.53). The ICH guidelines include a similar assertion, stating that investigators should be qualified by education, training, and experience to oversee the study and provide evidence of meeting all qualifications and relevant regulatory requirements (ICH, GCP 4.1). When the study intervention involves use of an investigational product (IP) or devices, then part of being qualified involves being familiar with that product. The investigator should be thoroughly familiar with the use of the IP as described in the protocol as well as having reviewed the Investigator's Brochure (for an unapproved product) or Prescribing Information (for approved products) which describe the pharmacological, chemical, clinical, and other properties of the IP. Appropriate general and protocol-specific training can help ensure that an investigator is adequately qualified to conduct the study. The FDA does not specifically require that a lead investigator have a medical degree (e.g., MD, DO), but often he or she does. If the PI is not a physician, one should be listed as a sub-investigator to perform trial-related medical decisions. This is consistent with GCP standards that state that medical care given to trial subjects (ICH GCP 2.7) and trial-related medical decisions (ICH GCP 4.3.1) should be the responsibility of a qualified physician.

Investigative Team Considerations

Investigator Equipoise

In research there is an expectation of equipoise or uncertainty about the effectiveness of the various intervention groups which is necessary to ethically run the trial. The nature of the relationship between a patient and physician changes once a physician enrolls a patient in a clinical trial, thereby creating a potential conflict of interest (Morin et al. 2002). For example, even if the physician believes that one of the treatment arms or groups is more likely to be successful, all investigators have a responsibility to follow the study protocol and most importantly the randomization plan. Physicians who have equipoise do not have an inherent conflict of interest when suggesting study enrollment and randomization to their patients. Those without equipoise may inject conscious or subconscious bias in treatment or protocol administration.

Investigator Motivation

Other investigator qualifications are more subjective in nature and difficult to quantify or document, such as motivation, leadership style, and investigator engagement. Motivation may arise from the desire to work on cutting-edge research or develop or test products that could ultimately improve the health of patients around the world. Other motivating factors include financial benefits as well as prestige and recognition in the professional and scientific community. Some have asserted that enthusiasm and scientific interest in the research question are the most important qualifications for potential principal investigators (Lader et al. 2004). A passionate PI leading the study team is likely to evoke enthusiasm and determination which will be valuable for successful implementation of the trial.

Site Team Dynamics

Sponsors and prospective investigative teams need to evaluate the dynamic characteristics among the study investigative team. In addition to motivation and passion, an investigator will typically need the assistance of several research staff members to successfully run a clinical trial.

Most studies will have a research coordinator who supports the daily operations of the study such as scheduling subjects for visits, interacting with subjects at the site and possibly conducting some of the assessments, ensuring data is accurately collected and reported, and maintaining the site regulatory files. Other site staff may include physicians and other medical clinicians, pharmacists, phlebotomists, counselors, and other support personnel. Investigators can increase the likelihood for a strong and productive team by fostering an environment of cooperation based on the site staff's shared mission of implementing a successful trial. Establishing clear roles and responsibilities for each staff member is also important, and investigators are required to maintain a list of all staff and their delegated trial-related duties (ICH GCP 4.1.5) in addition to ensuring that the activities are delegated appropriately to trained and qualified site staff members. An engaged investigator who spends sufficient time at the research site will be able to monitor and evaluate the group dynamics throughout the trial and ensure that morale remains high during difficult times (e.g., low subject recruitment rates) and that staff have sufficient time to complete their work. Other strategies for maintaining a strong site team include providing immediate feedback to staff about their performance, having backups for key staff roles, and providing opportunities for staff to review and provide input on the protocol and manual of operations prior to study start-up to ensure their input is incorporated in final versions.

Research Experience and Past Performance

Other metrics for evaluating site staff include previous experience. Site teams with little to no research experience may automatically be excluded from sponsor consideration for participation in a clinical trial. Concerns may arise regarding their abilities to recruit and retain subjects and understand fundamental ethical and regulatory requirements for participating in clinical research. A sponsor may debate whether research-naïve sites are worth the risk in financial and time investments. Then again, the extent of staff previous experience may not always be a good indicator of future performance. Moreover, extensive research experience may promote more rigidity ("I've been doing it this way for 20 years") and over-confidence, whereas a less experienced team may be more open to different approaches and perspectives.

Reputations and past performance of an investigative team can offer important information, but past performance is not necessarily predictive of future performance. There are many variables (e.g., medical condition, staffing resources and dynamics, access to the desired study subjects, trial design, sponsor/site dynamics, etc.) that can contribute to past and future site performance. It is important to take the time to understand what factors contributed to study performance and evaluate the advantages of site teams who achieved study goals versus the obstacles another site team may have encountered contributing to an inability to fully satisfy study goals. Even with this information, the dynamic nature of a site team can have significant influence on future studies.

Any change, in any area of the facility or team, will either negatively or positively impact site team performance; neither will ever be the same as before. If obstacles can be mitigated or overcome, there can be many advantages of selecting a site team with research history and experience. Such advantages include:

- Training from prior study participation may be transferrable, ultimately requiring less overall training time.
- Experienced researchers may have already established a flow and process for basic study requirements such as facilitating the consent process, collecting lab samples, or compiling a study research record. These may contribute to quicker, more efficient study implementation.
- The site team may already have thorough training, understanding, and experience in applying regulatory requirements within study processes that may result in lower risk of compromises in regulatory compliance.
- Site teams with prior experience in subject recruitment may have already determined effective outreach initiatives to increase potential to recruit members of the desired study population.

There may also be advantages in selecting site teams with limited or no previous research experience; these sites should not be overlooked based on this criterion alone. New research sites may:

- Be eager to learn and be compliant in following the study procedures because they do not have pre-conceived ideas about how things must be done
- Have an untapped pool of subjects available in their practice or within the referral regional area
- Have greater diversity within their populations

Site and Investigator Selection Methods

Once the ideal criteria and characteristics for a site and study team for a project have been determined, sponsors will need to find efficient and effective means to share information about the project and collect relevant information from site teams. This is often accomplished via a combination of utilities and interpersonal interaction.

There are several ways for sponsors to solicit site information about prospective study site teams. Sponsors may elect to cast a broad net and open the selection process to any study team interested in participation. They may also elect to implement a more strategic approach using some of the following resources:

- Sponsor databases
- Participation in similar studies listed on ClinicalTrials.gov (see Fig. 3)
- Research network memberships/registries
- Prior research partnerships
- Professional organization databases
- Literature searches

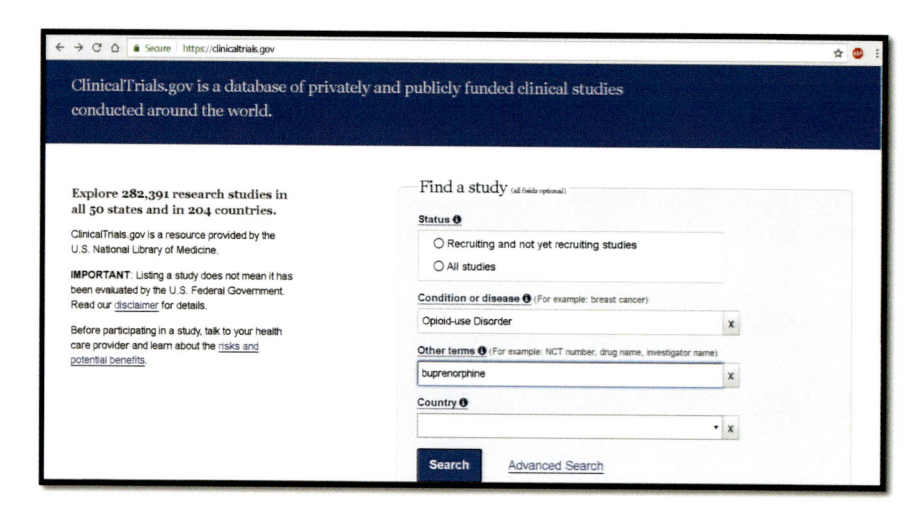

Fig. 3 ClinicalTrials.gov image

- Requests for proposals (RFPs)
- Colleague referrals
- Investigator selection services
- Public clinical trial databases/libraries
- Professional society membership databases
- Research professionals' societies

While a process that includes an "all are welcome" site recruitment approach may be an easy way to achieve a specific number of desired sites, and expedite study start-up, this may increase the risk of compromising longer-term goals of the study and can result in ineffective resource allocation. The site and investigator selection plan can help sponsors more clearly define the total number of sites, the type of site, site team, and corresponding qualifications and training expectations of ideal interest to support study activities.

With specified ideal qualifications, sponsors and site teams can conduct preliminary review of requirements to quickly determine "go/no go" conclusions for pursuing a study partnership. Once a site team elects to pursue study participation, they can highlight specific areas of their staffing, facilities, subject recruitment population, and any prior training and experience to illustrate why they are a good fit for the study. Sponsors can also compare the desired qualifications and characteristics for the study with submitted site application information to evaluate the site teams that are most compatible with study goals.

Surveys and Questionnaires

Common tools used to collect information about prospective study sites include surveys, questionnaires, and interviews. Depending on the design of the chosen method(s), the information collected can be integral in determining site team and study compatibility, or it can expend staffing time and resources without adding much value to the selection process. The tools intended to be used to collect information from sites should be included as part of the sponsor site and investigator selection plan.

The overall purpose of any method chosen needs to be clearly defined. This will help ensure that information relevant to study participation and to proposed outcome criteria will be offered by prospective study teams. For example, if a sponsor site selection plan indicates interest primarily in site teams with research experience in multiple sclerosis, but the method used to collect information from sites doesn't specifically address this level of detail, then the sponsor team may receive information from site teams that reflect research experience, but without specific reference to disease area expertise. Thus, the sponsor won't have a complete picture from which to determine whether a site team is compatible for the study. Additional time and effort for further clarification may be needed, or in the interest of time, the sponsor may move on to other proposals and overlook a potentially ideal site team because there wasn't sufficient detail in the information provided simply because of the design of the utility selected to solicit the information. The design of the collection tool will likely be a blend of both objective and subjective information. The questions posed should reflect the four primary areas discussed in section "Site Selection" of this chapter: facility resources, administrative considerations, recruitment potential, and regulatory and ethics requirements. The survey questions can be grouped by area for ease of completion and can include specific study-relevant items beyond the four primary areas described above.

A more objective design that corresponds with a scoring system for each type of response could limit potential bias in the site selection process. At the least, there should be a predetermined agreement on the particularly important items so that the sites can be appropriately scored or ranked based on those criteria (Figs. 4 and 5).

Examples of objective items include:

- Is there a $-80\,^\circ$F freezer on site for blood sample storage?
- How many feet is the freezer from where the samples will be collected?
- Are at least two members of the prospective study team available 24 h a day, 7 days a week?

On the other hand, subjective responses usually offer more insight into the dynamics of the site team that can offer information about the team's demeanor and motivation to participate in the study, empathy and compassion for the study population, and any creative means the site team has used to improve efficiencies and recruit and retain study subjects.

Examples of subjective items include:

- What challenges/risks do you anticipate should you participate in this study?
- Describe your thoughts on recommended subject recruitment and retention practices for this study at your site.

Clinical Practice Site Characteristics:

Q17 How many patients with the adolescent well visit CPT codes 99394 and 99384 have been seen by your providers
      in the past year? _____

Q18 How did you determine this number?

☐ Queried from patient billing records   ☐ Estimated from provider description
☐ Estimated from scheduling records   ☐ Other, describe below:

Fig. 4 Excerpt from Site Selection Survey: Site Characteristics

- Have any of the potential site staff worked together before? Share information about methods of communication at the site to ensure study requirements and updates are distributed.
- Describe a problem you encountered with a previous study and what approach was taken to address it.

Prior to distributing the information collection tool to the site team, sponsor teams should consider the process for how information from sites will be received and be reviewed for potential partnership. Consideration should be given to having sites provide masked information to the sponsor to eliminate as much bias in the selection process as possible. If this is clarified as part of the design process, the sponsor can be more forthright in advising prospective site teams of what to expect once a site proposal has been submitted. Some questions to consider include:

- Will the information collected be kept confidential solely with this sponsor team?
- How will the information be stored (e.g., paper/electronic files, a site database)?
- Will the information collected be considered for this study alone or for this study and other future potential studies with this sponsor?
- What process will be used to select site teams for study participation?
- Are additional activities expected after review of preliminary information (e.g., interviews, follow-up on site visits)?
- What process will be used to advise site teams of sponsor selections?
- What are the timelines for distribution and expected returned information from site teams?
- Who will be available to respond to inquiries from site teams as they attempt to complete the requested information?

Sponsors who approach prospective site teams as potential partners in their research, valuing the time and effort site teams will use to compile the information

Clinical Practice Site Physical Resources:

Q26 Does the clinical practice site have a <u>private</u> space (e.g., office, exam room, etc.) available to conduct interviews or other portions of the study?

☐ Yes   ☐ No

Q27 Does the clinical practice site have space for a locked filing cabinet to securely store participant records?

☐ Yes   ☐ No

Q28 Will the RA and study participants have access to a high-speed wireless internet connection? Note: The waiting room must have access.

☐ Yes   ☐ No

If Yes, describe how reliable the wireless internet connection has been over the past 6 months:

```



```

Q29 Does the site have access to IT support services?

☐ Yes   ☐ No

If No, describe who would be responsible for helping to resolve an internet outage:

```



```

Fig. 5 Excerpt from Site Selection Survey: Site Resources

and describing the process and expectations for evaluating prospective study partnerships, may be more likely to collect more timely, thoughtful, and comprehensive responses from site teams.

Site Qualification Visit

Despite all the effort that is required to compile a site information collection utility, and all the technology available to help people connect via phone, email, chat, social media, and video, in-person interactions offer the greatest opportunity to evaluate whether the sponsor and site teams can establish an effective partnership to conduct a study. On-site qualification visits are an invaluable way to gauge sponsor and site team dynamics that cannot be achieved via surveys, questionnaires, or interviews. Each party can better evaluate whether they are compatible and identify anticipated challenges in partnering together. An on-site visit also offers the opportunity for the site team to share perspectives in operations and logistics to which the sponsor team may be naïve. In-person site visits may be especially important in international studies where countries may differ in normative standards (e.g., what constitutes adequate research space for conducting a study). All partners can review and discuss anticipated areas of excellence and potential risks and work together toward mitigating risks. Items that were described in the "Site Selection" section above can be observed and evaluated "first hand" including:

- Facility organization/flow – sites can demonstrate what the subject experience may be like.
- Site team and subject access to the facility (i.e., public transportation, parking, accessibility for assistance devices, navigation from the entrance to the research site, location of labs, the pharmacy, etc. and other resources to the primary study location).
- Nonverbal cues/information.
- Storage locations/utilities.
- Equipment availability, calibration, and documentation.
- Subject recruitment and retention planning – site teams that devise a formal plan for recruitment in advance of site initiation that also includes timepoints for evaluation may be better equipped to evaluate the effect of planned initiatives and recalibrate initiatives as needed.

Summary

As has been described throughout this chapter, the site selection process is complex and dynamic. Sponsors and site teams who elect to conduct a trial together are entering, at minimum, into a short-term partnership with each other and must be interdependent to achieve the goals of the study. Sponsors must consider a variety of factors and embark upon both remote and in-person means to learn more about prospective study sites. Investigators who participate in a study have significant responsibility for ensuring appropriate staffing and corresponding training and qualifications, regulatory compliance, protocol compliance, and, most importantly, protecting the safety and rights of the subjects who participate in a study. Investigative teams must weigh their responsibilities with the study requirements provided by the sponsor. Ultimately, both sponsors and site teams must evaluate whether they can be compatible and can achieve the goals of the research project.

Key Facts

1. The sponsor and study teams should be viewed as partners with a common goal of identifying a good fit between a study and an investigator and site staff.
2. Some of the important considerations when selecting a site for a clinical trial include facility resources, administrative considerations, recruitment potential, and regulatory and ethics requirements.
3. Selection of an investigator may include objective quantifiable considerations such as previous studies and publications and specific area of expertise, as well as more subjective qualifications such as motivation and leadership style.
4. There are a variety of ways for sponsors to solicit site information about prospective study site teams, such as through site surveys and questionnaires and site qualification visits.

References

Anderson C, Young P, Berenbaum A (2011) Food and drug administration guidance: supervisory responsibilities of investigators. J Diabetes Sci Technol 5(2):433–438. https://doi.org/10.1177/193229681100500234

Lader MD, Cannon CP, Ohman EM et al (2004) The clinician as investigator: participating in clinical trials in the practice setting. Circulation 109(21):2672–2679. https://doi.org/10.1161/01.CIR.0000128702.16441.75

Morin K, Rakatansky H, Riddick F et al (2002) Managing conflicts of interest in the conduct of clinical trials. JAMA 287(1):78–84. https://doi.org/10.1001/jama.287.1.78

Design and Development of the Study Data System

13

Steve Canham

Contents

Abstract

The main components of a typical modern study data system are described, together with a discussion of associated workflows and the options for deployment, such as PaaS (platform as a Service) and SaaS (software as a service), and their implications for data management. A series of recommendations are made about how to create a study specific system, by developing a specification from the study

S. Canham (✉)
European Clinical Research Infrastructure Network (ECRIN), Paris, France
e-mail: steve.canham@ecrin.org

© Springer Nature Switzerland AG 2022
S. Piantadosi, C. L. Meinert (eds.), *Principles and Practice of Clinical Trials*,
https://doi.org/10.1007/978-3-319-52636-2_36

protocol within a multidisciplinary framework, obtaining formal approval of that specification, building prototypes, and then carrying out a detailed and systematic validation of the system before releasing it for use. The use of data standards is described and strongly encouraged, and the need for distinct development, test, and production environments is discussed. Longer term aspects of system management are then considered, including change management of the study data system and preparing the data for analysis, and managing data in the long term.

Keywords

Clinical Data Management System · CDMS · Study definition · Electronic remote data capture · eRDC · Functional specification · Validation · Data standards · Change management · Data extraction

Introduction

The study data system is designed to collect, code, clean, and store a study's data, deliver it for analysis in an appropriate format, and support its long-term management. In fact, a "study data system" is rarely a single system – it is normally a collection of different hardware and software components, some relatively generic and others study specific, together with the procedures that determine how those components are used and the staff that operate the systems, all working together to support the data management required within a study.

This chapter has three parts. The first provides a descriptive overview and looks at the typical components of a study data system, the associated data processing workflows, and the main options for deployment. The second is a more prescriptive account of how a data system should be designed, constructed, and validated for an individual study, while the third discusses two longer term aspects of system use: managing change and delivering data for analysis.

Descriptive Overview

System Components: The Naming of Parts

Any study data system has to be study specific, collecting only the data items required by a particular study, in the order specified by the assessment schedule. But any such system also has to meet a more generic set of requirements, to guarantee regulatory compliance and effective, safe, data management. The functionality required includes:

- The provision of granular access control, to ensure users only see the data they are entitled to see (in most cases, only the data of the participants from their own site).

- Automatic addition of audit trail data for each data entry or edit, with preservation of previous values.
- The ability to put logic checks on questions, so that impossible, unusual, or inconsistent values can be flagged to the user during data entry.
- Conditional "skipping" of data items that are not applicable for a particular participant, (as identified by data entered previously).
- Support for data cleaning – usually by built in dialogues that allow central and site staff, and monitors, to easily exchange queries and responses within the system.
- The ability to accurately extract part or all of the data, in formats that can be consumed by common statistical programs.

These requirements mean that a study data system almost always has as its core a specialist **Clinical Data Management System (CDMS)**, a software package that provides the generic functions listed above, but whose user interface can be adapted to reflect the requirements of specific studies. Such systems are usually purchased on a commercial basis and may be installed locally or hosted externally.

A single CDMS installation can and usually does support multiple studies. It makes use of a database for storing the data and provides a set of front-end screens for inputting and querying it. The database is normally one of the common relational systems (e.g., SQL Server, Oracle, MySQL), but it will be automatically configured by the CDMS to store both the study design details and the clinical, user, and audit data. The user interface screens are normally web pages, which means that as far as end users are concerned, the CDMS system is "zero-footprint": it does not require any local installation at the clinical sites or the use of a dedicated laptop. An end user at a clinical site accesses the system, remotely and securely, by simply going to a pre-specified web page. From there they can send the data immediately back to the central CDMS, where it is transferred to the database. For security and performance reasons, the database is normally on a different server, with tightly controlled access, whereas the web server is necessarily "outward facing" and open to the web (see Fig. 1).

The study-specific part of the system is essentially a definition and is often therefore referred to simply as the "**study definition**." It is stored within and referenced by the CDMS, and stipulates all the study-specific components, for example, the sites, users, data items, code lists, logic checks, and skip conditions. It also defines the order and placement of items on the data capture screens (usually referred to as "eCRFs," for electronic case report forms), and how the eCRFs are themselves arranged within the "study events" (or "visits"), i.e., the distinct time points at which data is collected. Even though a single CDMS installation usually contains multiple study definitions, it controls access so that users only ever see the study (or studies) they are working on, and the data from their own site.

Almost all systems also allow a study definition to be exported and imported as a file. This allows the definition to be easily moved between different instances of the same CDMS – for example, when transferring a study definition from a development to a production environment. If the file is structured using an XML schema called the Operational Data Model, or ODM (CDISC 2020a), an international standard developed by CDISC (the Clinical Data Interchange Standards Consortium), then it is

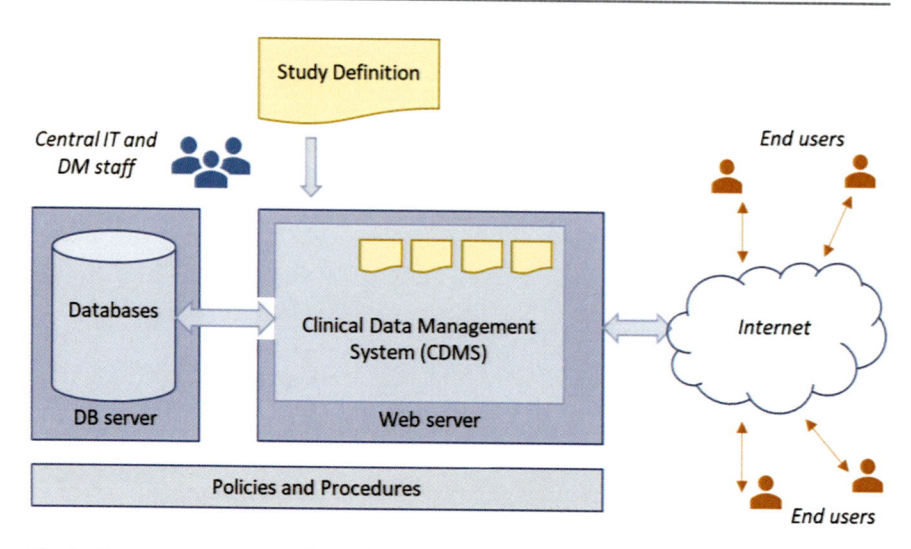

Fig. 1 The main components of a modern study data system. The CDMS stores one or more study definitions and is usually installed on a web server, which presents each study's screens to authorized users via a secure internet link. The CDMS is also connected to a database, usually on a separate server, for data storage

sometimes possible to transfer the study definition between *different* data collection systems, (e.g., between collaborators). Sometimes rather than always because, unfortunately, not all CDMS fully support ODM export/import and there are some elements of a study definition (such as automatic consistency checks on data) where ODM still only provides partial support.

In terms of features, almost all CDMS are *technically* compliant with clinical trial regulations, especially GCP and CFR21(11), e.g., they allow granular access control, they provide automatic audit trail data, the internal timestamps are guaranteed to be consistent, etc. Without this technical compliance, they would stand little chance in the marketplace. What makes a system fully compliant, however, is *the way in which it is used*: the set of standard operating procedures and detailed work instructions that govern how the system is set up and functions in practice, together with the assumed competence of the staff operating those systems. For this reason both 'policies and procedures', and 'central IT and DM staff' are included as elements within Figure 1.

The study-specific system that users interact with, the product of the study definition and the underlying CDMS, is sometimes known as a **Clinical Data Management *Application* (CDMA)**. Although in practice "study definition," or even "study database," is probably more common, in this chapter, the more accurate "CDMA" is used to refer to the software systems supporting a specific study, and "study definition" is restricted to the detailed specification that defines the CDMA's features.

Researchers are normally much more engaged with the details of the CDMA rather than the underlying systems, but they should at least be satisfied that the systems used for their trial are based upon an appropriate CDMS and that there is a mature set of procedures in place that govern its consistent and regulatory compliant use. This is one of the many reasons why the operational management of a trial is best delegated to a specialist trials unit, which might be a department within a university, hospital, research institute or company, or an independent commercial research organization, or CRO (for simplicity, in this chapter, all of these are referred to as a "trials unit"). Not only will such a unit already be running or managing one or more CDMSs, they will also be able to provide the expertise to develop the study specific part of the system safely and quickly.

CDMSs differ in their ease of use and setup, for instance, in creating study definitions, extracting data or generating reports, and the additional features that they may contain. The latter can include:

- Integrated treatment allocation systems, so sites obtain a randomization decision immediately they recruit a participant into a trial
- Built-in support for data standards, e.g., the ability to import/export CDISC ODM files
- Integrated coding modules (e.g., for MedDRA coding of adverse events)
- Supporting versions for tablets and mobile phones, especially for obtaining data directly from participants (ePRO or "electronic participant-reported outcomes")
- Built-in support for monitors and source data verification
- Integration with laboratory systems

The great majority of CDMSs in use are commercial systems, available from a wide variety of vendors. In early 2020, a search on a software comparison site listed 58 different systems that offered both electronic data capture and CFR21(11) compliance (Capterra 2020), and that list was far from comprehensive. Vendors range from large multinationals to small start-ups, and license costs vary over at least an order of magnitude, from a few thousand to several hundred thousand dollars per study, though as discussed below costs can also depend on the deployment models used. There are also a few open source CDMSs: OpenClinica (2020) and RedCap (2020) are the two best-known; both are available in free-to-install versions (as well as commercial versions that provide additional support), and both have enthusiastic user communities.

There are also some local CDMSs, built "in-house," particularly in academic units, although they are becoming less common. CDMSs are increasingly complex and costly to build and validate, and effective ongoing support requires an investment in IT staff that is beyond the budget of most noncommercial units. Local systems can also be over dependent on local programmers and become more difficult to maintain if key staff leave. Although there is no question that home-grown CDMSs can function well, there is an increased risk in using such systems. Sponsors and researchers who find themselves relying on such systems need to be confident that they are fully validated, and that they are likely to remain supported for the length of the trial.

The Rise of the eRDC Workflow

The dominant web-based workflow for collecting clinical trial data, as depicted in Fig. 1, is known as **electronic remote data capture**, or eRDC (EDC and RDC are also used, and in most contexts mean the same thing). Since the early 2000s, eRDC has slowly supplanted the traditional paper-based workflow, where paper CRFs were sent through to the central trials unit or CRO, by post or courier, to be transcribed manually into a central CDMS. Early papers extolling the benefits of eRDC were often written by the CDMS vendors (e.g., Mitchel et al. 2001; Green 2003), who had obvious vested interests. Despite this, the cost and time benefits of eRDC have driven gradual adoption, especially for multi-site trials and in geographical areas where reliable internet infrastructure is available. The advantages include:

- Removing the transcription step, and thus the time lag between the arrival of a paper CRF and loading its data into the system, and eliminating transcription errors. It therefore removes the need for expensive checks on data transcription, such as double data entry.
- Speeding up data queries – the "dialogue" between site and central data management can proceed securely on-line, rather than by sending queries and responses manually. This can be especially important when chasing down queries in preparation for an analysis.
- Allowing safety signals to be picked up more quickly. In addition, some systems can generate emails if adverse events of a particular severity or type are recorded.
- Making it possible to reject "impossible" data (e.g., dates that can never be later than the date of data entry) and thus force an immediate revision on data entry. In a paper-based system, the need to reflect a paper CRF's contents, however bizarre, means that this type of data error must be allowed and then queried, or subject to "self-evident correction" rules.
- Making it easier and clearer to tailor systems to the particular requirements of a site, or a particular study participant (e.g., based on gender, treatment, or severity of illness), by using skipping logic rather than sometimes complex instructions on a paper CRF.
- Avoiding CRF printing costs and time.
- Allowing the data collection system to be more easily modified, for instance, in the context of an adaptive trial.

By 2009, a Canadian study found 41% eRDC use for phase II–IV trials (El Emam et al. 2009), and anecdotal evidence suggests eRDC use has continued to rise considerably since then, with many units now only using eRDC for data collection. 42 of the 49 (86%) of the UK noncommercial trials units that applied for registration status in 2017, i.e., most of the university-based trials units in the country, explicitly mentioned using eRDC based systems, even if they did not always indicate they were using eRDC for every trial (personal communication, UKCRC, Leeds). Furthermore, empirical studies have now confirmed some of the benefits claimed for eRDC (Dillon et al. 2014; Blumenberg and Barros 2016; Fleischmann et al.

2017). Not all those benefits are relevant to single site studies, but even here the same systems can be used, albeit normally within an intranet environment.

The main disadvantage of eRDC is that it demands that a large group of staff, across the various clinical sites, are trained to use both the CDMS system and specific CDMAs, and there is a greater level of general user management. A user-initiated, automatic, "forgotten password?" facility in an eRDC system is a nontrivial feature of any CDMS, avoiding an otherwise inordinate amount of time spent managing requests to simply reenter the system.

Where paper-based trials are still run, they use essentially the same system for their data management, except that the CDMS's end users will be in-house data entry staff rather than clinical site staff. Paper-based trials are still used, for instance, in areas where internet access is patchy or unreliable, but eRDC is now the default workflow for collecting clinical site data. Participant questionnaires (e.g., on quality of life measures) have traditionally been collected on paper and then input centrally, though in recent years there has been much interest in replacing these with ePRO (electronic patient reported outcomes) systems, e.g., using smart phones, that can connect directly to a CDMS. A review is provided by Yeomans (2014), though some potential problems with ePRO, from a regulatory compliance perspective, are highlighted by Walker (2016).

Deployment Options and Implications

Traditionally, a CDMS would be installed and run directly by the trials unit or CRO, with hardware in server rooms within the trials unit's own premises or at least under their direct control. That scenario allows the unit to have complete control over their systems and infrastructure, making it much easier to ensure that everything is run according to specified procedures and that all staff understand the specialized requirements of clinical trials systems.

This can be a relatively expensive arrangement, however, and may not sit well with the centralizing tendencies of some larger organizations. It is also sometimes difficult to retain the specialist IT staff required. It has therefore become increasingly common to find the CDMS hosted in the central IT department of a hospital, university, or company. The trials unit staff still directly access the CDMS across the local network and can develop study definitions as well as oversee data management. They often also access and manage the linked databases, but data security, server updates, and other aspects of IT housekeeping are carried out by "central IT." The servers are provided as PaaS, or "platform as a service," i.e., they are set up to carry out designated functions, as database or web servers, and the customer, the department managing the trials, manages those functions (see Fig. 2).

This arrangement may be more efficient, but it does require that all parties are very clear about who does what and that clear communication channels are in place. From the point of view of trial management, the central IT department is an additional subcontractor supporting the trial. It shifts the day-to-day responsibility of many IT tasks (backups, server updates, firewall configuration, maintaining anti-

Fig. 2 A common PaaS eRDC architecture. The data is captured directly at the sites and transferred directly to a central CDMS. The trials unit (or CRO) manages that CDMS, including providing the study-specific definitions, though the system is embedded in an IT infrastructure managed by a central IT department, who provide the servers as "platforms as a service"

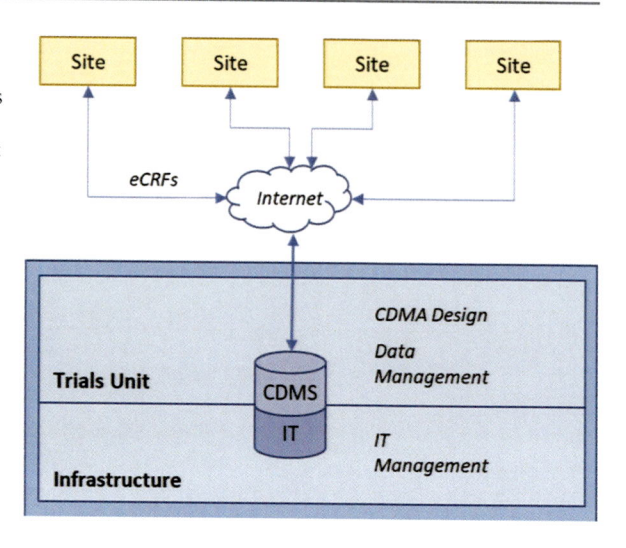

malware systems, user access control, etc.) out of the trials unit, but it does not change the fundamental responsibility of the unit, acting on behalf of the sponsor, to assure itself that those tasks are being carried out properly.

As stressed by the quality standards on data and IT management established by ECRIN, the European Clinical Research Infrastructure Network (ECRIN 2020), this oversight is not a "one-off" exercise – the requirement is for continuous monitoring and transparent reporting of changes (Canham et al. 2018). For example, trials unit staff do not need to know the details of how data is backed up but should receive regular reports on the success or otherwise of backup procedures. They do not need to know the details of how servers are kept up to date, or logical security maintained through firewalls, but they do need to be satisfied that these processes are happening, are controlled and documented, and that any issues (e.g., security breaches) are reported and dealt with appropriately.

This problem, of "quality management in the supply chain," becomes even more acute when considering the increasingly popular option of external CDMS hosting. In this scenario, the CDMS is managed by a completely different organization – most often the CDMS vendor. The trials unit staff now access the system remotely to carry out their study design and data management functions, with the external system presenting the CDMS to the unit as "software as a service" or SaaS. This scenario is popular with many system vendors, because it allows them to expand their business model beyond simple licensing to include hosting services, and in many cases offer additional consultancy services to help design and build study systems. It also means that they only have to support a single version of their product at any one time, which can reduce costs. In fact, some CDMS vendors now insist on this configuration, and only make their system available as SaaS.

But in many cases, the delegation chain is extended still further, as shown in Fig. 3, because the software vendor may not physically host the system on its own

Fig. 3 CDMS hosting by an external SaaS supplier. Three different organizations may be involved in supporting a study data system, with links mediated by the internet. Systems are physically located within a third-party data center, though the CDMS is managed by the software vendor. The trials unit, like the clinical sites, accesses the system via the internet

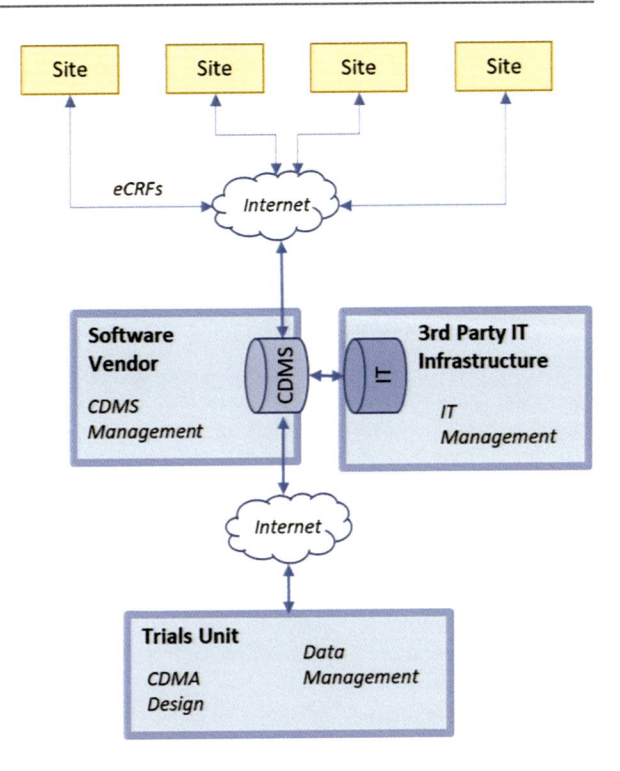

infrastructure. Instead it may make use of external IT infrastructure in a third-party data centre, or within one of the large commercial "cloud" infrastructures.

Using externally hosted systems has some advantages for trialists and trials units. For instance:

- It provides a very good way for trials units and CROs to experiment with different CDMSs, without the costs and demands of installing and validating them locally.
- The burden of validating the CDMS is transferred to the organization controlling its installation, usually the software vendor. The trials unit/CRO still needs to satisfy itself that such validation is adequate, but that is cheaper and quicker than doing it themselves.
- It empowers sponsors, who have greater ability to insist that a particular CDMS system is used, regardless of who is carrying out the data management.
- It removes any suspicion that the trials unit or CRO, and through them the sponsor, can secretly manipulate the data – data management is always through the CDMS' user interface, where all actions can be audited, and never by direct manipulation of the data in the database.

On the other hand, an externally hosted system can lead to difficulties in accessing and obtaining bulk data quickly (e.g., for analysis), and it can introduce substantial difficulties in maintaining quality control in what is now an extended supply chain. The trials unit is now dependent on the quality assurance processes and transparency of the CDMS provider, to make sure that not only the CDMS itself but also the IT provision is fit for purpose. A key point, if the CDMS provider uses a "cloud" infrastructure, is the need for the trials unit to be fully aware of exactly where the data, including the backup sets derived from it, is located. This will determine the legal jurisdiction that applies and dictate whether additional safeguards (e.g., Privacy Shield compliance in the USA for data on European citizens) need to be sought.

Contracts, information flows, and oversight processes need to be in place that ensure all users not only know that the CDMS is validated and secure, and continues to be through successive system changes, but are also aware of the underlying IT infrastructure, and are happy that the CDMS provider is itself carrying out proper oversight of that infrastructure. Too often, unfortunately, this is not happening. In 2018, the Inspectors Working Group of the European Medicines Agency listed a wide range of issues they had discovered in respect of subcontracted services, including:

- Missing or out-of-date contractual agreements
- Poor definition of the distribution of tasks
- Lack of understanding of the location of data
- A lack of understanding of GCP obligations by subcontractors
- Unwillingness to accept audits
- Poor understanding of reporting requirements
- Confusion over outputs and actions to be taken at the end of the trial

Sponsors, researchers, and trial teams, therefore, need to ensure that when functionality is subcontracted, these issues have been dealt with, so that they are confident that appropriate oversight is taking place all the way down the supply chain. This need not involve detailed scrutiny, but it does mean selecting and building up relationships and trust with a specialist trials unit or CRO, and being confident that they have not just good technical systems available but also a comprehensive quality management system in place.

Constructing the Study Definition

Overview

Whoever is managing and monitoring the CDMS and its underlying IT infrastructure, there is no doubt that the study-specific part of the study data system, the "study definition" or CDMA, is the responsibility of the study management team. The team aspect is important – even though the sponsor retains overall responsibility, successful development of a CDMA requires expertise and input from a wide variety of people: investigators, statisticians, study managers, data and IT staff, quality managers and site-based end users.

The process of creating a CDMA is summarized in Fig. 4. It has two distinct and clearly defined phases – development and validation – both of which involve iterative loops. The development phase takes the protocol and the data management plan as the main input documents and creates a full functional specification for the CDMA. It does so by organizing input from the various users of the system and consumers of the data, and iteratively developing the specification until all involved are happy that it will meet their requirements. Very often prototype systems are built against the developing specification to make the review process easier but, in any case, a system built to match the approved specification must be available at the end of the development phase. The validation phase takes that system and checks, systematically and in detail, that it does indeed match the agreed study definition. Once that check is complete, the CDMA can be released for use.

Both phases should be terminated by a formal and clearly documented approval process. At the end of the first, development, phase, all those involved in creating the specification should sign to indicate that they are happy with it – the result should therefore be a multidisciplinary and dated sign-off sheet for the specification. At the end of the second, validation, phase, someone (often a data manager or operational manager) needs to sign to indicate that the validation has been successfully completed and that the system can be released.

Working from the Protocol

CDMA development has to start with the study protocol, because that document specifies the key outcome and safety measures to be captured, implying the individual data points that need to be collected, and the assessment schedule that determines when the data should be collected.

One way to convert a protocol into a study definition would be to simply ask the investigator and/or statistician to specify the data points needed to carry out the required analyses, either by setting out a formal set of analysis data requirements, or more simply by annotating the protocol document. Perhaps because the time available to both investigators and statisticians is often limited, neither approach seems very common, though anecdotal evidence suggests that when it is used, it can be very effective. What often happens, in practice, is that experienced data management staff take the protocol and, sometimes using previous trials that have covered similar topics, construct either a spreadsheet with the data items listed, or mock paper CRFs, annotated with additional details such as the data item type or range limits for values, or – very often – both, with the spreadsheet providing more details than can be easily shown on an annotated paper form. These are then presented for review to the multidisciplinary study management team.

The use of mock paper CRFs is undoubtedly effective, not least because most people find it easier to review a paper CRF than a series of screens or a spreadsheet, especially in the context of a meeting. It can, however, increase the danger of

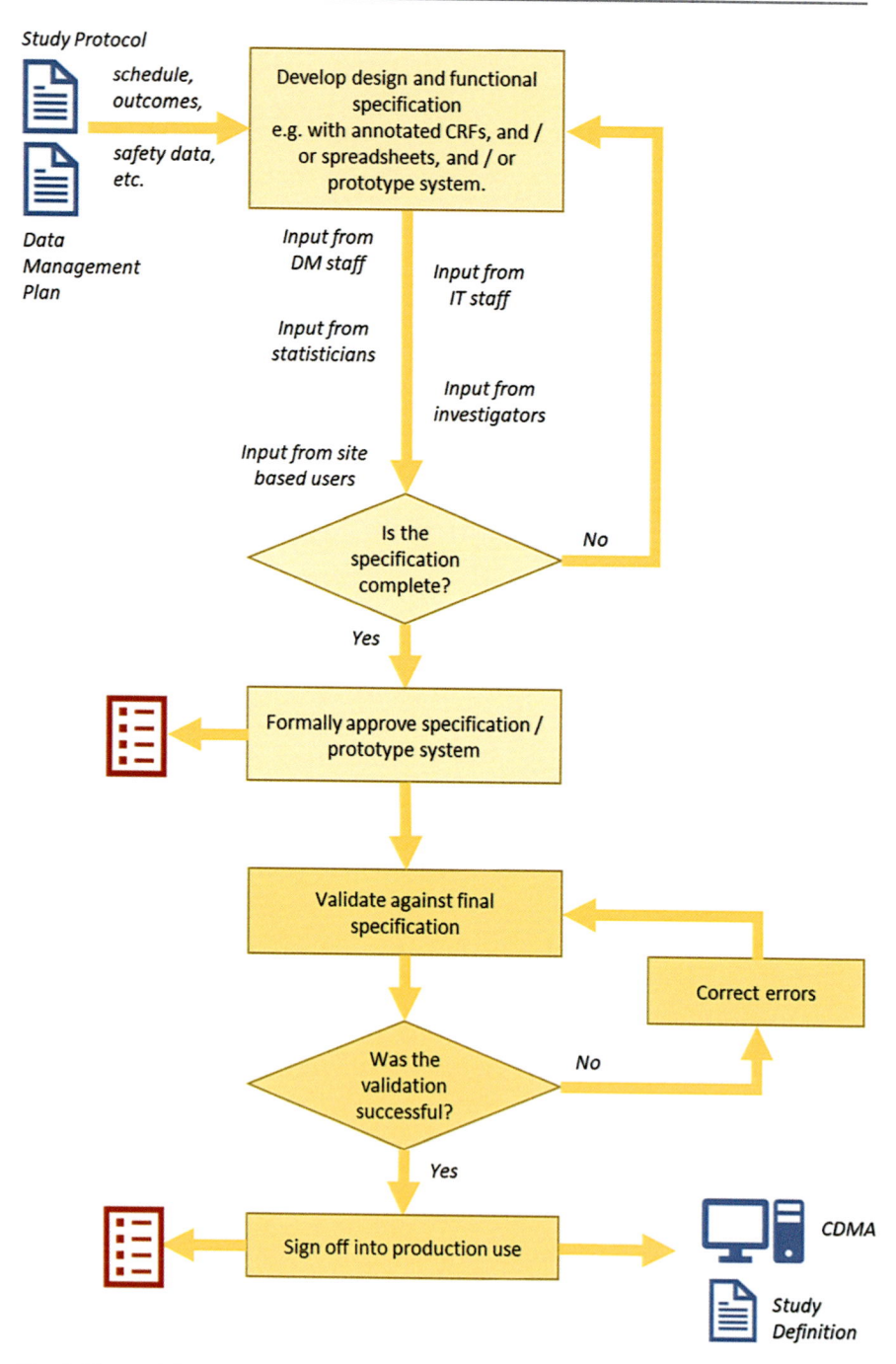

Fig. 4 The workflow for CDMA development. There are two iterative loops: the first, usually longer, results in the approval of a functional specification and the construction of a prototype system, and the second results in the approval of that system for production use once it has been validated. (Adapted from Canham et al. 2018)

collecting data that is not strictly required to answer the questions posed by a study, but which is included only because it was part of a previous, similar study, or because there is a vague feeling that it might be "possibly useful one day."

Collecting too much data in this way runs counter to *data minimization*, an important principle of good practice emphasized in the General Data Protection Regulations (GDPR) of the EU: "Personal data must be adequate, relevant and limited to what is necessary in relation to the purposes for which those data are processed" (GDPR Rec.39; Art. 5(1)(c)) (Eur-Lex 2020). At least within the EU, collecting unnecessary data may therefore be illegal as well as unethical.

There are circumstances where data can be legitimately collected for purposes other than answering the immediate research question – for instance, to obtain a disease-specific "core dataset," to be integrated with similar datasets from other sources in the future. But if that it is the case, it should be explicitly mentioned within study information sheets, so that a participant's consent is fully informed and encompasses the collection of such data.

One effective way of reducing the risk of collecting unused or unusable data is to ensure the study statistician reviews the CDMA's data points towards the end of the development process. Far better for spurious data points to be removed before the study begins, rather than being collected, checked, and queried, only for the statistician – after they receive the extracted dataset – to protest that they would never make use of that data.

A second document that feeds into CDMA design is the Data Management Plan, or DMP. All trials should have such a plan, either as a section within the Trial Master File (TMF) or as a separate document referenced from the TMF. Although a trials unit or CRO would be expected to have a set of generic SOPs covering different aspects of data management, there will almost always be study specific aspects of data management that need planning and recording, and these should be described within the DMP, which therefore forms part of the input to the design process.

A key aspect of study design is the balance between different methods of ensuring data quality. Modern CDMS can include sophisticated mechanisms for checking data, allowing complex and conditional comparisons between multiple data items on different eCRFs and study events, for instance, to check for consistency between visits, plausible changes in key values, and adherence to schedules. The fact that these complex checks can be designed, however, does not necessarily mean that they should always be implemented. The more complex a check, the more difficult it is to implement and the harder it is to validate. There is also a possibility that data entry may become over-interrupted, and take too long, if the system flags too many possible queries during the input process.

The alternative to checking data as it is input is to check it afterwards, by exporting the data and analyzing it using statistical scripts. For complex checks, this has several advantages:

- It usually allows simpler, more transparent design of the checks than the often convoluted syntax required within CDMS systems.
- It is easier for the checks to be reviewed, e.g., by another statistician, and validated.

- It gives the statisticians, as the consumers of the data, greater knowledge of and confidence in the checks that have been applied.
- Most importantly, it allows checks to be made *across* the study subject population, for instance, when identifying outliers (CDMS based checks can only usually be applied within a *single individual's* data).

The final point, coupled with the need for statistical monitoring to compare site performance (to help manage a risk based monitoring scheme), means that some level of "central statistical monitoring" of data quality is almost always required (an exploration of the use of central statistical monitoring is provided by Kirkwood et al. 2013). The question is how far it should be extended to include the checks that might otherwise be designed into the study definition. Clearly the availability of statistical resource to help design (if not necessarily run) the checks will influence the approach taken. There is also the issue that queries discovered using statistical methods need to be fed back into the CDMS system so that they can be transmitted to the sites, and few CDMS allow this to be done automatically. Whatever the decision of the study management team, it should be documented as part of the Data Management Plan and then taken into account during the development of the functional specification.

Working Up the Functional Specification

CDMA development needs to be a multidisciplinary, iterative process, as shown in Fig. 4. It will involve periodic reviews of the developing study definition, with data management staff adding and editing items after each review and then sending out updated documents. The staff involved in the process should always include, as a minimum, the coordinating investigator and the study statistician, as well as the trial's project manager, but can often also involve sponsor's representatives, quality assurance staff, data managers, IT staff, and a subsample of the end users for the system, the staff based at the clinical sites. Input from these different reviewers will be focused on different things and sought at different times, and different trials units will have different ways of coordinating the process and involving other groups around the core study team. That is not important as long as the goal of the development process – a full and approved functional specification for the CDMA – is met.

Many CDMS systems can generate detailed metadata of the systems they contain, including listing not just the study schedule and data items but also the details of derivations, skipping, and range and consistency checks that have been programmed into the study definition. Such data may be available as a set of standard reports, or it may be drawn directly from the database where the study definition is stored. This offers probably the most efficient way of developing a functional specification, which is to prototype it. After the initial specification has been created, by annotating the protocol or setting up mock paper CRFs, the IT and/or data management staff can create a first prototype of the CDMA within the CDMS. The prototype can then provide a detailed record of its own metadata, which is guaranteed to be an accurate representation of the developing system. This allows everyone involved in the review process to see the CDMA taking shape and inspect design elements like layout, colors, and prompts, as well as examining the more detailed specification generated by the system.

To be clear, this is not an "agile" development strategy, other than in the relatively minor sense that the visual layout of elements can be more easily negotiated. The user requirements for the system are fixed and are represented by the protocol and the context in which the CDMA will be delivered. Gradually building the CDMA by using a succession of prototypes simply offers an easier way for people to monitor development and check the specification is being interpreted correctly. It is more accurate and takes less work to document, than trying to use a paper specification on its own, but it should always be used in conjunction with review of the detailed metadata documents. In this approach, the final formal specification can be generated from the final version of the prototype.

If prototyping is not used, and the specification only exists on paper, then towards the end of the development phase, the system will need to be built from that specification, initially to allow end users to examine it (as part of the development phase, see the section below) and then, after any final changes, in order that it can be validated. Thus, even if working only from a document-based specification, the development phase should still end with an initial CDMA build.

"User Acceptance Testing"

The phrase "User Acceptance Testing" has been put into quotes to emphasize that it is such a misleading and potentially confusing phrase that it really should be avoided. There are three significant problems with the term:

- Different people refer to different groups as "users." IT staff often, but not consistently, refer to data management staff as the users, but the data management staff usually mean the end users of the system at the clinical sites.
- Whoever makes the final acceptance decision for a system, it is almost certainly not the users – it is more likely to be a sponsor's representative, the study project manager, or the unit's operational manager.
- Users, especially end users at the clinical site, rarely test anything. They may inspect and return useful feedback – about eCRF design, misleading captions, illogical ordering of data items, etc., but they can rarely be persuaded to systematically test a system, and one would not normally expect them to do so.

Having said all of that, "input from site-based users" can often be a useful thing to factor into the end of the development phase. The system obviously needs to be up and running and available to external staff, and system development should be in its final stages – there is little point in asking end users to comment on anything other than an almost completed system. Normally only a small subset of site-based staff should be asked to comment, drawn from those that can be expected to provide feedback in a timely fashion. Such feedback is best kept relatively informal – emails listing queries and the issues found are usually sufficient.

The decision to use end-user feedback should be risk based. A simple CDMA that is deployed only to sites that already have experience of very similar trials will have little or no need for additional feedback from end users. But a CDMA that includes novel features or patterns of data collection could benefit from site-user feedback. If new sites are being used for a trial, especially if they are from a different country or language group, then user feedback can be very informative in clarifying how the eCRFs will be interpreted and in identifying potential problems.

The key point is that this is late input into the *design and development phase* – it is not "testing." It is obtaining feedback from the final group of stakeholders. The difficulty that many trials units have is that they seek end-user feedback at the same time as beginning the testing and validation phase. They sign off the design as approved and start to test the system. Then feedback from end users arrives and results in changes (most commonly over design issues but more fundamental changes to data items may also be required) and then they have to start the testing again. The work, and its documentation, expands and risks becoming muddled. One of the basic principles of any validation exercise is that it must be against a fixed target – hence the need to garner all comments, from all stakeholders, and complete the entire design and development process before validation begins.

Final Approval of the Specification

As a quality control mechanism (and as evidence for external auditors), it is important to have a final sign-off from major stakeholders stating that they are happy with the final functional specification. This group should include as a minimum the chief or coordinating investigator, the study statistician, and the study's project manager. For commercially sponsored studies, a representative of the sponsor is also often included, and others (the QA officer, IT staff, data management staff) may be added according to local procedures.

Cross-disciplinary approval does not necessarily mean that all parties will check the specification for the same things. It is probably unreasonable to expect the chief investigator to look through every data item in detail, but they should at least be satisfied that the main outcome and safety measures are properly covered. As mentioned earlier, statisticians may be asked to check there is no unnecessary data being collected, as well as confirming that the collected data will be fit for their analysis. A trial manager will probably check the eCRFs in detail and confirm that feedback has been received from end users, while the unit's quality manager may also check for adherence to unit policies on CDMA design, use of coding systems, etc. Some of this assessment can be done by inspecting the system itself, but some of it will require checking of more detailed documents. The outcome of the approval process should be a suitably headed sheet bearing the required dated signatures.

Using Data Standards

One of the ways of making a study data system easier and quicker to develop, and of making the resulting system and the data exported from it easier to understand, is to establish conventions for the naming and coding of data items, and to stipulate particular "controlled vocabularies" in categorized responses. That can provide a consistency to the data items that can be useful for end users and a consistency to the data that can be useful for statisticians.

Consistency can be extended into a "house style" for the eCRFs, with a standard approach to orientation, colors, fonts, graphics, positioning, etc. (so far as the CDMS allows variation in these) and to the "headers" of the screens, that usually contain administrative rather than clinical data (e.g., study/visit/form name). This simply makes it easier for users to navigate through the system and more easily interpret each screen, and to transfer experience gained in one study to the next.

Establishing conventions for data items can provide greater consistency within a single trials unit, but at a time when there is increased pressure for clinical researchers to make data (suitably de-identified) available to others, the real value comes from making use of *global, internationally recognized* standards and conventions, which allow data to be compared and/or aggregated much more easily across studies.

Fortunately, a suite of such global standards already exists. These are the various standards developed by CDISC, the Clinical Data Interchange Standards Consortium. The key CDISC standards in this context are CDASH (CDISC 2020b), from the Clinical Data Acquisition Standards Harmonization project, and the TA or Therapeutic Area standards (CDISC 2020c). Both are currently used much more within the pharmaceutical industry than the noncommercial sector. The FDA, in the USA, and the PMDA, in Japan (though not yet the EMA in the EU), have stipulated that data submitted in pursuance of a marketing authorization must use CDISC's Study Data Tabulation Model (SDTM), a standard designed to provide a consistent structure to submission datasets. Creating SDTM structured data is far easier if the original data has been collected using CDASH, which is designed to support and map across to the submission standard.

Trials units in the noncommercial sector do not generally need to create and document SDTM files, and consequently have been less interested in using CDASH, although many academic units have experimented with using parts of the system. The system is relatively simple conceptually, but it is comprehensive and growing, and it does require an initial investment of time to appreciate the full breadth of data items that are available and how they can be used. The nature and use of data standards are treated in more detail in the chapter on the long-term management of data and secondary use. The key takeaway for now is that an evaluation of CDASH and its potential use within study designs is highly recommended.

Along with the CDISC standards and terminology, other "controlled vocabularies" can also help to standardize trial data. For the coding of adverse events and serious adverse events, the MedDRA system (MedDRA 2020) is a *de facto* standard. Drugs can also be classified in various ways, though the ATC (Anatomical

Therapeutic Chemical) scheme is the best known (WHO 2020). Other systems include the WHO's ICD for disease classification, and MESH and SNOMED CT for more general medical vocabularies, though in general, the larger the vocabulary system, the more difficult it is to both integrate it with a CDMS and ensure that staff can use it accurately.

MedDRA is the most widely used of all these systems and is, for example, mandated for serious adverse event reporting in the EU. Its effective use requires training, however, and a variety of study specific decisions need to be considered and documented (in the DMP). For instance, what version of MedDRA should be used (the system is updated twice a year) and how should upgrades, if applied, be managed? How should composite adverse event reports ("vomiting and diarrhea," "head cold and coughing") be coded? Probably most critically, which of the higher order categories, used for summarizing and reporting the adverse events, should be used when categorizing lower level terms? MedDRA is not a simple hierarchy, and a lower level term can often be classified in different ways. A "hot flush" (or "flash") can be related to the menopause, hyperthyroidism, opioid withdrawal, anxiety, and TB, among other things – so how should it be classified? The answer will normally depend on the trial and the participant population, but where there is possible ambiguity, a documented decision needs to be taken, so coding staff have the required guidance. Such ambiguity is also the reason why MedDRA auto-coding systems should be treated with caution, unless they can be configured or overridden when necessary.

Validating the Specification and Final Release

Once the functional specification has been approved, the prototype that has been built upon it needs to be validated. During the build, or during successive prototypes if that has been the approach taken, the basic functionality will have been tested by the staff creating the system, but this is normally an informal process and unlikely to have been documented. Validation, in contrast, requires a systematic, detailed, and documented approach to testing all aspects of the system. It is intended to verify that:

- The build has been implemented correctly – i.e., that it matches the specification, and is therefore fit for purpose.
- The detailed logic built into the system, e.g., the consistency checks between data items, or the production of derived values, works as expected.

Validation of a study definition is therefore essentially a *test and debugging* exercise. By default, validation should mean that all elements and all logic in the system are tested. That includes ensuring data types, captions, tab order, and code lists are all correct for each data item, and also systematically checking the skipping logic, derivation logic, and each of the data validation (range and consistency) checks.

Validation can therefore be a rather tedious, mechanical exercise, for example, when "walking through" each range limit check (inputting values just under the limit, at the limit and just above) to ensure that the system fires a warning message when appropriate and accepts a valid value without complaint. It may therefore be carried out by relatively junior staff, which is fine if the specification and any additional instructions are clear and there is sufficient supervision. Validation should *not* be carried out by anyone that constructed the system, because any misinterpretations of the original requirements will simply be repeated. In some cases, the data managers for the study are asked to carry out the validation exercise. This has the advantage that if they were not very familiar with the details of the system before they certainly will be after the exercise is completed, but it may not be the best use of skilled staff time.

The default validation strategy should be described in an SOP, but study-specific decisions may alter that strategy in any particular case. For instance, it may be decided to skip some checks if they have already been covered earlier. A check that a date entered is not in the future is a condition commonly applied to date data. If the date questions have been copied from a common precursor (most CDMS allow data items to be copied and pasted during the design process) that already included this test, it does not necessarily need to be checked for all the derived date items. Similarly, an eCRF representing a questionnaire, imported from another study where it had been used and tested previously, may not need such a detailed checking as a completely novel eCRF. Conversely, some CDMAs will require additional testing for functionality (like coding, or message triggering) that is specific to a study definition. The individual managing the validation process, e.g., the trial manager, should make risk-based decisions about the detailed strategy to be followed and document the justification for them (for example in the DMP).

Another approach to CDMA validation involves completing dummy paper CRFs, inputting them into the CDMA, and then exporting them again in a form that is readily comparable with the original data. This has the advantage of testing overall system usability as well as many of the functional components of the system, and also means that the extraction/reporting functions are tested as well. Unfortunately, unless a very large set of test data is prepared, not all components of the system will be tested in a systematic way. If used, this method should therefore probably be seen as an addition to the detailed testing of each component described above.

The bugs found in the exercise and their resolution should be documented, usually by the record of the relevant retests. At the end of the exercise, it should be possible to show the system does indeed meet its functional specification, and the validation should then be signed off. The signatures or initials of those who were actually doing the validation should be embedded in the test documents themselves. The sign off needs to be done by whoever is responsible for releasing the system into production, usually the manager responsible for the validation process, such as the trial's project manager, or the unit's quality or operations manager, who are in a position to judge that the validation has been successfully completed.

Development and Testing Environments

Systems used for CDMA development and those used for CDMA production use should be isolated from each other. Development and production environments have very different user groups and (assuming there is no real data in the development/test environment) different security requirements. The system should be developed on machines specifically reserved for development and testing, and there should be no possibility, however unlikely, of any problems in a developing CDMA spilling over to affect any production system. Similarly, there should be no possibility of users, including IT staff, inadvertently confusing development and production systems. This allows the production servers to be kept in as simple and as "clean" a state as possible, unencumbered by additional versions of the same study system, making their management easier and providing additional reassurance that their validation status is being maintained (see Fig. 5).

With the virtual machines that are now commonly used, "isolated from" means logically isolated rather than necessarily on different physical hardware. That means distinct URLs for the web-based components, distinct connection strings for database servers, and different users and access control regimes on the different types of server. It is also a good idea if development systems can be clearly marked as such on screen (e.g., by the use of different colors and labels).

Note that if end-user input is required, so also is remote access to the development and test system. In some IT infrastructures, this may be problematic and necessitate a separate, third, testing environment, specifically for external access to a copy of the developing system. This environment could therefore be used for the final stage of system development, but once this was complete and the specification approved, it would also be the obvious place in which to carry out validation.

This "Final Development" environment can also be useful for training purposes – giving external users access to the fully validated system so that they can familiarize themselves with it. Site-based users may want to input real data into the system during this training phase, one reason why it should be under the same tight access control within the IT infrastructure as the production system. The other benefit of a secure testing/training environment is that the system can also be used for "backfill" of data during revalidation exercises, as described in more detail in the section "Change Management."

Figure 5 illustrates such a combination of systems, but it is stressed that it is only an example of many possible ways of arranging development, test, and production environments. The optimum will depend on the server, security, and access options available. If the initial development environment can handle external users, then the A and B environments can be merged into one, as long as the possibility of that environment having sensitive personal data in it is fully considered.

It is possible to support training on a production server, by setting up a dummy site within that system and initially only giving site-based users access to that site. This can be simpler to manage than using a separate system, and it ensures that the

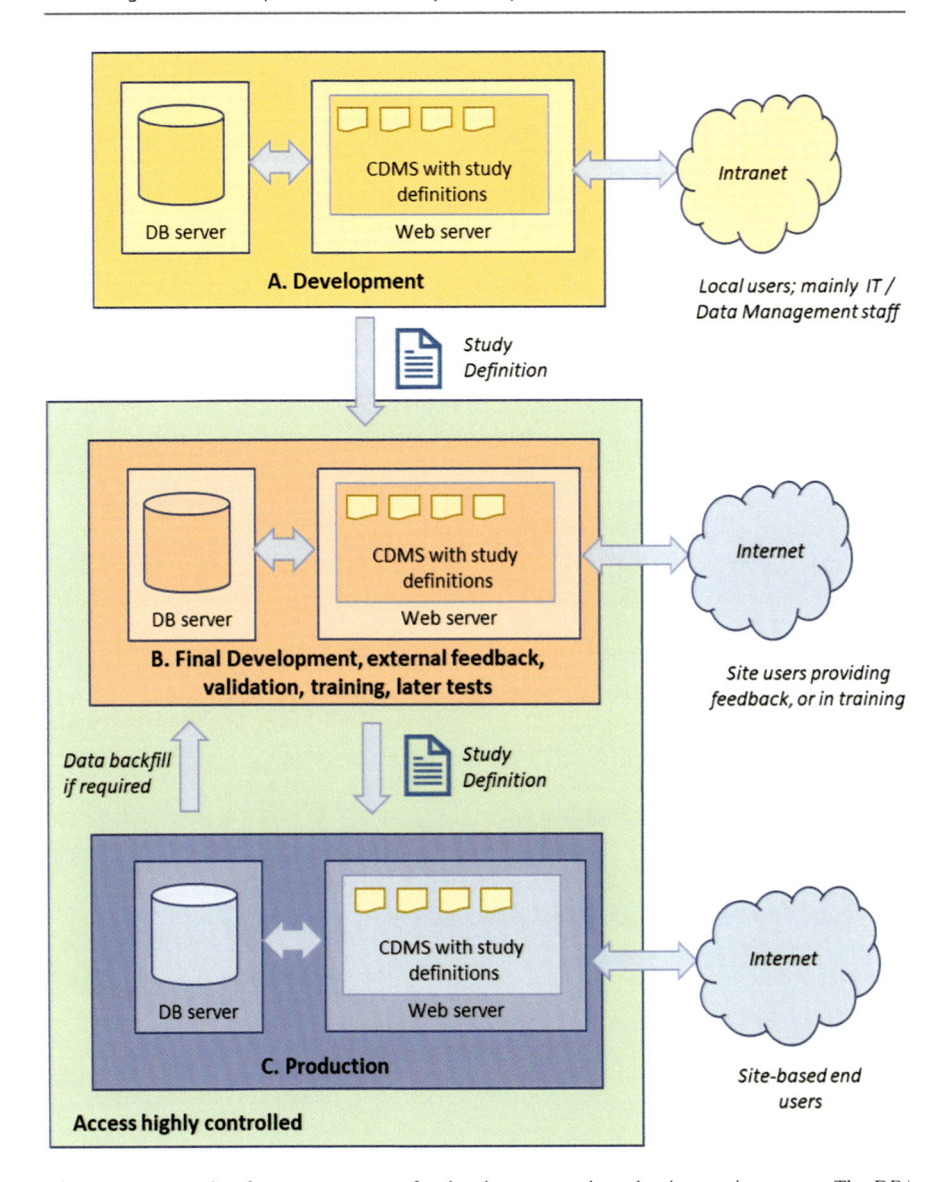

Fig. 5 An example of one arrangement for development and production environments. The DB/web server combination in A is used for most of the development process but never contains any real data. The test environment in B can be linked to external users and is used to complete development. It can also support validation and later testing when backfill with real data may be useful. C is the "clean" production environment. Both B and C have tightly controlled access

training system will exactly match the production system's definition. It has the disadvantage, however, that all the data from the training "site" need to be excluded from the analysis dataset (during or after the extraction process).

The Study Data System in the Longer Term

Change Management

Once the CDMA's final specification has been approved, any further changes to that specification will need to be considered within a formal change management process, to ensure that all stakeholders are aware of proposed changes and can comment on them, and that the changes are validated.

Any request for a change in the system should therefore be properly described and authorized, so a paper or screen-based proforma needs to be available, to be completed with the necessary specification and justification for the change. Changes may be relatively trivial (a question caption clarified) or substantial (additional eCRFs following a protocol amendment). Whoever initiates the change process, staff should be delegated to assess the possible impacts of the change and identify any risks that might be associated with it.

Risk-based assessment is the key to change management. The easiest way of handling and documenting that process is to use a checklist that considers the common types of potential impact. These can include:

- *Impact on data currently in the database.* Any change that dropped a data item or a category from the system and "orphaned" existing data would not normally be allowed and should be rejected. In fact, many CDMS would automatically block such a change, though many do allow a field to be hidden or skipped within the user interface.
  Other changes may have less obvious consequences. For instance, if new options are added to a drop-down to give a more accurate set of choices to the user, does the existing data need to be reclassified? If so, how and by whom?
- *Impact on validation checks and status.* If a new consistency test is added, how can the existing data be tested against it? If a new data item is added, does it need new consistency checks to be run against other data? Detailed mechanisms are likely to be system dependent but need to be considered and the resulting actions planned.
- *Impact on data extraction.* In many cases, extraction will use built-in automatic mechanisms, but if any processing/scripts are used within the extraction process, will they be affected by the change? If additional fields are added, will that data appear in the extracted datasets?
- *Impact on metadata.* A metadata file, or at least a "data dictionary," should always be available, for instance, to support analysis. Any change will render the current metadata out-of-date and require the production of a new version.
- *Impact on analysis.* If the statistician has already rehearsed aspects of analysis and has the relevant scripts prepared, how will any additional data items be included? Will any hidden, unnecessary fields still be processed?
  For example, changing an item's data type could make existing data invalid and is not normally allowed, or even possible in many CDMSs. If it transpires that an integer field needs to hold fractional values, and thus must be changed into a real

number field, it may therefore be necessary to add a new real field and hide or skip the original integer one. The database ends up with two fields holding data for the same variable, meaning that the statistician needs to combine them during the analysis.

- *Impact on site-based end users.* The staff inputting the data need to be informed of any change and its implications. When and how?
- *Impacts on system documentation and training.* For substantial changes, simply informing end users is unlikely to be enough. Study-specific documentation and training may need also need changing.

Considering possible risks in this systematic way provides a solid basis for identifying and documenting the possible sequelae of a proposed change, deciding if the change should be allowed and, if it is allowed, identifying the follow-on actions that will be required. Those actions are likely to include testing of the revised system, with the test results documented and retained. It also means that the change management process needs to involve statisticians as well as trial managers, and the IT and/or data management staff who usually implement the change. The key staff involved should explicitly "sign-off" the change.

Substantial system changes often result from protocol amendments and cannot be released into the production version of the system until those amendments have been fully approved. It can sometimes happen, though it is relatively rare, that a requested change implies a change in the protocol, even when it has not been presented or recognized as such. This is another reason for the change management process to include review by experienced staff (usually the trial manager and statistician), or even the whole trial management team, to ensure that any need for protocol amendment is recognized and acted upon before the change is implemented. In other words, change management should never be seen as a purely technical process.

Implementation of any change should always occur in *all* the environments being used – i.e., in the development environment, in any intermediate test and training environment, and finally in the production system. The flow of changes should be unidirectional, with in each case a revised study definition exported to the destination system. It can be tempting, for a trivial change, to shortcut this process and just (for example) change a caption in the production system. But this then risks being over-written back to the previous version, when, following a more substantial change elsewhere in the system, a new study definition is imported from the development environment.

The testing required will occur in the development and any test system. For some changes, it may be considered more realistic, and therefore safer, to test against the whole volume of existing data, rather than just the small amount of dummy data that usually exists within development environments. Backfilling the test/development server, or at least one of them if there are multiple development environments, with the current set of real data can therefore be a useful way of checking the impact of changes on the current system. This does depend, however, on the test server having a similar level of access control as the production system, otherwise there is a risk that sensitive personal data is exposed more widely than it should be, and that nonspecialist staff are unfairly exposed to sensitive data.

A coherent and consistent versioning system can help to support any change management process. All versions of the study definition should be clearly labelled and differentiated, for instance, by adapting the three part "semantic versioning" system used for software (Semver 2020). In this scheme,

- The specification as finally approved should be version 1.0.0 (while versions in development are 0.x.y).
- Changes that involve a protocol amendment should increment the first number.
- Changes that are not protocol amendments, but which include changes to the data in any way (including changes to the options available to categorized items), should increment the second number.
- Changes that do not include changes to the data – e.g., changes in presentation or to the logic checks used – should change only the third number.

Changing a study definition, even within a well-managed system, is an expensive process that can carry risks. All stakeholders need to be aware of that and so minimize the changes they request. The best way to do that is by the rigorous and collective development of an initial specification that accurately meets the needs of the study.

Exporting the Data for Analysis

At the end of a trial, the data needs to be extracted for analysis, usually in a generic format (csv files, CDISC ODM) or one tailored to a particular statistical package (e. g., SAS, Stata, SPSS or R). Because most statistics packages can read csv or similar text files, the ability to generate such files accurately is the key requirement.

Data extractions can take place before this of course, e.g., for interim safety analysis by a data monitoring committee, for central statistical monitoring, and to support risk-based monitoring decisions. In the noncommercial sector, trials may also be extended into long-term follow-up, so that data is periodically extracted and analyzed long after the primary analysis has been done and the associated papers published.

The extraction process, especially when supplying data for the main analysis, needs to be controlled and documented. An SOP should be in place outlining roles, responsibilities, and the records required, often supported by a checklist that can be used to document the readiness of the database for extraction. The checklist should confirm that:

- All data is complete, or explicitly marked as not available.
- Outstanding queries are resolved.
- All data coding is completed (if done within the CDMS).
- All planned monitoring and source data verification has been completed.

- All data has been signed off as correct by the principal investigators at sites.
- Serious adverse event data (transmitted via expedited reporting) has been reconciled with the same data transmitted through standard data collection using eCRFs.

Any exceptions to any of the above should be documented. Most CDMS include a "lock" facility which prevents data being added or edited, and this can be applied at different levels of granularity, e.g., from an individual eCRF, to a whole participant, to a clinical site, to the whole study. Once the issues listed above have been checked, one would expect the entire database to be locked (with any later amendments to the data rigorously controlled by an unlocking/relocking procedure which clearly explained why the data amendments were necessary).

The extraction process results in a series of files, with traditionally the data items in each file matching a source eCRF, or a repeating question group within a CRF. Although the data appears to be directly derived from the eCRFs, the extraction usually requires a major transformation of the data, because in most cases, the data is stored quite differently within the CDMS database. Internally most systems use what is called an entity-attribute-value (EAV) model, with one data row for each data item, and often with all the data, from all subjects, visits, and eCRFs, stored in the same table.

The EAV structure is necessary to efficiently capture the audit data that is a regulatory requirement, to more easily support various data management functions like querying, and to provide the flexibility that enables a single system to store the data from different studies, each with a wide variety of eCRF designs. It is almost never evident to the end users, who instead see the data points neatly arranged within each eCRF, the system consulting the relevant study definition to construct the screen and place the data items within it as required.

When the data is extracted, the audit and status data for each item is usually left behind, and the data is completely restructured as a table per eCRF or repeating group as described above. This underlines the need for the *validation* of data extraction, because not only is the output data central to the research, the process by which it is created is complex. Extraction mechanisms will usually be tested within the initial validation of the CDMS, but this often involves just a very small data load from a simple test CDMA. Extractions from real CDMAs should undergo a risk-based assessment of the need for additional, study specific, validation. The validation does not usually need to be extensive or burdensome, but it is worth checking (and documenting) that, for instance:

- The number of extracted study participants is correct.
- The data for the first and last participants appears correct (because extraction issues tend to affect the edges of data sets).
- Dates have retained their correct format.
- The correct version of (examples of) corrected data is extracted.
- Fields with any unusual (e.g., non-Latin) characters have been extracted properly.

As more extractions are performed and checked, the level of confidence in the system will grow, and the need for validation can become less, especially if a trial is similar in design to a previously extracted study. But if a CDMS update is applied, the risk may increase again and so should the inspection of the extracted data.

Once the data has been extracted, it is often combined with data from other sources, for example:

- From collaborators: Although sometimes such data may be imported into the CDMS, more often it will be imported by aggregating extracted records. Care must be taken that the extractions are fully compatible.
- From treatment allocation records: Up to this point, this data may have been kept separately to preserve blinding.
- From laboratories: It is usually simpler to add data from external laboratories at this stage rather than trying to import it into the CDMS, but this is a study-specific decision, and may depend on lab preference and the need to carry out range and consistency checks on the data.
- From coding tools, because in some trials units and CROs, coding is done on the extracted data rather than within the CDMS.

Exactly how this data is aggregated with that from the CDMS should be planned and documented within the data management plan. It is important that a description of the newly combined data is included within the metadata documents for the study, so in these cases, if metadata is normally generated by the CDMS, it will need to be supplemented by additional documents.

The final analysis dataset, comprising the data from the CDMS and any additional material integrated with it, needs to be safely retained. This is partly for audit or inspection purposes, and partly to allow the reconstruction of any analysis using the same extracted data, if that is ever required. In practice, it can be done by adding the analysis dataset, in a folder, clearly labelled and date stamped according to an agreed convention, into a read-only area of the local file system. A group (usually the IT staff, who are deemed to be uninterested in the data content) has to have write privileges on this area for the data to be loaded, but all other users, including the statisticians who need to analyze the data, must take copies of the files if they wish to work on them.

Though obviously not part of the CDMS, the procedures and infrastructure required to implement the safe storage of the output data, so it is protected from accidental modification, as well as any suspicion of intentional edit, are an important part of the total study data system. They form the final link in the chain that begins with the study protocol, stretches through system design, definition, and testing, moves on to months or years of data collection, with maximization of data quality, and finally ends with the primary function of the system – the delivery of data for analysis.

Summary and Conclusion

A study data system is centered around a specialist software tool – the Clinical Data Management System or CDMS – that provides the core functionality required to guarantee the regulatory compliance of data collection, plus the flexibility needed to support a wide range of different study designs and data requirements. CDMSs or, increasingly, externally hosted CDMS services, are usually purchased from specialist vendors. The CDMS is the core component but by no means the only one: supporting sub-systems, e.g., for coding, file storage, backup, and metadata production, may also be involved. The "system" also includes the competences of the staff that operate it and, crucially, the set of policies and procedures that govern workflow. It is these policies, more than the technical infrastructure, which determine the quality of any study data system.

Procedures are especially important for supporting the workflows around developing and then validating the systems constructed for individual studies, ensuring that these activities are done in a consistent, clear, reliable, and well-documented fashion. They are also key to the systematic consideration and application of (for example) data standards, systems for managing data quality, procedures for change management, import and aggregation of externally derived data, preparation for data extraction, and the extraction process itself.

The data flow of modern study data systems is now dominated by a web-based approach (eRDC) that removes the need to install anything at the clinical site or provide additional hardware, as was the case in the past. Over the last 20 years, eRDC has almost entirely supplanted traditional paper based data transfer. There is growing interest in extending this approach directly to the study participants, to capture directly from them using smart phones or portable monitoring devices. The major current trend in study data systems, however, is the growing use of externally hosted systems, so that the coordinating center or trials unit, as well as the clinical sites, access the system through the internet. This approach can bring greater flexibility and reduced costs, but it carries potential risks, for example, around communication, responsiveness, and quality control. Developing the technical and procedural mechanisms to better manage these risks is one of the biggest challenges facing vendors and users of study data systems today.

Key Facts

1. The core software component of any study data system is a specialist tool known as a Clinical Data Management System, or CDMS, usually purchased on a commercial basis.
2. A web-based data management workflow known as eRDC, for electronic remote data capture, is used in the great majority of clinical studies.
3. It should be noted that the data system also consists, in addition to the CDMS software, of the people managing it and the policies and procedures that govern workflows and data flows.
4. Increasingly, study data systems are provided remotely, as "software as a service" or SaaS.
5. SaaS offers advantages (e.g., reduced system validation load) but can carry risks. A range of communication problems have been identified in SaaS environments.

6. A trials unit retains the overall responsibilities for safe, secure, and regulatory compliant data management, as delegated from the sponsor, even when some of the functions involved are subcontracted to other agencies. Its quality management strategy therefore needs to include mechanisms for monitoring the work of these subcontractors.
7. Developing a successful study data system for any specific study requires a clear separation between the development of a detailed specification for the required system, requiring input and agreement from all important stakeholders, and a second validation step, requiring detailed, systematic testing of the completed system.
8. The use of data standards can reduce system development time and increase the potential scientific value of the data produced.
9. The production version of the study data systems should be maintained separately from the development and/or training versions of the same systems, and be accessed using different parameters.
10. Proposed changes in the study data system need to be managed using a clear and consistent risk-based change management system.

Cross-References

▶ Data Capture, Data Management, and Quality Control; Single Versus Multicenter Trials
▶ Documentation: Essential Documents and Standard Operating Procedures
▶ Long-Term Management of Data and Secondary Use
▶ Patient-Reported Outcomes
▶ Responsibilities and Management of the Clinical Coordinating Center

References

Blumenberg C, Barros A (2016) Electronic data collection in epidemiological research, the use of REDCap in the Pelotas birth cohorts. Appl Clin Inform 7(3):672–681. https://doi.org/10.4338/ACI-2016-02-RA-0028. https://www.ncbi.nlm.nih.gov/pmc/articles/PMC5052541/. Accessed 31 May 2020

Canham S, Bernalte Gasco A, Crocombe W et al (2018) Requirements for certification of ECRIN data centres, with explanation and elaboration of standards, version 4.0. https://zenodo.org/record/1240941#.Wzi3mPZZFw-U. Accessed 31 May 2020

Capterra (2020) Clinical trial management software. https://www.capterra.com/clinical-trial-management-software. Accessed 31 May 2020

CDISC (2020a) The operational data model (ODM) – XML. https://www.cdisc.org/standards/data-exchange/odm. Accessed 31 May 2020

CDISC (2020b) Clinical data acquisition standards harmonization (CDASH). https://www.cdisc.org/standards/foundational/cdash. Accessed 31 May 2020

CDISC (2020c) Therapeutic area standards. https://www.cdisc.org/standards/therapeutic-areas. Accessed 31 May 2020

Dillon D, Pirie F, Rice S, Pomilla C, Sandhu M, Motala A, Young E, African Partnership for Chronic Disease Research (APCDR) (2014) Open-source electronic data capture system offered increased accuracy and cost-effectiveness compared with paper methods in Africa. J Clin Epidemiol 67(12):1358–1363. https://doi.org/10.1016/j.jclinepi.2014.06.012. https://www.ncbi.nlm.nih.gov/pmc/articles/PMC4271740/. Accessed 31 May 2020

ECRIN (2020) The European Clinical Research Infrastructure Network. http://ecrin.org/. Accessed 31 May 2020

El Emam K, Jonker E, Sampson M, Krleža-Jerić K, Neisa A (2009) The use of electronic data capture tools in clinical trials: web-survey of 259 Canadian trials. J Med Internet Res 11(1):e8. https://doi.org/10.2196/jmir.1120. http://www.jmir.org/2009/1/e8/. Accessed 31 May 2020

Eur-Lex (2020) The general data protection regulation. http://eur-lex.europa.eu/legal-content/en/TXT/?uri=CELEX%3A32016R0679. Accessed 31 May 2020

Fleischmann R, Decker A, Kraft A, Mai K, Schmidt S (2017) Mobile electronic versus paper case report forms in clinical trials: a randomized controlled trial. BMC Med Res Methodol 17:153. https://doi.org/10.1186/s12874-017-0429-y. Published online 2017 Dec 1. https://www.ncbi.nlm.nih.gov/pmc/articles/PMC5709849/. Accessed 31 May 2020

Green J (2003) Realising the value proposition of EDC. Innovations in clinical trials. September 2003. 12–15. http://www.iptonline.com/articles/public/ICTTWO12NoPrint.pdf. Accessed 31 May 2020

Kirkwood A, Cox T, Hackshaw A (2013) Application of methods for central statistical monitoring in clinical trials. Clin Trials 10:703–806. https://doi.org/10.1177/1740774513494504. https://journals.sagepub.com/doi/10.1177/1740774513494504. Accessed 31 May 2020

MedDRA (2020) Medical dictionary for regulatory activities. https://www.meddra.org/. Accessed 31 May 2020

Mitchel J, You J, Lau A, Kim YJ (2001) Paper vs web, a tale of three trials. Applied clinical trials, August 2001. https://www.targethealth.com/resources/paper-vs-web-a-tale-of-three-trials. Accessed 31 May 2020

OpenClinica (2020). https://www.openclinica.com/. Accessed 31 May 2020

RedCap (2020). https://www.project-redcap.org/. Accessed 31 May 2020

Semver (2020) Semantic versioning 2.0.0. https://semver.org/. Accessed 31 May 2020

Walker P (2016) ePRO – An inspector's perspective. MHRA Inspectorate blog, 7 July 2016. https://mhrainspectorate.blog.gov.uk/2016/07/07/epro-an-inspectors-perspective/. Accessed 31 May 2020

WHO (2020) The anatomical therapeutic chemical classification system, structure and principles. https://www.whocc.no/atc/structure_and_principles/. Accessed 31 May 2020

Yeomans A (2014) The future of ePRO platforms. Applied clinical trials, 28 Jan 2014. http://www.appliedclinicaltrialsonline.com/future-epro-platforms?pageID=1. Accessed 31 May 2020

Implementing the Trial Protocol

14

Jamie B. Oughton and Amanda Lilley-Kelly

Contents

J. B. Oughton (✉) · A. Lilley-Kelly
Clinical Trials Research Unit, Leeds Institute of Clinical Trials Research, University of Leeds, Leeds, UK
e-mail: J.Oughton@leeds.ac.uk; A.C.Lilley-Kelly@leeds.ac.uk

© Springer Nature Switzerland AG 2022
S. Piantadosi, C. L. Meinert (eds.), *Principles and Practice of Clinical Trials*,
https://doi.org/10.1007/978-3-319-52636-2_37

Abstract

This chapter outlines the steps required to bring a protocol to life as a clinical trial. Developing the protocol is a multidisciplinary effort which must be approached in an ordered and logical way with clear leadership. Poor site feasibility is a common reason for trial failure when performed badly and is crucial to capture a generalizable population. The key site feasibility assessment issues are outlined. The chapter goes on to give advice on data collection and how this should be planned alongside developing the trial protocol. Trial processes must be adequately described and trial staff trained well to maximize efficiency and minimize error. Strategies to identify and mitigate risks to participant safety and trial integrity are discussed along with techniques that can be implemented to monitor the identified risks. Typical trial oversight groups and processes are provided to reach a structure that is effective and proportionate to the level of trial risk. Finally, suggestions for how to manage trial promotion to maximize engagement with investigators, potential participants and other stakeholders are discussed.

Keywords

Protocol · Feasibility · Monitoring · Oversight · Publicity · Training program · Competency

Introduction

This chapter attempts to bridge the gap between the finalized protocol and patient accrual. It outlines necessary considerations for identifying and selecting participating centers to optimize trial delivery. Similarly, it covers the vital task of risk assessment and monitoring and the establishment of effective oversight bodies. Finally, the topic of trial promotion is discussed, with suggestions based on the needs and resources of a trial.

Protocol Development

The protocol is the most important document in a clinical trial and sufficient time and expertise must be allocated to its development. The nature of the trial will dictate which specialties will contribute but typically this will include: clinical, regulatory, laboratory, statistical, operations, funder, and safety. A member of the coordinating team, for example, the project manager, should take responsibility for making sure each party has reviewed the protocol at the appropriate development stage. Omissions or mistakes can be costly in time taken making amendments and therefore it is useful to obtain a final review from a member outside of the immediate trial team.

The most appropriate protocol structure must be chosen at the start of development. For example, is it reasonable to contain all the required information in one protocol or should there be separate sub-protocols underneath a master protocol? In a platform trial (Park et al. 2019), for example, it is common to describe platform-wide processes in a master protocol and processes that only exist in certain groups of participants in a separate sub-protocol.

Site Selection, Feasibility, and Set Up

At an early stage of the development of a clinical trial, a decision must be made on the scale of the trial. Single-site trials have the advantage of being easier and cheaper to set up and a Chief Investigator (the person responsible for leading the clinical trial) can effectively oversee the entire trial conduct. However, single-site trials may return results that are less generalizable, are less free from systematic bias, and limit the number of available participants. Multisite trials reduce the impact of bias, improve generalizability, and allow access to increased number of participants. The loss of control in comparison with a single-site trial can be overcome with trial oversight strategies. Multisite trials require significantly more resources: both financial and staffing. International participation may also be desirable due to the rarity of the target condition, scarcity of equipment or to accelerate recruitment.

Every clinical trial requires a legal entity to be responsible for trial conduct. This legal entity is known as the sponsor. The sponsor is able to delegate responsibilities to other institutions to carry out the trial; for example, a contract research organization or academic coordinating center to develop the protocol or a participating hospital to collect the data.

Site Characteristics

Investigators can overstate their capabilities to secure opening a desirable trial, particularly with regards to recruitment projections. If there are more sites available than required to conduct the trial, site selection criteria should be developed. If the coordinating center has worked with the site before, suitability can be assessed from past performance (e.g., set up time, recruitment, data quality). Alternatively, self-assessment by the site using a questionnaire has the advantage of discovering an investigators commitment to the trial and collecting updated information. Often it can be helpful to request objective data to support a recruitment target. For example, by asking the site to review the last month's clinic list and count the number of patients with the target disease. The site should also provide the coordinating center with evidence of staff who are qualified and who have any additional appropriate training. This is usually achieved by reviewing copies of CV/resumes or training certificates. It may be necessary to request the completion of a questionnaire to address trial-specific issues; for example, where relevant, questions could include:

Is the investigator familiar with the proposed intervention?
Are there any competing trials open at that site?

Is there a facility to accommodate an overnight stay?
Is there a facility to prepare drugs under aseptic conditions?
Is it possible to review a CT scan and provide the report within 1 week?
Are there sufficient staff to facilitate the data collection?

The site must have sufficient staff (e.g., trial coordinators, research nurses, data managers, trial pharmacists) to deliver the trial. For some trials, it may be appropriate to recruit additional staff and time must be allowed for this. There must be sufficient enthusiasm from management and the site investigators for the trial to succeed. Sponsors should be sensitive to the motivations of a site to participate in research, be they prestige, financial, or patient-driven. Where there are likely to be barriers to set up or recruitment (for example, excess treatment costs in the UK), these should be highlighted by the coordinating center at an early stage in set up and addressed with appropriate guidance and mitigation.

For international trials, a range of issues may become relevant. Is the treatment environment (e.g., political, financial, or environment) likely to remain stable during the lifetime of the trial? Are there factors that will limit the delivery of a trial? For example, there are financial incentives towards hospital-based interventions in the United States or lack of refrigeration facilities in some settings for a vaccine trial. International trials also bring significant complexities due to multiple regulatory requirements; for example, in the United States, each recruiting institution may require separate ethics approval, although there has been a recent change for trials sponsored by the National Institutes of Health (NIH) where single IRBs are encouraged/required. More detailed information on setting up international trials is available elsewhere (Minisman et al. 2012; Croft 2020).

Timing of Site Activation

Once the sites have been selected, there needs to be a systematic approach to site set up based on the resource available. It may be necessary to take a phased approach rather than seeking to open all sites at the same time. This is often necessary because of finite resources to complete all necessary tasks, e.g., on-site training, intervention availability, or temporary low capacity at site.

It is important for sponsors and trial management teams to keep up to date and engage with such schemes for prompt set up. For example, in England, the Health Research Authority (HRA) made changes to the way research is initiated in the National Health Service (NHS). The approach now is that the HRA give permission on behalf of the NHS, potentially making it faster for individual hospitals to participate.

Trial-wide approvals from the ethics committee and/or regulatory authority must have been received before a site is permitted to start recruiting participants. Sponsors must have a robust process to ensure both site level and trial level approvals have all been received.

Registration/Randomization System

For a randomized controlled trial, it is crucial to present a transparent, robust, and reproducible technique to allocate participants to treatment groups. Most commonly this is via an automated telephone- or web-based service that can be accessed directly by participating sites. Access is restricted to sites that have been approved for the trial and staff that have undergone the required training. Alternatively, a paper-based randomization system could serve the same purpose.

Data Collection

All trials require a robust system for collecting the data in a format that is transparent and suitable for the analysis. Clinical trial data is almost always collated in an electronic database nowadays, and many trials also use electronic data capture systems to collect data from participating sites. It is necessary to have a firm idea of the data items required before developing the database, and this usually begins once the protocol has been finalized. The data collection process should be mapped out from the source data to the final analysis. The source of the data will dictate the format of data collection tools. For example, laboratory results can occasionally be provided electronically as a table to the sponsor, whereas a physical examination may require a paper/electronic form to report the result. The complexity of the database will be dictated by the sources of data and risk assessment. The database and data collection instruments should be finalized and fully tested before opening to recruitment.

Training

A key part of ensuring successful delivery of a trial is a clear training program to support the protocol. When developing a training program, there are many elements to consider, with initial focus on the target of the training – who will implement the protocol, and within which teams do they work?

It is essential to consider the structure of the team required to deliver the protocol, what expertise they have, and which elements of the study they will support. To do this, it is best to consider each element of trial delivery, usually summarized in a trial flow diagram (Fig. 1). The trial flow will determine which team members will support specific activities; for example, will a medic be required to identify potential participants and support the consent process, or will a research nurse carry out the screening and recruitment process? It is also important to consider the administration involved in all trial activities, for example, will a member of the trial team produce recruitment packs, request patient notes, screen participant admissions, and complete general administration activities or will a research nurse complete these tasks?

It is also important to determine research-specific training requirements. Are the team members delivering the project well versed in research, or are there basic

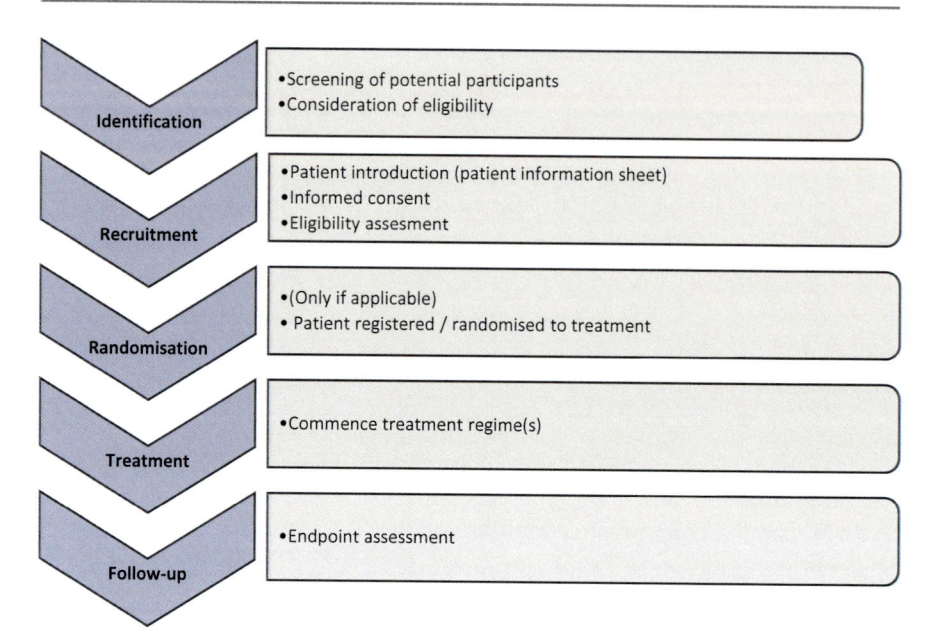

Fig. 1 Flow diagram showing the stages of a clinical trial (Collett et al. 2017)

principles that need to be covered to ensure the trial is conducted appropriately? For example, will the research team include clinical disciplines that are not often involved in clinical research, such as allied health professionals (e.g., paramedics, radiotherapists, or dieticians)? If so, should the training include an overview of Good Clinical Practice (GCP) to underpin their participation in trial activities?

Dependent upon the trial, there may also be a need to consider additional training requirements relevant to the trial population. For example, if participants will be recruited from an older population that may have a high incidence of cognitive impairment, it is important to provide an overview of any local legislation governing participants with limited cognitive capacity and the process of informed consent within a vulnerable population. Establishing expertise required is essential to the development of the content of training; however, it is important to be mindful of existing training programs available – balancing trial requirements with practicalities. It is often best practice to direct researchers to additional sources of information that can cover complex topics in greater detail than required for specific trials.

Once the team delivering the trial and the expertise and knowledge required has been defined, the content and structure of the training program can be developed. A key consideration for the content of the training is the time available to support training – how long will it take for each member of the team to be properly trained in their elements of the trial? If the trial involves frontline clinical staff, there may be a need to adapt training to accommodate other commitments. If there is a large team of clinicians that would like to train together, what is an acceptable / practicable duration? These considerations need to be balanced with the key components of

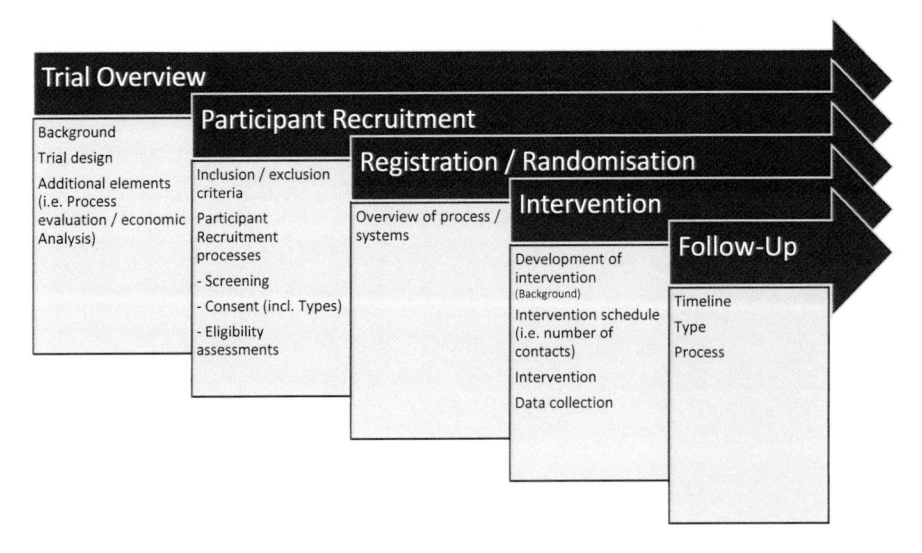

Fig. 2 Overview of training schedule

training, ensuring that topics are covered in order of priority, being mindful of the logical flow of information and the burden of training on the target audience.

To establish a logical flow of information, it is often best to link back to considerations of key trial elements (Fig. 2) and the relevant information around these topics. An example of these and associated topics to include are outlined in Fig. 2 – these broad topics should be tailored to include trial specifics and time allocated dependent on content. It is also important to consider the expertise required within the training team to deliver these sessions, potentially using changes in trainer as natural breaks to avoid audience burden. The content of training often evolves as the program develops, and it is beneficial to gain input from the wider trial team to review content as it develops.

Methods of delivery for the training should be considered during development of the training content, taking the audience and amenities available. Often a slideshow is developed that can be adaptable for presentations where facilities exist or as preprinted handouts if not. However, other options include online presentations that could be delivered remotely (i.e., webinars/video blogs) and which also have the added benefit of being reusable and readily available.

As part of the training program, materials need to be developed to support training. For example, training slides, reference data collection instruments specific to the trial, trial promotional materials, and site-specific documentation (i.e., Investigator Site File – ISF). Training development also often highlights procedures that are more complex and require additional supporting information to ensure standardized completion throughout the trial, in the form of a guidance manual or standard operating procedure (SOP) with these materials provided as part of the training pack.

Once the training package is developed, it is important to consider how attendance at training will be documented, and how robust this process needs to be. A list of attendees should be generated if attending in person or a system developed to monitor access to online training materials for self-training. In some situations, local investigator oversight of staff of listed on an Approved Personnel List (APL) may be sufficient. It is essential to have an audit trail of staff training and a clearly defined and reproducible training package to support the trial delivery. These training records should be retained for the duration of the trial, even if personnel change over time.

It is also essential to consider the on-going training and competency of site staff delivering the trial – how are new staff sufficiently trained in a timely manner? Often on-going training is trial specific and dependent upon things like trial design (i.e., number of sites/geographical location/duration), complexity of the trial (i.e., trial design and intervention delivery), and the impact of poor performance (i.e., maximizing competency of site staff to deliver an intervention). It may therefore be necessary to consider how to assess staff competency and identify additional training requirements for key elements of the trial. An example would be monitoring completion of key data collection instruments to highlight errors and disseminate feedback to the site and wider trial team. Additional methods to support sharing of best practice include regular teleconferences with trial teams, discussion boards, newsletters, and social media. However, the team needs to be mindful of site burden and consider the impact and benefits of these methods for site staff.

Risk and Monitoring

By their very nature, clinical trials contain an element of uncertainty. It is important that investigators identify any significant risks before commencing a trial protocol and develop effective strategies to mitigate such risks. The lowest risk trials contain interventions that are already licensed and used as part of standard care and the highest risk trials assess unlicensed interventions that are often earlier in the development pathway.

In an attempt to stratify risks in noncommercial trials, Brosteanu et al. (2009) developed the risk categories shown in Table 1.

The imminent European Union (EU) Clinical Trials Regulation No 356/2014 includes scope for central monitoring for low-intervention trials (EU Commission 2014). In the UK, the Medicines and Healthcare products Regulatory Agency

Table 1 Risk stratification in noncommercial trials. (Adapted from the Brosteanu article)

Trial categories based on associated risk		Examples of types of clinical trials
Type A:	No higher than the risk of standard medical care	Trials involving licensed products or off-label use if this use is established practice
Type B	Somewhat higher than the risk of standard medical care	Trials involving licensed products if they are used for a different indication, for a substantial dosage modification or in combinations where interactions are suspected
Type C	Markedly higher that the risk of standard medical care	Trials involving unlicensed products

already permits different approaches based on the level of risk inherent in an interventional drug trial (MHRA 2011). Risk adaptions can be made to the requirements for the original application and review process, drug labelling, drug accountability, and safety surveillance. The lowest risk trials can sometimes benefit from expedited regulatory approval.

Trial Risk Assessment

For every trial, there must be an attempt to identify the potential hazards and an assessment of the likelihood of those hazards occurring and resulting in harm. Risks fall into two main categories: those that affect patient safety and those that affect the integrity of the trial. Appropriate control measures should be documented for each risk. It may be appropriate to include key elements of the risk assessment as part of the trial protocol so that all stakeholders are fully informed. Key risks to participants should be explained in the patient information or consent form. The risks described in the patient information should be presented in the context of the disease and standard treatment. Generally only risks that are common (between 1/1 and 1/100) or thought to be particularly serious should be detailed in the patient information. Patient groups are valuable to ensure patient information is appropriate and directed towards the needs of patients.

Trial Monitoring Plan

The risk assessment should then be used to develop the trial monitoring plan. The level of monitoring will depend upon the level of risk and the resources available. Monitoring falls into two categories: on-site source data verification and central monitoring. Pivotal trials that will be used as evidence to support a marketing application and phase I trials will usually contain substantial on-site monitoring, whereas an interventional trial evaluating two interventions already used in standard care or where endpoints can be collected centrally from routine data may require none. On-site monitoring should be complemented by centralized monitoring, where the sponsor or delegate is provided with source data by the site (e.g., the laboratory or imaging reports) in order to validate key endpoints.

On-site monitoring can be separated again into two categories: planned visits and triggered visits.

Planned Monitoring Visits

Planned monitoring visits are usually scheduled to occur at key points of risk or vital data collection time points. For example, the monitoring plan may require a visit 1 week after the first drug dose in order to evaluate the appropriate reporting of adverse events or that the pre-dose assessments have been carried out correctly. Visits can be weighted in favor of the interventions that have greater risk or sites with the least experience.

Table 2 Example of triggered monitoring visit parameters

	Low (1)	Medium (2)	High (3)
Serious adverse event reporting	Within timelines	1 SAE outside of timelines	>1 SAE outside of timelines
Overall case report form compliance	>90%	70–90%	<70%
Recruitment	80–100% of target	50–79% of target	>50% of target
Problem data items	<1%	1–20%	>20%
Protocol violations	No violations	1 violation	>1 violation
Key personnel	No changes	Change to research nurse or other key staff in last 6 months	Change to investigator or high staff turnover in the last 6 months

Triggered Monitoring Visits

Before commencing a trial, it may be helpful to establish a list of parameters and a severity score, which collectively can highlight sites for a triggered monitoring visit. An example is presented in Table 2.

Each site is periodically scored and then ranked. The seriousness of any problems is weighted within the score (1 point for low and 3 points for high). Sites with the highest scores will pass the threshold for a triggered monitoring visit. Other options are available to address issues, such as suspending recruitment, but this method is a useful tool to identify sites that need extra support and monitoring. There is a risk of high percentages due to low denominators, rather than risky data. To prevent unnecessary action, consider setting a minimum threshold under which action will not be taken.

A comprehensive procedure for developing the monitoring plan has been published by others (Brosteanu et al. 2009), but recent evaluations suggest such procedures should be supplemented by centralized checking (von Niederhausern et al. 2017).

Trial Oversight

It is vital to establish appropriate oversight processes prior to opening to recruitment. The standard oversight groups for supervising a clinical trial are outlined here. The conventional oversight structure described below may be adapted in line with the level of trial risk, as discussed earlier. A phase I trial would convene more frequent oversight meetings than a phase IV observational trial. Responsibilities of the oversight groups should be decided and outlined in the protocol and group terms of reference. For a large research group, it may be efficient to review similar trials at the same meeting (i.e., review multiple trials using the same committee).

Project Team

The staff responsible for carrying out the day-to-day management of the trial should meet to review key performance indicators from accumulating data. The group would usually include the data manager, on-site monitor, trial manager, statistician/methodologist, and team leader.

Trial Management Group (TMG)

The TMG consists of the project team with the addition of the clinical investigators, patient representatives, and sub-study collaborators with the objective of reviewing a higher level summary than the project team meetings. As the TMG is made up of the staff running or leading the trial, it is not independent.

Independent Data Monitoring Committee (IDMC)

The IDMC periodically reviews accumulating summaries of data with the purpose of intervening in the interests of trial participants. Unlike the project team or the TMG, the IDMC may review data presented by study arm. The group consists of disease-specific experts and statisticians experienced with the trial design, none of whom have any involvement in delivering the actual trial.

To avoid any uncertainty, it is recommended that the trial team/sponsor prepare explicit guidelines outlining how the IDMC should operate (Sydes et al. 2004b). The use of an IDMC should be briefly described in the trial results. Notably only 18% of 662 RCTs in a review done in 2000 did so (Sydes et al. 2004a). However, this is likely to have improved substantially over the last 17 years with the advent of initiatives, such as CONSORT (Hopewell et al. 2008) which aim to standardize reporting.

Independent Trial Steering Committee (TSC)

The purpose of the TSC is to take advice from the IDMC and make key decisions for the trial. The TSC usually has the power to terminate the trial or require other actions to protect participants.

The Medical Research Council in the UK has published guidelines for appropriate oversight structures (MRC 2017), and a recent survey has suggested widespread compliance with academic trials units in the UK (Conroy et al. 2015). Members of the independent groups should generally not be involved with the trial

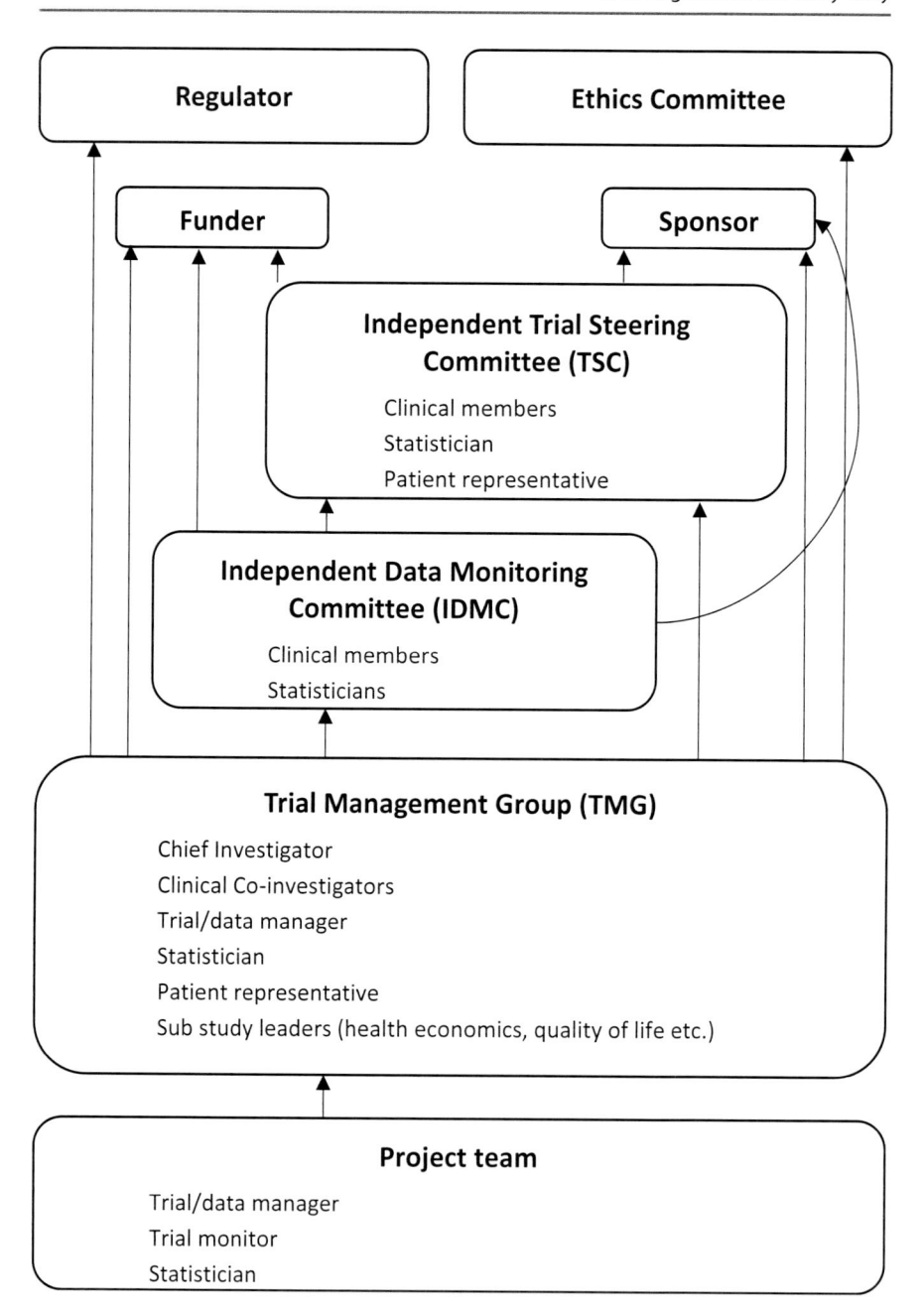

Fig. 3 Example trial oversight structure

in any way, be from outside the investigator's institution and ideally have an excellent knowledge of the relevant disease area. For large multisite trials, it may be necessary to consider international colleagues or those recently retired from practice (Fig. 3).

Trial Promotion

At the start of a project, and throughout delivery, it is important to consider the end impact of the results. Trial publicity and dissemination of information is essential to support publication in high-impact journals and ensure future research for patient benefit. The trial team, including any oversight committees, should develop a promotional strategy, which could include a schedule of press releases to support key milestones (i.e., launch/participant recruitment/analysis) disseminated by organizations associated with the trial (i.e., co-applicants/charitable organizations/disease-specific groups).

Large multisite trials often develop a brand identity. This starts with having a trial name that is an accessible shorthand for everyone to refer to the research trial quickly and easily. Trials with acronyms were more likely to be cited than those without (Stanbrook et al. 2006). Convention dictates that the name is an acronym using the letters from the trial's full title, ideally with some link to the subject area, though this is not essential. Others have written about what can be humorously known as acronymogenesis (Fallowfield and Jenkins 2002; Cheng 2006) but essentially avoid anything that could discourage potential patients (e.g., RAZOR) or that could be perceived as coercive (e.g., HOPE, LIFE, SAVED, CURE, IMPROVED).

Following the trial acronym is often the trial logo. Those with access to a graphic designer can have more elaborate designs but the trial acronym in a special font may be sufficient emphasis. A couple of examples of trial logos are displayed below in Figs. 4 and 5.

Trial Website

A trial website is a helpful way for people to access trial information. This can be targeted towards investigators, with password protection as required, and/or towards

Fig. 4 Example of trial logo

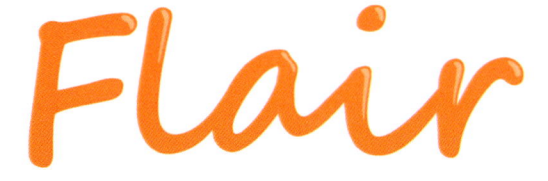

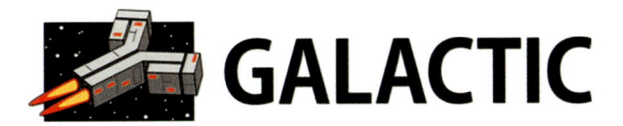

Fig. 5 Example of trial logo (Oughton et al. 2017) (N.B. that this was an antibody trial, hence the shape of the spacecraft)

patients to encourage interested patients to volunteer for the trial and/or an alternative means of providing information. It is very common for patients who have been invited into the trial to do their own internet research, so it is important that any online publicly available information compliment patient materials, such as the patient information sheet. Websites have more flexibility in methods for presenting the information than a paper information sheet. The website can aid the dissemination of the results to participants by linking to published results or lay summaries of the findings. An exemplar of good practice in this area can be found for the INTERVAL blood donation frequency study (University of Cambridge 2017; Moore et al. 2014). Websites can be a vital channel of communication for sites, patients, and the media. Contents of official websites may need to have to be approved by an Ethics Committee/Institutional Review Board depending on local requirements.

With appropriate access controls, there are potential gains to be made from having trial documents accessible to investigators via the website. The website can provide a link to remote data capture systems and online registration/randomization services. Training videos can be hosted from the website for investigators as can participant questionnaires.

Social Media

The use of social media has increased over the last two decades. Patients frequently use the internet and social media as a primary source of information. Patient support groups often have a significant online presence, with forums to facilitate discussions about a wide variety of topics. Some patients even blog about their experience as trial participants.

Some have expressed concern that there is potential to compromise the integrity of clinical trials. However, a review of more than one million online posts found that discussions of active clinical trials were rare and no discussions were identified that risked unblinding of clinical trials (Merinopoulou et al. 2015). The authors go on to recommend basic training for trial participants on the risks of social media discussions and also that sponsors should consider periodic monitoring of social media content.

There is the potential that participants may disclose adverse events on social media that would otherwise be unreported. A systematic review (Golder et al. 2015) review found that adverse events are identifiable within social media and that mild and symptom-related adverse events are overrepresented online when compared with traditional data sources, or perhaps alternatively that the lower end of side effects are underrepresented in trial reporting. Undoubtedly, pharmaceutical companies are working to develop tools to aggregate social media data, but at present, this approach is still in its infancy. There is currently only a regulatory responsibility to report events that are reported to a sponsor/Marketing Authorization Holder rather than to actively seek out events online. An active approach would also be confounded by the difficulty in matching a report to a specific research participant and there would be ethical issues of perceived intrusive monitoring.

Press

To accomplish wider reach, a press release for either regional or national news outlets could be considered. To maximize the chances of the story being published, it may be helpful to include a patient interest angle. For example, a trial patient that has done well in the phase I trial and is now excited that the trial has expanded to phase II. Photographs or willingness to be photographed/interviewed are key to success. Permission for the press release must be obtained from all those involved and an institution's press office will often be able to provide support. If the press release is directed towards recruiting patients, the relevant trial ethics committee should give approval beforehand.

Investigator Meeting

Investigator meetings are useful to provide information about the trial, to foster a collective commitment to the trial aims, and as a way of recognizing investigator's commitment. They are often timed to occur before recruitment commences but can also be valuable during the lifetime of the trial to provide updates or to help publicize the results. The organization and resources required to host an investigator meeting are significant, and it is therefore important to consider carefully what goals and achievements are important for the meeting and to select an appropriate venue. Costs can be minimized by holding investigator meetings alongside scientific conferences where investigators are already likely to attend.

Summary and Conclusion

Effective implementation of a clinical trial protocol requires the execution of the tasks described in this section. Careful attention to protocol implementation will maximize the likelihood of delivering an efficient and successful trial.

Key Facts

- A structured approach to identifying and selecting participating sites will translate to optimal participant accrual.
- The requirements of the trial must be communicated to participating investigators and staff in a format that meets their needs.
- Risks in a trial must be identified and mitigated using a proportionate monitoring program.
- A clear and effective oversight structure is necessary to ensure the interests of participants and funders are protected.
- Promotional strategies can optimize participant recruitment and retention.

Cross-References

▶ Centers Participating in Multicenter Trials
▶ Documentation: Essential Documents and Standard Operating Procedures
▶ Pragmatic Randomized Trials Using Claims or Electronic Health Record Data
▶ Principles of Protocol Development
▶ Qualifications of the Research Staff
▶ Selection of Study Centers and Investigators
▶ Trial Organization and Governance

References

Brosteanu O et al (2009) Risk analysis and risk adapted on-site monitoring in noncommercial clinical trials. Clin Trials 6(6):585–596

Cheng TO (2006) Some trial acronyms using famous artists' names such as MICHELANGELO, MATISSE, PICASSO, and REMBRANDT are not true acronyms at all. Am J Cardiol 98 (2):276–277

Collett L et al (2017) Assessment of ibrutinib plus rituximab in front-line CLL (FLAIR trial): study protocol for a phase III randomised controlled trial. Trials 18(1):387

Conroy EJ et al (2015) Trial Steering Committees in randomised controlled trials: a survey of registered clinical trials units to establish current practice and experiences. Clin Trials 12 (6):664–676

Croft J. International surgical trials toolkit. cited 2020. Available from: https://internationaltrialstoolkit.co.uk/

European Commission (2014) Risk proportionate approaches in clinical trials-recommendations of the expert group on clinical trials for the implementation of regulation (EU) no 536/2014 on clinical trials on medicinal products for human use. 2014 08/08/17. Available from: http://ec.europa.eu/health/files/clinicaltrials/2016_06_pc_guidelines/gl_4_consult.pdf

Fallowfield L, Jenkins V (2002) Acronymic trials: the good, the bad, and the coercive. Lancet 360 (9346):1622

Golder S, Norman G, Loke YK (2015) Systematic review on the prevalence, frequency and comparative value of adverse events data in social media. Br J Clin Pharmacol 80(4):878–888

Hopewell S et al (2008) CONSORT for reporting randomised trials in journal and conference abstracts. Lancet 371(9609):281–283

Merinopoulou E et al (2015) Lets talk! Is chatter on social media amongst participants compromising clinical trials? Value Health 18(7):A724–A724

MHRA (2011) Risk-adapted approaches to the management of clinical trials of Investigational Medicinal Products Ad-hoc Working Group and the Risk-Stratification Sub-Group. 2011. cited 2019. Available from: https://assets.publishing.service.gov.uk/government/uploads/system/uploads/attachment_data/file/343677/Risk-adapted_approaches_to_the_management_of_clinical_trials_of_investigational_medicinal_products.pdf

Minisman G et al (2012) Implementing clinical trials on an international platform: challenges and perspectives. J Neurol Sci 313(1–2):1–6

Moore C et al (2014) The INTERVAL trial to determine whether intervals between blood donations can be safely and acceptably decreased to optimise blood supply: study protocol for a randomised controlled trial. Trials 15:363

MRC Guidelines for Management of Global Health Trials Involving Clinical or Public Health Interventions. Medical Research Council (2017) https://mrc.ukri.org/documents/pdf/guidelines-for-management-of-global-health-trials/

Oughton JB et al (2017) GA101 (obinutuzumab) monocLonal Antibody as Consolidation Therapy in CLL (GALACTIC) trial: study protocol for a phase II/III randomised controlled trial. Trials 18:1–12

Park JJH et al (2019) Systematic review of basket trials, umbrella trials, and platform trials: a landscapanalysis of master protocols. Trials 20(1):572

Stanbrook MB, Austin PC, Redelmeier DA (2006) Acronym-named randomized trials in medicine – the ART in medicine study. N Engl J Med 355(1):101–102

Sydes MR et al (2004a) Systematic qualitative review of the literature on data monitoring committees for randomized controlled trials. Clin Trials 1(1):60–79

Sydes MR et al (2004b) Reported use of data monitoring committees in the main published reports of randomized controlled trials: a cross-sectional study. Clin Trials 1(1):48–59

University of Cambridge (2017) Interval study website 2017. Available from: http://www.intervalstudy.org.uk/

von Niederhausern B et al (2017) Generating evidence on a risk-based monitoring approach in the academic setting – lessons learned. BMC Med Res Methodol 17(1):26

Participant Recruitment, Screening, and Enrollment

15

Pascale Wermuth

Contents

P. Wermuth (✉)
Basel, Switzerland
e-mail: pascale.wermuth@intergga.ch

© Springer Nature Switzerland AG 2022
S. Piantadosi, C. L. Meinert (eds.), *Principles and Practice of Clinical Trials*,
https://doi.org/10.1007/978-3-319-52636-2_38

Abstract

Participant recruitment and retention are key success factors in a clinical trial. Failure to enroll the required number of participants in a timely manner can have significant impact on trial budget and timelines, and data gaps due to under-recruitment or early dropout of participants may lead to misinterpretation or unreliability of trial results.

Prior to the start of a trial, a thorough recruitment plan should be set up, considering the screen failure rate, the potential need to replace early dropouts, and the geographical distribution of participants, timelines, and budgetary constraints. Understanding how to calculate the recruitment rate based on the number of enrolled participants per site per month will help in assessing the probability of successful recruitment. In addition, recruitment planning tools and services such as comparison with benchmarking data from analogous historical or ongoing trials, simulation tools, and specialist service agencies may support the setup of a robust recruitment plan. Risk factors with the potential of leading to under-recruitment, over-recruitment, or recruitment of unsuitable participants should be identified upfront to allow risk mitigation as far as possible, e.g., through protocol amendments or increasing the number of participating centers. Evaluation of the most appropriate channels to identify and contact trial candidates will ensure optimal turnout in relation to the financial and resource investments. Strategies for participant screening, enrollment, and retention are reviewed in this chapter.

Keywords

Recruitment · Recruitment plan · Screening · Enrollment · Recruitment rate · Retention · Benchmarking · Simulation · Recruitment issues

Introduction

Once the design of a clinical trial has been defined and the final trial protocol has received all required approvals, after participating centers have been set up and trained appropriately, and when all trial supplies (including study drug) are available, the trial is ready to start being populated with participants.

Studies conducted on metadata or on data obtained from local or national registries do not require the active involvement of any individuals, and recruitment as such will not be needed for these studies. However, most studies, interventional and non-interventional, require the identification and enrollment of individual trial participants, carefully selected according to trial-specific eligibility criteria, to allow collection of relevant data that will address the objective of the trial. Failure to get the right participants enrolled into a trial, or to retain participants in the trial, may have significant impact on the quality of the trial results, as reliability and power of the trial outcome may decrease (Little et al. 2012). Likewise, failure to enroll within an appropriate time frame can have significant impact on the trial budget if additional costs and resources are required to bring recruitment back on track and, in the case of new therapies being investigated, can cause costly delays in time to market for these therapies. Consequently, planning for successful recruitment and participant retention will need to start at the very beginning of the conceptualization of a clinical trial.

This chapter looks into the details of recruitment including planning tools such as benchmarking and simulation, highlighting the various challenges that are so often experienced in recruitment and how to avoid them, and how to identify candidates for a trial. It also describes methods that can be applied to support the accrual of participants and their retention in the trial until its completion. For further reading refer to Anderson (2001), Bachenheimer and Brescia (2017) and Friedman et al. (2015).

Definitions

Recruitment

Describes the overall process from the point of identifying a candidate for a clinical trial (either a volunteer or a person diagnosed with the disease or condition under investigation), through the steps of obtaining their informed and written consent and verifying their eligibility ("screening"), up to the candidate's inclusion into the clinical trial (including randomization and/or treatment assignment where applicable).

Consenting

Describes the process of informing a candidate of the specifics of the clinical trial (including the objectives of the trial, potential benefits and risks, the assessments and procedures involved and their impact on the participant, and the participant's rights and responsibilities) and of obtaining the candidate's (or their legal representative's) consent to collect personal data and biological samples and to analyze and publish the derived data. This process is mandatory according to ICH GCP E6(R1).

Screening

Describes the process of ensuring an identified candidate meets all trial inclusion and exclusion criteria, including obtaining written consent and confirmation of the candidate's willingness and ability to adhere to the trial requirements. Screening assessments requiring any type of intervention not considered routine procedure or standard of care can only be performed after a participant's consent has been obtained. Candidates not meeting *all* of the eligibility criteria are considered *screen failures* and cannot be enrolled into the trial.

- The terms *pre-screening* or *pre-identification* can be used to describe the process of identifying potential candidates from sources such as registries or medical records of investigational sites, without necessarily directly contacting the candidates. This may be applicable in trials with small numbers of highly selected participants, in which screening slots are assigned to participating sites.
- The term *rescreening* is used when trial candidates who fail one or several eligibility criteria at a given time point are reconsidered for participation at a later time point (e.g., after successfully addressing the eligibility criteria previously not met), where and as allowed by the trial protocol.

Enrollment

Enrollment is the process of actually including an individual into the trial after their identification and verification that all trial-specific eligibility criteria are met. This can include randomization and/or treatment assignment where applicable and usually marks the point from which on data can be collected (both pro- and retrospectively). The number of enrolled participants typically does not include screen-failed individuals, but will include participants that drop out of the trial for any reason at any time after enrollment (Fig. 1).

Planning Recruitment

During the conduct of clinical trials, recruitment has shown to be a common challenge, with estimates of up to 80% of trials facing recruitment issues. Therefore, setting up a recruitment plan including thorough investigation of the trial landscape and detailed scenario and risk mitigation planning is key for successful recruitment. See e.g. Thoma et al. (2010).

A recruitment plan should describe the assumptions used for calculations and simulations, the planned budget, and, importantly, the risk mitigation and issue management plans for the trial. These should include pre-defined trigger points for escalation steps to be kicked off, and a detailed action and communication plan for escalation, should recruitment issues occur during the trial. For multinational and multicenter trials, setting up recruitment plans on country and/or site level will help identify and address potential recruitment issues with high granularity, allowing targeted and individualized mitigation or escalation. Also, recruitment plans should be adapted on an ongoing basis as changes occur to the trial (e.g., protocol amendments), the environment (e.g., start of new competitive trials), or the logistics (e.g., closedown of participating centers).

The following are the main points to be considered during recruitment planning:

- **Numbers**: The trial protocol will define the number of participants required according to the statistical sample size calculations. In addition, the expected *screen failure rate* will need to be established as the number of candidates to be

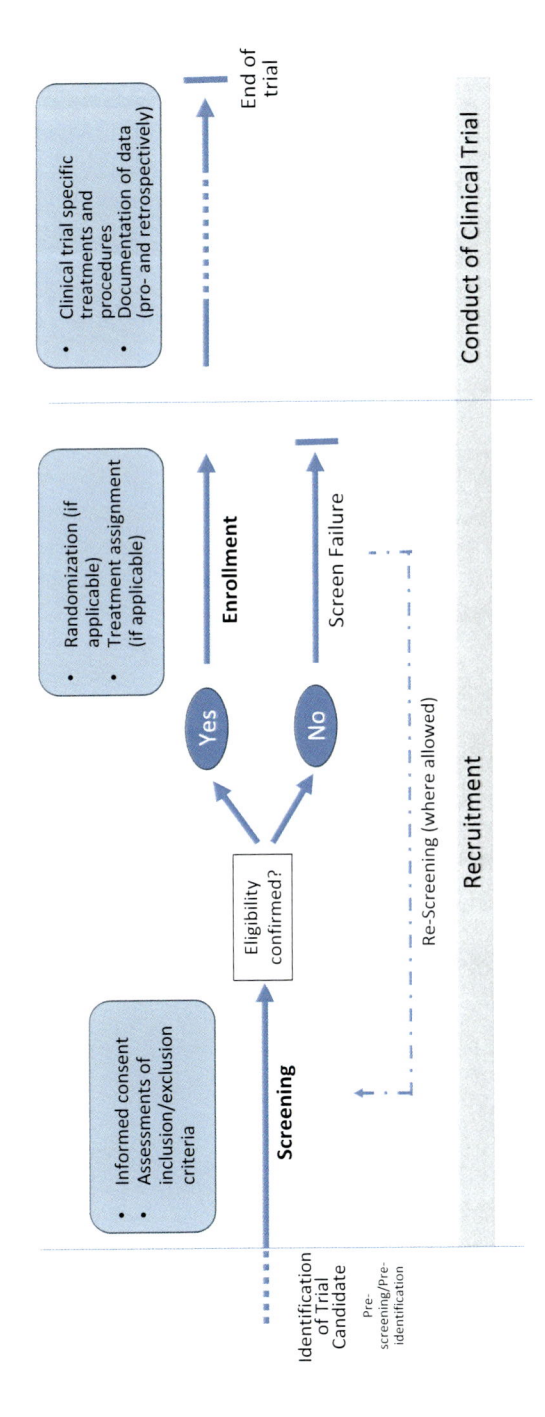

Fig. 1 Overview of the recruitment process for enrolled participants documentation of reportable adverse events may be required from the beginning of screening (retrospectively), up to the end of the clinical trial

screened in total will need to include the candidates not subsequently enrolled. Also, the protocol may require replacement of enrolled participants who drop out of the trial prior to reaching a specific milestone (e.g., the end of a certain observation/treatment period or exposure duration). In this case, the expected *dropout rate* should also be assessed, and the number of enrolled participants increased accordingly (Fig. 2).

- **Timelines**: Restrictions on duration of the recruitment period can be defined by budget and/or resource limitations, by ethical and/or regulatory requirements (e. g., post approval commitments to health authorities), or by statistical requirements (e.g., occurrence of endpoints to be observed within a specific time frame). Planning of timelines should also take into consideration the time needed to identify and screen candidates (i.e., how often are candidates seen by trial investigators; how long do trial-specific screening assessments take).

- **Geographical distribution**: Is the trial a single- or a multicenter trial, a local, national, or international trial? Are there any specific geographic considerations from an epidemiological stand point? Are there any logistical restrictions to the distribution of the trial such as language constraints, limitations in clinical research associate (CRA) monitoring resources, challenges in supply of the investigational medicinal product, or differences in standard of care (e.g., availability of comparator treatment) that would influence the geographical spread of the trial? Are there any regulatory requirements for acceptance of data for licensing or marketing considerations (e.g., minimum number of participants from a certain country required to allow filing)?

Example: some countries tend to be strong and fast recruiters but may have long start-up timelines, potentially precluding their involvement in trials where the overall recruitment period is expected to be short. On the other hand, other countries may be included due to short start-up timelines, despite a perhaps limited enrollment potential.

- **Budgeting**: Recruitment contributes significantly to the costs of a clinical trial; hence, the trial budget will often influence the recruitment strategy of a trial. The decision on how many sites to be included in which countries may not only be based on the sites' potential to contribute but also on how much it will cost to run the trial in specific countries. Also, while generally the more sites are opened for a trial the shorter the enrollment duration will be, opening up sites is costly in resources as well as in pass-through costs (e.g., fees for contracts, IRB/EC submissions, etc.). Therefore, a balance will need to be found between the costs of adding more sites and the savings of having a shorter enrollment duration.

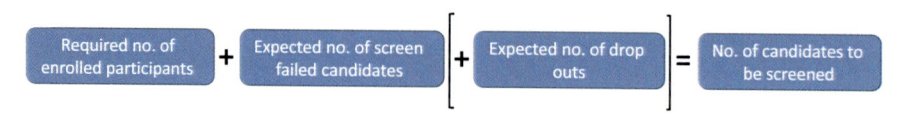

Fig. 2 Calculation of the number of patients to be screened

- **Protocol feasibility outcome**: Well-conducted protocol feasibility will help establish the enrollment potential of investigational sites and will provide information on how capable sites are to conduct the trial (e.g., logistical infrastructure at a site, their experience in conducting clinical trials, resources available to support the trial, commitment/interest of the investigator, competitive trials run at the site). The information obtained through feasibility will indicate if the planned sites will be sufficient to conduct the trial or if additional or different sites will need to be approached.
- **Recruitment challenges**: Experience from comparable trials and feedback received from investigators during protocol feasibility can help in identifying potential recruitment challenges. Addressing these proactively as much as possible will minimize the risk of missed recruitment goals. Early identification might allow implementation of actions that are more difficult later on during the trial such as amending the protocol (e.g., to relax eligibility criteria or to reduce the frequency of trial assessments). Other preparatory steps might include proactive tailored training of site staff and the preparation of supportive material for sites (e.g., medical equipment, trial-specific "pocket summaries").
- **Advisory boards**: Where available the benefit of consulting with scientific advisory boards or with individual medical experts should be considered, as input from such groups or individuals may help ensure trial assessments are in accordance with current standard of care and/or feasible for the participants and investigators.
- **Patient involvement**: Similarly, seeking input from patient representative groups may support the development of a "patient-friendly" trial. Ensuring a trial is manageable and relevant for the participants will go a long way in ensuring successful enrollment and retention. This can include aspects of the clinical trial design (e.g., frequency of blood sampling), terminology used (e.g., potentially inappropriate use of the word patient versus participant or person), reimbursement of expenses, and understandability of consent (i.e., ensure all participants are informed in language and terms they are able to understand).

The "Recruitment Funnel"

Typically, it has to be expected (and planned for) that not all identified candidates will end up being enrolled into a clinical trial, and similarly, not all enrolled participants will complete the trial. The phenomenon of the number of candidates decreasing between pre-screening and enrollment, and again after randomization, is often referred to as the "recruitment funnel."

The first sweep of candidates will fall off the radar during the pre-screening phase. Often site staff overestimate the number of potential trial participants they can contribute to a trial, not fully taking into consideration competitive trials being conducted at their site on a similar patient population, or the site's resource constraints and the related limitations in their ability to oversee the often time-intensive management of participants in a clinical trial. A further proportion of candidates will drop out during the actual screening and consenting phase, as not

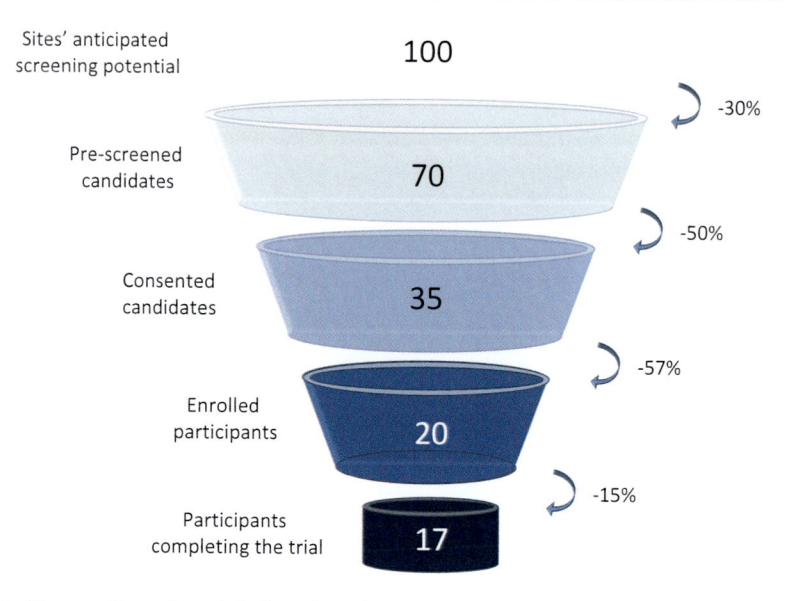

Fig. 3 The recruitment funnel (indicated numbers and percentages are examples)

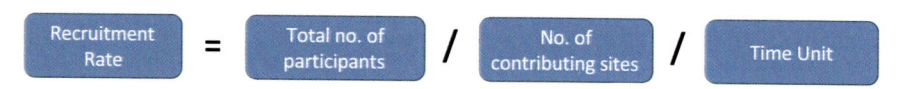

Fig. 4 Calculation of the recruitment rate

all candidates will meet all the eligibility criteria and/or are willing to enter a trial. A reason for this is that during initial protocol review, investigators might underestimate the stringency of the trial's eligibility criteria. For potential enrollment barriers, see Brintnall-Karabelas et al. (2011) and Lara et al. (2001). Thirdly, even after randomization, the number of participants is likely to decrease over time, through early dropouts due to various reasons such as adverse reactions experienced during the trial, withdrawal of consent, or participants being lost to follow-up. The dropout rate generally increases with the longer duration of a trial (Fig. 3).

The Recruitment Rate

The most often used metric in recruitment is the recruitment rate. The recruitment rate of a clinical trial, both for single-center and for multicenter trials, is defined by the following factors (Fig. 4):

- Total number of enrolled participants
- Number of contributing sites (will be 1 in single-center trials)
- Required enrollment duration (mostly indicated in months)

Example: In a phase II trial, 80 participants were enrolled by 12 contributing sites, over the course of 8 months. Hence, the recruitment rate of this trial was 80 participants divided by 12 sites divided by 8 months = 0.83 participants per site per month.

Breaking down recruitment into these factors allows a standardized quantification of enrollment, irrespective of the trial specifics such as design or indication. However, recruitment rates vary vastly between different disease areas, from a two- (or more) digit rate for trials in common indications to rates lower than 0.1 in rare diseases, and therefore recruitment rates should be interpreted carefully when used to compare recruitment in different trials.

Fine-Tuning the Recruitment Rate

The recruitment rate provides an indication of the average recruitment speed across all sites and over the full recruitment period. However, in reality, recruitment is rarely linear over the course of the trial, and breaking it down to an individual site level and/or to specific phases during the enrollment period will provide a more realistic picture of what recruitment may actually look like.

One factor to consider is the ramp-up period at the beginning of a trial, taking into account the time needed to have all sites activated and ready to start enrollment. During this ramp-up period, fewer sites will be contributing to enrollment as not all might be able to start recruitment at the same time.

Example: Estimation of recruitment during ramp-up period: x weeks with 25% of sites activated and contributing, y weeks with 50% of sites enrolling, and z weeks (the remaining recruitment period) with 90% of sites contributing to recruitment. Calculating with 90% instead of 100% of planned sites allows for the possibility of some sites not enrolling any participants (e.g., approvals not received in time, no candidates available).

Another factor impacting the recruitment rate may be decreased site activity during holiday seasons, and being aware of the various holiday customs within the participating countries will allow planning for potential dips during recruitment.

Recruitment Planning Tools

There are different methodologies and tools available that can be used to generate a differentiated approximation of the estimated recruitment rate for a planned trial. Ideally two or more of these are used in combination as this will allow the most complete coverage of possible eventualities and the development of the best possible recruitment strategy.

Benchmarking

Researching the trial landscape by identifying clinical trials (either historical or currently running) that are analogous to the trial at hand will provide benchmarking data on what can be expected with regard to recruitment metrics. Benchmarking data of clinical trials can be obtained either from government-mandated reportable trial registries (e.g., ClinicalTrials.gov, EudraCT, EU PAS) or from data collected by specialized service providers from pharmaceutical companies through anonymized methods. Some of these are publicly accessible; others require purchase of licenses.

By extracting the key recruitment metrics for each identified analogous trial, i.e., number of enrolled patients and of participating sites and recruitment start and end date, the recruitment rate of each trial can be calculated. This can then be used as a starting point for the planning of the own trial but will need to be adjusted for any variables not matching well. For example, if the treatment under investigation is considered promising by the community, the recruitment rate might need to be increased. Likewise, a decrease of the recruitment rate might be applicable if there is a high density of concurrently running competing trials.

The research of such data will also provide information on the number of trials run in the field and how many and which countries participated in these trials, indicating both recruitment potential and competitive pressure in a given field and region. However, data will be limited to indications, treatment classes, etc. as previously or currently investigated, and it might not always be possible to find relevant historical matches.

Simulation

Another useful tool is the simulation of recruitment by feeding different sets of variables into a model and thus imitating different potential scenarios. Modifying factors such as number of sites, recruitment rates, ramp-up times for individual sites, etc. will help visualizing their impact on the recruitment duration and will allow refinement of one's assumptions (DePuy 2017) (Fig. 5).

Patient Recruitment Service Agencies

There are a number of service providers in the industry specializing in the planning, support, and conduct of recruitment into clinical trials. Services provided range from provision of benchmarking data for recruitment planning, to simulation tools, and to the preparation of study material and tools supporting recruitment and retention.

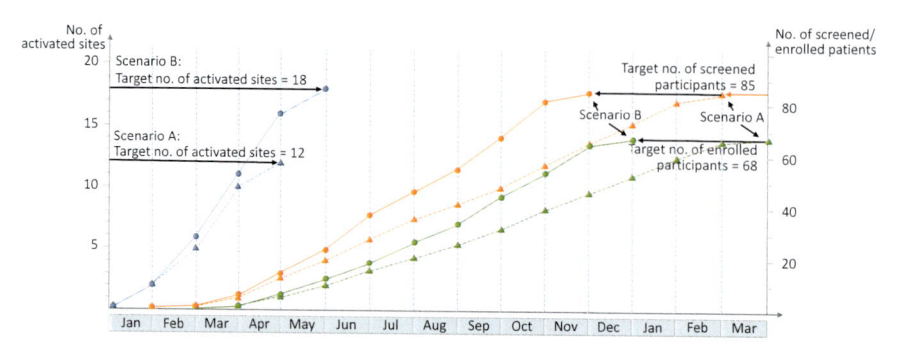

Fig. 5 Visualization of simulation outputs for two different scenarios: scenario A = 12 activated sites; scenario B = 18 activated sites. Target sample size = 68; assumed screen failure rate = 20%

Identifying Trial Candidates

Tailoring recruitment-related communication to the protocol-defined target population, identifying the right sources, and being able to access the right candidates will ensure optimal enrollment outcome in relation to cost and resource investments (see, e.g., Graham et al. 2017; National Institute on Aging 2018). The questions that should be asked when defining the recruitment communication strategy are where can candidates matching the protocol requirements be found (sources) and who will the trial team be communicating to.

Potential sources of candidates can include:

(a) Health-care professionals: e.g., hospitals, health centers, and general practitioners
(b) Real-world data sources: e.g., patient registries and genomic profiling databanks
(c) Participant community: e.g., patient advocacy groups and individuals of the target population directly (community reach)

With the advance and increasing dispersion of genomic profiling and personalized health care, the concept of finding a trial for a patient rather than finding patients for a trial will become more prevalent, with computational platforms allowing real-time matching of patients to trials using genomic and clinical criteria (Fig. 6).

Recruitment Material

Once the source (or sources) and contact points have been established, communication material to support recruitment can be developed accordingly. Content as well as review and approval processes will differ depending on who the targeted recipients are.

Note: any patient-facing material needs to be approved by IRBs/ECs.

Examples of written material for the *promotion of a trial* include flyers, cards, posters, or ads with a trial overview and trial contact details. Target audiences can be participating centers, referring physicians, the broad community, and/or preselected trial

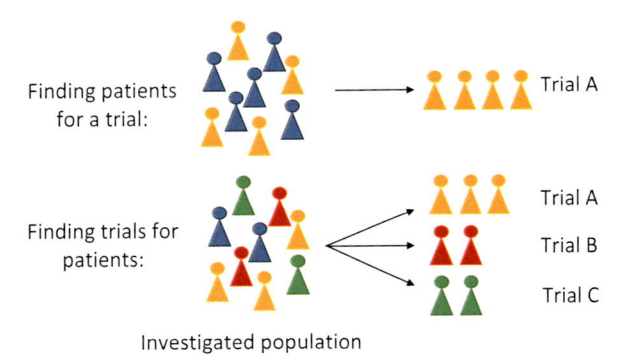

Fig. 6 Illustration of how personalized health care may affect trial recruitment

candidates. Material *supporting the informed consent process* can be booklets or cards, or short videos, with explanations and schemas of the scientific or medical background of the trial, the underlying disease, or the treatments/medical procedures in question.

Other means of outreach include printed media (such as newspapers and magazines), television, and radio broadcasts, as well as multimedia and online platforms such as community web sites, forums, social media, apps, etc. (see, e.g., Katz et al. 2019) (Table 1).

The choice of formats used in a trial often depends on the budget and available resources (e.g., consider the need for translations in multinational studies) but should also reflect the specifics of the target audience to allow maximization of the uptake of the information. To increase the success of the communication campaign, it is often useful to use more than one means of communication (see, e. g., Kye et al. 2009).

It should be noted that the choice of communication pathway could have a pre-selective impact on the trial candidates identified (e.g., limited access to online media for certain social or age groups).

Table 1 Overview of different communication formats

Format	Examples	Advantages	For consideration
Printed material	Flyers, posters, cards, booklets	Neither cost nor resource intensive Can be easily distributed	Risk of getting lost or not receiving much attention
News media	Ads in newspapers, magazines, in public areas (incl. public transport), on TV, or radio	Very broad outreach possible Often not costly	May be more useful for trials with broad eligibility criteria
Online media	Ads on dedicated web sites, forums, or chat rooms, in apps or search engines	Can reach very specific target audience	Legal restrictions to be adhered to when posting information online IRB/EC approval required for patient-facing content prior to posting – may lead to delays globally, or the need for geofencing (i.e., blocking content for users with certain IP addresses) Uptake limited to web-literate audience
Other	Mass letters, "cold calls," e.g., to all GPs in a certain area	Broad outreach possible	Risk of relatively low turnout in relation to invested effort

Examples:

- For a single-center phase I study with healthy volunteers, a useful approach could be to hand out study flyers and hang up posters in close-by universities or sport centers.
- For a global phase III study in hemophilia (a well-connected and well-informed community), ads on dedicated web sites such as association portals or patient forums could be useful.

Often, recruitment material will be the primary tool to promote the clinical trial, and therefore the relevance of the trial should be included in the communication. Where possible a visual identity (e.g., trial logo) can be used that will help the trial in standing out from others. However, it is important that the material, texts, and visuals strictly promote only the trial and not the therapy or treatment under investigation. There are a set of legal regulations that need to be followed when authoring communications around clinical trials. These regulations may vary locally but in general include points such as:

- Must use language that can be understood by lay people
- Must not promise a cure or other benefit (including free treatment) beyond what is outlined in the protocol
- Must not be unduly coercive
- Should not include logos, branding, or phraseology used (or planned to be used) for marketing of the therapy

Screening

The objective of the screening process is to ensure only eligible candidates enter the trial. Therefore, the assessments required to identify eligibility of candidates will need to be defined, and the necessary processes and systems will need to be set up accordingly. Questions to be addressed include the following:

- Are the required screening assessments standard of care and can be expected to be performed as part of routine clinical practice, or are they trial specific and will require prior consenting by the candidates? Will eligibility tests be performed locally at the sites or will they need to be performed centrally (e.g., due to limited availability of technology or the need for standardization for comparability)?
- What is the time frame in which screening assessments need to be performed? Are there any time constraints in having to get the candidate's eligibility confirmed (e.g., is there a maximum time window between diagnosis and start of therapy during which screening will need to be completed)?

Screening activities need to be documented for all candidates (e.g., by use of a screening log to be maintained by the participating sites), both for candidates ending up being enrolled and for screen failures (including the reason for screen failure). Also, especially for multi-site trials, a method on how to track screening activities should be implemented, allowing (ideally real-time) monitoring of progress against projections.

Planning the Screening End

The aim is to hit the protocol required number of enrolled patients as closely as possible, for budgetary reasons, but also in order not to unnecessarily expose participants to experimental therapy. Toward the end of the enrollment period for a trial, screening should be monitored carefully, as, for ethical reasons, all informed, screened, and eligible candidates should be allowed to enter the trial. Therefore, screening activities should stop once a sufficient number of candidates are in the screening pool to fill the remaining enrollment slots. Especially in fast- recruiting trials, this requires extrapolation of the screen failure rate observed previously.

Example: If the screen failure rate during the last period of enrollment in a trial was 10%, and 9 participants are still required to complete the trial, screening should stop when 10 candidates are in screening.

Screening Tools

- While for small trials screening progress can be tracked manually, larger trials with several participating sites are often managed with the support of an *Interactive Voice or Web Response System (IxRS)*. This will allow sites to enter into the system when a candidate has been identified ("screening call") and then again when the outcome of the screening assessments is established, either leading to enrollment or to screen failure. Screen failure reasons, usually in categories, can also be tracked this way. The use of an IxRS allows real-time tracking of screening progress but can be costly and time-intensive to set up.
- A tool allowing close control of screening activities is the *screening request form*: this is to be completed by a site once a candidate has been identified and to be sent to the central trial team for approval. Screening assessments for a candidate can only start once the screening request is approved by the central team. Screening request forms are typically used in trials requiring only small numbers of participants (e.g., phase I cohort studies with less than ten participants per cohort) or when a certain lag time is required between enrollment of individual participants (e.g., where tolerability of a treatment needs to be established prior to enrollment of subsequent participants).
- The allocation of *screening slots* can also be useful in trials with small numbers of participants. Here, the central trial team will allocate individual screening slots to a small number of sites at a time, allowing only these sites to screen one candidate at a time. Once a candidate is either enrolled or screen failed, a next screening slot will be allocated to another site.

Enrollment

Enrollment Strategies

Enrollment is often straightforward, with participants being entered into a trial as they get identified and screened. However, there might be considerations to a trial that warrant the definition of a specific enrollment or recruitment strategy.

- Competitive versus allocated enrollment (applicable to multicenter studies only): competitive enrollment means that all sites can enroll participants as and when they are identified, until the overall sample size has been reached. However, it may be necessary to restrict the number of enrolled participants by individual sites or countries, even if these could contribute more and the overall sample size has not yet been reached. This might be the case if a certain distribution of enrolled participants is required (e.g., where a minimum number of participants per site or country are needed).
- Enrollment in batches versus ongoing enrollment: enrolling in batches may be required in trials where resource-intensive therapy is required that is best applied to several participants at a time or if there has to be a time lag after enrollment of a certain number of participants to allow observation prior to subsequent enrollments (e.g., enrollment into cohorts).

Enrollment Procedures

- Where applicable *randomization* (blinded or open, including stratification and treatment assignment as needed) will occur during the enrollment process. In smaller studies, these steps can be managed manually; however, in larger, multicenter trials, it is common to use an interactive voice or web response system (IxRS). Sites will access the system to report an enrollment and to request a randomization or participant ID which the system will link with the assigned treatment code and where applicable with a medication or biological sampling material kit number.
- Enrollment approval: in early phase studies in which participants' safety might be of particular concern, a process may have to be set up to allow central trial team review of a candidate's screening data prior to enrollment. This will allow the central trial team to confirm that the candidate meets the trial's entry criteria.

Monitoring Enrollment

- Close monitoring of enrollment progress on study and site level, and comparison with projections as defined at trial start, will allow early detection of any deviations from the recruitment plans. The setup of appropriate reports (e.g., through the IxRS if used) should be included in the trial preparation activities as they should be available early on. Such reports will also be useful for regular reporting of enrollment progress to trial stakeholders, e.g., participating sites, sponsor management, and regulatory authorities.

- Specific attention should be given when getting close to the end of recruitment. As described under the screening procedures, over-enrollment should be avoided, both for budgetary reasons and to avoid unnecessary exposure of participants to the treatment under investigation.

Retention

In trials with single observation points or very short follow-up participant, retention will not be an issue. However, for trials with longer observation or follow-up, plans on how to limit the number of missed individual assessments during the trial, and to keep participants in the trial for as long as required by the protocol, will need to be put in place at study start-up. Participants have the right to withdraw from a trial at any time; however, participants with a good understanding of the objectives of a trial are less likely to drop out. Therefore, participant education of their responsibilities in achieving these objectives, including adherence to the schedule of assessments until the end of the trial, should be part of the consent process.

- *Partial withdrawal*: Should a participant wish to discontinue the trial-specific treatment under investigation, they should be encouraged to remain in the study for follow-up and to complete all remaining visits and assessments (without continuing with the treatment). This will allow collection of outcome data. However, if a participant withdraws their consent for the entire study, no further data can be collected.

Reasons for participants to drop out include:

- Participant has not met the eligibility criteria (protocol deviation/violation).
- Consent withdrawal from either study treatment only or from the entire study.
- Death and adverse events.
- Pregnancy.
- Perceived or real lack of efficacy.
- Physician decision.
- Unwillingness or inability to comply with the protocol-mandated assessments.
- Logistical reasons such as translocation and changes in personal circumstances.
- Participant is lost to follow-up.

If a participant is *lost to follow-up*, every effort should be undertaken to locate the participant. It might be useful to set up a clear definition of actions to be taken by a site before a participant is considered lost to follow-up (e.g., at least three attempts to contact the participant through different communication means at different time points throughout a minimum period of 3 weeks).

Retention Strategy

A retention strategy should aim at positively influencing the trial experience for participants and at establishing a rapport between the participant and the trial and/or the trial team. An integral part of the retention strategy will therefore include communication with the trial participants beyond their enrollment into the trial, ideally through different pathways and at various time points throughout the trial duration.

Being the main trial contact point for participants, keeping local site staff engaged, well informed of the global trial progress, and fully trained on trial processes is key.

Examples of Retention Support

Supporting participant directly:

- Visit reminders (e.g., phone calls, email notifications, or alerts through mobile apps)
- Educational material on the underlying disease or the treatment under investigation
- Communication aiming to establish a sense of community, including layman summaries of the trial results and thank you letters at the end of the trial
- Reimbursement of expenses incurred for travel to the trial site (**note**: local regulations need to be considered for the management of travel reimbursement, as some IRBs/IECs may require out-of-pocket expenses to be reimbursed to participants, whereas others will prohibit it)
- Logistical support for participants (e.g., home nursing, possibility to report data electronically rather than having to go to the site)
- Trial treatment supporting gadgets (e.g., pillows or blankets)

Note: any material distributed to participants will need prior approval by IRBs/IECs. Also, local regulations will apply, including that the material cannot promote the treatment under investigation, only the trial itself, and that the value of the material cannot be seen as persuasive to participation in the trial. The material should be strictly trial related and not exceed a certain financial value.

Supporting site staff:

- Participants' visit reminders (e.g., phone calls or email notifications)
- Template forms to capture participant's contact details (including those of close relatives where provided by the participants)
- Pocket summaries, schedules, and charts providing an overview or quick reference to the protocol procedures

Recruitment Issues and Their Impact

Recruitment has been one of the most common challenges in clinical trials in the past, and the changing environment is not making it any easier. Factors contributing to the increased complexity are an increasingly demanding regulatory environment and competitive pressure caused by the increasing number of clinical trials being run. Also, the tendency to tailor studies to more and more specific target populations (i.e., the trend toward individualized health care), as well as the patients' increased literacy and desire to be involved in their treatment decisions, requires differentiated planning of recruitment.

Recruitment issues can be grouped into the following three categories:

- **Slow/under-recruitment**: if this happens, the estimated enrollment potential of the contributing sites was too high, and participants are either enrolled at a lower rate than expected (leading to longer recruitment and therefore longer trial duration) or cannot be enrolled at all. Common reasons for lower than expected recruitment rates are too restrictive eligibility criteria and unanticipated or underestimated concurrent trials run at the participating sites, affecting both the number of trial candidates as well as site resources and engagement of site personnel. Other possible reasons include logistical factors such as issues with access to comparator treatment, unplanned unavailability of site staff (e.g., due to illness or transfer), and changes in the regulatory environment (e.g., approval of new competitive treatment decreasing the interest in the trial). Patient-related reasons might include limited patient access to the trial sites and too high burden of the protocol.
- **Over-recruitment**: while this tends to be a less frequently experienced issue, it can also have significant negative impact on the success of a clinical trial. If participants are enrolled into a trial faster than anticipated (*higher recruitment rate*), this can impact trial resources both at the site level and at the central trial team level, potentially limiting the ability to ensure adequate medical oversight of the participants (caused by delayed data reporting and review). Also, the quality of the collected data may suffer through insufficient trial oversight, putting the trial outcome at risk. Recruiting more participants into a trial than anticipated (*increased sample size*) can lead to budgetary constraints and can be ethically problematic as more participants than statistically needed are exposed to experimental treatment.
- **Low quality of recruitment:** in this case, recruitment may seem to be on track; however, the participants enrolled into a trial may not necessarily be the right ones. This can happen if, often due to lack of oversight, participants not fully meeting the eligibility criteria are enrolled into a trial (resulting in the so-called protocol violations or deviations). Once identified, continuation of these participants in the trial will need to be assessed carefully, and they may need to be excluded from the trial for safety and/or efficacy reasons (risk due to exposure to investigational treatment may not be justified given the potential lack of response). The trial team will then need to decide if exclusion of these participants will impact the power of the trial outcome and if they need to be replaced by additional participants.

Risk Mitigation

Some potential risks to the planned recruitment can already be identified prior to the start of a trial, during comparison with analogous trials (e.g., spread of competitive trials), during protocol feasibility (e.g., sites' capability to run the trial), and during interaction with patient advocacy groups, scientific experts, and advisory boards (e.g., trial alignment with current standard of care), see e. g. National Institute of Mental Health (2005). While not all risks can be avoided fully, some mitigating actions can be implemented, either through modifications of the protocol or by adding (or exchanging) countries and sites to the trial.

Examples of risks that may require mitigation:

- Exclusion of patients with active, controlled hepatitis will significantly reduce the participant potential in some countries.
- High frequency of radiology assessments or too high blood sample drawing burden might not be approved by some IRBs/ECs

The common need for a speedy study setup also bears risks that can lead to an enrollment backlog from the very beginning of the trial, including starting trial recruitment preparations with a nonfinal protocol version, underestimating the time needed for the setup of sites (e.g., contract negotiations taking longer than anticipated), and not having contingency plans in place early on. Also, ensuring all involved stakeholders such as different departments of a hospital and referring institutions are informed of the upcoming trial and are able to communicate with each other will help in avoiding any delays.

Engaging participating investigators early on in trial planning can positively impact recruitment. Key opinion leaders, by their reputation in the community, may influence their colleagues to promote the study protocol and enrollment into the trial. Also, additional motivation might be gained if there are opportunities for authorship on study-related publications for participating investigators (in alignment with applicable publication authorship guidelines).

Issue Management

Once recruitment is at risk of getting off track or is off track already, different corrective actions can be taken, with often a combination of several actions being the most successful approach. Ideally, these actions (as well as the trigger points for their implementation) are defined in the recruitment plan, but there should also be flexibility to adapt the corrective actions to the current situation (Bachenheimer 2016).

Possible measures to address delays in recruitment include:

- Increase/change of communication (e.g., newsletters to sites, investigator meetings/teleconferences, trial promotional, and recruitment supporting material)
- Engage key opinion leaders or trial steering committee members to help promote the trial in their community
- Opening up of new sites (ideally already "pre-initiated" as far as possible as part of the recruitment plan) or expansion into other countries

- Review of the protocol to identify areas that could hinder recruitment and assess if these can be modified (e.g., less stringent eligibility criteria, simplified, and/or less frequent study assessments)
- Increase incentive for participating investigators where and as possible (payment, authorship on planned publications)
- Facilitate study participation for participants (e.g., payment where allowed, reimbursement of expenses, material to help understand the informed consent form, and the study specifics; see Fiminska 2014; Kadam et al. 2016)

Possible measures to address too fast recruitment include:

- Implement the assignment of screening/enrollment slots to individual sites (i.e., restrict the number of participants that can be enrolled per site or per country).
- Implement a temporary recruitment hold for all sites (although sometimes it can be difficult to get sites restarted at the same rate of recruitment as before).

Possible measures to address enrollment of wrong participants include:

- Retrain site staff of trial specifics.
- Investigate possibilities to increase resources at sites (e.g., hiring of temporary contractors dedicated to the study).
- Implement recruitment stop at individual sites.

Summary and Conclusion

Recruitment has been the main challenge in the management of clinical trials in the past and is expected to become even more difficult with an increasing regulative environment and more trials being run in highly specified populations. Therefore, thorough upfront planning of recruitment is key to ensure enrollment of the right participants in time and within budget. The factors to be considered include evaluation of the quality and number of sites needed, feasibility of the protocol, and mitigation of any potential risks as much as possible through communication with the key stakeholders. The recruitment plan should also include a strategy to access candidates, to monitor enrollment progress, and to retain participants in the trial. The use of supporting tools such as benchmarking and simulation should be factored in when setting up the trial budget.

Key Facts

Recruitment of trial participants consists of identification, assessment, and enrollment of trial candidates. A basic metric to quantify enrollment is the recruitment rate, defined as the number of participants enrolled per site per time unit (usually months). Factors influencing recruitment are related to the availability of appropriate sites, the protocol design, and the communication with key stake-holders of the trial. Retention of trial participants for as long as mandated by the protocol is important to minimize gaps in data collection.

Cross-References

▶ Advocacy and Patient Involvement in Clinical Trials
▶ Consent Forms and Procedures
▶ International Trials
▶ Selection of Study Centers and Investigators

References

Anderson DL (2001) A guide to patient recruitment: today's best practices and proven strategies. CenterWatch, Boston

Bachenheimer JF (2016) Adaptive patient recruitment for 21st century clinical research. Available via Applied Clinical Trials. http://www.appliedclinicaltrialsonline.com/adaptive-patient-recruitment-21st-century-clinical-research. Accessed 08 Jan 2019

Bachenheimer JF, Brescia BA (2017) Reinventing patient recruitment: revolutionary ideas for clinical trial success. Taylor and Francis BBK Worldwide, Needham MA, USA

Brintnall-Karabelas J, Sung S, Cadman ME, Squires C, Whorton K, Pao M (2011) Improving recruitment in clinical trials: why eligible participants decline. J Empir Res Hum Res Ethics 6 (1):69–74. https://doi.org/10.1525/jer.2011.6.1.69

DePuy V (2017) Enrollment simulation in clinical trials. SESUG Paper LS-213-2017. Available via https://www.lexjansen.com/sesug/2017/LS-213.pdf. Accessed 08 Jan 2019

Fiminska Z (2014) 5 tips on how to facilitate clinical trial recruitment. EyeForPharma. Available at https://social.eyeforpharma.com/clinical/5-tips-how-facilitate-clinical-trial-recruitment. Accessed 08 Jan 2019

Friedman LM, Furberg CD, DeMets D, Reboussin DM, Granger CB (2015) Fundamentals of clinical trials. Springer International Publishing, Cham

Graham LA, Ngwa J, Ntekim O, Ogunlana O, Wolday S, Johnson S, Johnson M, Castor C, Fungwe TV, Obisesan TO (2017) Best strategies to recruit and enroll elderly blacks into clinical and biomedical research. Clin Interv Aging 2018(13):43–50

Kadam RA, Borde SU, Madas SA, Salvi SS, Limaye SS (2016) Challenges in recruitment and retention of clinical trial subjects. Perspect Clin Res 7(3):137–143

Katz B, Eiken A, Misev V, Zibert JR (2019) Optimize clinical trial recruitment with digital platforms. Dermatology Times. Available via https://www.dermatologytimes.com/business/optimize-clinical-trial-recruitment-digital-platforms. Accessed 08 Jan 2019

Kye SH, Tashkin DP, Roth MD, Adams B, Nie W-X, Mao JT (2009) Recruitment strategies for a lung cancer chemoprevention trial involving ex-smokers. Contemp Clin Trials 30:464–472

Lara PN Jr, Higdon R, Lim N, Kwan K, Tanaka M, Lau DHM, Wun T, Welborn J, Meyers FJ, Christensen S, O'Donnell R, Richman C, Scudder SA, Tuscana J, Gandara DR, Lam KS (2001) Prospective evaluation of cancer clinical trial accrual patterns: identifying potential barriers to enrollment. J Clin Oncol 19(6):1728–1733

Little RJ, D'Agostino R, Choen ML, Dickersin K, Emerson SS, Farrar JT, Frangakis C, Hogan JW, Molenberghs G, Murphy SA, Neaton JD, Rotnitzky A, Scharfstein D, Shih WJ, Siegel JP, Stern H (2012) The prevention and treatment of missing data in clinical trials. N Engl J Med 367 (14):1355–1360

National Institute of Mental Health (2005) Points to consider about recruitment and retention while preparing a clinical research study. Available via https://www.nimh.nih.gov/funding/grant-writing-and-application-process/points-to-consider-about-recruitment-and-retention-while-preparing-a-clinical-research-study.shtml. Accessed 08 Jan 2019

National Institute on Aging (2018) Together we make the difference – National Strategy for recruitment and participation in Alzheimer's and related dementias clinical research. Available via U.S. Department of Health & Human Services. https://www.nia.nih.gov/sites/default/files/2018-10/alzheimers-disease-recruitment-strategy-final.pdf. Accessed 08 Jan 2019

Thoma A, Farrokhyar F, McKnight L, Bhandari M (2010) How to optimize patient recruitment. Can J Surg 53(3):205–210

Administration of Study Treatments and Participant Follow-Up

16

Jennifer J. Gassman

Contents

J. J. Gassman (✉)
Department of Quantitative Health Sciences, Cleveland Clinic, Cleveland, OH, USA
e-mail: gassmaj@ccf.org

© Springer Nature Switzerland AG 2022
S. Piantadosi, C. L. Meinert (eds.), *Principles and Practice of Clinical Trials*,
https://doi.org/10.1007/978-3-319-52636-2_39

Abstract

After clinical trial participants have consented, provided baseline data, and been randomized, each participant begins study treatment and follow-up. This chapter covers administering a participant's randomly assigned treatment regimen and collecting the participant's trial data through the end of their time in the study, along with tracking and reporting data on timeliness and quality of treatment administration and of follow-up visit attendance and trial data collection. Treatment administration can include providing study medications or, in a lifestyle intervention trial, teaching the participant to follow a diet, exercise, or smoking cessation intervention. Trial data collection includes, for example, questionnaires completed via smartphone, laboratory sample collection details and results of lab analyses, imaging data, treatment adherence data, measurements taken at clinic visits, and adverse event data. Monitoring participant follow-up and capturing reasons why patients discontinue treatment or end follow-up early can aid in interpretation of a trial's results. Treatment administration, treatment adherence, and participant follow-up metrics should be captured in real time, with the Data Coordinating Center (DCC) providing continuous performance feedback to study leadership and to the participating sites themselves. These aspects of trial conduct are described in the context of a multicenter trial in which two or more clinical sites enroll participants and study data are managed in a centrally administered database. Timeliness and accuracy of study treatment administration is key to the success of a trial. Participants providing required data according to the protocol-defined schedule allow a trial to attain its goals.

Keywords

Run-in · Pill count · Treatment crossover · Unblinding · Treatment discontinuation · Visit schedule · Visit window · Close out · Drop out *(no longer attending clinic visits)* · Withdrawal of consent *(no longer willing to provide data)*

Introduction

The success of a multicenter-randomized clinical trial depends on valid study design and study conduct. Valid study design starts with the requirement that all specified baseline data be captured prior to randomization /registration and that treatment commence as soon as possible after randomization. Once trial randomization begins, recruitment, adherence, and retention are the keys to study success. This chapter addresses *administration of study treatments* and *participant follow-up* in the context of a multicenter trial where two or more clinical sites enroll participants and study data are managed in a database administered by a Data Coordinating Center (DCC) at an academic site or a commercial site such as a CRO.

Study treatments in a trial may include, for example, active and placebo medication in the form of pills, liquids, injections, or IV drugs; methods of surgery; and systems by which patients are taught or encouraged to follow diet, exercise, or smoking cessation regimens. Observation (no intervention) can also be a study "treatment" in a trial with multiple arms. Interventions chosen for a trial should be considered acceptable by physicians treating patients with the condition under study; this can be evaluated by survey prior to study initiation, as was done in the NIDDK FSGS Clinical Trial (Ferris et al. 2013) or discussed during physician training. Appropriate study conduct requires monitoring initial and subsequent treatment administration, and treatment adherence data can be important for interpretation of trial results.

Participant follow-up includes postrandomization/enrollment data collection including patient-reported outcome questionnaires completed via smartphone, laboratory sample collection details and results of lab analyses, imaging data, treatment adherence data, and measurements taken at clinic visits. Monitoring participant follow-up and capturing reasons why patients discontinue treatment or end follow-up early are useful for assessing bias and for interpretation of a trial's results. A well-designed and well-conducted trial will have high rates of participant follow-up. An appropriate study protocol is key here; the protocol's defined visit schedule must include contact with patients sufficiently frequently so that patients are unlikely to move or change phone numbers between visits, and sufficiently infrequently so that patients do not become burned out by having to constantly fulfill study requirements for questionnaires, phone calls, lab sample collections, and visits. The intent-to-treat data analyses that make trial conclusions valid benefit from high rates of participant follow-up and data collection completeness (Byar et al. 1976).

Treatment administration, treatment adherence, and participant follow-up metrics should be captured in real time, with the Data Coordinating Center (DCC) providing continuous performance monitoring of these data to study leadership and to the participating sites themselves. Methods for this feedback include frequently updated routine reports posted on a study website and/or pushed to study leadership and participating sites via e-mail as weekly reports.

Administration of Study Treatments

Introduction to Administration of Study Treatment

Immediate and per-protocol administration of study treatment is essential. Any steps that can be taken that will facilitate a participant starting study treatment as soon as possible after randomization and stay on treatment per protocol will enhance study validity. If the treatment requires a drug, starter supplies of the medication should be available at each clinical site. If this is not possible, the study should have a system in place such that the participant can receive their treatment in an expedited way. The study treatment administration goal is that all participants start treatment soon after randomization, remain on treatment throughout their assigned study follow-up period, and comply as described in the study protocol.

Training

During staff training, study coordinators and other team members should be taught how treatment is administered and the importance of treatment adherence (as well as study visit schedule implementation and the importance of retention, covered in section "Participant Follow-Up" of this chapter). Study coordinators and investigators experienced with the treatment being studied should be invited to present segments of training related to treatment administration including blinding and treatment challenges.

Regarding blinding, the training should include (1) Who will know what treatment each participant receives, particularly with regard to whether the study be unblinded/open label; single blinded, where the participant does not know their treatment but members of the study team do; or double-blinded, where neither the participant nor any member of the study team knows the participant's treatment assignment, (2) managing unblinding (see ▶ Chaps. 43, "Masking of Trial Investigators," and ▶ 44, "Masking Study Participants"), and (3) a discussion of the role of study blinding in preventing subconscious bias in outcome assessment.

Regarding challenges which are associated with the study treatment, study coordinators who are less familiar with the trial treatment will benefit from hearing from those with on-the-ground experience using this treatment or similar treatments. For lifestyle intervention trials, the systems in place implementing the experimental and control treatment arms should be covered in detail, including the study coordinators' role in encouraging adherence to the intervention. For medication trials, coordinators should be trained to teach participants requirements for their assigned treatment, e.g., whether a study drug should be taken on an empty stomach or with a meal as well as how and when dosage is to be increased or reduced. At training, study coordinators should also be informed of the study plans for monitoring and reporting treatment adherence. The Data Coordinating Center (DCC) team should present templates of treatment administration and treatment adherence-related tables from planned feedback reports/electronic weekly reports.

Once the trial is under way, coordinators at one site may be able to offer valuable tips to those at other sites based on their experience with participants who have had difficulties with treatment adherence. Study coordinators and other participating site team members can learn additional strategies for improving treatment adherence informally, as part of a structured routine study coordinators' web meetings or calls, and at annual training/retraining meetings.

Study coordinators should be fully engaged in helping to ensure participants receive their treatments on schedule and maintain the trial's treatment blinding as they work to enhance treatment adherence. Coordinators should also be encouraged to engage and garner support from the participant's family when possible.

Training should also include a description of closeout in which a participant's treatment ends, remaining medications – if any – are returned, and study visits cease.

Verification of Site Readiness

Before a participating site's subjects are enrolled and randomized, site readiness should be assessed. A site "Ready to Enroll" table should be included in trial monitoring (e.g., in the weekly report) showing whether each site has met requirements to begin consenting participants. These requirements will vary from study to study but should include IRB/ Ethics Committee approval, completion of staff training requirements, capture of needed site delivery addresses and staff contact information, and (for medication trials that include a starter supple of medication) receipt of the initial supply of medication, or information on how study drug is ordered, and clear plans for appropriate secure storage of medication and participant study documents as required by local regulations. Participants should not be consented until a site is ready to begin randomization/recruitment. Site initiation visits are sometimes conducted to ensure site-readiness.

Inclusion and Exclusion Criteria Focused on Treatment Administration

The trial protocol should ensure that participants who consent and are randomized to study treatment are likely to be able to comply to study treatment. Treatment-related inclusion and exclusion criteria can help ensure participants who are not likely to be able to comply with study treatment requirements are not randomized. A first step in this process is to ensure that the potential participant can safely follow the treatment; participants who are allergic to or have had side effects when on the study treatment will generally be excluded, as will participants who require treatment with a concurrent medication that is contraindicated for a participant on the active treatment arm. A second step would be to ensure that the participant is likely to follow the treatment regimen; participants who have a history of nonadherence to the type of treatment being administered will generally be excluded. A third step would be to ensure that the participant will be available to take the treatment; for many studies, participants who spend several months each year away are problematic. Study investigators should consider whether, for example, a participant who spends winter in Florida or a participant who is away at school during the academic year would be appropriate for randomization and should adjust exclusion criteria accordingly. (Note that this third criterion is also important for complete participant follow-up, i.e., retention, as described in section "Participant Follow-Up.")

Eligibility Checking and Randomization

Informed consent is, of course, part of a participant's time line in a trial. Study procedures may not be performed and data may not be submitted to the DCC until the participant has consented. The timing of informed consent is covered

in this book's ▶ Chap. 21, "Consent Forms and Procedures." A trial participant's data collection time line generally consists of screening, a baseline visit
or visits, eligibility confirmation, randomization, and subsequent follow-up
visits. Ideally, the participating site's team will have at least two contacts
with a potential enrollee prior to randomization (Meinert 2012). This will
allow time for the participant to be certain they understand the requirements
of the trial and are fully on board and have had all their trial-related questions
answered, and time for the study team to fully consider the participant's
suitability for the trial.

Trials in which the protocol includes baseline visits allow an opportunity to
test the participant's ability to follow trial requirements during a run-in, or test,
period, and many trials include a run-in trial of patient requirements, as
described in this book's ▶ Chap. 42, "Controlling Bias in Randomized Clinical
Trials." For example, in the Frequent Hemodialysis Network Daily Trial, the
experimental treatment arm featured 1 year of six shortened dialysis sessions per
week versus the usual care control arm (three standard sessions per week).
During baseline, participants were required to visit the dialysis unit daily for 6
consecutive days. Three participants dropped out or were excluded (FHN Trial
Group et al. 2010) because of unanticipated difficulties in getting to their dialysis
unit 6 days a week. In the Frequent Hemodialysis Network Nocturnal Trial, each
participant's home water supply needed to be evaluated for appropriateness of
use of in-home hemodialysis (Rocco et al. 2011). In FONT II (Trachtman et al.
2011), each participants' Angiotensin Converting Enzyme (ACE) inhibitor/
Angiotensin Receptor Blocker (ARB) was followed through a series of baseline
visits to ensure the regimen was effective and stable. In medication trials,
participants sometimes take placebo medication during Baseline. A run-in period
is particularly useful if the treatment may be unacceptable to some patients
because of pill/capsule size or the number of pills that must be taken each day.
Such a Baseline run-in period may include specified adherence criteria such as
"Pill count must show 80% adherence to treatment during run-in," as was
required in the COMBINE Trial (Ix et al. 2019) or may include a check-in
with the participant and a record of whether the participant reported any difficulties taking the study medication. Once the Baseline period is complete, the
participant will be randomized to treatment if study eligibility confirmation, e.g.,
a "Ready to Randomize" interactive program, has verified that all required
baseline data have been collected and the site has verified that, logistically, the
participant is available to start their randomized treatment, e.g., the participant is
not currently traveling or hospitalized. At this point, the participant is randomized and irrevocably part of the study, and the site is notified of the patient's
treatment assignment; in a blinded medication trial, the site would receive the
bottle or bin number of the medication to be provided to the participant. In
studies where randomization is carried out online, the treatment assignment
should be e-mailed to the study coordinator in addition to being displayed on
the randomization screen to ensure that the study coordinator can easily confirm
the assignment.

Getting the Treatment to the Participant

In studies with drug treatments, each participating site will provide an address for shipment of drug; at many sites, this will be the address of a hospital's research pharmacy. Drugs will come from their manufacturer or a study's central pharmacy (as described in this book's ▶ Chap. 7, "Centers Participating in Multicenter Trials") and may be provided to the sites in bulk (for local blinded distribution) or in coded, numbered bins or numbered bottles. Details on how drugs come to the participating sites are in this book's ▶ Chap. 11, "Procurement and Distribution of Study Medicines." On-site options for getting the treatment to the participant include, having the participant pick their medications up from the site's pharmacy, or having the study coordinator pick the medication up for the patient so the coordinator can hand the medication to the participant. When possible, handoff by the study coordinator is easier for the participant and ensures that the participant leaves the site with study drug.

Participants should begin treatment as soon as possible after randomization. In studies with a baseline period, final baseline eligibility data and baseline values for study outcomes including, lab results or imaging, must be captured prior to randomization, so the participant timeline will include a final baseline visit shortly prior to randomization. If all required results are expected to be available before the participant leaves the clinic and arrangements can be made such that study drug is available on-site at the clinic, it may be possible for a participant to be randomized at the end of this last baseline visit and go home with medication that day. If inclusion criteria include data resulting from images or lab tests done at the last visit of baseline, eligibility cannot be determined until after the final baseline visit. In such a case, procedures should include randomizing the participant as soon as possible, but at a time when the participant can begin taking drug (i.e., when the participant is in town and not in the hospital) and getting the treatment to the participant as soon as possible after randomization. A participant's appointment schedule will be based on the date of randomization, not on the day he or she started treatment, i.e., the target date for a 1-year follow-up visit should be 1 year from randomization. The study protocol may include a visit held shortly post-randomization in which the participant receives their study medication (often referred to as the "Follow Up 0" or the "Week 0" visit as in the AASK Trial (Gassman et al. 2003) or FSGS Trial (Gipson et al. 2011)). A face-to-face visit will be required if the treatment must be delivered under medical supervision, i.e., an IV infusion. Alternatively, the protocol may allow for the treatment being delivered to the participant or the participant picking the drug up from the site's research pharmacy. It may be helpful for a participant to interact with a study team member when a treatment is provided, particularly under protocols in which there is some complexity to treatment administration, e.g., in the case of double-dummy system where the participant must take two different types of medication or in the case where it is critical that the medication be taken under specific circumstances, such as on an empty stomach or with a meal. Whichever method is used, the date the participant begins taking medication should be captured in the study database.

Table 1 Time from randomization to initiation of treatment

Participating Site	Randomized	Initiated Treatment	Median time from randomization to treatment initiation (days)
1 California	20	20	2.2
2 Colorado	48	46	1.3
3 Connecticut	17	17	1.0
4 Delaware	34	33	1.0
5 Florida	47	45	1.6
6 Georgia	16	15	1.8
7 Illinois	7	7	2.4
TOTAL	189	183	1.5

Time from randomization to initiation of treatment (overall and by participating site) is a useful metric to track. An example is shown in Table 1.

Promoting Treatment Adherence

It may be shocking for those new to the conduct of clinical trials to learn that sometimes participants who are randomized to a study treatment do not adhere to their treatment assignment. A trial's Coordinating Center and Steering Committee should implement multiple systems to enhance treatment adherence. As a first step for any medication trial, efforts should be made to ensure that the participant does not simply forget to take their pills. This can be customized to the treatment requirement. For example, if a pill is to be taken in the morning, the study coordinator might review the participant's morning routine and determine where the study medication should be kept, e.g., next to the coffee pot. If a pill is to be taken multiple times a day, it may be useful to provide the participant with a pillbox; 2×7 and 4×7 weekly pillboxes are readily available. Smartphone applications for reminders are available (Dayer et al. 2013; Ahmed et al. 2018; Santo et al. 2016) and have been used successfully in randomized clinical trial settings (Morawski et al. 2018). Some medications have clear requirements for successful administration. For example, phosphate binders must be taken with a meal containing phosphorus in order to reduce the possibility of GI side effects, and all patients randomized to the COM-BINE Study (Isakova et al. 2015) were reminded at each visit to make sure to take their blinded study medication with a meal. Ensuring requirements such as this are met can also prevent treatment unblinding; e.g., a participant who takes placebo phosphate binders on an empty stomach will not experience GI side effects where as a patient who takes active phosphate binders on an empty stomach likely will.

Study protocols and manuals of operations will include steps related to reducing or temporarily stopping medication when a participant reports mild side effects potentially related to treatment, seeing if the side effect goes away, and then up-titrating back, possibly to a lower dose. Reducing or temporarily stopping medication may also be helpful for a participant who suspects a symptom he or she is experiencing is caused by the study medication, even if the study team sees no pathway by which the drug in use could cause that symptom.

In a long-term study, investigators might consider studying coordinators suggesting a brief "pill holiday," to allow participants who are at risk of ending participation to take a week or a month off their study drug. In long-term studies, when participants have stopped medication (treatment discontinuation) for reasons unrelated to the study drug and continue attending study visits, it is useful to ask the participant at subsequent visits if he or she might now consider going back on the medication, perhaps at a lower dose than previously.

Participants may refuse the treatment to which they have been randomized or become a treatment crossover, i.e., a participant who has switched to another study treatment arm. Such a participant is sometimes called a drop-in, defined by Piantadosi (2017) as a participant who takes another treatment that is part of the trial instead of the treatment he or she was randomized to, and can be followed for study outcome. Drop-ins cause treatment effect dilution whereby the estimate of the difference between the effect of experimental treatment and the control treatment is reduced.

Finally, for many types of participants (e.g., adolescents, the elderly) and many types of treatments (e.g., antihypertensives, antirejection drugs, retroviral drugs, and dietary interventions), there is a full body of research on barriers to adherence. This is beyond the scope of this chapter, but the DCC and the study leadership should be aware of the literature on adherence related to the participant group and the treatment under study.

Monitoring Treatment Adherence

Drugs do not work in participants who do not take them. – C. Everett Koop, M.D., US Surgeon General, 1985 (Osterberg and Blaschke 2005).

A variety of methods are available for treatment adherence monitoring, and the method selected depends on the type of study and the type of information required (Zulig and Phil Mendys 2017). Medication electronic monitors, also called MEMS or "smart bottles," are expensive but can provide precise information on when a pill bottle or a particular section of a pillbox is opened, allowing investigators to assess adherence to days and adherence to times of day pills are taken (Schwed et al. 1999). Methods such as pill counts and weighing medication bottles require participants to remember to return their "empty" bottles and are logistically cumbersome for the site staff, and these methods are easily influenced by participants who know their adherence will be monitored in this way (Meinert 2012), a phenomenon sometimes referred to as "piles of pills in the parking lot," i.e., participants who have not taken their study meds and want to please their study team will discard pills before coming in to a visit so their adherence by pill count is high. Medication diaries may also be utilized (Farmer 1999). An example report of adherence by pill count by site is shown in Table 2. Only those who brought in their pills for counting and had a pill count done are generally included in pill count denominators, which could cause pill counts to be biased upward, i.e., those who do not bring in pills for counting may have taken fewer pills on average than those who did bring pills in for counting. Rates of pill count completion and implications of missing pill counts should be included in the discussion section of papers that include information on adherence. Note that taking more than 100% of prescribed medication is another form of nonadherence, and consideration should be given to how rates over 100% should be handled in calculations of adherence; a participant who sometimes takes 80% of required medications and sometimes takes 120% of required medications should not be considered to be 100% compliant over time. Consider capping adherence estimates at 100% when evaluating adherence, as was done in Table 2. The DCC should also provide Participating Sites with feedback on numbers and proportions of participants with adherence over a threshold, e.g., over 100%, so the sites can work with their participants on this. Because adherence and treatment crossover vary over time in a long-term study, adherence should be considered as a continuum (Meinert 2012), so a participant has a percent compliance in a trial, not a dichotomous classification as a complier or noncomplier.

When treatment and visits are both discontinued (e.g., because a participant has become lost to follow-up or withdrawn consent for follow-up), this is reported as a study discontinuation, and as with those who did not provide pills for counting, the participant is removed from the denominator of reports of adherence to treatment.

Medication interview questions are less cumbersome than pill counts for participants and staff. Questions must be chosen with care; good interviews, or "medication interrogation," can yield results similar to those obtained from pill counts. Stewart (1987) found that a single question could identify 69.8% of compliers and

Table 2 Adherence at 3 months by Pill Count

Participating Site	Randomized 3 months ago plus 14 day lag time for data entry	Number with 3-month visit documented	Number with 3-month pill count	3-month Pill Count Mean +/- SD, min, max	% of participants with 80%+ Adherence (out of participants with pill counts)
1 California	19	16	15	89.9 +/- 14.7, 56.7, 100.0	86.67
2 Colorado	52	49	40	87.5 +/- 13.5, 48.6, 100.0	77.50
3 Connecticut	18	16	15	95.1 +/- 9.4, 66.7, 100.0	93.33
4 Delaware	41	38	36	90.9 +/- 10.0, 62.9, 100.0	83.33
5 Florida	49	45	39	88.3 +/- 18.0, 21.9, 100.0	84.62
6 Georgia	18	16	13	86.8 +/- 14.7, 50.0, 100.0	76.92
7 Illinois	7	7	5	82.1 +/- 24.2, 45.7, 100.0	60.00
Total	204	187	163	89.2 +/- 14.3, 21.9, 100.0	82.21

80% of noncompliers if pill count is used as a gold standard. Stewart's question was phrased as "How many doses might you have missed in the 10 days?" and was asked as follow-up to an affirmative answer to a nonjudgmental question regarding whether the participant might have missed some doses. It is important that medication interrogation be carried out in a nonjudgmental way. Kravitz, Hays and Sherbourne (1993) reported that when a cohort of 1751 patients with diabetes mellitus, hypertension, and heart disease was surveyed on their adherence to medications, more than 87% reported they had taken their medications as instructed by their doctors "all of the time. A review by Garber et al. (2004) found a wide range of level of agreement between participant-reported adherence by interview, diary, or questionnaire and more objective measures of adherence such as pill count, canister weight, plasma drug concentration, or electronic monitors.

In a pragmatic trial, a participating site may be able to track whether a participant has picked up their treatment or refilled their prescription.

Direct signs of treatment adherence include laboratory measures of levels of the drug itself or of one of its metabolites (Osterberg and Blashchke 2005). Biomarkers of treatment response may also be useful as an indirect sign of treatment adherence.

When monitoring treatment adherence, it is traditional to report adherence on those for whom the adherence was measured. That is, if 100 participants were assigned to a treatment and pill counts are available for 50 of these participants, treatment adherence is reported for the 50 who provided pill count data. The "zero" pill count adherence for those who did not return their pills to the participating site, or those whose pills were not counted for some other reason, is discussed in a nonquantitative way rather than being "averaged in" as pill counts of zero.

Monitoring Early Treatment Discontinuation and Tracking Reasons for Discontinuation

Early treatment discontinuation and treatment crossover can dilute the estimate of a true treatment effect. In early discontinuation, a participant stops taking their assigned treatment. With early discontinuation of active treatment, the treatment effect crosses over to a different treatment effect which may be less than or equal to the treatment effect observed in the study's placebo group. Treatment crossover is worrisome when a participant randomized to the placebo group seeks out and begins taking the treatment being used in the active treatment group. Discontinuations and treatment crossovers can lead to effective interventions being found ineffective and should be carefully tracked to allow for sensitivity analyses and to inform investigators planning future trials of similar treatments.

Sometimes, early treatment discontinuation is clearly related to an adverse event (AE) or a serious adverse event. Examples include AEs related to lab values or symptoms. Lab Value AEs requiring treatment discontinuation may be specified in the study protocol. For example, in the AASK Study, participants (who may have been randomized to Lisinopril) discontinued their ACE inhibitor arm if their serum potassium was over 5.5 (Weinberg et al. 2009). In situations such as this, a physician may choose to stop study treatment if a participant is near the protocol-required cut-point as well. Either way, the primary reason for such treatment discontinuations should be tracked in the study database and should be tracked separately as treatment stopped due to lab value as defined by protocol, or treatment stopped due to lab value observed, physician judgment. Similarly, treatments stopped due to the appearance of specific symptoms or potential medication side effects could be categorized as having been stopped due to symptoms with separate categories for protocol-defined discontinuation, physician judgment, or participant preference.

Other reasons for treatment discontinuation include a participant becoming burnt out by the medication requirements of a study in the absence of abnormal lab values or side effects. Such discontinuations may be flagged as discontinuation due to "pill burden." The study database should explicitly track the Participating Site's evaluation of the primary and secondary reason a participant stopped taking study drug. These data should be captured in real time.

When participants stop taking medications because they have stopped coming to visits, this should also be tracked. Table 3 shows an example of tabulation of the **Primary reason a study participant was not on study medications at the final study visit** including both cases thought to be related to study medication (stopped drug due to lab adverse event, stopped drug due to patient-reported side effects, stopped drug due to patient-reported pill burden) versus cases where a patient stopped attending visits early but did not withdraw consent (discontinued active study participation, allowing for passive follow-up only) or declared withdrawal of consent (would no longer provide study data) or can no longer be located or contacted.

Regarding the topic of adherence in statistical analyses of clinical trials, the reader is referred to the ▸ Chap. 93, "Adherence Adjusted Estimates in Randomized Clinical Trials" in the **Analysis** section of this book authored by Sreelatha Meleth.

The Role of the Study Team in Enhancing Treatment Adherence

Every member of the clinical trial team has a role in enhancing treatment adherence. Treatment adherence issues should be discussed on study coordinators conference calls; it is particularly useful for coordinators who have had success in adherence-related issues to share their experiences with those who have had less success. Principal investigators (PIs) should become personally involved in providing positive feedback for high adherence, as well as encouraging and strategizing with participants who have had difficulties with adherence. PIs should routinely discuss each participant's adherence with the team. An adherence committee made up of study coordinators, physicians, and data-coordinating center staff members may be able to come up with suggestions as a brainstorming group. Treatment adherence should be a topic on the agenda of every steering committee meeting. The data coordinating center should ensure that the trial's manual of operations includes strategies that will assist with adherence for the treatments being studied, and the DCC is responsible for providing feedback on every aspect of adherence and

Table 3 Primary reason a study participant surviving to final visit (end of study) was not on randomized study medication at final visit

Participating Site	Participant ID	Reason not on randomized study medication
1 California	10003	Patient reported side effect (skin rash)
	10015	Lost to follow up
2 Colorado	20023	Patient reported pill burden
	20039	Discontinued active study participation
	20041	Lost to follow up
3 Connecticut	30006	Lab-related adverse event
	30014	Attending visits but quit study meds (noncompliant)
4 Delaware	40015	Side effect (GI symptoms)
	40024	Lost to follow up
	40037	Patient report: pill burden
5 Florida	50005	Withdrawal of consent
	50027	Patient reported side effect (skin rash)
	50040	Withdrawal of consent
6 Georgia	60009	Lost to follow up
	60013	Attending visits but quit study meds (noncompliant)
7 Illinois	70004	Lost to follow up
Number for each reason		
Attending visits but quit study meds (noncompliant): 2		
Discontinued active study participation : 1		
Lab-related adverse event: 1		
Lost to follow up: 5		
Patient reported side effects: 3		
Patient reported pill burden: 2		
Withdrawal of consent: 2		
Total not on randomized treatment at final visit: 16		

treatment discontinuation in an easy-to-read manner. Finally, in their role of monitoring study conduct, a trial's Data Safety and Monitoring Board (DSMB) should track study treatment adherence throughout the study and should note issues related to treatment adherence in its reports back to the study leadership and DSMB.

More work is needed in the area of predictors of or antecedents to adherence. In an early review, Sherbourne and Hays (1992) noted interpersonal quality (having a good social support system) of care and satisfaction with financial aspects of cases stood out as potential predictors of adherence. Different antecedents appear predictive in different studies, and Dunbar-Jacob and Rohay (2016) noted that different methods of measuring adherence yield different predictors of adherence. They looked for predictors in two trials and observed indications of gender and race being more associated with electronically monitored adherence and a participant's self-efficacy being more associated with self-reported adherence.

The End of Treatment

For each trial participant, the last on-treatment-study visit marks the participant's closeout, and remaining medications should be collected at the participating site. If the participant forgets to bring their medications in to their last visit, effort should be made to collect these medications.

Many trials include an off-treatment observation period after treatment ends. If a lab test is to be taken at the end of a specified observation period (a final off-treatment visit) to check for the persistence of a biomarker after treatment ends, as in the BASE Trial (Raphael et al. 2020), the target date for the final off-treatment visit may depend on the date the last dose of study medication was taken. For example, a month 13 final off-treatment visit may have a target date of 4 weeks after the month 12 visit, rather than 13 months after randomization, to allow for reduction of biomarkers or signs 4 weeks after treatment. This should be considered during protocol development and incorporated into the participant appointment schedule described in section "Participant Follow-Up" below.

Participant Follow-Up

Introduction

Every trial has a goal of complete follow-up for all participants, and complete collection of the primary outcome for the study intent-to-treat analysis is the goal. In order to achieve this goal, the participant follow-up visit schedule must be well-defined and reasonable from both the patient and the participating site team's point of view, and the team will need to focus on visit attendance and prevention of incomplete follow-up throughout the course of the trial. For a full discussion of intention to treat analysis, see this reference book's Analysis Section's chapter ► Chap. 82, "Intention to Treat and Alternative Approaches" by J. Goldberg. Incomplete follow-up carries with it a risk of bias in the primary outcome, particularly when the number lost is substantially different between the two treatment groups and the question of whether the experimental intervention influenced attrition (Fewtrell et al. 2008). Even when retention rates are the same in two treatment groups, if retention is not high, study power is reduced and generalizability can be harmed (Brueton 2014). The **Special Topics** section of this reference book includes the chapter on Issues in ▶ Chap. 113, "Issues in Generalizing Results from Clinical Trials" by Steve Piantadosi. Statistical methods are available to handle missing data and are discussed in this book's Analysis Section's ▶ Chap. 86, "Missing Data" by A Allen, F Li, and G Tong, but clearly prevention of missing data is the goal and the impact of some missing data in the middle of a patient's follow-up is less of an issue than the loss of a patient's final data. Results from trials with retention rates of 95% or greater will generally be considered to be valid, particularly when retention is similar in all treatment groups. Retention rates of 80% or lower call into question the validity of results (Sackett et al. 1997). During trial design, staff training, and throughout participant follow-up, retention is key.

Planning the Follow-Up Schedule During Trial Design

The follow-up schedule requires careful consideration during study design. Visits held prior to randomization include screening visits and baseline visits. Visits held after randomization (when a randomized treatment is allocated to the patient from the study's randomization schedule) are designated as follow-up visits. If the treatment is provided to the patient on the day of randomization, the visit may be referred to as the "randomization visit." The number of visits and other contacts included in a trial's visit schedule must be frequent enough to allow for treatment administration and, where necessary, dose adjustment, as well as patient training and collection of needed adherence, process, safety, and outcome data. Trials sometimes have more visits early in follow-up as participants learn to follow their assigned intervention and/or ramp up dosages.

The visits should therefore be often enough but not too often, and in cases where no hands-on data collection is required, phone or electronic contact can be substituted for visits. If participant contact or participant visits occur only once a year, more participants will become difficult to locate or contact because they have moved or changed phone numbers since their last contact. Infrequent visits also make it difficult to capture complete and accurate information on adverse events (AEs) and serious adverse events (SAEs). On the other hand, if participant contact or participant visits occur frequently (e.g., weekly) throughout a trial, this may be too much for a participant to bear. This is particularly true if a number of participants have long travel times due to distance or traffic; it is useful to collect information on participant travel time to the clinic so that if during study conduct, visit adherence becomes an issue, the site can check on the relationship between travel time and visit attendance and, if necessary, limit enrollment of participants who live in areas that are problematic for follow-up visits. The schedule of follow-up visits will depend on the complexity of the study intervention and the disease being studied.

All participants should have the same visit schedule; this will prevent bias in AE and SAE detection ["The more one looks, the more one sees" (Meinert 2012)] and will reduce follow-up bias associated with more time and attention spent on intervention group participants. The duration of the visit schedule should be well-defined;

follow-up either continues until a common calendar date for all patients or continues to a common time point for each patient, e.g., 24 months postrandomization. Follow-up should continue according to protocol regardless of patient adherence to treatment or patient attainment of a given outcome.

Making Trial Data Collection as Easy as Possible for the Participant

As noted, once a study begins, recruitment, retention, and adherence are key. The plans for visits and collection must be safe for the patient and should be kept as easy as possible for the participant. When multicenter trials are being designed, steering committees balance their hopes for pragmatism with special research interests, and a study protocol may be full of visit requirements including, questionnaires, lab tests, physical function tests, imaging, and clinical measurements.

The desire to capture a large amount of data is sometimes addressed by having shorter routine visits and collecting more data remotely and collecting more data at annual visits. Collecting more data remotely is helpful. Questionnaires can be completed from home during the week before a visit, online via smartphone, tablet, or computer, or can be sent and returned by mail. Collecting more data at annual visits can cause annual visits to be overwhelmingly long. The steering committee should think outside the box. In a trial with brief quarterly visits, it may be possible to collect some of the "annual extra data" at months 0, 12, 24, and 36 and other data at, say, months 0, 9, 21, and 33. If participants decide that their visits are too long, they will be less likely to attend all of their visits.

Reminders can help with visit attendance. Coordinators can customize reminders prior to visits to the participant; some participants will prefer reminder via text message rather than phone call, for example. Reminders are also helpful when a patient must bring along a sample (24-hour urine jug, for example) or their pill bottle(s) for counting or weighing.

Consideration should be given to ensure that requirements are convenient and that participants will be comfortable. The site should consider not only covering parking expenses but also making sure the participant can park in a convenient area. Childcare expenses could be covered. Holding evening and weekend visits will be helpful for working participants. If, for example, a visit includes a test that requires a 12-hour fast, visits should be scheduled in the morning. If a trial requires going to a distant part of the medical campus, the study coordinator should arrange for a shuttle ride. Making visits as convenient as possible for participants will pay off in retention.

Training the Participating Site Staff on Follow-Up

Initial site-staff training, and retraining at staff annual meetings, should include a review of the trial's visit schedule and the trial's retention plan as well as training in methods known to facilitate retention. The expectation should be that each participant will attend all visits, with a recognition that of course some participants will miss some visits. When a participant is randomized, the DCC should provide the site with the participant's appointment schedule showing both the target date for each visit (e.g., the target date for the 12-month visit is 12 months postrandomization) and the study-specified visit window (e.g., plus or minus 1 week of the target date). It is also helpful to have a master schedule with the start of visit windows and target appointment dates for each participating site.

Methods to facilitate retention that should be covered at training could include as examples:

- Procedures should be established such that prior to randomization, participating site teams discuss each eligible participant's suitability for a trial. During recruitment, sites may feel considerable pressure to enroll more participants. Care must be taken that the site has thought about whether each participant they consider is likely to comply with treatment and to attend required visits/to provide required data.
- Participating site team members who recruit participants should try to collect data at study and start on alternative ways to contact a participant should he or she become unreachable (e.g., changes their phone number).
- The study coordinator should set up systems for visit reminders that are appropriate for the participant. Automated text messaging is a good way to reach smartphone users. Automated or coordinator-initiated phone calls may be better for those who do not routinely text.
- The participating site team members should engage with the participant in ways that make them feel valued. In studies where participants are not paid, the participants may appreciate birthday cards. In long-term studies, sites might consider annual incentives such as grocery store vouchers or small gifts such as fleece blankets or tote bags. Thank you notes signed by the study team make a participant feel appreciated at little cost to the study and should be considered in cases where tangible incentives are not funded or are not permitted. Sometimes, smaller rewards are provided for questionnaires or short visits and larger rewards are provided for longer visits or for a study's final visit.

In a long-term study in which patients may become burned out over time, training in retention should include prioritization for outcome measures. The study will always accept whatever data a not-fully-adherent participant is willing to provide, and obtaining the primary outcome measure for each patient will always be top priority. However, if there are multiple secondary measures, the study leadership should provide guidance to the sites on the relative importance of each planned measure or the value of a surrogate for the primary outcome if the primary outcome is not available. Such prioritization will help the site team negotiate with patients who reach a point in a long-term study where they will no longer comply with all of the study requirements.

As an aside, trial leadership should also ensure that study coordinators and other participating site personnel feel valued and appreciated.

Retention Monitoring

The DCC should design their retention monitoring feedback at the start of study and provide an example retention table at training and review how to read it. It may be helpful for the feedback to include missingness for a single visit and a summary of those who have missed their last two (or more) visits; the first is noteworthy but may be easily explained by the circumstances of the participant, e.g., they were on vacation or hospitalized for much of the visit window, but the participating site team expects them back for their next visit. The second note, of one who has missed their past two or more visits, flags a participant at risk of becoming lost to follow-up.

It is helpful to report on missed visits both looking at each visit (month 6, month 12) and looking overall (across all visits). An example of a table monitoring missed visits by visit and by site is shown in Table 4. The first column would list the participating sites. The second column would show how many randomized participants would have been expected to have that visit, i.e., the number of randomized participants who have been in follow-up through the end of that visit window as of a data entry lag time such as 2 weeks previous to the report being run. The third column shows the number and percent of expected visits held. The fourth column shows the number of visits known to have been missed, based on site reporting; it is useful to have an item at the beginning of a study's visit form on status of visit – held or missed to document the cases where the visit window is past and the form is not pending; the site confirms that the visit was not held. A fifth column can be used to document cases where the site has submitted a form for that visit but the visit was held so far outside of the window that it is unlikely to be used in analyses, e.g., the visit intended for Month 3 was held in the beginning of the Month 6 target window. The sixth column would show counts of participants with an unknown visit status, flagging cases where the visit form has not yet been submitted. This table is appropriate for the study-wide weekly report; site personnel will also need the details for columns 4–6, so they are reminded of which participants missed the visit

Table 4 3-month visit held and missed

Participating Site	Randomized 3 months ago plus 14 day lag time for data entry	Number with 3-month visit form documenting visit held	Number with 3-month visit form documenting visit missed	Number with 3-month visit form showing visit held outside window	Number with 3-month visit form not yet submitted
1 California	19	16 (84.2%)	1	1	1
2 Colorado	52	49 (94.2%)	2	0	1
3 Connecticut	18	16 (88.9%)	1	0	1
4 Delaware	41	38 (92.7%)	1	0	2
5 Florida	49	45 (91.8%)	1	2	1
6 Georgia	18	16 (88.9%)	1	1	0
7 Illinois	7	7 (100%)	0	0	0
Total	204	187 (91.7%)	7	4	6

Table 5 Participants missing two most recent protocol visits

Participating Site	Randomized ≥73 Days ago	Missing F1 and F2 Visits	Randomized ≥104 Days ago	Missing F2 and F3 Visits	Randomized ≥196 Days ago	Missing F3 and F6 Visits
1 California	19	0	19	0	19	0
2 Colorado	47	0	44	0	37	0
3 Connecticut	16	0	16	0	15	1
4 Delaware	33	0	32	1	22	1
5 Florida	46	0	42	0	41	1
6 Georgia	15	0	13	0	13	0
7 Illinois	6	0	6	0	5	0
Total	182	0	172	1	152	3

(column 4), know the IDs of those whose visit was done so outside the window that it cannot be used as data for that visit (column 5), and have a pending visit form (column 5). If a study's recommended visit windows are strict and the report shows a high proportion of visits as having been missed, it is useful for the weekly report to include two versions of these tables, one showing visits missing under the study's strict visit window limits and one showing visits missing under a broader window indicating that the data are close enough to the target date to be used for some statistical analyses.

Early detection of patients at risk for becoming drop outs (randomized patients who have stopped attending study visits) is critical. It is helpful to report on those who have missed their last two visits. Table 5 shows an example tallying this by site and identification of the last two visits missed. The IDs of those who have missed the last two visits should be provided to each site. Participants will "fall off" Table 5 and the listing when they resume visit attendance. Participants who have died (or been censored) are reported separately rather than in these tables, which are focused on dropouts.

It is helpful to have participating site personnel investigate and provide an explanation of why a participant has missed the last two visits. The process used to get this information from the site ensures that the site realizes that the participant has missed two visits and requires the site team to investigate. This can help detect cases where a participant has moved, had an extended hospitalization or rehab visit, or died and will focus the site on retention of participants at the individual participant level.

Factors Related to Predicting Retention

Sites should publish efforts taken to enhance retention. They are more likely to be applicable to other trials in other populations or other disease areas than methods used to enhance recruitment and adherence (Fewtrell et al. 2008).

When reporting on retention, if the number of patients available through the end of a trial for full analysis of study safety and other outcomes (treatment adherence, quality of life) differs from the number of patients available for the trial's primary outcome, both should be reported as was done in the BID Trial (Miskulin et al. 2018); in this study, fewer patients had data for the primary outcome of change in LV Mass than were available for other study measurements because of difficulties with scheduling and measurement of baseline and month 12 MRI. In studies with mortality outcomes, trialists may be able to capture the primary outcome in more patients than one can evaluate for other outcomes.

The Role of the Study Team in Promoting Retention

Each member of the Study team has a role in promoting retention. At the participating site, study coordinators should engage the patient. As noted, the study coordinators and site investigators could set up a system such that reimbursement for expenses such as parking and payment, gift cards, and other incentives are provided to the patient. The data coordinating center should provide retention feedback and facilitate discussion of retention on study coordinator calls and at Steering Committee meetings, and the Study DSMB should highlight retention issues and emphasize the importance of retention in its recommendations back to the steering committee.

Interrelationship Between Treatment Discontinuation and Dropouts

The challenges in getting the participant to comply with their study treatment (section "Administration of Study Treatments") and getting the participant to attend study visits and provide data (section "Participant Follow-Up") are related. These are directly related on a patient level in that a patient who misses visits may also be noncompliant to treatment. Difficulties with these two may go hand in hand at the study or site level as well. A trial or a participating site in a trial that is having significant trouble with adherence may also have difficulties in retention and vice versa. Of course, it is hoped that those who discontinue treatment remain available for follow-up and obtaining the primary result variable, but studies with a higher number of patients who do not comply to treatment may also have more patients who stop attending visits and providing follow-up data. Site personnel should be reminded often that if a patient says they will no longer follow study treatment per protocol, they should be encouraged to follow any level of treatment. If the patient will no longer accept any study treatment, they should be counseled on the importance of continuing to provide follow-up data. As noted, it may be helpful for the study leadership to provide a prioritized list so patients who are reluctant to provide full data care can be asked to provide as much as possible, in the order of importance. Every study should follow up on drop outs in any way possible, even if all that can be done is to check for vital status at the end of the study. Unless a patient has withdrawn consent and refuses to allow the study to capture any information, it is likely that at least some data will be available on most patients who drop out, and, as noted, patients who stop attending visits may be quite willing to allow for passive follow-up whereby their local medical charts are used to provide information on blood pressure, lab measures, and hospitalizations, for example. The DCC should take care to report on two types of protocol nonadherence as separate issues, so the study leadership and DSMB can consider why participants are not following treatment or why they have stopped attending visits so it is clear which patients who have discontinued treatment are available for continued follow-up for the primary outcome variable (and have the potential to return to adherence) and which patients are no longer willing to attend visits.

Summary and Conclusion

All of the steps in study design and organization leading up to the initiation of a study are critical, yet once trial randomization begins, achieving the study's planned recruitment, adherence, and retention and accurately capturing data on these factors are key to meaningful study results. Training sessions, meetings, and conference calls of the Steering Committee, subcommittees, and study coordinators should include agenda items focused on these areas of trial conduct. Treatment administration, treatment adherence, and participant follow-up data should be shared using metrics and should be captured in real time, with the Data Coordinating Center providing continuous performance monitoring of these data to study leadership and to the participating sites themselves to optimize performance for valid study conduct and complete and accurate data capture.

Key Facts

- Study coordinators and site investigators should be trained that it is important to get the primary outcome variable for intent to treat analyses in all patients whether they adhere to treatment or not.
- The schedule for study visits and the system for collection of data should not be too hard on patients, and sites should engage patients and provide incentives and rewards as permitted.
- If a participant drops out, he or she may still be agreeable to passive follow-up through their chart; the trial leadership should consider which data would be useful to capture for a patient who will no longer attend visits.
- The DCC should provide performance data on adherence, treatment discontinuation, missed visits, and dropouts. These reports should be continuously updated and should show data site by site.
- Categorization of reasons why patients discontinued treatment or dropped out should be captured in real time and included in reports.

Cross-References

▶ Adherence Adjusted Estimates in Randomized Clinical Trials
▶ Intention to Treat and Alternative Approaches
▶ Missing Data
▶ Procurement and Distribution of Study Medicines

References

Ahmed I, Ahmad NS, Ali S, George A, Saleem-Danish H, Uppal E, Soo J, Mobasheri MH, King D, Cox B, Darzi A (2018) Medication adherence apps: review and content analysis. JMIR Mhealth Uhealth 6(3):e62. https://doi.org/10.2196/mhealth.6432

Booker C, Harding S, Benzeval M (2011) A systematic review of the effect of retention methods in population-based cohort studies. BMC Public Health 11:249. https://doi.org/10.1186/1471-2458-11-249

Brueton VC, Tierney JF, Stenning S, Meredith S, Harding S, Nazareth I, Rait G (2014) Strategies to improve retention in randomised trials: a Cochrane systematic review and meta-analysis. BMJ Open 4(2):e003821. https://doi.org/10.1136/bmjopen-2013-003821

Byar DP, Simon RM, Friedewald WT, Schlesselman JJ, DeMets DL, Ellenberg JH, Gail MH, Ware JH (1976) Randomized clinical trials – perspectives on some recent ideas. N Engl J Med 295:74–80. https://doi.org/10.1056/NEJM197607082950204

Dayer L, Heldenbrand S, Anderson P, Gubbins PO, Martin BC (2013) Smartphone medication adherence apps: potential benefits to patients and providers. J Am Pharm Assoc (JAPhA) 53 (2):172–181. https://doi.org/10.1111/j.1547-5069.2002.00047.x

Dunbar-Jacob J, Rohay JM (2016) Predictors of medication adherence: fact or artifact. J Behav Med 39(6):957–968. https://doi.org/10.1007/s10865-016-9752-8

Farmer KC (1999) Methods for measuring and monitoring medication regimen adherence in clinical trials and clinical practice. Clin Ther 21(6):1074–1090. https://doi.org/10.1016/S0149-2918(99)80026-5

Ferris M, Norwood V, Radeva M, Gassman JJ, Al-Uzri A, Askenazi D, Matoo T, Pinsk M, Sharma A, Smoyer W, Stults J, Vyas S, Weiss R, Gipson D, Kaskel F, Friedman A, Moxey-Mims M, Trachtman H (2013) Patient recruitment into a multicenter randomized clinical trial for kidney disease: report of the focal segmental glomerulosclerosis clinical trial (FSGS CT). Clin Transl Sci 6(1):13–20. https://doi.org/10.1111/cts.12003

Fewtrell MS, Kennedy K, Singhal A, Martin RM, Ness A, Hadders-Algra M, Koletzko B, Lucas A (2008) How much loss to follow-up is acceptable in long-term randomised trials and prospective studies? Arch Dis Child 93(6):458–461. https://doi.org/10.1136/adc.2007.127316

FHN Trial Group, Chertow GM, Levin NW, Beck GJ, Depner TA, Eggers PW, Gassman JJ, Gorodetskaya I, Greene T, James S, Larive B, Lindsay RM, Mehta RL, Miller B, Ornt DB, Rajagopalan S, Rastogi A, Rocco MV, Schiller B, Sergeyeva O, Schulman G, Ting GO, Unruh ML, Star RA, Kliger AS (2010) In-center hemodialysis six times per week versus three times per week. N Engl J Med 363:2287–2300. https://doi.org/10.1056/NEJMoa1001593

Garber M, Nau D, Erickson S, Aikens J, Lawrence J (2004) The concordance of self-report with other measures of medication adherence: a summary of the literature. Med Care 42(7):649–652. https://doi.org/10.1097/01.mlr.0000129496.05898.02

Gassman J, Agodoa L, Bakris G, Beck G, Douglas J, Greene T, Jamerson K, Kutner M, Lewis J, Randall OS, Wang S, Wright JT, the AASK Study Group (2003) Design and statistical aspects of the African American Study of Kidney Disease and Hypertension (AASK). J Am Soc Nephrol 14:S154–S165. https://doi.org/10.1097/01.ASN.0000070080.21680.CB

Gipson DS, Trachtman H, Kaskel FJ, Greene TH, Radeva MK, Gassman JJ, Moxey-Mims MM, Hogg RJ, Watkins SL, Fine RN, Hogan SL, Middleton JP, Vehaskari VM, Flynn PA, Powell LM, Vento SM, McMahan JL, Siegel N, D'Agati VD, Friedman AL (2011) Clinical trial of focal segmental glomerulosclerosis (FSGS) in children and young adults. Kidney Int 80(8):868–878. https://doi.org/10.1038/ki.2011.195

Isakova T, Ix JH, Sprague SM, Raphael KL, Fried L, Gassman JJ, Raj D, Cheung AK, Kusek JW, Flessner MF, Wolf M, Block GA (2015) Rationale and approaches to phosphate and fibroblast growth factor 23 reduction in CKD. J Am Soc Nephrol 26(10):2328–2339. https://doi.org/10.1681/ASN.2015020117

Ix JH, Isakova T, Larive B, Raphael KL, Raj D, Cheung AK, Sprague SM, Fried L, Gassman JJ, Middleton J, Flessner MF, Wolf M, Block GA, Wolf M (2019) Effects of nicotinamide and lanthanum carbonate on serum phosphate and fibroblast growth factor-23 in chronic kidney disease: The COMBINE trial. J Am Soc Nephrol 30(6):1096–1108. https://doi.org/10.1681/ASN.2018101058

Kravitz RL, Hays RD, Sherbourne CD (1993) Recall of recommendations and adherence to advice among patients with chronic Medical conditions. Arch Intern Med 153(16):1869–1878. https://doi.org/10.1001/archinte.1993.00410160029002

Meinert CL (2012) Clinical trials: design, conduct and analysis, 2nd edn. Oxford University Press, New York

Miskulin DC, Gassman J, Schrader R, Gul A, Jhamb M, Ploth DW, Negrea L, Kwong RY, Levey AS, Singh AK, Harford A, Paine S, Kendrick C, Rahman M, Zager P (2018) BP in dialysis: results of a pilot study. J Am Soc Nephrol 29(1):307–316. https://doi.org/10.1681/ASN.2017020135

Morawski K, Ghazinouri R, Krumme A et al (2018) Association of a smartphone application with medication adherence and blood pressure control: the MedISAFE-BP randomized clinical trial. JAMA Intern Med 178(6):802–809. https://doi.org/10.1001/jamainternmed.2018.0447

Osterberg L, Blashchke T (2005) Adherence to medication August 4, 2005. N Engl J Med 353:487–497. https://doi.org/10.1056/NEJMra050100

Piantadosi S (2017) Clinical trials a methodologic perspective. Wiley series in probability and statistics, 3rd edn. Wiley, New York

Raphael KL, Isakova T, Ix JH, Raj DS, Wolf M, Fried LF, Gassman JJ, Kendrick C, Larive B, Flessner MF, Mendley SR, Hostetter TH, Block GA, Li P, Middleton JP, Sprague SM, Wesson DE, Cheung AK (2020). A Randomized Trial Comparing the Safety, Adherence, and Pharmacodynamics Profiles of Two Doses of Sodium Bicarbonate in CKD: the BASE Pilot Trial. J Am Soc Nephrol 31(1):161–174. https://doi.org/10.1681/ASN.2019030287

Rocco MV, Lockridge RS, Beck GJ, Eggers PW, Gassman JJ, Greene T, Larive B, Chan CT, Chertow GM, Copland M, Hoy C, Lindsay RM, Levin NW, Ornt DB, Pierratos A, Pipkin M, Rajagopalan S, Stokes JB, Unruh ML, Star RA, Kliger AS, the FHN Trial Group (2011) The effects of nocturnal home hemodialysis: the frequent hemodialysis network nocturnal trial. Kidney Int 80:1080–1091. https://doi.org/10.1038/ki.2011.213

Sackett DL, Richardson WS, Rosenberg W (1997) Evidence-based medicine: how to practice and teach EBM. Churchill Livingstone, New York

Santo K, Richtering SS, Chalmers J, Thiagalingam A, Chow CK, Redfern J (2016) Mobile phone apps to improve medication adherence: a systematic stepwise process to identify high-quality apps. JMIR Mhealth Uhealth 4(4):e132. https://doi.org/10.2196/mhealth.6742

Schwed A, Fallab C-L, Burnier M, Waeber B, Kappenberger L, Burnand B, Darioli R (1999) Electronic monitoring of adherence to lipid- lowering therapy in clinical practice. J Clin Pharmacol 39(4):402–409. https://doi.org/10.1177/00912709922007976

Stewart M (1987) The validity of an interview to assess a patient's drug taking. Am J Prev Med 3:95–100

Trachtman H, Vento S, Gipson D, Wickman L, Gassman J, Joy M, Savin V, Somers M, Pinsk M, Greene T (2011) Novel therapies for resistant focal segmental glomerulosclerosis (FONT) phase II clinical trial: study design. BMC Nephrol 12:8. https://doi.org/10.1186/1471-2369-12-8

Weinberg JM, Appel LJ, Bakris G, Gassman JJ, Greene T, Kendrick CA, Wang X, Lash J, Lewis JA, Pogue V, Thornley-Brown D, Phillips RA, African American Study of Hypertension and Kidney Disease Collaborative Research Group (2009) Risk of hyperkalemia in nondiabetic patients with chronic kidney disease receiving antihypertensive therapy. Arch Intern Med 169 (17):1587–1594. https://doi.org/10.1001/archinternmed.2009.284

Zulig LL, Phil Mendys HB (2017) Bosworth, Medication adherence: A practical measurement selection guide using case studies. Patient Educ Couns 100(7):1410–1414. https://doi.org/10. 1016/j.pec.2017.02.001. ISSN 0738-3991

Data Capture, Data Management, and Quality Control; Single Versus Multicenter Trials

17

Kristin Knust, Lauren Yesko, Ashley Case, and Kate Bickett

Contents

Abstract

Data capture, data management, and quality control processes are instrumental to the conduct of clinical trials. Obtaining quality data requires numerous considerations throughout the life cycle of the trial. Case report form design and data capture methodology are crucial components that ensure data are collected in a streamlined and accurate manner. Robust data quality and validation strategies must be employed

K. Knust (✉) · L. Yesko · A. Case · K. Bickett
Emmes, Rockville, MD, USA
e-mail: kknust@emmes.com; lyesko@emmes.com; acase@emmes.com; kate.bickett@gmail.com

© Springer Nature Switzerland AG 2022   303
S. Piantadosi, C. L. Meinert (eds.), *Principles and Practice of Clinical Trials*,
https://doi.org/10.1007/978-3-319-52636-2_40

early on in data collection to identify potential systemic errors. Data management guidance documents provide an opportunity to set clear expectations for stakeholders and establish communication pathways. These tools need to be supplemented with adequate training and ongoing support of trial staff. Trials may be conducted in a single or multicenter setting, which has implications for data management. Risk-based monitoring is one approach that can help data managers target quality issues in a multicenter setting. Evolving technologies such as electronic medical record and electronic data capture system integration, artificial intelligence, and big data analytics are changing the landscape of data capture and management.

Keywords

Data management · Data collection · Data quality · Multicenter trial · Case report form (CRF) · Risk-based monitoring (RBM) · Data review · Electronic medical record (EMR) · Electronic data capture (EDC)

Introduction

One of the key components to a successful clinical trial is a strong foundation of quality data. Data management and quality control measures ensure the accuracy and reliability of the database used in analyses, which are imperative to the outcome of a clinical trial. The goal of a data management program is to produce a clean dataset containing no data entry errors or unexplained missing data points and assure that all the necessary data to analyze the trial endpoints are collected consistently. The consequences of a poorly designed or improperly implemented data management and quality control program are manifested in additional burdens of time, resources, trial costs, and, perhaps most importantly, in a failure to produce an accurate database for analysis.

Some important considerations for designing a data management program include the method of data capture, design of case report forms and edit checks, implementation of data management reporting tools to assess data quality, setting clear expectations based on trial objectives and sponsor/investigator goals, development of training and reference tools for trial stakeholders, and strategies for conducting data review. In addition, the context of the trial must be considered, such as whether it is conducted in a single center, multicenter, or network setting and the platform, format, and methods for sharing trial data.

Data Capture

Data Management Life Cycle

Data management activities span the life cycle of a clinical trial. Ideally, data management teams are integrated into the protocol development phase, during which case report form (CRF) development and database design may begin. Review and input from data managers (DMs) during this crucial stage may help identify and reduce extraneous data collection and anticipate potential data management challenges.

During implementation, data management documents are developed in conjunction with other trial management processes, and site training materials should be developed. Data managers may be involved in the creation of system or CRF user guides, in addition to establishing data management and data validation plans to inform the collection and management of data throughout the trial.

At the time of activation and accrual, data management includes implementation of data collection tools and early monitoring of data to identify potential trends or issues. During trial maintenance, data management and quality control activities are ongoing, and data managers typically utilize tools to detect anomalies, resolve queries, retrieve missing data, and ensure the integrity of the trial database.

In preparation for trial analysis, data quality and cleaning activities may become more targeted or focused on trial endpoint data to ensure the analysis can be completed. During trial closure or in preparation for data lock, all remaining data quality items are resolved or documented.

Data Capture Methods

The method of data capture and data storage should be considered during the design of the trial and prior to the development of CRFs to ensure that information is efficiently collected. Potential data capture methods include traditional paper-based data collection, electronic data capture (EDC), electronic health record (EHR) integration, and external data transfer/upload or any combination of these methods. While clinical trials historically used paper CRFs, there has been an increasing trend toward digital integration due to the enhanced quality control and real-time communication features available. EDC offers centralized data storage which will speed analysis and distribution of results at the end of a trial. Additionally, the availability of tablets and other portable devices has made this a cost-effective and practical option.

An EDC system has become the gold standard for use in clinical trials, where site staff or participants enter the data directly into the system, staff collect data on paper CRFs and then enter data in the system, or data is transferred through an upload into the system. Many EDC systems contain additional tools for managing data quality, including features for real-time front-end data validation, shipment and specimen tracking, transmission of non-form or imaging data (e.g., blood/tissue samples, X-rays), report management and live data tracking, query resolution, adjudication of trial outcomes, scheduling for participant visits, and other trial management tools (Reboussin and Espeland 2005). Having a direct data entry system reduces the potential for transcription errors when the data are recorded in EDC and provides the ability to perform real-time data checks such as those for values outside the expected ranges (e.g., a weight of 950 pounds). As worldwide availability of internet capabilities and prevalence of EDC systems have expanded over the years, traditional paper CRF data entry has diminished. In circumstances where EDC is the preferred method of data capture but internet access is unreliable or limited, offline data entry may be used to collect data and then transmit once an internet connection is established.

The technological enhancements available through EDC systems have a significant advantage for multi-center trials in that it provides a mechanism for Data Managers (DMs) to view the data across all sites in real-time and perform quality control checks such as identifying missing values, performing contemporaneous data audits, or issuing queries. Specifically, it allows the DM to review current data across all sites to identify trends or potential process issues earlier in the data collection stream.

A variety of commercial EDC applications are available for use. Some are available as "off the shelf" software and are free of charge, although features may be limited. Other proprietary systems are available and may be customizable to the needs of a client. Many factors go into choosing the appropriate application, including the complexity of the trial and the number of participants and sites. It is often more appropriate for a multi-center trial to choose a customizable EDC, as it offers additional flexibility and reliability in data collection, storage, review, retrieval, validation, analysis, and reporting as needed. A small, less complex single site or limited resource trial may use a free commercial off the shelf (COTS) solution, as it still offers some of the important features such as front-end validation but may not have the capability for more complex reporting or customizations.

The design of the database will depend on the specific method of data capture and encompasses a wide range of activities. However, it is important to evaluate whether the database structure is both comprehensive enough to ensure all trial objectives are met while minimizing the amount of extraneous data that may be captured. The volume and complexity of data collected for a given trial should be weighed against the relative utility of the information. If the data point being collected is not essential to the outcome of the trial, consider the cost of the data collection burden to site staff, in addition to the cost of cleaning the data, before including it.

Case Report Form (CRF) Development

A CRF, also sometimes known as a data collection form, is designed to collect the participant data in a clinical trial. The International Conference on Harmonization Guideline for Good Clinical Practice defines the CRF as "a printed, optical or electronic document designed to record all of the protocol-required information to be reported to the sponsor on each trial participant." (ICH 2018). When implemented in an EDC system, CRFs may be referred to as data entry screens or electronic CRFs (eCRFs).

The thoughtful design of CRFs is fundamental to the success of the trial. Many challenges in data management result from poor CRF design or implementation. Designing a format for CRFs or data entry screens is important, and the basic considerations are the same with paper or eCRFs. CRF development is ideally performed concurrently with protocol development to ensure that trial endpoints are captured and will yield analyzable data. Ideally, the statistical design section of the protocol (or statistical analysis plan) will be consulted to map all data points to the analysis to confirm the data required will be available.

At a minimum, CRFs should be designed to collect data for analysis of primary and secondary outcomes and safety endpoints and verify or document inclusion and exclusion criteria. When developing a schedule of assessments (i.e., visit schedule), the feasibility of data collection time-points should be evaluated. The schedule should include all critical time-points, while ensuring that the frequency of visits and anticipated participant burden is considered. Furthermore, the impact of data collection on site staff should be assessed. When possible, soliciting input on form content from individuals responsible for entering data may identify problematic questions and clarify expectations.

While the content is crucial for analysis, structure and setup of the CRF is vital to collecting quality data. There are no universal best practices for form development, although the Clinical Data Interchange Standards Consortium (CDISC) has made significant progress toward creating tools and guidelines (Richesson and Nadkarni 2011). CDISC has also implemented the Clinical Data Acquisition Standards Harmonization (CDASH) project, which utilizes common data elements and standard code lists for different therapeutic areas to collect data in a standardized approach (Gaddale 2015).

The primary objective of CRF design is to gather complete and accurate data. This is achieved by avoiding duplication of data elements and facilitating transcription of data from source documents onto the CRF. Ideally, it should be well structured, easy to complete without much assistance, and should collect data of the highest quality (Nahm et al. 2011).

Some basic principles in CRF development and design include the following:

- Identify the intended audience and data entry method (e.g., trial staff direct data entry or electronic participant reported outcomes/ePRO) and style of the CRF (interview, procedural, or retrospective). This will determine the question format and reading level of the question.
- Standardize CRF design to address the needs of all users such as investigator, site coordinator, trial monitor, data entry personnel, medical coder, and statistician (Nahm et al. 2011). Review by all affected parties before finalization confirms usability and ensures complete data elements.
- Organize data in a format that facilitates and simplifies data analysis (Nahm et al. 2011).
- Keep questions, prompts, and instructions clear and concise to assure that data collection is consistent across all participants at various sites.
- Group-related fields and questions together.
- Use consistent language across different CRFs in the same protocol and across protocols. Avoid asking the same question in different ways (e.g., a field for "date of birth" as well as a field for "participant age") as data provided for these fields may be inconsistent and creates additional work for the clinical sites.

- Avoid capturing the same information more than once (duplication).
- Include clear and concise instructions regarding skip patterns and the characteristics of the expected data.
- Make the CRF easy to follow. Avoid information clutter.
- Version control all CRFs.
- Use consistent formatting across all CRFs.
- Specify the unit of measurement, including decimal places.
- Use standard date format throughout the CRFs.
- Provide CRFs with coded field responses (e.g., "Yes," "No" checkboxes) rather than open text fields when possible to aid in analysis. Codes should be consistent throughout a CRF set (e.g., "Yes" should always be coded as "1").
- Avoid the use of negatively phrased questions. For example, instead of "Did the participant fail to sign the informed consent document?" use "Did the participant sign the informed consent document?"
- Avoid phrasing statements in such a way that leads the participant to a specific response.
- Avoid collecting extraneous or excessive data that are not described in the protocol, as this may distract sites from considering only the data related to trial outcomes.
- Consider the flow of the clinical setting in which data will be collected (e.g., vital sign fields may not be appropriate on a urinalysis CRF).
- Avoid collection of derived data on the CRF to minimize calculation errors. For example, age can be calculated using date of birth. Body mass index can be calculated using height and weight of the participant; only the latter two should be captured (Nahm et al. 2011).
- Avoid creating fields designed to collect information in which a participant's identity can be determined in trial data (e.g., name, initials, phone number, address). In such instances where this information is integral to the trial objectives, appropriate security and privacy measures per regulatory guidelines must be implemented.

Data Management and Quality Control

Risk-Based Monitoring in Data Management

Once data collection begins, the management and quality control of data become the primary focus. However, the volume and pace of data collection may require data managers to target data quality efforts, particularly when a trial is conducted in a multicenter or network setting.

In the Food and Drug Administration Guidance for Industry "Oversight of Clinical Investigations- A Risk Based Approach to Monitoring" (August 2013), the agency acknowledges that some data have more impact on trial results; therefore a risk-based approach can be used. These critical data points include informed consent, eligibility for the trial, safety assessments, treatment adherence, and maintenance of the blind/masking (FDA 2013).

Risk-based monitoring (RBM) creates a framework for managing risks through identification, classification, and appropriate mitigation to support improved participant safety and data quality. Adopting a targeted RBM approach to data management may be appropriate in some settings and can provide significant advantages, including more efficient use of resources, without compromising the integrity of the clinical trial. In this approach, a range of metrics known as key risk indicators (KRIs) may be used in real-time to identify areas of critical importance and are tracked to flag data that may need additional attention (may be participant, site, or trial level). KRIs may include protocol deviations, adverse events, missing values, missing CRFs, or other areas of concern. An example of a report for monitoring KRIs and identification of performance issues is shown in the Fig. 1 below. In this table, the values are programmatically compared to pre-determined standards and given a color code of green (indicating good performance), yellow (problem areas identified), or red (remedial action required). This allows for continuous monitoring in real time and increases responsiveness by the clinical team in identifying patterns or trends that may impact risk assessment of a site or trial, as well as quickly correct and prevent further issues.

A sample report provides a framework for the general timeline and major milestones throughout the protocol life cycle, from the time of protocol approval to the publication of the primary outcome manuscript. This high-level overview compares data from each trial to the defined expectations of the sponsor to highlight trial performance (i.e., column displaying initial proposed dates versus column for actual milestone dates). A column for current projections shifts in relation to current data such as number of participants enrolled. Significant deviations from this timeline highlight performance issues and identify the need for additional monitoring (Fig. 2).

While review of all KRIs is important in a risk-based approach, RBM has significant implications for data management, as data quality metrics may be used to identify higher-risk sites or data management trends that warrant more frequent onsite monitoring.

These might include percent of missing CRFs, missing data fields, outstanding data queries, availability of primary outcome, and number of protocol deviations. If any of these metrics lie outside the normal range, more frequent review of data should be performed to determine if there are additional issues.

In an example of how RBM may be used to identify issues, a DM noticed that a site had exceeded the KRI metric for missing CRFs. Upon further investigation of the site's existing CRFs, several other issues were identified. CRFs had been completed at incorrect visits, and the audit history showed that site staff had completed ePRO assessments, instead of being entered directly in the ePRO system by the participant. The DM revealed that the site staff had been completing the CRFs on behalf of the participants, which was a protocol violation. By using KRIs to flag a high-risk site, the DM was able to identify and mitigate greater process issues, which could have had a significant impact during analysis.

Flags and Triggers: Overall and by Site
Monday, Septembr 17, 2018 9:26 PM ET

Site	Recruitment		Missing Forms	Audits	Regulatory issues	Availability of Primary Outcome Data		Treatment Exposure	Follow-up Visit Attendance
	Recruitment: Overall	Recruitment: Prior 3 Months[1]				Primary Outcome: Overall	Primary Outcome: Prior 90 days		
Site #1	90%	78%	0.0%	0.13%	None	66%	73%	66%	71%
Site #2	100%	180%	0.0%	0.49%	None	61%	58%	70%	72%
Site #3	70%	63%	0.1%	0.60%	None	65%	78%	73%	61%
Site #4	84%	42%	0.0%	0.29%	None	41%	50%	64%	59%
Site #5	100%	69%	0.2%	0.31%	None	79%	71%	71%	70%
Site #6	90%	115%	0.0%	0.50%	None	73%	89%	77%	82%
Site #7	60%	43%	1.5%	0.27%	None	85%	91%	95%	81%
Site #8	150%	100%	0.0%	0.93%	None	71%	78%	60%	45%
Overall	88%	79%	0.5%	0.45%	None	69%	72%	71%	68%

[1] Update on the 1st of the month to show percent of expected to actual randomizations over the previous 3 calender months.
[2] Primary outcome availability for only the prior 90 days calculated as the percentage collected to expected UDS in the past 90 days.
See next page for color definitions

Fig. 1 Example of report for monitoring key risk indicators

Study Number/Title
Basic Protocol Information and Timeline [Updated Monthly]
Tuesday, August 28, 2018 9:31 PM ET

	Initial Proposal	Current Projection	Actual
N (Sample size)	420	450	229
Number of Sites	7		8
Number of Nodes	5		5
Concept Approval Data			9/15/2015
Protocol Approval Date			3/16/2016
Date First Participant Enrolled			11/15/2016
Publication Plan Submitted to Pub. Com.	11/15/2017		2/13/2018
Date Last Participant Enrolled	9/11/2018	11/19/2018	#
Date Trial Completed (Last Follow-up at Last Site)	11/20/2018	1/28/2019	#
Date of Database Lock	1/21/2019	3/31/2019	#
Date of Final Study Report to Sponsor	5/23/2019	7/31/2019	#
Date of Submission of Primary Outcome Paper	7/24/2019	10/1/2019	#
Date of Acceptance of Primary Outcome Paper	9/24/2019	12/2/2019	#
Date to Data Share	7/23/2020	9/30/2020	#

These cells will remain blank until actual occurrence
1 "Initial Proposal" column reflects the plan at the time of first randomization
2 "Current Projection" date are based on the actual average randomization rate over the past 5 months
3 "Actual" N (Sample Size) represents the total number of participants randomized as of last month, and "Actual" number of sites includes both active sites and those closed for new enrollment.

Fig. 2 Example of report for monitoring trial performance

Data Quality Control Tools

In addition to using RBM, there are several different types of data management tools that should be implemented to ensure the validity and integrity of data collected, including a variety of reports and edit checks.

Reports are often developed to track trial metrics for data quality and assess progress and can provide both real-time and summary information. These reports can provide high-level data quality information to both the data management team and site staff collecting the data. While the reports can be made available for review at any time (e.g., via a website or EDC system), they should also be discussed or sent to staff collecting the data points on a set schedule or at pre-determined time-points so that site staff can address discrepancies identified and the data management team can provide feedback and/or training for collection of data.

Reports used to track missing CRFs, missing data points, or numeric data entered outside of an expected range (e.g., an unexpected date or a lab value that is not compatible with life) should be implemented as standard tools to assist with data management review (Baigent et al. 2008). These should be integrated within an EDC system whenever possible to facilitate real-time review.

Edit checks (also called validation checks or queries) are another tool to look for data discrepancies. These are employed as a systematic evaluation of the data entered to flag potential issues and alert the user. Ideally, these checks should be issued to site staff in real time or on a frequent basis, to facilitate timely resolution. Data managers are instrumental in writing edit check messages, which should include a clear description of the issue and the fields (variables) involved in the check, the reason it was flagged as potentially inconsistent, and indicate the steps required for resolution. An edit check program can look at a single data point within a single assessment, multiple data points within a single assessment, or multiple data points across multiple assessments. These checks should be run frequently (or on a set schedule) to identify inconsistencies in the data or data that is in violation of the protocol (Krishnankutt et al. 2012; Baigent et al. 2008).

Edit checks are typically conceptualized during CRF design, as it is important to identify potential areas for discrepant data and minimize duplicate or potentially conflicting data collection. Implementing edit checks early on in active data collection phase will allow detection of trends that may warrant changes to data entry or retraining of site staff. A high priority early in the trial is to develop edit checks to query baseline assessments and enrollment data. These discrepancies may uncover problems with CRFs, misunderstandings at clinical sites, or problems with the trial protocol that are critical to address. During the conduct of any trial, new checks are often identified and programmed due to protocol changes, CRF changes, findings during a clinical monitoring visit, or anomalies noted in trial-related reports.

Data Review

Throughout the conduct of a trial, it is expected that there is ongoing review of data. This may be conducted by different stakeholders, with the goal of monitoring and evaluating data collected in a contemporaneous fashion to identify potential concerns.

Initiating communication with site staff following the enrollment of the first participant is a simple review strategy to increase the likelihood of accurate and timely data entry. It is during the first participant enrollment that sites first enact the written protocol and trial procedures at their institution. Despite discussions regarding implementation and training prior to activation, the first participant enrolled is often when sites first experience any challenges with the integration of trial procedures into their standard practice. This is a critical time for the data manager to be engaged with the rest of the site team to be sure that any issues are resolved and that all necessary data are captured. Follow-up contact with site staff in this timeframe provides an opportunity to communicate parts of the enrollment process that went well and those that would be helpful to adjust. Immediately following the first participant enrollment, the site staff is more likely to recall issues and any missing or difficult information. This feedback is extremely valuable to the data management team, particularly in multicenter trials. The challenges encountered at one institution may be shared across multiple sites. Discussing with sites allows for the trend to be identified and potentially adjusted in real time so that other sites may avoid the same problems. Additionally, touching base with the site at this early time-point provides the opportunity to communicate reminders for upcoming assessments and trial requirements.

Another strategy for data review includes performing a data audit after a milestone has been met, such as a percentage of accrual completed or a certain number of participants reaching an endpoint. In this type of review, a subset of participants is identified, and data cleaning procedures are performed to ensure all data submitted through the desired time-point are complete and accurate. The subset of data may be run through statistical programs or checks to verify the validity of the data collected thus far. The goal of this type of review is to identify any systematic errors that may be present. If any errors are identified, there is an opportunity to review the potential impact and determine whether any changes to the CRFs or system are required.

Endpoint or data review committees may also be convened to provide an independent assessment of trial endpoints or critical clinical or safety data. For some trials where endpoints are particularly complex or subject to potential bias, an independent review committee may provide additional assurance that trial results are accurate and reliable. In the FDA's Guidance for Industry: Clinical Trial Endpoints for the Approval of Cancer Drugs and Biologics, it is noted that an independent endpoint review committee (IRC) can minimize bias in the interpretation of certain endpoints. If an endpoint committee is determined to be necessary for a trial, a charter or guidance document should be in place prior to the start of the trial to outline the data points that will be adjudicated by the committee, how the data will be distributed for review, and when the data review will occur. In addition, the charter should specify how "differences in interpretation and incorporation of clinical data in the final interpretation of data and audit procedures" will be resolved (FDA 2018).

Depending on the duration of the trial, endpoint adjudication may occur on an ongoing basis (e.g., as participants reach an endpoint that will be adjudicated) or may be conducted at the end of the trial (e.g., once a predetermined number of participants reach an endpoint). The scope of the review is typically limited to the primary or secondary endpoints of a trial but may include other clinically relevant data points. A risk-based approach can also be taken for the endpoint review, with a subset of cases reviewed and the committee adjourned if a certain concordance with the reported data is met. For example, if independent review of an endpoint demonstrates that committee review of data agrees with site-reported assessment in 95% of cases, it may not be necessary to review data for every participant in the trial. When this approach is used, the proposed concordance rate should be included in the charter. To provide data for independent review, a data listing or similar format is typically used to incorporate relevant information. Source documents (e.g., imaging, clinical records) may be included as part of the review but must be appropriately de-identified to protect participant information.

When used as a component of a data management program, independent endpoint review can ensure efficient and unbiased evaluation of key trial data.

Data Management Plan/Data Validation Plan

A comprehensive Data Management Plan (DMP) provides a blueprint for ensuring quality data throughout the life cycle of a trial. The DMP specifies the tools and processes that will be utilized in the management of clinical, laboratory, and pharmacovigilance databases prior to trial initiation through the final database lock or clinical trial report. The plan outlines database management and implementation, defines processes for training and certification of data entry staff, describes clinical data review, monitoring, and validation guidelines, and sets expectations for review and transfer of data at the completion of a trial. The DMP serves to combine the various methods that will be employed for data management and details how data will be entered and which stakeholder is responsible for entering data. Any relevant standard operating procedures (SOPs) for data collection, upload, and transfer process are specified. The consolidation of the strategy into one overarching document ensures that all stakeholders are aware of the plan and new staff can be trained.

A data validation plan (DVP) may be used to supplement the DMP or integrated as a component of the DMP. The DVP further outlines the processes for the quality control measures that will be utilized in the trial (e.g., front-end validation of electronic data capture systems, edit checks or manual queries, quality assurance reports, medical or clinical review, reconciliation of external data sources). This plan may also contain information about the criticality of the data collection points to support a risk-based monitoring approach, as well as outline the frequency of data monitoring.

CRF Completion Guidelines

Several resource documents should be created at the start of the clinical trial that will provide guidance to trial staff on expectations of the data capture system, collection of data within each of the forms/assessments and general guidelines not captured in the trial protocol. These documents should be available to trial staff prior to the start of the trial and should be maintained and updated throughout the trial using version control to address frequently asked questions and guidance or decisions on how to enter specific data as needed (Nahm et al. 2011; McFadden 2007).

Ideally, the CRF completion guidelines should contain a table reflecting the expected list of assessments per the schedule specified in the protocol (Nahm et al. 2011). There should be a section that clarifies when each assessment is expected, the source data for the assessment, and how data entry will be completed. These sections should also describe the intricacies of the CRF that are not immediately obvious by reviewing the questions. This includes explaining any fill/skip patterns or logic that may be used. For example, if a date is expected for an event, but several dates *could* be applicable, the CRF completion guidelines should identify clearly how the correct date should be determined and reported (McFadden 2007).

Having a central resource for all trial staff will help ensure that data are collected in a consistent manner across participants and sites.

System User/Quick Reference Guides

When electronic systems are utilized in the conduct of a trial, a system user guide should be provided to assist staff with guidance on how to access and navigate through the system. The guide should include a high-level overview of any data collection system or other tools that will be used and provide more in-depth detail about specific aspects of the data collection system (e.g., enrolling a participant using an EDC system) or how to administer a specific assessment tool.

Depending on the complexity of the system being used, or for multicenter trials which may have many participating institutions, it may be necessary to provide additional resources or "quick reference guides" to facilitate data submission. This is typically a short document that provides specific guidance on one or a few specific tools, assessments, or systems, for example, a quick reference guide on how to upload files to an electronic data capture system. The guide should provide specific details but supplements more in-depth documents like a user's guide or a CRF completion guide. The goal is to ensure that any system user can quickly understand key system features and expedite the training process.

Training Site Staff

Another area of data management support includes training of staff and system users. Data management training may include instruction on CRF completion, data entry or system navigation, query resolution, and trial-specific guidance. Training is an ongoing activity; initial training is typically conducted at site initiation visits, investigator meetings, or through group training or recorded module/webcast training modalities. There are many aspects to data collection, including regulatory documents, safety, the method of data collection, biological and other validated assessments, and possibly trial drug/intervention. At the beginning of the trial, stakeholders involved in the creation of the protocol, assessments, system, and overall trial guidelines should set up a detailed training for all site staff that will be collecting data and administering the assessments.

Providing a training module for each area can provide a structured training to staff before the trial start (Williams 2006). It is recommended that comprehension evaluations are completed for each module and question and answer sessions are provided to allow trial staff time to review training and ask questions. Providing trial staff with certification of completion on each module they are trained on for their records helps ensure that trial staff are prepared for data collection (Williams 2006).

As the trial progresses, it will be necessary to train additional site personnel and perhaps provide retraining as data quality issues are identified or there are changes to the trial due to protocol amendments or other updates. All initial training modules and evaluations should be recorded and readily available for new staff or as a refresher to existing staff throughout the protocol. Any supplemental training provided should also be recorded and readily available.

Training documentation includes the management of system access and maintenance of user credentials, when electronic systems are used. It is important to ensure that all users have appropriate access for their role and departing staff can no longer access systems.

Traditionally, clinical research associates (CRAs) are involved in training of site staff and perform on-site reviews to compare source documents to entered data, monitor data quality, and verify training and regulatory documentation. They serve as a front line resource to sites to help address any concerns early on and prevent them from occurring through the life of the protocol. Errors in data collection or sample storage are often identified and corrected during monitoring visits and should be communicated to data management staff to determine whether any changes to CRFs or guidance documents are warranted. Repeated issues may also lead to updates to training or user materials. Data managers and CRAs provide ongoing training support throughout the trial and work closely together to manage the overall integrity of data collection at sites.

Site and Sponsor Communication

A successful data management program requires setting clear expectations with sponsors or investigators on the format for data collection, acceptable data quality metrics, pathways for communication and escalation of data quality issues, and alignment on trial objectives and goals. Having regular meetings with data management and sponsor staff throughout the trial will help keep these goals in mind as the trial progresses, and questions are raised by trial staff. This also provides a mechanism to determine if protocol-specified assessments are aligned with current practice at sites. These types of issues should be discussed to decide whether additional training of site staff is needed, modifications to assessments are needed, or if clarification of data collection should be provided.

Data management staff are frequently a point of contact for trial personnel seeking assistance. Formal communication with sites is crucial to developing productive relationships with personnel and providing support for data quality or management issues that may arise. Impromptu calls, regularly scheduled meetings, or email communication are all potential avenues to provide ongoing data management support. Expectations regarding frequency and types of communication should be established during the training phase of the trial and should be frequently stated throughout the life of the protocol.

In addition to regular calls with both the sponsor and trial staff, clear guidance on the point of contact for the following areas should be established prior to the first enrollment of a participant: data quality or management issues, safety events that may arise, concerns or issues related to trial medication, or intervention or technical issues with the EDC system. Additionally, the sponsor and data management team should evaluate the locations of trial centers and ensure that an escalation plan is in place. If trial centers are in different time zones from data management staff or sponsor, consider having a help line or a designated staff member available during "off" hours to provide timely support to trial site personnel.

A potentially overlooked aspect of communication is the trial portfolio that is ongoing at a site. Many sites participate in multiple trials at the same time, which may stretch limited resources and lead to challenges with collecting quality and timely data. It is important to recognize the environment in which the site staff are operating and attempt to work within these constraints. When communicating with sites on data quality items, clearly state priority items and set concrete deadlines. If sites are unresponsive, enlist the support of CRAs or other team members to understand the site challenges and identify potential solutions.

Data Management in Single Versus Multicenter Trials

Data management is structured differently depending on whether the trial is conducted in a single center or a multicenter setting, but the overall goal of collecting quality data remains the same.

A single center trial generally relies on an individual institution or site to enroll participants and collect data for a trial. There are some advantages to a trial run at a single center, such as having personnel located in proximity and having more homogeneity in data collection techniques and participant population. However, multicenter trials (utilizing more than one site and/or having a central coordinating center or other shared resource to administer the trial) have the benefit of utilizing more than one site to enroll participants, yielding larger and potentially more diverse participant populations which expedites accrual and may enhance the generalizability of trial results (Meinert and Tonascia 1986). The multicenter trial is particularly important when the therapeutic area is for a rare indication or small population, but there are unique challenges as well.

From the data management perspective, a multicenter trial requires coordinated efforts to ensure quality data are received from all participating sites and that data management expectations are clearly communicated to all stakeholders. Multicenter trials rely on shared resources, such as the protocol, guidance documents, and standard operating procedures to ensure data are collected as uniformly as possible.

Managing multiple sites requires an understanding of local site standards for data collection. Sites may be academic institutions or participating hospitals which have varying standards of care, may be subject to institutional restrictions and procedures, and are utilizing laboratories or other facilities that have unique reporting techniques. Whenever possible, this information should be gathered during site selection and taken into consideration when implementing a CRF or process. For example, a CRF collecting lab information on an international trial needs the flexibility to capture lab values in varying units of measurement from different countries.

Managing data at a single center still requires a focus on completeness and accuracy, but it is also important to ensure there are no systemic errors in data entry, as these may be more difficult to detect without a comparison. When managing data across sites, there is an increased ability to detect outlier data or differences between sites, which can highlight issues for data management staff. Utilizing a data review process may assist with this potential risk.

Future Data Management Considerations

The advancement of technologies such as electronic medical record (EMR) integration, artificial intelligence, and cognitive computing, has the potential to revolutionize how data are collected, shared, and understood and will impact the landscape in which data management practices are deployed.

There are significant efforts to drive the integration of EMR and EDC, reducing or eliminating the need for time-consuming and error-prone transcription between local databases at the trial sites and central clinical databases. EMRs have become a pervasive part of the everyday experience of medicine, and many organizations are seeking to integrate EMR into their clinical trial collection processes. Data can be imported into the trial database directly from the electronic medical record (EMR), erasing traditional transcription and interpretation errors. However, barriers continue to exist to the widespread adoption of the automatic transfer of EMR to EDC, including the lack of standardization for data format, privacy concerns, and difficulty extracting data from the EMR (Goodman et al. 2012).

Artificial intelligence, machine learning, and big data analytics provide opportunities to analyze aggregated data to facilitate participant enrollment and site selection, identify potential fraud or data anomalies, and improve decision-making in clinical trials (Johnson et al. 2018). The ability to collect, store, and analyze massive amounts of data will intensify the need for a structured approach to data management and data quality to ensure outcomes can be distinguished from the noise (Chen et al. 2016). These approaches are not without concern; the challenges to security and privacy that face any electronic system are exacerbated in a rapidly evolving and shifting field. Precautions for each step of the data lifecycle should be taken when implementing an automated or integrated system (Khaloufi et al. 2018).

The impact of this digital transformation, combined with availability of enhanced computing power and storage is continually developing, but the principles of data management and database development are centered in a planned and comprehensive evaluation of available tools and careful selection of appropriate technologies for a clinical trial.

Summary and Conclusion

The role of data management in clinical trials is essential. Setting up a trial to obtain quality data begins early with the protocol, SAP, and data capture method selection and design. Errors or poor judgment at this stage have a significant impact on the process and may result in systematic errors that can compromise analysis and trial results. Thoughtful case report form design is one of the most important aspects of data management. Following commonly accepted principles of CRF creation and utilizing standard CRFs whenever possible ensures streamlined data capture and minimizes negative downstream effects.

Once the trial begins, the implementation of appropriate data quality tools such as risk-based monitoring, reports, data validation checks, and data review are crucial components to the data management program. These tools aid in identifying problematic data, provide information to support sites, ensure the consistency of data collected, and provide an unbiased assessment of trial endpoints. Data quality reports and checks should be updated frequently and implemented early. Additionally, periodic data review is recommended as a method to ensure the integrity and validity of data collected.

Setting clear expectations for all stakeholders is an important part of data management. Data management and validation plans, as well as CRF and system guidance documents, help provide valuable information regarding the flow of data for the trial and how data should be entered correctly. These documents should be supplemented by comprehensive training and a clear communication plan to ensure understanding and agreement on data collection and quality control measures.

Open and ongoing communication with sponsors and sites is necessary to establish rapport and encourage collaboration for the duration of the trial. Scheduled and ad hoc calls and meetings are helpful to build trust and facilitate discussion regarding data quality issues. CRF and system training must be prioritized at the start of a trial and is expected to continue throughout as new staff join or as there are changes to CRFs or system features.

Clinical trials may be conducted in a variety of settings, depending on the nature of the protocol and the trial objectives. There has been an increase in the number of trials that are conducted through a multicenter approach to capitalize on centralized resources and a larger participant population. Although the goal of a data management program may remain the same, there are different considerations for single center versus multicenter or network-conducted trials.

With advancements in technologies such as EMR-EDC integration, artificial intelligence, and big data analytics, the landscape of data management is changing rapidly. Utilizing principles of data quality assurance to manage new data sources and applying understanding of data to large volumes of information will be imperative to future data management programs.

Key Facts

- Quality data is critical
- Robust and reproducible quality control systems need to be developed
- Design step is very important to minimize changes after activation
- Aim for complete, timely and consistent data

Cross-References

▶ Design and Development of the Study Data System
▶ Implementing the Trial Protocol
▶ International Trials
▶ Multicenter and Network Trials

References

Baigent C, Harrel F, Buyse M, Emberson J, Altman D (2008) Ensuring trial validity by data quality assurance and diversification of monitoring methods. Clin Trials 5:49–55

Chen Y, Argentinis JD, Weber G (2016) IBM Watson: how cognitive computing can be applied to big data challenges in life sciences research. Clin Ther 38(4):688

Food and Drug Administration (2013) FDA guidance oversight of clinical investigations – a risk-based approach to monitoring. https://www.fda.gov/downloads/Drugs/Guidances/UCM269919.pdf

Food and Drug Administration (2018) FDA guidance clinical trial endpoints for the approval of cancer drugs and biologics: guidance for industry. https://www.fda.gov/downloads/Drugs/Guidances/ucm071590.pdf

Gaddale JR (2015) Clinical data acquisition standards harmonization importance and benefits in clinical data management. Perspect Clin Res 6(4):179–183

Goodman K, Krueger J, Crowley J (2012) The automatic clinical trial: leveraging the electronic medical record in multi-site cancer clinical trials. Curr Oncol Rep 14(6):502–508

International Conference on Harmonisation (2018) Guideline for good clinical practice E6(R2) good clinical practice: integrated addendum to ICH E6(R1) guidance for industry. https://www.fda.gov/downloads/Drugs/Guidances/UCM464506.pdf

Johnson K, Soto JT, Glicksberg BS, Shameer K, Miotto R, Ali M, Ashley E, Dudley JT (2018) Artificial intelligence in cardiology. J Am Coll Cardiol 71:2668–2679

Khaloufi H, Abouelmehdi K, Beni-Hssane A, Saadi M (2018) Security model for big healthcare data lifecycle. Procedia Comput Sci 141:294–301

Krishnankutt B, Bellary S, Kumar N, Moodahadu L (2012) Data management in clinical trial: an overview. Indian J Pharmacol 44(2):168–172

McFadden E (2007) Management of data in clinical trials, 2nd edn. Hoboken, NJ: Wiley-Interscience.

Meinert CL, Tonascia S (1986) Clinical trials: design, conduct, and analysis. New York: Oxford University Press.

Nahm M, Shepherd J, Buzenberg A, Rostami R, Corcoran A, McCall J et al (2011) Design and implementation of an institutional case report form library. Clin Trials 8:94–102

Reboussin D, Espeland MA (2005) The science of web-based clinical trial management. Clin Trials 2:1–2

Richesson RL, Nadkarni P (2011) Data standards for clinical research data collection forms: current status and challenges. J Am Med Inform Assoc 18:341–346

Williams G (2006) The other side of clinical trial monitoring; assuring data quality and procedural adherence. Clin Trials 3:530–537

End of Trial and Close Out of Data Collection

18

Gillian Booth

Contents

Abstract

Trial closure refers to the activities that take place in preparation for the cessation of trial recruitment through to archiving of the trial. Trial closure can be notionally divided into five stages: End of Recruitment; End of Trial Intervention; End of

G. Booth (✉)
Leeds Institute of Clinical Trials Research, University of Leeds, Leeds, UK
e-mail: G.Eddison@leeds.ac.uk

Trial; Trial Reporting and Publishing; and Archiving. The length and scheduling of each stage of trial closure is determined by the trial design and operating model. As trial closure approaches there is an increased emphasis on monitoring and controls to ensure the correct number of participants is recruited and data collection and cleaning in preparation for final database lock and analysis is complete. The End of Trial is a key ethical and regulatory milestone defined in the approved trial protocol and has associated time-dependent notification and reporting requirements to the independent ethics committee and, for regulated trials, the regulator(s). Key steps of trial closure, reporting, publishing, and data sharing are important mechanisms to support transparency in clinical trials. A Trial Closure Plan can be used to support the activities that ensure appropriate control over the final stages of the trial.

Keywords

Analysis · Archiving · Close out · Database lock · Data sharing · End of Trial · Public registry · Publishing · Reporting · Transparency · Trial Closure Plan

Introduction

Trial closure refers to the activities that take place in preparation for the cessation of trial recruitment through to archiving of the trial. During this period a range of different tasks take place at each of the physical locations (institutions) where the trial is being conducted in order to:

- Complete the protocol specified intervention and assessments
- Finalize the study data and documentation ready for analysis and reporting
- Close down investigator sites and notify trial participants, funders, regulators, and ethics committees of the trial results

The specific trial closure activities at each institution will depend upon the trial design and the role of each institution; however, the overarching aims remain the same.

Clinical trials each have different designs, participant pathways, and risk profiles therefore the trial closure activities undertaken can be adapted to ensure a risk proportionate approach appropriate to the trial design and operating model (MRC et al. 2012). Where risk proportionate approaches are utilized, these should be documented with the associated decisions in the trial risk assessment. It is also possible for many typical trial closure activities to be undertaken either remotely rather than "on site," thereby permitting the most appropriate method to be utilized and ensuring the most efficient and effective use of resources.

Planning for Trial Closure

Conducting methodologically sound, safe, ethical, and regulatory compliant trials requires careful planning and control, thus it follows that the trial closure activities and the timing of these will be carefully preplanned. The monitoring of timelines in the lead up to trial closure and the development of a Trial Closure Plan is critical to ensure appropriate control over the final stages of the trial. A Trial Closure Plan will include key milestones and deadlines relating to the responsibilities of each institution, with details of data items for on-site or central monitoring which can inform the trial closure and analysis timelines.

However, it is not uncommon for trial timelines to change; for example, as a result of slower than anticipated recruitment resulting in a delay to the recruitment closure date. Some trial designs also include predefined stopping rules which allow the trial to be stopped early; although the outcome of these prespecified reviews cannot be predicted, planning for the various outcomes can and should still take place. It is less common, but not unknown, for trials to be closed for unplanned reasons where the opportunity for preplanning can be greatly reduced.

Trial closure activities (for all institutions involved in the trial) take place between the cessation of trial recruitment to archiving and can be broadly divided into five stages of activity (Fig. 1). While it is helpful to think about the stages of trial closure in a linear, predictable way for planning purposes, in practice the design of the trial may influence the length of each stage and whether the stages overlap. The period of time between each stage will vary depending upon the length of time the trial is open to recruitment and also the length of the individual participant intervention, data collection, and follow-up periods. The design of the trial will also impact the overlap between the different stages of trial closure; for example, in the case of an adaptive platform multi-arm-multi-stage (MAMS) trial. A MAMS trial is a platform clinical trial with a single master protocol where multiple interventions are evaluated at the same time. Adaptive features enable one or more interventions to be "dropped" (e.g., due to futility) or added during the course of the trial. Different "arms" of the trial

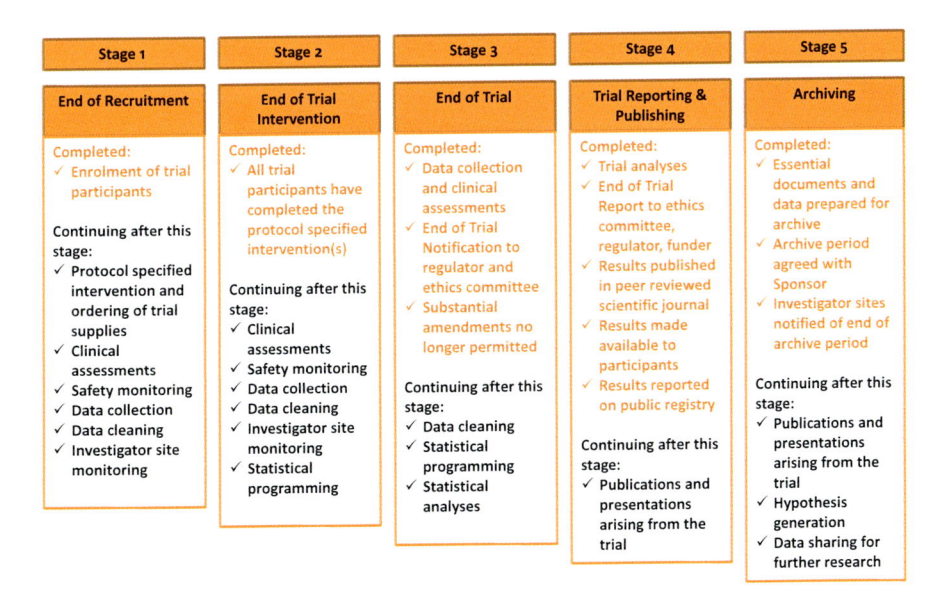

Fig. 1 Stages of Trial Closure

will remain open to recruitment and intervention, while others are closed and there may be protocol defined analyses performed and reported prior to the End of Trial thereby resulting in overlap of the different stages of trial closure.

Stage 1: End of Recruitment

The end of recruitment is the point at which all trial sites are no longer permitted to enroll participants into the trial. The trial protocol will specify the sample size, the number of participants to be enrolled to achieve the sample size, and will describe the recruitment pathway and related processes to achieve this. In most trials there will still be participants receiving the intervention and undergoing clinical assessments, safety monitoring, and data collection after the trial has closed to recruitment.

Stage 2: End of Trial Intervention

The End of Trial intervention is the point at which all participants enrolled into the trial have completed the trial intervention as specified by the approved trial protocol. Depending upon the trial design, it is likely that trial participants will be undergoing clinical assessments, safety monitoring, and data collection after this time.

Stage 3: End of Trial

The End of Trial is a key ethical and regulatory milestone with associated time-dependent notification requirements to the independent ethics committee and, for regulated trials, the regulator(s). There may also be specific contractual requirements for notification to other bodies, such as funders, at this time.

The End of Trial will be defined in the approved trial protocol; typically this will be the date of the last "visit" of the last participant or at the time the last data item is collected for the trial, that is, the point at which all clinical assessments, safety monitoring, and data collection stops, although there may be different regulatory requirements in different regions or countries. Preparatory activities for the End of Trial will therefore focus on monitoring key data associated with the countdown toward the End of Trial in addition to completing the data collection and cleaning required for final database lock and analysis.

Stage 4: Trial Reporting and Publishing

Trial reporting and publishing of the trial results follow completion of the protocol specified trial analyses. These are two discrete activities:

- **Trial reporting** is a requirement of regulators and involves reporting summary results to the independent ethics committee, regulator(s), and/or trial registry –

typically within 12 months of the End of Trial. Where a trial is intended to support a regulatory submission (e.g., in support of a manufacturer's license for a drug or medical device) the final report will take the form of a Clinical Study Report with supporting documentation and detailed datasets as required by the regional/country regulator.

- **Publishing** refers to publishing trial results, irrespective of the trial outcome, in a peer-reviewed scientific journal and tends to be an activity primarily, although not exclusively, associated with academic-led research.

Trial reporting and publishing of the trial results are two of the four key mechanisms to support transparency in clinical trials (Box 1). The overall aim of transparency in clinical trials is to ensure that the participants of trials, doctors, the scientific community, and the public have access to information about which trials have been conducted, how they have been conducted, and the outcomes of those trials. This builds trust with patients and the public, informs clinical practice by allowing access to all of the available evidence about a particular treatment, and minimizes research waste by ensuring the same trials are not repeated. Transparency is fundamental in meeting the expectations of research participants, regulators, and the wider scientific community.

Transparency in clinical trials is typically understood to mean registering, reporting, publishing, and making data from the trial available for further analyses or for the purpose of undertaking an independent analysis of the trial results (Box 1).

Transparency measures are a regulatory requirement for some trials and a prerequisite for publishing in many high-profile scientific journals, for example, to publish in some high impact journals (ICMJE 2019) the trial must be registered in a Primary Public Registry prior to the start of recruitment.

Box 1 Transparency in Clinical Trials

What does Transparency mean in practice?

- **Registering a trial in a public registry and/or regulatory database**

   The World Health Organisation considers trial registration to be not only a scientific but also an ethical and moral responsibility and has set out the International Standards for Clinical Trial Registries. Trial registration is defined by the World Health Organisation as the publication of an internationally agreed set of information about the design, conduct, and administration of clinical trials (WHO 2012). These are published on a publicly accessible website managed by a registry conforming to WHO standards. Registries which meet the WHO Registry Criteria and have at least a national remit are called WHO Primary Registries; an example of a Primary Registry is the EU Clinical Trials Register.

(continued)

– **Reporting a trial in a public registry or regulatory database**

Regulatory requirements specifying which registry or database to use when registering or reporting a trial differ by country, therefore the relevant laws and guidance for that country/region should be referred to.

– **Publishing the trials results in scholarly journal and presenting at professional society scientific conferences**

Regardless of the outcome of the trial it is important to make those results available to others. For regulators, doctors, patients, and participants of trials this enables them to make decisions based on the most up-to-date information about a treatment. For other researchers this avoids the same research questions being investigated again unnecessarily.

– **Making data from the trial available for further research purposes (Data Sharing)**

The quality control and curation of clinical trial datasets typically means these are valuable resources which can be used for further research, such as meta-analyses. Any further use of clinical trial datasets must be in line with participant expectations and always legally compliant; this typically means taking steps to anonymize a dataset prior to releasing to a third party.

For trial integrity reasons, data is not usually made available for further research purposes until the protocol specified analyses have been completed and reported/published.

Stage 5: Archiving

Archiving is the storage and retention of the trial essential documents (ICH 2016) and data produced in the trial. Retention periods may vary and are dictated by regulators, sponsors, funders, or institute policies. For regulated trials, the purpose of archiving is to ensure the records which demonstrate how the trial was conducted and the compliance of all individuals and institutions involved in the trial with good clinical practice (ICH 2016) and all relevant laws are available for audit or inspection purposes.

Trial Closure Activities

Developing a Trial Closure Plan

There can be many different types of institutions, groups, and individuals involved in the day-to-day conduct of a trial, for example, pharmaceutical companies, clinical trials units (CTUs), contract research organizations (CROs), laboratories, investigators, investigator sites, suppliers/vendors, and independent oversight committees.

Each institution, group, or individual will have agreed role(s) and an agreed set of responsibilities which are usually defined in contracts, the trial protocol, and other working documents. As trial closure approaches the lead institution responsible for trial conduct will instigate the development of a detailed Trial Closure Plan (Box 2) to ensure appropriate planning and control over the final stages of the trial.

When developing a Trial Closure Plan it is important to consider:

- **Who does the Plan need to include?**
  Consider who will use it. Depending upon the complexity of the trial, there may need to be detailed sub-plans for certain institutions, groups, or individuals which feed into a master plan controlled by the lead organization responsible for trial conduct.
- **What resources are needed to deliver the plan?**
  The workforce or other resources needed to deliver the trial closure activities will need to be identified. When considering the workforce planning implications at the end of the trial there may be contracts that will need to be terminated or the movement of people onto other projects.
- **Does the Plan include timelines and key milestones?**
  In a well-managed trial, the key milestones will have already been identified in the master trial project plan, as dictated by the protocol, contracts, and regulators. However, there may be milestones which can only be defined and agreed as the trial closure period approaches, such as scheduling the analysis to be completed by a specific date in order to present at a key professional society scientific conference.
- **What communication is needed, to whom, and when?**
  A communication plan should consider how communication strategies will need to change to ensure timely communication, which institutions, groups, and individuals need to be communicated with at each stage of trial closure and the best routes for communication.
- **Are there specific legal, protocol, or contractual obligations which need to be met?** (Box 2)
  Typically trials include many contracting partners. It is good practice to review the contracts regularly to ensure ongoing compliance. Contracts will usually include specific reporting and communication requirements relating to the end of trial; any contractual obligations should be built into the Trial Closure Plan so that they are not missed.

Box 2 Typical elements of a Trial Closure Plan to ensure legal, protocol, and contractual obligations

A Typical Trial Closure Plan will include detailed procedures to ensure legal, protocol, and contractual obligations are met at each Stage.

At Stage 1: Recruitment Closure:

(continued)

- The appropriate number of trial participants are recruited and removal of access to the trial systems for recruitment and randomization at the appropriate time.

At Stage 2: End of Trial Intervention:

- Trial supplies are appropriately controlled, accounted for, destroyed and removal of access to the trial systems for managing trial supplies at the appropriate time.
- Appropriate communication to trial participants about next steps and options once their trial treatment ends.

At Stage 3: End of Trial

- End of Trial notification requirements of the independent ethics committee and regulator are met.
- Data collection and cleaning is timed appropriately to meet database lock, analysis and reporting deadlines, and removal of access to the trial database for data entry at the appropriate time.
- Where required by the trial protocol, key data are signed off by the Site Investigator and independent adjudication of endpoint data are completed to meet database lock, analysis, and reporting deadlines.
- Final investigator site monitoring activities are completed according to the trial monitoring plan.
- Trial samples are destroyed or have the necessary approvals to be stored beyond the end of the trial.
- All final substantial amendments to the protocol or supporting documents are made.
- Final payments to investigator sites, vendors, suppliers, and contractors are made.

At Stage 4: Trial Reporting and Publishing

- Ethical and regulatory reporting requirements and timelines are met.
- A publication plan is developed to ensure timely publication and presentation of the trial results.

At Stage 5: Archiving

- Completion of the Trial Master File and Investigator Site File essential documents and preparation of these and any data files (paper and/or electronic) for archive.

Communication

Good communication between the different institutions involved in the trial is key to a successful trial closure; as such it is typical to see the frequency and format of communications between the different institutions, groups, and individuals increase and change in the run up to trial closure (Box 3).

Box 3 Illustrative Communication at Trial Closure

Newsletters and Websites

In the months before the end of the recruitment period, newsletters, websites, and other publicity information for the trial which are aimed at recruiting site staff and/or potential participants are updated with the confirmed or indicative recruitment closure date.

Project Planning Meetings

As trial closure approaches, to facilitate more detailed planning activities and timely decision making, the institutions responsible for the overall management of the trial agree to increase the frequency of project planning meetings.

Notification of Closure to Recruitment

The organization primarily responsible for trial conduct writes to all relevant organizations/groups/individuals involved in the trial including the funder, Sponsor, Independent Oversight Committees, Investigator Sites, and suppliers to inform them that the trial has closed to recruitment. The letter includes information such as:

- The date the trial closed to recruitment and the reason for the end of recruitment
- A summary of overall recruitment for the trial and, where writing to an individual investigator site, the recruitment summary for that individual site
- Key dates, such as the planned end of intervention period and the End of Trial date
- A reminder of ongoing activities/obligations such as the management of trial supplies and data collection

Institutions Involved in the Day-to-Day Conduct, Funding, and Independent Oversight of the Trial

Institutions, groups, and individuals involved in the day-to-day conduct, funding, and independent oversight of the trial might include investigator sites, suppliers,

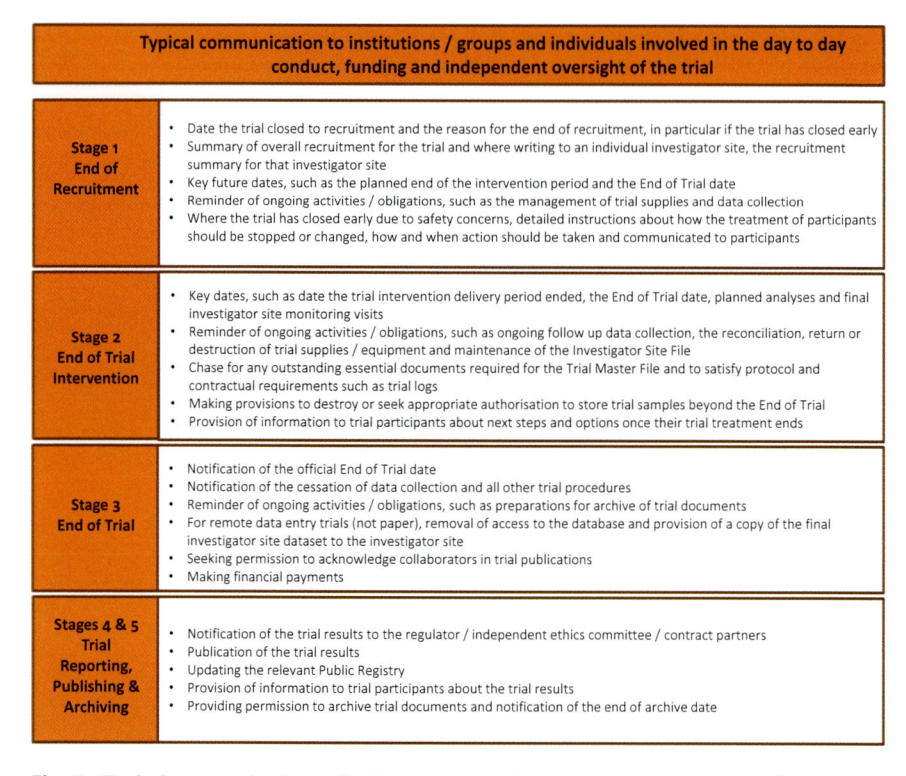

Typical communication to institutions / groups and individuals involved in the day to day conduct, funding and independent oversight of the trial	
Stage 1 **End of** **Recruitment**	• Date the trial closed to recruitment and the reason for the end of recruitment, in particular if the trial has closed early • Summary of overall recruitment for the trial and where writing to an individual investigator site, the recruitment summary for that investigator site • Key future dates, such as the planned end of the intervention period and the End of Trial date • Reminder of ongoing activities / obligations, such as the management of trial supplies and data collection • Where the trial has closed early due to safety concerns, detailed instructions about how the treatment of participants should be stopped or changed, how and when action should be taken and communicated to participants
Stage 2 **End of Trial** **Intervention**	• Key dates, such as date the trial intervention delivery period ended, the End of Trial date, planned analyses and final investigator site monitoring visits • Reminder of ongoing activities / obligations, such as ongoing follow up data collection, the reconciliation, return or destruction of trial supplies / equipment and maintenance of the Investigator Site File • Chase for any outstanding essential documents required for the Trial Master File and to satisfy protocol and contractual requirements such as trial logs • Making provisions to destroy or seek appropriate authorisation to store trial samples beyond the End of Trial • Provision of information to trial participants about next steps and options once their trial treatment ends
Stage 3 **End of Trial**	• Notification of the official End of Trial date • Notification of the cessation of data collection and all other trial procedures • Reminder of ongoing activities / obligations, such as preparations for archive of trial documents • For remote data entry trials (not paper), removal of access to the database and provision of a copy of the final investigator site dataset to the investigator site • Seeking permission to acknowledge collaborators in trial publications • Making financial payments
Stages 4 & 5 **Trial** **Reporting,** **Publishing &** **Archiving**	• Notification of the trial results to the regulator / independent ethics committee / contract partners • Publication of the trial results • Updating the relevant Public Registry • Provision of information to trial participants about the trial results • Providing permission to archive trial documents and notification of the end of archive date

Fig. 2 Typical communication to institutions involved in the day-to-day conduct, funding, and independent oversight of the trial

independent oversight committees, and funders. Good communication will ensure that those institutions, groups, and individuals are aware of the planned and final timing of each stage in the days, weeks, and months leading up to the event. It is good practice, and indeed an essential part of the audit trail for regulated trials, to write to the institutions, groups, and individuals involved in the day-to-day running, funding, and independent oversight of the trial at each stage of trial closure to keep them appraised of key dates, decisions, and as a reminder of any ongoing activities or obligations (Fig. 2).

Organizations Involved in the Authorization of the Trial

The organizations involved in the authorization of the trial, such as regulators and independent research ethics committees, will have their own trial authorization systems, processes, and timelines which will need to be followed. It is not usually necessary to notify the regulator(s) or independent ethics committee(s) of the End of Recruitment or End of Intervention unless recruitment has been terminated early and this was not prespecified in the trial protocol, for example, where a trial has been closed early for participant safety reasons. However, it is prudent to check the requirements of regulators and independent research ethics committees as these differ between regions and countries and can change over time.

Stage 1 End of Recruitment

Planning and Controlling the End of Recruitment

As the point at which the total number of participants to be recruited approaches, the frequency of monitoring recruitment will increase so as to ensure compliance with the approved trial protocol. Different systems for monitoring recruitment may be used, for example, spreadsheets or electronic trackers. Whichever system is used, close communication with the institutions and individuals involved in recruitment is critical to ensure an appropriate level of control over the number of participants recruited.

Specific communication with the investigator(s)/recruiting team(s) in order to prevent uncontrolled over-recruitment will be required and different approaches may be taken such as restricting the number of participants being approached to consent to the trial as the end of recruitment nears. It may also be necessary for the investigator(s)/recruiting team(s) to adjust the communication with potential participants to explain that the trial is nearing the point of closure and how this might impact on whether they can ultimately participate in the trial.

Interim Recruitment Stopping Rules

The overall total number of participants to be recruited, as detailed in the approved trial protocol, may not be achieved in cases where it becomes apparent ongoing recruitment into the trial is not feasible and cannot be met within an acceptable period of time. Where a risk of poor recruitment has been anticipated, the approved trial protocol may include a recruitment stopping rule, that is, a planned interim review of the trial recruitment rate and total to determine the feasibility of continuing to recruit into the trial. Trial closure planning activities would be expected to take place in preparation for review of any protocol specified stopping rules, particularly where early trial closure is considered likely (see "Early Trial Closure" Section).

Closing Enrolment Systems

Once the protocol defined recruitment period has ended the trial enrolment systems are closed. Trials commonly use phone or web-based systems for recruitment, that is, where an Investigator phones or logs into a website to enroll the participant into the trial; these are called interactive voice or web response systems (IVRS/IWRS). IVRS/IWRS are also commonly used for other associated trial management activities such as randomization, completing participant diaries, ordering trial supplies and in the case of blinded trials, un-blinding activities. Where an IVRS/IWRS is in use, permission to enroll participants into the system will be physically revoked while leaving permissions active for other associated ongoing trial activities where such functionality is provided by the IVRS/IWRS, for example, in relation to management of trial supplies.

Stage 2 End of Trial Intervention

Planning the End of the Trial Intervention Period

The activities associated with the end of trial intervention, once all participants have completed the protocol specified intervention, will depend upon the nature of the trial intervention(s). Common across all trials will be the careful monitoring of timelines and the availability of the intervention as the final trial participants complete the protocol specified intervention. In a well-managed trial, consideration of the impact of delays earlier in the trial such as a slower recruitment rate on the availability of trial supplies will have been identified during the trial with the planned mitigating action being taken in preparation for the stage, for example:

- For interventions which rely on the employment of certain healthcare professionals, for example, therapists; undertaking extensions to the contracts of employment
- For drug trials; where the delay has impacted on the expiry dates undertaking authorized extensions to the expiry or sourcing additional supplies

In trials involving supplies, such as drugs and devices, planning during trial setup will ensure there are sufficient trial supplies for each participant to receive the intervention as specified in the protocol. Indeed, any risks to the trial supplies could be classed as a reportable event to the independent ethics committee or regulator particularly where participant safety or the trial integrity are compromised as a result of poor trial supplies management (in the European Union and United Kingdom such events which occur in regulated drug trials are called Serious Breaches and required expedited reporting to the regulator (MHRA 2018)). Although careful monitoring and management of each individual participant and trial supplies is important during trial recruitment, this will become more important toward the end of the intervention period to ensure efficient use of the trial supplies and to avoid over-ordering and waste, and this can be particularly important where there are limited trial supplies.

Controlling the Ordering of Trial Supplies

IVRS/IWRS systems can be used to manage the ordering, receipt, accountability, and ultimately the return or destruction of trial supplies but simpler risk proportionate processes and systems are also used, particularly in the case of noncommercial or single site trials using a low-risk intervention where the trial supplies are available as part of routine clinical care.

For regulated trials with limited supplies towards the end of the trial intervention period, it may be necessary to restrict the amount of supplies each Investigator Site can order or have each supply authorized by the Sponsor or delegate prior to distribution because the expectation of some country regulators is that the transfer of trial supplies between trial research sites is not routinely permitted, other than in exceptional circumstances. Once all participants have completed the protocol defined intervention schedule, access to the systems for ordering new trial supplies will be revoked.

Trial Supplies Accountability and Reconciliation

The protocol or contract should detail how surplus trial supplies or specialist trial equipment left at the investigator site should be managed. It is not usually permitted for trial supplies to enter routine supply chains, nor to be used for non-trial participants. Typically contracts will specify one of the following scenarios:

- Ring fence and retain the remaining trial supplies until remote or on-site monitoring activities have been completed to confirm correct use and accounting of the trial supplies (Box 4). After any monitoring activities have been successfully completed and any arising issues resolved, the Sponsor (or delegate) will give permission to the investigator site(s) to either destroy or return unused trial supplies to the Sponsor or supplier for destruction.
- In the case of low-risk trials (i.e., where the intervention was of no higher risk than standard of care) there may be no accountability logs to monitor in which case the investigator site(s) will be instructed to destroy surplus supplies or return them to the Sponsor or supplier for destruction.
- The return of any specialist equipment to the Sponsor or supplier.

Box 4 Typical monitoring activities to confirm correct use and accounting of trial supplies

Typical examples of monitoring activities to confirm the correct use and accounting of trial supplies include:

- Checking storage locations and temperature logs to verify that trial supplies were stored and handled according to the manufacturers' recommendations and any deviations were notified to the Sponsor.
- Checking the records which detail the traceability and accountability of the trial supplies, ensuring that trial supplies were not used for participants who were not enrolled onto the trial.
- Checking logs and other records which verify that any equipment used was appropriately calibrated and maintained.

Such activities may take place at the Investigator site or written confirmation or evidence in the form of logs or other paperwork from the Investigator Site Pharmacist may be requested for remote review by the Sponsor or delegate.

Provision of Information to Participants at End of Intervention

It should be made clear to participants at the point of consent whether access to the intervention they receive during the trial will be made available to them after the trial has closed, or how their treatment options may change as a result of participation in the trial. Depending upon the nature of the intervention and the length of the intervention period, it can be a long time between the point of consent and the end of treatment for an individual participant therefore it is good practice to prepare information at the end of intervention for individual participants to serve as a reminder of what will happen to them in terms of changes to their treatment, ongoing clinical monitoring and how they can find out about or opt out of receiving information about the trial results. This is also a good point in time to thank participants for their contribution to the research.

Stage 3 End of Trial

Planning for the End of Trial

Preparatory activities for the End of Trial are dictated by the End of Trial definition as specified in the approved trial protocol, the regulatory required timeframe and activities post End of Trial for analysis and reporting and the fact that further substantial amendments to the trial protocol are not permitted after the End of Trial. The activities will therefore largely be focused on:

- **Meeting Ethical and Regulatory Requirements:** Monitoring the trial data or other trial information which indicates that the End of Trial has been reached and initiates the regulatory required timeframe for End of Trial Reporting.
- **Retention or destruction of research samples:** Ensuring appropriate authorization is in place for the retention of research samples (e.g., blood and tissue) collected within the trial which are intended to be held after the End of Trial.
- **Preparation for database lock.** Ensuring data collection, cleaning, monitoring, and any independent arbitration of endpoint data is timed appropriately to meet database lock, analysis, and reporting deadlines and removal of access to the trial database for data entry at the appropriate time.
- Completing final contractual close out activities such as making final payments to investigator sites, vendors, suppliers, and contractors.

Ethical and Regulatory Requirements

Although the definitions for End of Trial and the associated timelines and mechanisms for notification differ by country and region, there are consistencies in the general concept of defining the point in time at which a clinical trial ends "End of Trial" and the principle that the End of Trial date effectively "starts the clock" for reporting of the final summary clinical trials results. Typically in the United Kingdom and European Union, the definition of End of Trial will be the date of the last "visit" of the last participant or at the time the last data item is collected for the trial, that is, the point at which all clinical assessments, safety monitoring, and data collection stops (Official Journal of the European Union 2010). While in the United States two dates are used: Primary Completion Date (pertaining to completion of the intervention and clinical assessments for the purpose of data collection relating to the primary outcome) and Study Completion Date (pertaining to completion of the intervention and clinical assessments for the purpose of data collection relating to all protocol specified outcomes) with the Study Completion Date being equivalent to the UK/EU definition.

Depending upon the design of the trial, the End of Trial may occur many years after the end of recruitment and intervention stages have been completed. As a key regulatory milestone, the End of Trial must be notified to the relevant oversight body (ies) (usually the independent research ethics committee and for regulated trials the country specific Regulator) within a defined period of time after it occurs, therefore it is necessary to monitor the data and other trial information which indicate that the End of Trial has been reached in the run up to the End of Trial definition being met. This may require a change to the frequency of data collection, cleaning, or monitoring activities, for example:

– In trials where the timing of the analysis is linked to the event rate; as the target approaches the frequency of data collection or monitoring at the investigator sites may need to increase, with a greater focus on individual research site compliance of the relevant data collection forms.

The mechanisms for reporting also differ by oversight body, region, and country; this may be via a dedicated reporting system such as the European Union Portal/ EudraCT System, a registry or database such as ClinicalTrials.gov or simply a standard form completed and emailed to the oversight body.

In practice the End of Trial notification does not mean that ethical and regulatory oversight ends immediately at this point; there is an obligation for the Sponsor to provide a written report within a fixed period of time to the independent ethics committee, and for regulated trials the regulator. In addition active regulatory inspection or contractual audit periods may extend many years after the End of Trial.

The End of Trial, regardless of definition, only occurs once; thus it follows that for multicenter trials the End of Trial notification is made once the End of Trial has occurred in all participating research sites and for multinational trials the notification is made once the End of Trial has occurred in all participating countries.

Once the official End of Trial notification has been made substantial amendments are no longer permitted; therefore any amendments to the protocol or other authorized documents must be completed prior to the End of Trial being reached.

The End of Trial will be communicated in writing by the Sponsor or delegate to all of the institutions and individuals which have been involved in the conduct of the trial. There may also be specific contractual requirements for notification to other bodies such as funders at this time.

Research Samples

Many trials include the collection of research samples, such as tissue, blood, or urine samples which will be used for protocol defined analyses. Trial participants may also be asked to consent to any samples which are collected being held in a tissue bank and used for further research projects. The plan for the research samples after the End of Trial will have been originally approved by the independent research ethics committee and this approval must be adhered to. Where the plans have changed, an amendment to the original ethical approval or alternative authorization by the appropriate Authority/Regulatory Body will be needed in order to continue holding the samples after the End of Trial. Depending upon the specific authorizations in place, samples may need to be physically moved within or between institutions, for example, to an authorized tissue bank.

Close out of Data Collection and Preparation for Database Lock

Trial data is expected to be of high quality (in terms of accuracy and completeness) with data entered into the trial database contemporaneously to the associated protocol activity and rigorous processes in place to collect, clean, and monitor the quality of the data therefore data cleaning is not a one off activity and takes place through the trial. The activities undertaken to collect and clean trial data are typically documented in a Data Management Plan which is a comprehensive document detailing all aspects of the data handling parts of the trial and which provides reference for staff working on the trial, organizational memory and is a controlled document which supports the reconstruction of the trial for audit/inspection purposes.

Database lock is the action taken to "freeze" or take a final copy of the trial dataset in order that it can be used in the final trial analysis. Database lock ensures that a copy of the final dataset and statistical code used in the analysis of the trial are retained, so that analyses can be repeated and independently verified at a later date, if necessary.

In a well-managed trial, defining and detailing the plans for the data collection and cleaning period in the run up to Database Lock will have taken place at the time of developing the Data Management Plan and Trial Monitoring Plan. However, it is good practice to revisit the Data Management Plan in preparation for trial closure and database lock to ensure that the priorities are right and that resources are being used in the most efficient way (Box 5), for example:

– In trials where there are multiple different analyses taking place, or the analyses only involve subgroups of participants, developing specific data management plans directed to each trial analysis may be necessary. This could involve identifying the specific data items and case report forms required for each analysis and directing the investigator sites to prioritize certain case report forms for completion or responding to certain data queries.

Ultimately Database Lock will be the culmination of many years work in collecting and cleaning the clinical trial data to ensure the quality of the trial data for the trial analyses. If this is not well-managed, the timeliness of availability and quality of the data in the run up to database lock can adversely impact the timing of the trial analyses, reporting, and publication.

Box 5 Preparatory Steps for Database Lock

Typical checks in the run up to database lock include ensuring that:

- Data items have been received and where they have not, there is a documented reason why.
- Discrepant data have been queried with the investigator site and the queries have been resolved.
- All on-site and remote monitoring activities have been completed as per the Trial Monitoring Plan and any outstanding issues have been resolved.
- That the essential documents held at the investigator site are complete in case of future audit or inspection.
- The site investigator(s) have confirmed the accuracy and completeness of key data from their site.
- Any data coding, for example, of free-text fields and adverse events has been completed.
- The linkage, cleaning and reconciliation of datasets generated by other collaborators or parties, for example, laboratories, routine data providers have been completed.
- Where required by the trial protocol, independent verification/adjudication of outcome measures, for example, interpretation of clinical results has been completed.

Operationalizing Database Lock

How final "database lock" is practically implemented can differ between organizations and will usually be specified in a Standard Operating Procedure. Practical implementation can also differ depending upon the design of the trial; for example, there may be interim or other analyses prior to the End of Trial which require the database to be temporarily locked, a snapshot of the database to be taken at that time, and then the database unlocked in order that data collection and cleaning can continue. This is a feature of some adaptive trial designs (e.g., multi-arm, multi-stage trials, platform trials) and one which is likely to require careful consideration when determining the End of Trial definition in the protocol for those types of trial design.

Database lock is usually carried out through the temporary or permanent revocation of access rights to the trial database system by those individuals who are responsible for data entry and cleaning activities. At the time of full database lock, no further amendments are permitted to the database – the dataset will be the final dataset used by the Statistician for the trial analysis. The complexity of this exercise will depend upon the number of different individuals and institutions involved and whether the trial uses paper or electronic data capture technologies.

In common with all previous stages of trial closure; clear responsibilities and communication is critical in achieving a successful database lock and the institution responsible for data management for the trial will take responsibility for this. For trials with large and complex datasets it may be necessary to implement a step-wise approach to final database lock such as:

- Halting further data collection at investigator sites and focusing only on data query responses
- Where remote data entry systems are in use, locking individual data collection forms, participants or investigator sites to prevent further data entry or cleaning activities at the investigator site level whilst continuing to permit time-limited cleaning activities by the organization/individual responsible for data cleaning, for example, a Data Manager to complete their activities.

For data integrity reasons, it is important to ensure that when locking the database in a remote data entry system that each individual research site retains read only access to the database for their data (MHRA 2018).

Stage 4 Trial Reporting and Publishing

Trial Reporting

The End of Trial starts the clock for reporting the summary results of the trial; the typical expectation being that these are reported onto the relevant public registry / regulator portal within 12 months of the End of Trial date in the United Kingdom and European Union and Primary Completion Date (onto ClinicalTrials.gov 2017) in the United States. There may be exemptions to the requirement or timeframe for reporting certain trials, for example, to protect commercial interests. In some countries there are also financial penalties for delays to reporting or not submitting the report.

The content of the End of Trial Report (sometimes called the Clinical Trial Summary Report) will take the form as dictated by the regional/country regulator or independent ethics committee and will typically include information such as:

- Title of the trial and key objective(s)
- Key dates and milestones
- Any substantial amendments
- Results including safety data

Reporting summary results via an End of Trial report onto a public registry is an important mechanism to support clinical trials transparency (Fig. 1). Within the United Kingdom and European Union emphasis is also placed on the importance of providing trial results in an appropriate format to the participants of the trial and the wider general public via a lay-summary (European Commission 2017; HRA 2014).

Publication and Dissemination

It is typical to see publication policies established at the beginning of the trial and documented in the trial protocol and contracts. Toward the end of the trial the Sponsor, Chief Investigator or other institution with responsibility for performing the trial analyses will prepare a publication and dissemination plan. The publication and dissemination plan will set out a schedule of key outputs (typically publications in peer-reviewed scientific journals and presentations but may include other publicity outputs such as via social media or other media outlets). For each output a suitable individual will identified to lead it. In some trials there may be only one or two planned publications, whereas in others there could be significantly more; arising over future years as a result of sub-protocol and further exploratory analyses.

One of the most important aspects of dissemination is ensuring that participants on the trial are informed of the trial results and that these are also made available to other patient groups and communities, engaging with patient groups and communities can also be helpful in further disseminating the results of the trial.

Data "Sharing" for Further Research

The data generated from clinical trials are typically high quality and valuable datasets, with the potential to be used for further research and hypothesis generation. For legal or philanthropic reasons, many organizations now provide access to data generated in their clinical trials; making data available for other high-quality research projects. In most cases a controlled access approach is used; where an oversight committee reviews applications made to access the clinical trials data and makes a decision, based on the organization's data release policy (Box 6) as to whether the data will be released to the applicant. In some cases the committee members are independent of the organization who owns the clinical trial data; in this case the approach would be called an "independent controlled access approach" (MRC 2015). Some regulators, such as the European Medicines Agency, also publish anonymized clinical data submitted by pharmaceutical companies to support their regulatory applications for human medicines (EMA 2016).

Given the highly sensitive nature of clinical trials data it is essential that any data sharing takes place:

- In accordance with the expectations of the trial participants, for example, it is good practice to inform trial participants that further data sharing will take place in future via the participant information leaflet.
- In accordance with all relevant data protection laws.

In most cases data will only be released in an anonymized form and where released to another organization, further protected by a legally binding data release agreement.

Making clinical trials data available for further research and hypothesis generation is an important mechanism to support clinical trials transparency (Box 1). It is a regulatory requirement in some countries for certain types of trials and an approach also supported by the International Committee of Medical Journal Editors which require a data sharing statement to be included at the point of registering the trial on a public registry (ICMJE 2019).

Box 6 Key elements of a data release policy

Recommended elements of a clinical trial data sharing policy:

- The scope of data sharing
- The request and decision process including guiding principles or criteria to be used in making the decision
- The process for data release including preparing the data and associated data pack and signing an appropriate contract

Data release criteria should include:

- The data release is lawful and in line with participant expectations.
- The data release is in line with all contractual and licensing agreements including periods of exclusivity.
- The timing of data release will not adversely interfere with the integrity of the trial objectives as set out in the approved protocol.
- The proposed research project has clear objectives and will use appropriate research methods.
- The proposed research project will be carried out by a reputable organization that can demonstrate appropriate IT security standards and will comply with all relevant legal and contractual arrangements.
- The resources are available to satisfy the request.

Stage 5 Archiving

The documents collected throughout the life of a clinical trial which individually and collectively permit the evaluation of the clinical trial and the quality of the data produced are defined as essential documents (ICH 2016). These essential documents serve to demonstrate the compliance of the Chief Investigator, Investigators, Sponsor, and other organizations, groups, and individuals involved in the conduct of the trial with the standards of Good Clinical Practice (GCP) and with all applicable regulatory requirements. They are therefore required to be archived for a period defined by law (for regulated trials) or by the Sponsor (for all other trials) once the trial has ended.

Planning for Archive

Clinical trials can be very complex and involve many different institutions; this means the essential documents generated during a trial could be held in different institutions, which may be in different countries and the documents may be held in either paper or electronic form. In a well-managed trial how and where essential documents are stored will have been planned and documented up front and organized in line with standard operating procedures dictating paper or electronic file structures or by using an online document management system with a standard file structure. A standard approach, particularly when used across all contributing institutions in the clinical trial, mitigates the risk of documents being lost, unavailable for audit or inspection during or after the trial or documents being archived or destroyed too early. This approach also makes planning for archive significantly easier because documents are able to be easily located, collated, and organized prior to being put into the archive.

The Sponsor, or other organization, responsible for trial conduct will manage the overall planning for archive, which will typically involve:

- **Nominating a suitable archivist** – an individual qualified by training and experience to manage the archiving of trial documents, agree the start and end of archive period, maintain a record of what is archived and where, control access to the archive or documents held therein and authorize destruction at the end of the archive period.
- **Identifying a suitable archive** – where a third-party specialist archive company is used, it may be deemed necessary to undertake vendor selection to verify the suitability of the vendor's facilities, systems, and processes and that these are in line with relevant contractual or regulatory requirements.
- **Communicating with other Institutions** – notifying all relevant institutions involved in the conduct of the trial of the archive period and providing authorization to archive documents held at the various different institutions. Not all documents and data need to be archived directly by the Sponsoring organization; indeed, it is expected by regulators in order to ensure the integrity of the trial dataset, that source data from an investigator site are retained in the control of that investigator site.

Challenges Associated with Archiving

Archive periods differ by country, region, and trial type but are typically lengthy periods requiring retention of essential documents over several years. This leads to a number of challenges when planning for archive in relation to:

- The high costs associated with storing significant quantities of paper documents over long periods of time
- Storage life, compatibility and accessibility of data, software, and information technology in the future
- Factors outside of the Sponsor's control which might lead to an increase in the archive period such as the risk of future litigation arising from the trial, where the results are contentious/controversial or may inform national policy and so will be likely to undergo greater independent scrutiny over an extended period of time

Early Trial Closure

Many trial protocols and designs will include provisions for monitoring the safety, efficacy, or feasibility of the trial at pre-scheduled time points to inform whether it is safe, ethical, and feasible to continue the trial beyond that point. Examples include:

– Dose escalation review in phase I trials
– Interim safety or futility monitoring by an Independent Data Monitoring Committee
– Recruitment feasibility
– New adverse safety information about the treatment under investigation which significantly alters the risk: benefit balance of the trial and the safety of current or future participants of the trial

The Sponsor may decide to close a trial early for various reasons, including poor recruitment, withdrawal of the intervention, or safety/ethical concerns. The decision to close a trial will usually include some form of independent oversight such as that provided by an Independent Data Monitoring Committee or even in some cases the regulator, depending upon the reason for closing the trial early.

Planning for Early Trial Closure

Although it is not possible to always predict exactly if and when a trial will close early, it is usually possible to undertake some planning activities in the run up to protocol defined stop: go points such as dose escalation or interim analyses in case the decision is to temporarily or permanently halt the trial at that time. Early planning allows for the different scenarios to be worked through for each likely scenario and can be particularly helpful where a plan of action will require rapid operationalization to protect the safety of participants on the trial (Box 7). The short timeframes involved when managing early trial closure arising as a result of interim safety or efficacy monitoring or new adverse safety information which alters the risk: benefit balance of the trial and safety of current or future trial participants mean careful preplanning activities cannot always take place; however, the typical planning activities detailed in Box 7 would still be applicable.

Communicating with Trial Participants Following Early Trial Closure

The most important consideration following early trial closure is to assess the impact on previous, current, and future participants of the trial and understand how their further participation in the trial will be affected by the decision and how quickly.

Where a trial closes early as a result of a safety concern, the communication to site investigators and participants would be expedited and carefully consider the most appropriate mechanism for communicating any new information to participants in a clear and sensitive way. Depending upon the risk involved, immediate action may need to be taken to withdraw the trial intervention; changes to the intervention and communication may need to be made to site investigators and participants immediately, that is, before seeking ethical or regulatory approval for the changes to be made. In the European Union and United Kingdom such actions are reportable post the event as an Urgent Safety Measure, where ethical or regulatory approval for the actions is obtained within a defined period of time after the action has been taken.

In all cases where a trial is closed early, participants should be provided with clear information about what is happening, why, further treatment options (where appropriate), and ongoing follow-up data collection.

Box 7 Checks when preparing for early trial closure

- Where multiple institutions, groups, or individuals need to be involved in the decision, establish a communications plan between the key decision makers to facilitate timely decision making.
- Establish a communication plan to disseminate the decisions made and resulting actions. This might include:
  - The independent ethics committee and/or regulator (be aware that where a trial is closing early for participant safety reasons this may constitute an Urgent Safety Measure or require shorter timelines for End of Trial notification)
  - The funder
  - Other institutions, groups, or individuals involved in the trial (information about how the decision impacts their activities and funding contract)
  - Previous, current, and future participants
  - Trial websites and public registry information
- Consider whether a substantial amendment to the trial protocol or supporting documents will be required and when.
- Consider whether urgent action needs to be taken to protect the safety of participants on the trial and whether this is reportable to the independent ethics committee and / or regulator (e.g., as an Urgent Safety Measure or End of Trial notification).
- For blinded trials, determine whether it may be necessary to un-blind some, or all of the trial participants.

Individual Site Closure

Trials usually include more than one investigator site; these trials are called multicenter trials. Prior to the End of Trial an individual investigator site may choose to close or be closed following a decision by the Sponsor, independent ethics committee, or regulator; the reasons for this are varied; this is called individual site closure.

Site closure is achieved at an individual investigator site when (at that trial site):

- Participant enrolment has stopped
- The data collection and cleaning activities are complete
- Any trial supplies have been accounted for and returned or destroyed, as per the protocol and contract
- All trial payments have been made
- For remote data entry trials, the site staff have been provided with a copy of the data for that investigator site
- Any final monitoring visits have taken place and issues arising have been closed out
- The Investigator Site File is complete

Summary and Conclusion

In a well-managed trial preparation for trial closure is key to ensure appropriate control over the final stages of recruitment and data cleaning for database lock and analysis. Preparation for trial closure can be supported through a comprehensive Trial Closure Plan which considers communication, project management including key milestones, and the roles and responsibilities of each organization, group, or individual involved in the conduct of the trial.

There are a number of important trial closure milestones which require careful monitoring and control, such as the end of recruitment to prevent too many participants being recruited. From a regulatory perspective possibly the most important milestone is that of the End of Trial, which is a key ethical and regulatory milestone defined in the approved trial protocol and has associated time-dependent notification and reporting requirements to the independent ethics committee and, for regulated trials, the regulator(s).

Notably, several of the key steps of trial closure; reporting, publishing, and data sharing are important mechanisms to support transparency in clinical trials.

Key Facts

- Trial closure refers to the activities which take place in preparation for the cessation of trial recruitment through to archiving of the trial.
- Trial closure can be notionally divided into five stages: End of Recruitment; End of Trial Intervention; End of Trial; Trial Reporting and Publishing, and Archiving.
- The End of Trial is a key ethical and regulatory milestone defined in the approved trial protocol and has associated time-dependent notification and reporting requirements to the independent ethics committee and, for regulated trials, the regulator(s).

– Registering, reporting in a public registry, publication of trial results, and making clinical trial data available for further research purposes are important mechanisms to support transparency in clinical trials.

Cross-References

▶ Administration of Study Treatments and Participant Follow-Up
▶ Archiving Records and Materials
▶ Data and Safety Monitoring and Reporting
▶ Data Capture, Data Management, and Quality Control; Single Versus Multicenter Trials
▶ Documentation: Essential Documents and Standard Operating Procedures
▶ Institutional Review Boards and Ethics Committees
▶ Interim Analysis in Clinical Trials
▶ Investigator Responsibilities
▶ Long-Term Management of Data and Secondary Use
▶ Participant Recruitment, Screening, and Enrollment
▶ Regulatory Requirements in Clinical Trials
▶ Responsibilities and Management of the Clinical Coordinating Center

References

Clinical Trials.gov (2017) FDA 42 CFR Part 11 Final Rule for Clinical Trials Registration and Results Information Submission. Available via https://prsinfo.clinicaltrials.gov/ Accessed 17 October 2020

European Commission (2017) Summaries of Clinical Trial Results for Laypersons. Available via https://ec.europa.eu/health/sites/health/files/files/eudralex/vol-10/2017_01_26_summaries_of_ct_results_for_laypersons.pdf Accessed 17 October 2020

European Medicines Agency (2016) Clinical data publication. Available via https://www.ema.europa.eu/en/human-regulatory/marketing-authorisation/clinical-data-publication Accessed 17 October 2020

International Committee of Medical Journal Editors (2019) Clinical Trials Registration and Data Sharing Policies. Available via http://www.icmje.org/recommendations/browse/publishing-and-editorial-issues/clinical-trial-registration.html Accessed 17 October 2020

International Council for Harmonisation of Technical Requirements for Pharmaceuticals for Human Use (ICH) (2016) Guideline for Good Clinical Practice. Available via https://www.ich.org/page/efficacy-guidelines Accessed 17 October 2020

Medical Research Council/Department of Health/Medicines and Healthcare products Regulatory Agency (2012) Risk-adapted approaches to the management of clinical trials of investigational medicinal products. Available via https://assets.publishing.service.gov.uk/government/uploads/system/uploads/attachment_data/file/343677/Risk-adapted_approaches_to_the_management_of_clinical_trials_of_investigational_medicinal_products.pdf Accessed 17 October 2020

Medicines and Healthcare products Regulatory Agency (2018) 'GXP' Data Integrity Guidance and Definitions. Available via https://mhrainspectorate.blog.gov.uk/2018/03/09/mhras-gxp-data-integrity-guide-published/ Accessed 17 October 2020

MRC Methodology Hubs for Trials Methodology Research (2015) Good Practice Principles for Sharing Individual Participant Data from Publicly Funded Clinical Trials. Available via https://

www.methodologyhubs.mrc.ac.uk/files/7114/3682/3831/Datasharingguidance2015.pdf Accessed 17 October 2020

Official Journal of the European Union (2010) Detailed guidance for the request for authorisation of a clinical trial on a medicinal product for human use to the competent authorities, notification of substantial amendments and declaration of the end of the trial. Available via https://ec.europa.eu/health/documents/eudralex/vol-10_en. Accessed 17 October 2020

UK Health Research Authority (2014) Information for participants at the end of a study: Guidance for Researchers. Available via https://www.hra.nhs.uk/media/documents/information-partici pants-end-study-guidance-researchers.pdf Accessed 17 October 2020.

World Health Organisation (2012) International Standards for Clinical Trial Registries WHO Public Registries. Available via https://apps.who.int/iris/bitstream/handle/10665/76705/9789241504294_eng.pdf?sequence=1 Accessed 17 October 2020

International Trials

19

Lynette Blacher and Linda Marillo

Contents

Abstract

The number of international clinical trials being activated has increased greatly over recent years. There are valid reasons for this global expansion, including a need for greater numbers of subjects enrolled in as short a time as possible, application to diverse populations, and the potential for cost reduction. However, conducting trials internationally involves its own set of challenges related to every aspect of trial conduct, from site activation to data management. Challenges

L. Blacher (✉) · L. Marillo
Frontier Science Amherst, Amherst, NY, USA
e-mail: blacher@frontierscience.org

© Springer Nature Switzerland AG 2022
S. Piantadosi, C. L. Meinert (eds.), *Principles and Practice of Clinical Trials*,
https://doi.org/10.1007/978-3-319-52636-2_44

are primarily related to cultural, procedural, and regulatory differences between countries. The new General Data Protection Regulation (GDPR) (eugdpr.org/) in Europe is also affecting the conduct of these trials. This chapter details these challenges, as well as offering possible mitigation strategies.

Keywords

International clinical trials · General Data Protection Regulation (GDPR) · Regulatory approval · ClinicalTrials.gov

Introduction

Conducting clinical trials internationally involves many of the same components as conducting a trial in the United States, or in any single country. The trial requires regulatory approval, the protocol and case report forms (CRFs) need to be developed, investigational drug needs to be acquired, sites need to be selected, data need to be captured accurately, bio-specimens need to be obtained, and monitoring and auditing need to be performed. The critical aspects of conducting trials internationally are the cultural, procedural, and regulatory differences between countries. This chapter addresses the rationale for conducting trials globally; the challenges posed by these cultural, procedural, and regulatory differences, as well as the challenges resulting from implementing the new European General Data Protection Regulation (GDPR) in the international clinical trials arena; and possible mitigation strategies.

Background

Expanding the conduct of clinical trials to the international setting has increased greatly over recent years. ClinicalTrials.gov, a database of privately and publicly funded clinical trials conducted globally, lists 298,104 registered clinical trials conducted in 209 countries, with almost 16,000 trials including both US and non-US participants, and over 143,000 non-US trials (clinicaltrials.gov) (Fig. 1).

There are several benefits to conducting trials globally. Conducting trials in multiple countries allows access to a greater number of potential trial participants. This is particularly important now that research has become more targeted – in other words, tailored to a population with specific characteristics (such as a certain gene combination). Identifying participants with these characteristics may be challenging, and expanding the potential pool to multiple countries helps to alleviate this issue.

Having access to a larger participant pool should speed up recruitment, which in turn should lead to quicker realization of trial results, and ultimately benefit to the greater population. Having participants from multiple countries allows greater diversity in terms of ethnicity and disease characteristics and susceptibilities, allowing the results to apply to a broader population. In some cases, participants that may not

Fig. 1 Percentage of
registered studies by location

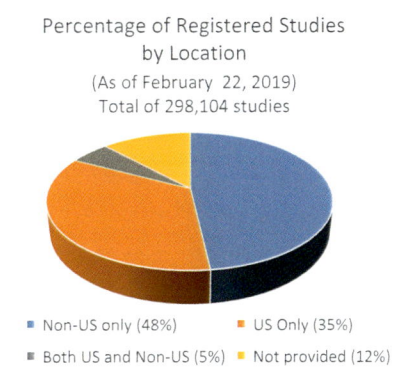

Percentage of Registered Studies
by Location
(As of February 22, 2019)
Total of 298,104 studies

- Non-US only (48%)   ■ US Only (35%)
- Both US and Non-US (5%) ■ Not provided (12%)

have had access to a certain treatment in their country can benefit by trial participation (Minisman et al. 2013).

Additionally, in theory, the cost of conducting the trial should decrease with quicker recruitment. Bringing a new drug to market can cost between $161 million to $2 billion (Sertkaya et al. 2014). A reduction in these expenses would make resources available for additional or new research.

Challenges of Conducting Trials Internationally

Challenges can present themselves in all areas and stages of the trial. This chapter will focus on the areas of Trial Coordination and Data Management.

Trial Coordination

Trial coordination refers to the oversight and coordination of the logistics of trial activities. Challenges can arise in several areas.

Procedural Differences

Earlier in this chapter it was discussed that conducting trials internationally could potentially reduce costs. However, costs can vary between different countries, making it much more expensive to include certain countries rather than others. This can be attributed to many factors, including research staff salaries, equipment expenses, fees for submission to Ethics Committees, and many more.

Infrastructure can also vary between countries. Areas that can pose challenges should be evaluated when considering sites from a country for participation (Garg 2016). For example, do they have access to the proper equipment; is the equipment in good condition and of the needed standard? Do they have appropriate storage procedures and facilities for the study drug, including a secured area, a reliable freezer; and a tracking process for receipt, distribution, and destruction or return of drug?

Quality standards must also be evaluated, as there can be variance between countries. Do the normal SOPs and procedures in place meet the standard expected for the trial? Does staff receive adequate training and guidance during trial conduct? Are staff fully qualified and skilled to perform the necessary procedures and document the research?

And most importantly, does the standard of care in the country lend itself to the trial requirements? (Bogin 2016) If certain procedures dictated by the protocol are not standard, will the principal investigator and research staff be able to perform them? Will enough participants be willing to undergo nonstandard procedures?

Regulatory Approval

The area that presents one of the more time-consuming challenges is "activating" a site to be able to participate in a trial. Activation involves many steps, including obtaining approval of the protocol and its related documents from regulatory bodies for each site. Various regulatory bodies may be involved including Ethics Committees (ECs)/Institutional Review Boards (IRBs), which are independent bodies that review and approve/disapprove research proposals for human participants. For certain countries, the trial protocol may also need to be submitted to/receive approval from Competent Authorities (CA)/Health Authorities (HA) (authorities that review submitted clinical data and those that conduct inspections), Data Protection Agencies (authorities responsible for upholding the right of data privacy), and/or individual Hospital Management. Additional review may be needed depending on the trial treatment or procedures (e.g., if the trial involves radioactive substances or transplant) (campus.ecrin.org).

There may be multiple ECs/IRBs involved as well. Some countries (or states/ regions) have a Central or Lead EC/IRB that performs complete review of the protocol, and the local ECs can adopt the decision of the Central/Lead EC. In other cases, local EC approval may be required in addition to the approval of the Lead EC, though this is usually a simplified review involving site-specific aspects.

Submission to ECs and CAs may occur in parallel or sequentially, depending on the country. The timeline for review and the fees associated with submission also vary. Even the submission platforms are different, from paper to CD to entry in an official database. Table 1 demonstrates these variances between a subset of European countries (campus.ecrin.org):

To illustrate the process in more detail, we will take Switzerland as an example. The CA for Switzerland is Swissmedic. (An additional CA, Bundesamt für Gesundheit (BAG)/Federal Office of Public Health (FOPH), is involved for trials with radioactive substances or transplant products.) The EC, Swissethics, is an association of the 9 cantonal (i.e., regional) ECs within Switzerland. Some cantonal ECs are

Table 1 Country-specific clinical trials submission

Country	HA/ CA	National/ central/ lead EC	Local/ regional EC	DPA	CA submission platform	General EC timeline (days)	Review order
Austria	X	X	X		CD/USB with hard-copy cover letter	60	
Belgium	X	X	Local	X	Electronic file with hard-copy cover letter	28	Parallel or sequential
Denmark	X		Regional	X	Online portal, or CD with hard-copy cover letter, or email	60	Parallel or sequential
Hungary	X	X			2 copies on CD	60	Parallel
Italy	X	X	Local		Online portal	60	Parallel
Portugal	X	X		X	CD with hard-copy cover letter	30	Parallel or sequential
Serbia	X		X		Hard-copy of all, or electronic file with hard-copy cover letter		EC then CA
Switzerland	X	X	X		Hard-copy in binder and CD	45	Parallel
United Kingdom[a]	X	X			Online Portal	30	Parallel or sequential

[a]The National Health Service Research and Development Forum is also involved in the approval process

responsible for several cantons. The submission application is submitted electronically through a portal to the Lead EC (the EC responsible for the site of the coordinating investigator) to check for completeness. At the same time the application is submitted to the ECs concerned for the participating sites, which evaluate local aspects. The Lead EC performs a complete review and informs the applicant, local ECs, and CA of its approval/disapproval. Local ECs can agree/disagree with the Lead EC's decision and may also add minor site-specific additions (campus. ecrin.org).

Table 2 Research groups and sites

Research group	Location	Sites
Breast cancer trials	Australia	Australia, New Zealand
EORTC: European Organization for Research and Treatment of Cancer	Belgium	Europe, Africa
IBCSG: International Breast Cancer Study Group	Switzerland	Europe, Australia, South America, India, New Zealand, Africa
GOIRC: Gruppo Oncologico Italiano di Ricerca Clinica/Italian Oncology Group of Clinical Research	Italy	Europe (Italy only)
JBCRG: Japan Breast Cancer Research Group	Japan	Japan
SOLTI: Grupo Español de Estudio, Tratamiento y Otras Estrategias Experimentales en Tumores Sólidos	Spain	Europe

One often thinks of international trials being conducted by pharma or industry, but it is important to note that Research Groups are involved in these trials as well. There are several Research Groups that act as a sponsor of clinical trials and/or participate in these trials. Research Groups are responsible for protocol development, trial management, and coordinating and overseeing the participation of several sites, which may be in the country of the Research Groups, or may be located within multiple countries. Table 2 demonstrates these variances between a subset of these groups in the breast cancer arena.

Each Research Group has its own procedures in place for trial conduct. Not only can there be group-specific variances in logistics, but country-specific variances within the groups as well. Responsibilities and the scope of work must be clearly defined between the sponsor (if the Research Group is not sponsor), Research Groups, and participating sites. Some items to consider: Will communication be through the group or directly to the sites? Will the site perform their own enrollments, or will the group act on their behalf? Will the group monitor their sites, or will this be the responsibility of the sponsor? If the sponsor is working with multiple Research Groups, the scope of work could vary greatly between them.

Investigational Medicinal Product Supply

The process to provide an Investigational Medicinal Product (IMP) to the site, and ultimately the participant, involves a series of steps, as well as several parties. This process is referred to as the clinical supply chain and follows the IMP from manufacturer, distribution center, local depots, sites, and participants. It is estimated that supply chain logistics account for 25% of pharmaceutical research and development costs, in part due to the globalization of trials (Fisher Clinical Services). Adding an international component can increase the complexity of the process, and issues can develop at or between any of these locations (Arnum 2011).

Appropriate logistics are essential to ensure the timely delivery of the IMP and any comparator product (current standard of care therapy). All parties involved must have the knowledge, experience, and imprint to meet the needs of a global setting. Any delay or shortage can cause delay of the start of a trial, or potentially even halt an ongoing trial. This, in turn, can affect the well-being and safety of participants.

It is important to start planning early, but not too early. Logistics should be discussed while the protocol is under development (Fisher Clinical Services). However, implementation should begin once it is relatively certain there will not be changes to the protocol and contracts with Research Groups or sites. For example, if a country decides not to participate, or a new country is added, and you have already planned the labels, distribution routes, and depots, these areas will need to be re-planned. Labels that included IMP dose would also need to be changed if the IMP dosage was changed in the protocol.

Logistical hurdles are many. Differing regulations between countries impact all areas of the process and considerations must be given to a variety of factors:

Availability of IMP – Sometimes a drug may have approval for the indication in certain countries and not in others. This could limit the number of countries that participate in the trial, as the patients already have access to the drug. This may result in slower recruitment, or not enough potential patients to conduct the trial. In other cases, the IMP may receive indication approval in one or more countries during the conduct of the trial, and these sites may cease recruitment.

There can also be the special case when a trial has concluded and the participant is still doing well, but drug is no longer supplied by the trial. In countries where it has been approved for the indication, the participant will be able to receive drug through standard mechanisms. In countries where the IMP does not have indication approval, an avenue of compassionate use may have to be pursued for these participants. Compassionate use allows individuals who are seriously ill and have no standard treatment options available to be treated with an IMP.

Forecasting – Underestimating need for drug (e.g., in case of faster recruitment or higher retention than expected) leads to participants without supply, whereas overestimating (in case of slower recruitment or lower retention) leads to unused material that is ultimately wasted, and again, is a cost issue. The differing infrastructure and working patterns within the countries can impact forecasting as well (Fisher Clinical Services). If proper procedures are not in place, the sites may not relay the necessary supply information to the sponsor and/or supplier to accurately calculate the IMP need.

Package Labeling – When planning labeling, participating countries must be selected early enough to ensure they are included on the IMP label in time for printing. The proper languages for each country must be determined, and translations validated. Additionally, authorities in each country may require specific terms to be used (Miller 2010).

If there are multiple countries, booklet labels to hold the volume of information may be useful, though they require additional time for production and printing. "Back-up" countries should also be anticipated in case one or more countries decide not to participate. Should this happen and no back-up countries have been planned, the labels/booklets would have to be revised and reprinted. Alternatively, a separate label could be created only for the new country(ies); however, this requires an additional supply pool. Either avenue can be quite costly.

There are several country-specific regulations regarding the information that needs to be included in the labeling. For example, in some countries, the local representative must be listed on the label/booklet. Sometimes even the comparator may need re-labeling (Weyermann 2006).

Packaging and Shipping – Proper packaging has become even more important due to the growth of biologics in research. It is necessary to transport and store biologics at proper cold temperatures (this is called cold-chain logistics). Specialized packaging is required, including insulated boxes and temperature-controlled containers (Fisher Clinical Services). The packaging materials must be assessed in relation to the weather conditions (e.g., temperature and humidity) of each country, including seasonal changes. Transport delays can occur at the border, with couriers, and at the site. Country infrastructure can affect the amount of time it takes to transport the medication to the site. In cases of longer timelines, it will be necessary to select a shipping vendor which is validated to maintain the required temperature for longer periods. Shipments also need to be planned around site working patterns, holidays, and religious observances, so as not to deliver product when responsible staff are not available to accept the package (Bioclinica).

Distribution – Multiple countries may translate to multiple depots. Whereas in the European Union one depot can function for all countries, in many other areas of the world, a separate depot is required for each country. This in turn leads to additional depot costs and a separate supply for each country.

Regulations and Documentation – Regulations are continuously being updated by governments and industry. Goods and service taxes to import drugs are levied across borders and differ between countries. Suppliers must be aware of these taxes, as well as country-specific documentation requirements. Original documents (rather than copies) may be required for some countries, and specialized documents or specialized versions for others, such as import permits and licenses (e.g., for Russia, an umbrella license from the Ministry of Health is necessary to ship supply, and a Certificate of Analysis is needed to grant the license). Another variance between countries relates to the Importer of Record, which is the legal body responsible for ensuring imported goods comply with local laws and regulations. In some countries only the sponsor can serve in this capacity; in others a Clinical Research Organization, distributor, or site may fill this role (Fisher Clinical Services).

Additionally, if the process for Ethics Committee/Competent Authority approval of the trial is extensive and time-consuming in some countries (e.g., it can take 12–16 months for approval in China) (George Clinical 2016), the expiration date of the IMP (and comparator, if applicable) must be considered. It must be ensured that the drug will be viable for the treatment of the participants.

Destruction and Return – At the end of trial, and upon expiration of drug, the IMP must be destroyed or returned to the sponsor. Which of these options is chosen and how it is accomplished can vary greatly by country due to country-specific regulations. Destruction can be done at the trial site or off-site. Some sites are not allowed to destroy product locally. If drug must be returned to the sponsor or dedicated vendor (e.g., pharma or supplier), an importation license into the country of destruction is usually required (Global Health Trials). Additionally, a certified carrier will need to be hired to transport the drug. Some countries, such as Serbia, may mandate drug is destroyed at a government-regulated location. Involving additional specialized companies and government authorities makes the return process more complex and costly (Mongan 2016).

Bio-materials

Collection of bio-materials (e.g., pathological tissue, blood serum, and plasma) is a component of many international trials. These materials may be required for:

- Central review: A central laboratory designated by the sponsor reviews materials to ensure the materials were categorized correctly by the local laboratory; this is often a factor in confirming eligibility.
- Translational research: Often referred to as "bench to bedside," this term refers to using results of research performed in laboratories to develop new methods of diagnostics and new therapies, and translating findings from clinical trials to everyday practice.
- Future research: In addition to the primary use of bio-material for the trial, material may be requested for future yet unknown research projects.

Challenges related to use of these bio-materials include:

- Obtaining materials: Each trial will have specific requirements for the materials. However, each country has specific regulations regarding the type of materials that can be provided to another entity, and specification may differ even between hospitals/medical institutions within the same country. For example, a block of tumor may be required for review, analysis, and/or bio-banking for a trial, but some countries may be allowed to provide only slides of the tumor material. In this case the material would not be sufficient to meet the requirements of the trial, and patients from these countries would be excluded from participation.
- Shipping materials: Materials are required to be sent to a central laboratory or biobank. As was seen with the IMP supply chain process, issues may arise due to the shipping regulations for each country, including special requirements; for example, the Ministry of Health must provide permission in Australia, Russia, and Brazil (export.gov; Fisher Clinical Services). Some countries, such as China, do not allow export of bio-materials. There can also be confusion regarding the classification of the material, for example, misconception from the courier that pathology material is hazardous.
- Retaining materials: Length of pathology material storage differs by trial. Materials may be needed only for central review (in which case the materials would be returned after a specified period), or for future use (in which case materials would

be stored indefinitely). Some countries and institutions do not allow indefinite storage and require materials to be returned within a specified timeframe.

Monitoring/Auditing

The goals of site monitoring and auditing are to ensure:

- Compliance with Good Clinical Practice (GCP) and regulatory requirements (ich. org)
- Compliance with the trial protocol and procedures
- Accurate and timely data collection
- Appropriate facilities, staff qualifications, and investigator oversight
- Communication between stakeholders
- Protection of patient safety and well-being

Although monitoring and auditing have the same goals, there is a key difference between them, in that monitoring is a quality control function and auditing is a quality assurance function. Monitoring refers to the performance of ongoing oversight and operational checks to verify processes are working as intended and in accordance with the protocol, standard operating procedures (SOPs), GCP, and the applicable regulatory requirements. Auditing refers to the systematic and independent examination of all trial-related activities and documents, to determine if they were conducted according to the protocol, SOPs, GCP, and the applicable regulatory requirements. An audit is designed to improve the effectiveness of processes (Ruppert 2007).

The international setting presents several similar challenges to both monitoring and auditing. Both processes rely heavily on communication, and language barriers can be an issue. If the trial is not conducted using a primary language, there may be the need for a monitor/auditor to be fluent in multiple languages in order to cover multiple countries; these qualified staff may be more costly and/or more difficult to find. If multilingual staff are not available, alternatives include hiring several monitors/auditors, each fluent in a different language, or hiring translators.

Scheduling visits may be problematic due to work patterns, holidays, and religious observances. Additionally, the need to be sensitive to cultural differences is even more important in the type of face-to-face interaction that takes place during an on-site monitoring or audit visit. Monitors and auditors also need to be aware of country-specific regulations regarding how GCP is interpreted and implemented.

Site monitoring can account for up to 40% of the cost of a clinical trial (Sprosen 2017). The cost of on-site visits particularly can be exacerbated in the international arena due to the extensive travel. There has been a shift to risk-based monitoring approach due to increased number, complexity, and globalization of clinical trials (Beauregard et al. 2018). This approach involves assessing risk, impact, and mitigation of the monitoring strategy. The goal is to focus on critical areas that relate to patient well-being, safety, and privacy. A risk-based monitoring plan often employs the use of more centralized monitoring (i.e., remote evaluation) where appropriate, to reduce the frequency and cost of on-site visits.

Although there are several benefits to central monitoring, one potential drawback can be that site personnel may believe they are not receiving the same level of support as provided during an on-site visit. It is much easier to develop a rapport with face-to-face interaction rather than through phone calls and email.

The concept of the remote "visit" has extended to auditing as well (Cobert 2017). Several considerations need to be given to up-front preparation, including:

- **Communications**: Remote audits are generally conducted via teleconference; therefore, local information technology support needs to be confirmed for the length of the audit, and communication should be tested in advance. Videoconferencing could also be employed to enhance the communication.
- **Documentation**: A means to access documentation (e.g., essential, regulatory, and Investigator Site File documents, as well as SOPs and any other relevant document) needs to be determined. Possibilities include uploading documents to a Trial Master File (TMF) structure within a web-based content management system. Or, more ideally, into an eTMF if available. This would be done in advance of the audit. Scans of source data or other necessary paper documents would be included as well.
- **Facilities**: In order to review facilities, creative measures, such as the use of digital photos or a video tour of the work environment, could be employed.
- **Systems and processes**: Screen-sharing technology could be used to demonstrate computer systems and processes.

Though the cost of travel is reduced with remote monitoring and auditing, there are still inherent costs in arranging and conducting remote visits.

Data Management

Challenges and costs can arise during data management activities as well.

Enrollment

Time and Date

Given the time differences between the various countries, the sponsor or data collection agency may not be located in the same time zone as the participating site or sites. To accommodate for these differences, a series of questions can be asked in the enrollment checklist regarding current time at the site, which are then put through validation checks to ensure the enrollment is happening within 24 h of the completion of the checklist.

Race and Ethnicity

The collection of race and ethnicity has been mandated by United States (US) standards as put forth by the Food and Drug Administration (FDA) for clinical trials conducted domestically and abroad (fda.gov). These minimum standards are for US Federal reporting purposes. The categories are social-political constructs only and are not scientific or anthropological in nature. They are to provide a common framework for uniformity and consistency in the collection and use of data on race and ethnicity by US Federal agencies.

Questions about race and ethnicity should be self-reported to the extent possible and never presumptively completed by site staff. The participant may identify with more than one racial group or choose not to report race or ethnicity.

Ethnicity choices are Hispanic/Latino, or Not Hispanic/Latino.

Race options are based on the following primary racial groups:

- **American Indian or Alaska Native**: having origins in any of the original peoples of North, Central, and South America, and who maintains tribal affiliation or community attachment.
- **Asian**: having origins in any of the original peoples of the Far East, Southeast Asia, or the Indian subcontinent, including Cambodia, China, India, Japan, Korea, Malaysia, Pakistan, the Philippine Islands, Thailand, and Vietnam.
- **Black or African American**: having origins in any of the black racial groups of Africa.
- **Native Hawaiian or Other Pacific Islander**: having origins in any of the original peoples of Hawaii, Guam, Samoa, or other Pacific Islands.
- **White**: having origins in any of the original peoples of Europe, the Middle East, or North Africa.

If additional granularity or more detailed characterizations of race or ethnicity are collected to enhance understanding of the trial participants, the FDA recommends these characterizations be traceable to the five minimum designations for race and the two designations for ethnicity as listed above (US Food and Drug Administration 2016).

A hurdle with trials conducted in Sub-Saharan Africa, Brazil, and India is that these guidelines cause confusion for participating sites and their diverse populations. In trials conducted by the International Maternal Pediatric Adolescent AIDS Clinical Trials Network (IMPAACT) and AIDS Clinical Trials Group, to counter the conflict, each trial site provided a list of acceptable racial categories for their anticipated participants (impaactnetwork.org).

Since data are collected at the time of enrollment, these choices are provided only to those specific sites. On the backend, the selections are collapsed into the five primary racial categories as well as the designations of multiracial or choosing not to report. The specific selections are still kept in the study database and available to the study team if requested.

Trial Designs and Populations

In the following list of potential protocol design populations, it is imperative to develop a tracking table to identify the links between the individuals. In many of these cases, the same treatment or observational arm will need to be assigned to the pairs or groupings.

- Discordant couples
- Index Case/Households
- Index Case/Caregiver
- Perinatal (Mother/Child)

Unique to the IMPAACT Network are trials involving perinatal populations in sub-Saharan Africa, Brazil, India, and Thailand. To accomplish the rigors of enrollment and follow-up, the mother and her fetus generally enroll between 28 and 35 weeks gestation. Both the mother and fetus are assigned a unique participant ID that keeps personally identifiable information to a minimum. The fetus is automatically assigned the same race and ethnicity as the mother. The fetus is considered on study at the time of enrollment, but the clock does not start for the baby until birth, whereas data collection on the mother begins from time of enrollment. If the birth outcome is not viable only the date of miscarriage or stillbirth is collected for the baby; all other information is collected as adverse events for the mother (impaactnetwork.org).

Data Collection Strategies

The development of well-designed case report forms (CRFs) or electronic CRFs (eCRFs) is integral to the collection of quality study data. These include eligibility and screening logs, participant questionnaires, clinic staff completed study forms, laboratory results, and adverse events reports. Data should be collected in the language of the sponsor, DMC or CRO, most of the time in English or French. NIH sponsored or supported studies will be collected in English. The expectation is that study site staff will understand and write in English.

The technical capabilities of participating sites will determine the best method to collect the study data. If Internet access is limited or nonexistent, paper CRFs should be provided to the sites and mailed back to the data center for centralized entry. The central data center reviews the records and communicates via mail with the site staff regarding errors and other questionable items.

When Internet access is at least minimally reliable, the sites are capable of keying their own data into a dedicated electronic data collection (EDC) package. With appropriate training, site staff are willing and able to manage their own data, thus allowing them real-time or near real-time access to their records. They are able to take ownership of the quality of the data and respond to data queries in a timely manner.

Study CRFs are designed to be completed by site staff and incorporate only elements necessary to meet trial design questions. These should be developed in the primary language of the protocol and the protocol team members, usually English. Care should be taken to minimize repetitive questions on separate CRFs thus avoiding potential inconsistencies between responses. The placement of questions should also be considered to provide a logical flow of responses and grouping of like data elements.

Participant questionnaires should be presented in the language of the enrolled participant. There are qualified translation services available but mostly for European, Chinese, and Japanese languages. For other ethnic or tribal languages, there would be reliance on local staff to provide the translation and back translation, utilizing separate staff to perform these activities. This can be tedious, repetitive, and time-consuming for both the sites and for the DMC staff required to verify the translations, but aids in maintaining a consistent method of presenting study concepts and questions, and eliciting responses from participants. One problem to avoid is asking open-ended questions that would require text replies which have to be translated back into English before being entered into the study database. This is particularly important to maintain privacy when collecting sensitive information the participant would not expect to be shared with site staff.

Questionnaires may be collected on paper and submitted to the data center via mail or facsimile for data keying, or through an online Internet package that prompts the user to provide responses to the questions – these responses are saved and downloaded to the database. Since the completed local language form will be submitted, the formatting of the questions and responses should align with the English versions to ensure the data are entered into the study database appropriately.

Laboratory test data CRFs should be designed to capture the units of measurements used in local laboratory, allowing for each site to report results as collected and measured. Upper and lower limits of normal as well as results should have data fields large enough to capture abnormally high or low results.

Ultimately, careful thought should go into the design of the data collection instruments to mitigate confusion about the goals of the study and minimize repetitive questions. The database should be developed in conjunction with the designing of the CRFs. A robust EDC system will have built-in validity and QA/QC checks, whereas data submitted via paper will be centrally checked further downstream in the data submission process.

Mitigation of Issues

At the beginning of this chapter, we discussed that the potential for reduced cost was one of the factors leading to the globalization of clinical trials. However, the numerous challenges of the global arena come with costs of their own. One needs to employ various mitigation approaches to balance these costs.

It is important to begin with a proactive risk-based strategy for conduct and monitoring of the trial. This allows any potential hurdles to be identified in advance, and plans put in place to reduce or eliminate their impact. A risk-based strategy will also lessen the chance of emergency or crisis situations arising; and if they do arise, there will already be a plan for addressing them.

Methods to mitigate risk include, wherever possible, creating simplified protocols, employing user-friendly data collection tools, and developing streamlined procedures for trial activities. It is extremely important to train – and re-train – the research team in these areas. This will ensure everyone has the same interpretation of the protocol and procedures. Requiring a primary language be used for the conduct of the trial, and mandating that all sites have at least one person on the trial team that speaks this language, can also reduce the potential for misunderstandings.

The proper selection of partners and collaborators is also important for risk mitigation. A site feasibility evaluation should be conducted before accepting a site for the trial, and vendors should be thoroughly researched and vetted. Partnering with experienced and dedicated collaborators allows for more efficient trial conduct.

A quality management system should be put in place to monitor each area of trial conduct. The use of technology can greatly aid in this oversight. For example, tracking systems can be utilized for IMP and bio-materials, and metrics reports can be created for areas in site performance, such as length of time to activation, data submission timeliness, query resolution, critical data items, protocol deviations, etc.

The most important facet of risk mitigation, which should be started at the very beginning of the trial, involves communication. It is critical to develop a rapport and understanding with all stakeholders. Establishing a clear communication pathway is key to the conduct – and ultimately the success – of the trial.

European Union General Data Protection Regulation

A chapter on international clinical trials would not be complete without some discussion of the General Data Protection Regulation (GDPR). The GDPR came into effect for the European Union (EU) May 2018, replacing the previous EU Directive 95/46/EC regarding data protection (eur-lex.europa.eu). The primary purpose of the regulation is to harmonize data protection and privacy laws across EU countries. The regulation covers the protection of natural persons with regard to the processing of personal data and on the free movement of such data and applies to all organizations who process personal data of EU subjects, even if the organization is not in the EU.

The main principles of the regulation emphasize transparency of data processing, legitimate use of data, minimization of data collected (e.g., minimum required for legitimate use), accuracy of data, security of data, subject consent to use of data, and limitation for data retention (e.g., retain data only for the length of time required for purpose of use) (eugdpr.org).

The GDPR strives to protect subjects by outlining their rights in regards to the processing of their data. Rights of data subjects include:

- **Right to Access** – right to a copy of their data
- **Right to Rectification** – right to correct their data
- **Right to Information** – right to know how their data are being used

- **Right to be Forgotten** – right to have the data erased/destroyed
- **Right to Restriction** – right to restrict data processing
- **Right to Portability** – right to take data from controller and/or transfer to another entity
- **Right to Object** – right to object to data processing (eugdpr.org/)

The GDPR also stresses the accountability of the data controller (person or entity which determines the purpose and manner of processing personal data, for example, a sponsor) and the data processor (person or entity that processes data on behalf of the controller, for example, an organization responsible for quality control or statistical analysis of the data), including strengthening enforcement and penalties (Yeomans and Abousahl 2017). Each EU member state must appoint an independent supervisory authority to enforce GDPR compliance; these authorities cooperate with each other and report to the European Data Protection Board. The data subject has the right to lodge complaints against these authorities and/or data controllers and to receive compensation. Fines may be levied against member states and/or controllers. Noncompliance to GDPR can lead to fines up to 10,000,000 EUR or a percentage of an organization's annual turnover (gdpreu.org).

There are many challenges in interpreting and implementing the regulation. The sponsor and any other data controllers or processors must determine how to uphold this regulation in the context of clinical trials. A first step is defining personal data, which is considered to be data that relate to an identified or identifiable individual (Advarra Regulatory Team 2018). The regulation applies to the processing of said data if it is either processed in an automated manner, or processed in a nonautomated manner such that it becomes part of a filing system (which is considered to be a system organized by specific criteria).

If there are no identifiers that can link or relate that data to an individual, the data can then be considered anonymized. Anonymized data are not considered personal data. On the other hand, pseudonimyzed data are personal data that can no longer be attributed to a specific individual without the use of additional information, but are still considered personal data (eugdpr.org/). In order to determine whether pseudonimyzed data are personal, it must be determined if there is information or means available to identify the participant, and whether these means/information are readily available. In terms of a clinical trial, participant data is usually coded (e.g., participant identification number, randomization code, site identification number) and would therefore be considered pseudonimyzed (Advarra Regulatory Team 2018).

The concept of personal data applies not only to participants in clinical trials, but also employees of the sponsor, site staff, and collaborators as well (Gogates 2018). The collection of names and contact information from these individuals is necessary for the conduct of the trial. The GDPR does state that the legitimate interests of the controller may provide a legal basis for processing data, especially if there is a relevant relationship between the controller and the subject, provided the rights of the data subject are still upheld.

According to Article 89 of the regulation, there is also some allowance for derogation regarding rights of data subjects (e.g., rectification, erasure, right to be forgotten, restriction of processing, portability, objection) when data are processed for scientific or historical research or statistical purposes, and Recital 156 refers to clinical trials as such research. Note derogation is allowed only in the case where complying with these provisions would make it impossible, or would significantly hinder, the fulfillment of the purpose of the research. Also, the research must still comply with GCP and appropriate safeguards must be put in place.

The rights of clinical trial participants can be upheld by ensuring the informed consent clearly states what data are being collected, why it is being collected, and by whom it will be processed or used (including whether it will be transferred to a third country) (Gogates 2018). Internally, sponsors, processors, and controllers should ensure appropriate security measures (including technology, processes, and training) are in place to maintain the privacy of the data. Data protection impact assessments should be conducted for each data process (Gogates 2018), to determine its purpose, management, and risks to rights of data subjects, as well as whether additional safeguards need to be established.

A Data Protection Officer (DPO), who will serve as the point person to ensure GDPR compliance, may also need to be appointed (HIPPA Journal 2018). A data privacy notice should be created and readily available to data subjects and should include contact information for the data controller (and DPO if applicable), categories of data that are collected, information regarding data transfer and retention, and data subject rights as outlined in the GDPR. The means by which requests or complaints can be made should be indicated (gdpr.eu).

Despite best efforts to ensure data protection, a data breach is still possible. Should this occur, the controller must inform the authorities within 72 h, unless the breach is unlikely to result in a risk to the rights and freedoms of natural persons (data.europa.eu/eli/reg/2016/679/oj). The controller must keep a record of all breaches and the resulting investigations, regardless of whether they were reported.

If the breach is likely to result in such risk, the controller must communicate the breach to the subject, including the likely consequences of the breach and steps taken to mitigate the effects (data.europa.eu/eli/reg/2016/679/oj). Of course in the case of a clinical trial the controller usually does not have direct contact with the participants or access to their information, so the communication would be handled by the site investigator, based on information provided by the controller.

Upholding the principles of GDPR within the clinical trial arena involves and impacts many stakeholders, including the sponsor and other controllers, data processing organizations, investigators and site research staff, and data subjects. The measures undertaken to understand the regulation and implement it often involve more complex processes and more personnel, which is an added cost to the conduct of the trial.

Summary and Conclusion

This chapter has provided information on the challenges involved in conducting clinical trials internationally. When planning an international trial, every area of conduct must be carefully assessed to determine how country-specific procedures and regulations can impact each area. Extra care must be taken to vet and establish communication pathways with all partners, from site staff to vendors. Risk assessment and mitigation strategies must be put in place. Though implementing these measures may be costly, the hoped-for benefit of conducting clinical trials globally is the quicker realization of trial results, and ultimately benefit to the greater population.

Key Facts

The benefits to conducting trials globally include access to a greater number of trial participants; greater diversity in terms of ethnicity, disease characteristics, and susceptibilities; faster recruitment; and quicker realization of trial results.

The challenges involved in conducting international clinical trials are primarily related to cultural, procedural, and regulatory differences between countries.

Regulatory bodies vary across countries and may include Ethics Committees/Institutional Review Boards, Competent Authorities, Health Authorities, Data Protection Agencies, and/or individual Hospital Management.

Logistical variances between countries in the clinical (drug) supply chain include approval for indication of the investigational medicinal product, impact of infrastructure on forecasting, languages and terminology on package labels, weather conditions for cold-chain logistics (packaging), requirements for multiple depots, goods and services taxes and permits, and local or off-site destruction of unused product.

Country-specific restrictions apply to the use of biomaterials in clinical trials, such as type of material that can be provided (if provided at all), export regulations, and length material that can be retained.

The challenges in auditing and monitoring international sites include language barriers; scheduling visits due to work patterns, holidays, and religious observances; and the cost of the visit due to international travel.

Challenges in data management of global clinical trials include time differences, interpretation of race and ethnicity, language issues, and technical capabilities of the sites (which affect whether paper-based or electronic data capture is possible).

Several considerations must be taken into consideration in terms of Case Report Form design for international trials, including minimal data collection, participant questionnaires in the language of the participant, and laboratory units in local measurements.

The challenges of conducting international clinical trials can be mitigated by developing a proactive risk-based strategy. Risks can be mitigated by simplified protocols, user-friendly data collection tools, streamlined procedures, training, and establishing a clear communication pathway.

The European General Data Protection Regulation (GDPR) strives to protect subjects by outlining their rights in regard to the processing of their data. Rights of data subjects include:

Right to Access – right to a copy of their data
Right to Rectification – right to correct their data

Right to Information – right to know how their data are being used
Right to be Forgotten – right to have the data erased/destroyed
Right to Restriction – right to restrict data processing
Right to Portability – right to take data from controller and/or transfer to another entity
Right to Object – right to object to data processing

Cross-References

▶ ClinicalTrials.gov
▶ Data Capture, Data Management, and Quality Control; Single Versus Multicenter Trials
▶ Documentation: Essential Documents and Standard Operating Procedures
▶ Implementing the Trial Protocol
▶ Institutional Review Boards and Ethics Committees
▶ Multicenter and Network Trials
▶ Procurement and Distribution of Study Medicines
▶ Qualifications of the Research Staff
▶ Responsibilities and Management of the Clinical Coordinating Center
▶ Selection of Study Centers and Investigators
▶ Training the Investigatorship

References

Advarra Regulatory Team (2018) The GDPR and its impact on the clinical research community (including non-EU researchers. In: Advarra. Available via https://www.advarra.com/the-gdpr-and-its-impact-on-the-clinical-research-community-including-non-eu-researchers/
Arnum P (2011) Managing the global clinical-trial material supply chain. In: Pharmtech. Available via http://www.pharmtech.com/managing-global-clinical-trial-material-supply-chain
Beauregard A et al (2018) The basics of clinical trial monitoring. In: Applied clinical trials. Available via http://www.appliedclinicaltrialsonline.com/basics-clinical-trial-centralized-monitoring
Bogin V (2016) Feasibility in the age of international clinical trials. In: Applied clinical trials. Available via http://www.appliedclinicaltrialsonline.com/feasibility-age-international-clinical-trials
Cobert B (2017) Remote PV Audits & Inspections. In: C3i Solutions. Available via https://www.c3isolutions.com/blog/remote-pv-audits-inspections/
European Clinical Research Infrastructure Network. Available via http://campus.ecrin.org/
Export.gov Brazil – Import Requirements and Documentation. In: Brazil Country commercial guide. Available via https://www.export.gov/article?id=Brazil-Import-Requirements-and-Documentation
Fisher Clinical Services Managing Complex Global Drug Distribution and Expiry. Available via http://info.fisherclinicalservices.com/clinical-supply-optimization-global-distribution-case-study-box
Fisher Clinical Services New Challenges for Global Clinical Trials: Managing Supply Logistics in an Expanding Clinical Trial Universe. Available via http://info.fisherclinicalservices.com/white-paper-global-clinical-trial-challenges

Fisher Clinical Services The Challenges of Cold Chain Management. Available via http://www.
    fisherclinicalservices.com/content/dam/FisherClinicalServices/Learning%20Centre%20Images/
    Latest%20Article%20Images/Latestarticlespdf/CTP012_Fisher%20Clinical_TRIM%20DPS.
    PDF
Fisher Clinical Services What Clinical Teams Should Know About Changing Trial Logistics and
    How they Will Affect Development. Available via http://info.fisherclinicalservices.com/log
Garg S (2016) An auditor's view of compliance challenges in resource-limited clinical trial sites. In:
    Applied clinical trials. Available via http://www.appliedclinicaltrialsonline.com/auditor-s-view-
    compliance-challenges-resource-limited-clinical-trial-sites?pageID=4
Gogates G (2018) How does GDPR affect clinical trials? In: Applied clinical trials. Available via
    http://www.appliedclinicaltrialsonline.com/how-does-gdpr-affect-clinical-trials
HiPAA Journal (2018) GDPR: what is the role of the Data Protection Officer. Available via https://
    www.hipaajournal.com/gdpr-role-of-the-data-protection-officer/
International Council for Harmonisation of Technical Requirements for Pharmaceuticals for Human
    Use (ICH). Available via https://www.ich.org/home.html
Miller J (2010) Complex clinical trials are posting new challenges across the clinical supply chain.
    In: BioPharm. Available via http://www.biopharminternational.com/complex-clinical-trials-are-
    posing-new-challenges-across-clinical-supply-chain
Minisman et al (2013) PMC US National Library of Medicine National Institutes of Health
    implementing clinical trials on an international platform: challenges and perspectives. J Neurol
    Sci. Available via https://www.ncbi.nlm.nih.gov/pmc/articles/PMC3254780/
Mongan A (2016) Three factors impacting on the destruction of IMP material. In: Clinical trials
    arena. Available via https://www.clinicaltrialsarena.com/uncategorized/clinical-trials-arena/
    three-factors-impacting-on-the-destruction-of-imp-material-4839806-2/
NIH U.S. Library of Medicine ClinicalTrials.gov. Available via https://clinicaltrials.gov
Regulation (EU) 2016/679 of the European Parliament and of the Council of 27 April 2016 on the
    protection of natural persons with regard to the processing of personal data and on the free
    movement of such data, and repealing Directive 95/46/EC (General Data Protection Regula-
    tion). Available via http://data.europa.eu/eli/reg/2016/679/oj
Ruppert M (2007) Defining the meaning of 'auditing" and 'monitoring' & clarifying the appropriate
    use of the terms. Available via https://ahia.org/assets/Uploads/pdfUpload/WhitePapers/
    DefiningAuditingAndMonitoring.pdf
Sertkaya A et al (2014) Examination of clinical trial costs and barriers for drug development.
    Available via https://aspe.hhs.gov/report/examination-clinical-trial-costs-and-barriers-drug-
    development
Sprosen T (2017) News: does cutting trial costs by reducing monitoring visits also reduce quality?
    In: MoreTrials. Available via https://moretrials.net/news-cutting-trial-costs-reducing-monitor
    ing-visits-also-reduce-quality/
The International Maternal Pediatric Adolescent AIDS Clinical Trials (IMPAACT). Available via
    https://impaactnetwork.org/
U.S. Department of Health and Human Services Food and Drug Administration (2016)
    Collection of race and ethnicity data in clinical trials. Available via https://www.fda.gov/
    regulatory-information/search-fda-guidance-documents/collection-race-and-ethnicity-data-clini
    cal-trials
Web learning resources for the EU General Data Protection Regulation; Fines and penalties.
    Available via https://www.gdpreu.org/compliance/fines-and-penalties/
Weyermann A (2006) Labelling requirements for IMPs in multinational clinical trials: bureaucratic
    cost driver or added value? Available via https://dgra.de/media/pdf/studium/masterthesis/mas
    ter_weyermann_a.pdf
Yeomans A, Abousahl I (2017) Preparing for the EU GDPR in clinical and biomedical research.
    Available via https://www.viedoc.com/site/assets/files/1323/preparing_for_the_eu_gdpr_in_
    clinical_and_biomedical_research.pdf

Further Reading

About NIAID Division of AIDS (DAIDS). Available via https://www.niaid.nih.gov/about/daids

ASPE U.S. Department of Health and Human Services (2014) Examination of clinical trial costs and barriers for drug development. Available via https://aspe.hhs.gov/report/examination-clinical-trial-costs-and-barriers-drug-development

Ayalew K (2015) FDA perspective on international clinical trials. Available via https://www.fda.gov/downloads/Drugs/NewsEvents/UCM441250.pdf

Bioclinica (2017) Collaboration between clinical operations and the logistics and supply chain teams is key to trial success. Available via https://www.bioclinica.com/blog/collaboration-between-clinical-operations-and-logistics-and-supply-chain-teams-key-trial

Clinical Trials Guidance Documents. Available via https://www.fda.gov/RegulatoryInformation/Guidances/ucm122046.htm

ClinRegs. is an online database of country-specific clinical research regulatory information designed to assist in planning and implementing international clinical research. Available via https://clinregs.niaid.nih.gov/index.php

Collection of Race and Ethnicity Data in Clinical Trials. Available via https://www.fda.gov/downloads/RegulatoryInformation/Guidances/UCM126396.pdf

DAIDS Regulatory Support Center (RSC). provides support for all NIAID/DAIDS-supported and/or sponsored network and non-network clinical trials, both domestic and international. Available via https://rsc.niaid.nih.gov/

Department of Health and Human Services Office of Inspector General (2001) The globalization of clinical trials a growing challenge in protecting human subjects. Available via https://oig.hhs.gov/oei/reports/oei-01-00-00190.pdf

Division of AIDS Clinical Research Policies and Standard Procedures Documents. Available via https://www.niaid.nih.gov/research/daids-clinical-research-policies-standard-procedures

European Commission, Enterprise and Industry (2009) EU guidelines to good manufacturing practice medicinal products for human and veterinary use. Available via http://www.gmp-compliance.org/guidemgr/files/2009_06_ANNEX13.PDF

Foust M (2014) Strengthening the links in the clinical supply chain: aim for transparency throughout the process. In: Applied clinical trials. Available via http://www.appliedclinicaltrialsonline.com/strengthening-links-clinical-supply-chain-aim-transparency-throughout-process

George Clinical (2016) Regulatory timelines in the Asia-Pacific. Available via https://www.georgeclinical.com/resources/research/regulatory-timelines-asia-pacific

Global Health Trials (2012) Destruction of investigational medical product following trial termination. Available via https://globalhealthtrials.tghn.org/community/groups/group/regulations-and-guidelines/topics/172/

Henley P (2016) Monitoring clinical trials: a practical guide. In: Tropical medicine and international health. Available via https://onlinelibrary.wiley.com/doi/full/10.1111/tmi.12781

Leyland-Jones B et al (2008) Recommendations for collection and handling of specimens from group breast cancer clinical trials. J Clin Oncol. Available via https://www.ncbi.nlm.nih.gov/pmc/articles/PMC2651095/

Mattuschka J (2016) Clinical supply chain: a four-dimensional mission. In: BioProcess international. Available via https://bioprocessintl.com/manufacturing/supply-chain/clinical-supply-chain-a-four-dimensional-mission/

Muts V (2018) International patient recruitment: the grass is not always greener abroad. In: Applied clinical trials. Available via http://www.appliedclinicaltrialsonline.com/international-patient-recruitment-grass-not-always-greener-abroad

National Cancer Institute Division of Cancer Treatment and Diagnosis (2018) Biorepositories and Biospecimen Research branch best practices. Available via https://biospecimens.cancer.gov/bestpractices/2016-NCIBestPractices.pdf

Pharmaceutical Engineering (2016) Clinical labeling of medicinal products: EU clinical trial regulation. Available via http://www.pharmtech.com/managing-global-clinical-trial-material-supply-chain

Research Conducted in NIAID Labs. Available via https://www.niaid.nih.gov/research/research-conducted-niaid

The Clinical Data Interchange Standards Consortium (CDISC) is an open, multidisciplinary, neutral, 501(c)(3) non-profit standards developing organization. Available via https://www.cdisc.org/

U.S. Department of Health and Human Services Food and Drug Administration (2013) Guidance for industry oversight of clinical investigations – a risk-based approach to monitoring. Available via https://www.fda.gov/downloads/Drugs/Guidances/UCM269919.pdf

World Courier (2015) Managing the myths. Available via https://www.worldcourier.com/insights/managing-the-myths

World Health Organization (WHO). Available via https://www.who.int/topics/epidemiology/en/

Documentation: Essential Documents and Standard Operating Procedures

20

Eleanor McFadden, Julie Jackson, and Jane Forrest

Contents

E. McFadden (✉)
Frontier Science (Scotland) Ltd., Kincraig, Scotland, UK
e-mail: eleanor.mcfadden@frontier-science.co.uk

J. Jackson · J. Forrest
Frontier Science (Scotland) Ltd, Grampian View, Kincraig, UK
e-mail: julie.jackson@frontier-science.co.uk;
jane.forrest@frontier-science.co.uk

© Springer Nature Switzerland AG 2022
S. Piantadosi, C. L. Meinert (eds.), *Principles and Practice of Clinical Trials*,
https://doi.org/10.1007/978-3-319-52636-2_45

Abstract

Documentation is a critical component of clinical trials. There are requirements not only to be able to verify that the data being analyzed is accurate but that it was collected and processed in a consistent way. Anyone involved in a trial has to recognize the documentation requirements and ensure that they are met. The International Conference on Harmonization (ICH) Guidelines on Good Clinical Practice E6 provides details of standards to be met along with relevant definitions. This chapter provides guidance on identifying essential documents for a trial and also on how to develop and maintain systems for standard operating procedures.

Keywords

Documentation · Standard operating procedures · Trial master file · Essential documents

Introduction

Documentation is now a fact of life for everyone involved in the conduct of clinical trials. The Sponsor, the Funder, the Trials Unit coordinating the trial, the investigator at the site, and often the trial subjects themselves have a responsibility to ensure that complete and accurate documentation is kept relating to their role in the trial. The conduct of clinical trials is now a highly regulated industry, and there are many people who are employed to maintain and oversee the quality of the trial documentation. The basic rule of regulators and other auditors is that if it is not written down, then it didn't happen, and they expect to be able to reconstruct the exact conduct of the trial from the documentation, including source documentation.

As well as creating and revising the documentation, there is a requirement to keep all documentation and archive it securely for lengthy time periods, which can vary depending on the type of trial and where it is being conducted. This chapter will outline requirements for essential documentation for sites, for coordinating centers, and for the Sponsor. It also includes some guidance for monitors and independent statistical centers (ISC) if relevant to the study.

The chapter also addresses the need for standard operating procedures (SOPs) ensuring that routine procedures are always carried out in the same way. We discuss the types of procedural documentation that are needed, and give suggestions for systems for the preparation and maintenance of trial documentation. This chapter will close by providing an overview on the use of document management systems.

Terminology

As there are several different models possible for running a clinical trial, we describe the model which we will use in this text for explanations. The hypothetical trial is a multicenter trial with several hospitals/clinics entering patients. The trial has oversight by a study Sponsor. Data is submitted to a coordinating center (on either paper case report forms (CRFs) or electronically via a remote data capture system), and the coordinating center is responsible for randomization/registration of patients, quality control of the data, queries to sites, statistical design and statistical analysis, and the management of those trial-related services. There is a separate independent statistical group responsible for preparing reports for the independent data monitoring committee. Site monitoring, including source data verification (SDV), is done by a separate organization contracted by the Sponsor. The Sponsor is responsible for provision and distribution of study medications/devices, oversight of the trial and all trial documentation. The collection of essential documentation required for this trial will be referred to as the trial master file (TMF). Where relevant, we will describe how other trial models would address some of the documentation requirements.

Background

In the early days of "modern" clinical trials, there was very little documentation maintained. Case report forms (CRFs) were relatively short and were all paper-based. Investigators and their staff at the sites completed them manually with source data being the patient's medical record. Sometimes they were signed – by the investigator, sometimes by a member of the investigator's staff or a rubber stamp signature, sometimes not signed at all, but it really didn't matter – the data was entered into the computer and used in analysis. This is just one example of how things have changed over the last 30–40 years, and there are many others.

Why have things changed so substantially?

One reason was the detection of cases of fraudulent data on cancer trials being submitted to a central trials office in the late 1970s. A result of an investigation into submission of fraudulent data by one of the US National Cancer Institute-funded cancer trials groups, the Eastern Cooperative Oncology Group (ECOG), was the establishment of an ECOG audit process where all sites were visited on site at regular intervals, and CRFs compared against source data on a random selection of cases. The US cancer cooperative group program implemented this approach across the board with involvement from the National Cancer Institute (NCI), and, while it has been refined and strengthened over the years, this program is still very much in place for NCI-sponsored clinical trials, and source data verification is now a routine practice in clinical trials (Ben-Yehuda and Oliver-Lumerman 2017; Weiss 1998).

Another completely different dynamic was the difficulty of doing clinical trials across borders because of the different regulations and practices around the world. Sponsors of international trials in the 1970s and 1980s were finding it challenging to deal with these variations, yet the urge to complete large trials more quickly meant an increase in companies and researchers wanting to use this cross-border model and to be able to use the same standards when submitting new drug applications in separate countries.

The biggest influence in addressing this has come from the International Conference on Harmonization, starting as a meeting in 1989 in Brussels of representatives from the pharmaceutical companies and regulatory authorities from Europe, Japan, and the USA. This followed early work to harmonize procedures in the European Union and strengthening of regulatory requirements by the US Food and Drug Administration (FDA). This conference generated a set of guidelines for clinical trials which have been widely adopted throughout the world as standards for the conduct of clinical trials (Good Clinical Practice Guidelines, E6 (R2) 2016). The ICH organization is still in place and constantly working to update and improve their guidelines.

In parallel, we saw the growth of an industry of contract research organizations (CROs) providing support services to the pharmaceutical industry in the conduct of clinical trials, including on-site monitoring and source data verification. The rapid and constant development of relevant technology has also had a huge impact as it is now feasible to collect and manage data and documentation electronically rather than on paper.

ICH Guidelines on Documentation

The version of ICH E6 Guidelines on Good Clinical Practice (GCP) published in November 2016 defines *Documentation* as "*All records in any* form *(including, but not limited to, written, electronic, magnetic, and optical records, and scans, x-rays, and electrocardiograms) that describe or record the methods, conduct, and/or results of a trial, the factors affecting a trial, and the actions taken.*" The definition given for *Essential Documents* is "*Documents which individually and collectively permit evaluation of the conduct of a study and the quality of the data produced.*"

These definitions are important as they are very comprehensive, cover all aspects of the trial and, as mentioned, have been accepted in many (and certainly all major) countries in the world involved in the conduct of clinical trials. There is a lot of information in ICH E6 revision 2, and we recommend that anyone involved in clinical trials become familiar with its contents. For this particular chapter, the key section of ICH E6 is Sect. 8, Essential Documents for the Conduct of a Clinical Trial. ICH E6, Sect. 8 groups its overview of documents by timing, before the trial commences, during the clinical conduct of the trial and after completion or termination of the trial. We will not reproduce the list of essential documents but will refer to some of the documentation types in our chapter.

One of the GCP principles, in ICH E6, Sect. 2, is that systems should be implemented with procedures that assure the quality of every aspect of the trial. This principle is expanded in ICH E6, Sect. 5.1 where it is stated that it is the responsibility of the Sponsor to implement and maintain quality assurance and quality control systems with written standard operating procedures (SOPs). We will explore SOPs later in this chapter.

Another principle to follow has become known as ALCOA. Documents should be:

- **Attributable**: can the data be traceable to the person responsible for recording a patient visit/event, along with the relevant date and time?
- **Legible:** can the data/information be easily read?
- **Contemporaneous:** was the data recorded at the time (or close to the time) that it happened, and not recorded a long time after?
- **Original:** is the source or first-captured data available for review?
- **Accurate:** are the details recorded complete and correct?

Attributes added to this list are:

- **Enduring:** is the information recorded in a way that is durable and long-lasting? (Ink can fade and electronic media become obsolete!)
- **Available and accessible:** is the data easily available for review or retrievable within a reasonable time frame?
- **Complete and credible:** is the data based on real and reliable facts and complete to that point in time?
- **Consistent**

We will refer to the complete list of attributes as ALCOA+.

The above are general guidelines to follow for all study documentation to meet compliance reconstruction requirements. Document quality can be determined by the degree to which documentation meets these ALCOA+ attributes. Other good documentation practices include document naming and versioning for ease of document identification and retrieval. This chapter considers the kind of documentation that is needed for various constituencies in a clinical trial. Documentation in general can be split up into two primary types, those which are instructional (e.g., plans, procedures, specifications, agreements) and records/reports.

Sponsor

The Sponsor of a clinical trial has ultimate responsibility for ensuring that all required documentation is available at the end of the trial. In addition, during the trial conduct period, the Sponsor usually has primary responsibility for the trial protocol, the Informed Consent Form and any patient information sheets, the Investigator's Brochure (if relevant), and some oversight plans for the conduct of the trial, such as a communications plan which documents communication pathways between all parties involved in the trial.

For the overall TMF contents, there are templates available which specify TMF requirements by category, and many Sponsors (especially pharmaceutical companies) will use a version of such a template to provide a standardized structure and content for the TMF. One such commonly used reference model is published online by the Drug Information Association (DIA Trial Master File Reference Model v3.1.0, 2018). Not all documents will be required for all trials, but this provides an excellent starting point for defining study-specific requirements. This model includes the minimum ICH E6 GCP essential document set and additional documentation commonly created to support trial activities. While the Sponsor has overall responsibility for the entire TMF, they will normally delegate responsibility for specific documents to other parties involved in the trial. In our hypothetical model, the sites, coordinating center, ISC, and the monitoring organization will all be responsible for aspects of the TMF.

During the trial or at the end of the trial (or phase of a trial), the Sponsor is responsible for collection of all the documents from all the involved parties and for integrating them into a manageable TMF. The responsibility can be delegated, but any delegation of this responsibility should be clearly defined and documented.

For all parties involved in the trial, these requirements are relevant:

1. Training records have to be maintained and updated over time to show that all staff involved in the trial have the appropriate training and qualifications to fulfil their trial-related responsibilities. This is required to meet one of the ICH GCP key principles. Training records for former staff involved in the trial should be maintained.
2. Retention of trial-related records is critical, and guidance should be sought from the Sponsor about the retention period. In many instances, this can be for a minimum of 25 years or until 2 years after the "last" regulatory submission involving trial data. As it is very difficult to assess whether a submission will be the "last" one, this effectively means that the records should be retained until the Sponsor has said they can be destroyed. Remember that records have to remain legible and accessible, to ensure that ink is not fading on handwritten documents and that electronic media can still be read. If copies are made of original paper records, the copies must be certified as exact copies of the original.
3. There must always be a complete audit trail of any changes made to clinical trial CRF data. With electronic remote data capture systems, this type of audit trail is usually built in, and a record will be kept of the original value, the new value, the name of the person making the change, and the date and time stamp of the change. Any eCRF system which does not meet these criteria should probably not be used for any trial where regulators may eventually review and adjudicate the data and the trial conduct. With paper records, the same level of information should be recorded on the paper record to ensure transparency, with a single line through an original value so that the value is not obliterated; the new value clearly written beside the original, along with initials/name of the person making the change; and the date and time of the change being made. The change must be supported by source data.

4. Electronic trial data handling systems used in support of clinical trial activities must be validated including those handling essential documents. A validation document set confirming the systems fitness for purpose should be created; ICH E6 GCP Sect. 5.5 provides detail on the documentation and SOPs required.

The following sections describe the responsibilities of each component of the trial management team, but it is the Sponsor who defines these study-specific responsibilities and also the Sponsor who should have systems to ensure that the required documentation is created and available for review and inspection.

Participating Sites

Relevant trial-related documents should be kept at each participating site in an Investigator Site File. These site files are part of the TMF but are usually held separately from the main Sponsor TMF. The staff at the participating sites have primary responsibility for ensuring that the required trial data is collected, recorded, and transcribed accurately on to the CRF. They are also responsible for ensuring that the original Informed Consent Form signed and dated by the patient entered on the trial is available. For many drug trials, sites are periodically visited by trial monitors who check the availability, completeness, and accuracy of the trial documentation, as well as performing source data verification (SDV) on trial data entered in CRFs and on pharmacy records (where relevant). Good organization at the sites is key to success in these monitoring visits. They can also be seen as good practice for any Sponsor audit or regulatory inspection of the site! The following points are intended to help sites with their organization and address issues commonly found at site monitoring visits or audits:

1. Most "formal" medical records do not contain sufficient information to allow the complete reconstruction of a patient's journey through a clinical trial. In such a situation, the site should maintain a "research record" containing documentation for the trial which is not recorded in the medical record. Information recorded should follow the ALCOA+ rules defined above.
2. The principal study investigator at the site is responsible for all the trial activities at that site. However, responsibilities can be delegated to other staff at the site. It is essential that all such delegations be written down in a log, showing the name of the person to whom a responsibility is delegated, the delegated responsibility and the relevant dates. Lack of a delegation log is a common finding at site monitoring visits/audits. Figure 1 shows an example of a site delegation log.
3. As well as CRF data, the site will be responsible for ensuring that all required documentation is available for the specific trial. This could include some or all of the following:
   (a) Approved informed consent forms and original signed patient consent forms
   (b) Ethics/Institutional Review Board (IRB) approvals
   (c) Contracts, agreements, indemnity, insurance, financial aspects of the trial

Site Signature and Delegation Log

Study Title: Study Number/ Short Name: Site Number:

PI Name: PI Signature: Start Date: End Date:

Name (Print)	Role in Study	Signature	Tasks Delegated*	Start Date	End Date	PI Signature	PI Date

*Fill in code for delegated task from list below

1.Obtain Informed Consent	8.Processing study samples	15.Reporting SAEs to sponsor
2.Obtain Medical History	9.Completion of CRFs	16.Report deviations/ violations
3.Perform Physical Exam	10.Signature of CRF	17.Prescription of study treatments
4.Assess eligibility	11.Data QC check	18.Dispensing study treatment
5.Confirm eligibility	12.Respond to Data Queries	19. Drug accountability
6.Medical oversight of trial patients	13.Assessment of AE	20.Maintenance of Site File
7.Collection study specific samples	14. Causality assessment for SAE	21. Other (specify)

Fig. 1 Site delegation log

(d) Protocol and amendments

(e) Investigator's brochure

(f) Sponsor correspondence

(g) Relevant emails about the study

(h) Any surveys/questionnaires completed by the site or by patients

(i) Minutes of any trial-related meetings

(j) Training materials used for staff training, training records, and curriculum vitae (CVs)

(k) Delegation of tasks

(l) Site selection and closure documentation/correspondence

(m) Any monitoring visit reports or audit certificates

(n) Any serious adverse event (SAE) reports and follow-up

(o) Details of any protocol deviations

(p) Details of local review of adverse events (AEs/SAEs)

(q) Pharmacy records for drug trials of receipt, storage, dispensing, and destruction of trial supplies

(r) Laboratory accreditation and sample management procedures

(s) Records of receipt and subsequent disposition of any other trial materials provided to the site

Very often, the Sponsor will provide a site binder for the participating sites to use for documentation, with instructions on the documentation to be maintained and stored in the binder. If none is provided, it would be beneficial for the site to create their own prior to the start of the trial. There are also now electronic site binders being used so that all documents are organized and stored electronically rather than on paper.

Procedural documentation (or SOPs) is relevant to all parties involved in a trial and is covered in a separate section in this chapter.

Coordinating Center

Our hypothetical trial has a coordinating center which is responsible for data collection, quality control, randomization/registration, trial management, and statistical design and analysis. As well as development of SOPs (see section in this chapter), what other documents will be needed for the TMF? The following is a summary of typical documentation needs by function.

Data Collection

To collect data, a case report form (CRF) must be designed, tested, and implemented. If the CRF is electronic, validation documentation of its design and implementation should be maintained. Key correspondence relating to the design and content of the CRF should be kept in an organized way such that it is easily retrievable at any time. If a CRF is updated after data collection begins, the CRF should be version controlled with dates of implementation and a record kept of all changes made as this could be important when using data for reporting and analysis. The statisticians need to know which version was being used when data was collected. It would also be important to document whether changes made were to be applied for all patients (including those already entered) or applied prospectively for new data only. There will also be a need for procedural documentation to provide guidance on CRF completion. Much of this can be covered in a data management plan for a study.

Edit Checks

Whether data is collected via an electronic data capture (EDC) system or on paper, the coordinating center will develop edit checks on the data as part of its quality control process. The edit checks can be either electronic (programmed to run automatically) or be manual checks implemented on review of the data or be a combination of both. The suite of edit checks will almost certainly evolve over time, and again, it is essential to maintain documentation on the edit checks which are implemented (including the testing and validation process), when they were implemented and on which subjects they apply (all or only prospectively entered).

Trial Management

Much of the documentation around trial management will revolve around project and quality process documents and can include topics such as risk, communication, training, and TMF management and is covered later in the chapter. As with the sites, the coordinating center will maintain contractual documents including documentation of responsibilities delegated by the Sponsor.

Statistics

The documentation required from the statistical team includes the following:

- Details of sample size calculation.
- All versions of the statistical analysis plans (SAPs).
- Statistical programs along with specifications, testing, and validation plans and results. Statistical programs and associated validation documents should be version controlled.
- Outputs from all protocol-defined analyses or analyses/simulations which led to a change in protocol design.
- Details of any randomization system used, which can be covered in a randomization plan, along with any relevant system validation documents.

Independent Statistical Center

Most Phase III trials have an independent data monitoring committee (IDMC), also referred to as a data and safety monitoring committee, to review study data and progress periodically. This committee is independent from the Sponsor. The role and responsibilities of the IDMC are well described in other publications (Ellenburg et al. 2003). The IDMC meets periodically and reviews reports prepared by one or more statisticians who are not involved in the conduct of the study. The reports for the IDMC are confidential and not seen by the Sponsor and are usually prepared by statistician(s) who are independent of the Sponsor *and* independent of the protocol statisticians. We refer to these independent statisticians as the independent statistical center (ISC) in this chapter.

The IDMC has a very important role in the trial and can make recommendations to modify or to stop a trial based on the information with which they are presented. They make these decisions based on the data prepared for them by the ISC. The ISC therefore has to maintain documentation of all the reports prepared for the IDMC along with corresponding statistical programs and datasets. Quality control records and validation reports on the programs should also be maintained for each version. Minutes of the closed and open sessions of the IDMC meetings would also need to be saved and all documentation available for inclusion in the TMF. The role and responsibilities of the ISC and the IDMC will often be documented in an IDMC Charter. The documents maintained by the ISC are usually kept confidential from the Sponsor until the end of the trial.

Trial Monitors

In our hypothetical trial, monitors visit sites to complete source data verification (or carry out remote monitoring visits, depending on the model in place for the trial) and check essential documents. Monitors may also visit sites during the site selection process for a new trial to see whether a site is suitable for trial participation, for a site initiation visit to ensure that all necessary documentation and processes are in place, and for a site close-out visit to close down the site at the end of trial participation. The role of the monitor and monitoring activities in a trial is usually defined in a study-specific monitoring plan.

Site Binder

As mentioned, it is common practice in drug trials for the trial Sponsor to create a site binder for each participating site to assist them in maintaining and organizing the necessary trial documentation which is required for the TMF (see above under Participating Sites). On a visit to the site, the monitors will routinely check the site binders to ensure that they are complete. The site binder would usually contain copies of all versions of the protocol used at the site, all relevant Ethics and Regulatory approvals, plus any other required local approvals, site staff curriculum vitae, training records, delegation logs, and study procedure documentation. It may also contain copies of signed patient consent forms, depending on the local procedures. Monitors will use this documentation prior to a site activation to verify that a site can be activated to accrue patients and then, during the trial, to ensure that the site is compliant with all study requirements.

Source Data Verification

One of the primary responsibilities of the monitors is to verify that the data entered into the CRF is accurate and complete. This is done by comparing the CRF entries to the data at its source. This could be the patient's medical or clinic record, a separate file with original documents relating to the patient's participation in the trial but not part of the official medical record, and ancillary records such as pharmacy inventory and dispensation records. A log of each monitor visit (on-site or remote) should be maintained along with details of what was checked and any findings. Monitors would also follow up to ensure that any deficiencies were appropriately corrected.

Monitoring Reports

These monitoring reports are written after each monitoring visit and submitted to the Sponsor or the coordinating center. The reports will also be maintained as part of the TMF.

Standard Operating Procedures

From the previous section about documentation requirements, it is clear that all parties maintain trial-specific plans and associated records/reports. In this section of the chapter, we consider instructional/process documents in the form of SOPs.

As mentioned previously there is a requirement to document not only what was done but how it was done and to show that a task was done in a consistent way throughout the trial, no matter who was doing it.

All of the entities involved in trials will follow SOPs. Procedures form the foundation of a good quality system and describe how to perform a repetitive trial activity. Procedures are often based on a standard policy which is more of a high-level statement of intention to satisfy requirements. Details of the standard process to comply with the policy that defines what needs to be done and why are operating procedures.

SOPs are essential documents and, like those covered in previous sections, should include records to demonstrate that compliance with the procedure has been measured and the procedure has been followed. The protocol document itself can be considered a procedure document for the selection, entry, and treatment of a patient entered on the trial. It may also contain instructions on trial related activities such as ordering trial medication, submitting materials for central review, randomization of patients, and other essential trial activities.

The philosophy behind SOPs is that they should be general enough to apply to all clinical trials being done by an entity and not be trial-specific. Depending on the entity organization, SOPs may be at a global or local level. If there are certain activities that are specific only to one trial, then a separate document should be created to describe that procedure. A common approach for this type of document is to call it a trial-specific work instruction rather than an SOP.

Clinical trial staff should be trained in applicable SOPs. Sometimes an entity will follow Sponsor or other collaborator procedures, and there is a need to ensure at the start of a trial that all parties are aware of the SOPs that are being followed. If external/Sponsor SOPs are used, it is key to ensure good communication between parties about procedure distribution and training. The entity that owns the SOPs should provide training on the procedures. As procedures set out the standard to work to, it is advisable that they are subject to periodic or scheduled review to ensure they reflect the current practice. The quality system should include a process on how to handle deviations from procedures.

How do you decide what procedure documentation is needed? The UK Clinical Research Collaboration has developed a process for assessing competency of clinical trials units (CTUs) as part of a CTU registration process. They have developed a list of areas of expertise which they consider essential for a CTU (McFadden et al. 2015) and recommend that SOPs be developed to cover these areas. The names of the SOPs can vary, but this list describes the basic topics which should be covered in SOPs in a coordinating center.

We have updated this list to reflect recent changes in legislation and present it as a table showing recommendations for documentation for each of our entities involved in a trial. Table 1 shows recommended topics for procedure documentation by entity.

Table 1 Recommended topics for standard operating procedures by entity

Topic area	Sponsor	Site	Coordinating center	Independent statistical center	Monitors
SOP on SOPs	√	√	√	√	√
Protocol development	√		√		
Risk assessment and monitoring	√	√	√	√	√
Trial master file/site file (investigator and pharmacy)	√	√	√	√	√
Regulatory approvals	√	√			
Trial initiation and site set up	√	√	√	√	√
Data management	√	√	√		
Trial supplies	√	√	√		√
Safety reporting/pharmacovigilance (if IMPs)	√	√	√		√
Quality management systems	√	√	√	√	√
Informed consent/patient information	√	√			
Training	√	√	√	√	√
Registration/randomization (if randomized trials)	√	√	√		
Statistics	√		√	√	
IT systems/databases	√		√	√	
Trial closure	√	√	√	√	√
End of trial reporting	√	√	√		
Archiving	√	√	√	√	√
Deviations, misconduct, and serious breaches of GCP and/or the protocol	√	√	√	√	√
Sponsorship, contracts/agreements, and indemnity	√	√	√	√	√
Data protection and confidentiality	√	√	√	√	√
Document control	√	√	√	√	√

Sponsor

The Sponsor has ultimate responsibility for ensuring that all necessary procedures and documentation are in place and maintained throughout the course of the trial. The Sponsor can audit sites, coordinating centers, ISC, and monitors to check for that assurance. The Sponsor should ensure that each participating party or entity understands their responsibilities for preparation and maintenance of trial documents and development and implementation of study procedures. It is also important to establish which SOPs are to be used for the conduct of the study – is it the Sponsor SOPs regardless of who is doing the specific task, or is it the SOPs of the entity to which the task has been delegated?

Participating Site

The site should have their own hospital/clinic SOPs for trial-related activities or follow those provided by the Sponsor (or a combination of both).

Coordinating Center

Depending on the responsibilities delegated to the coordinating center, there will be a variety of procedure documentation required, much of it relevant to any trial coordinated by the same unit.

Independent Statistical Center

The ISC will require procedure documentation for preparation of reports, interactions with the IDMC members, secure transfer of reports, minute taking, and archiving. There is usually also a study-specific charter for the IDMC activities developed as part of the overall study governance documents.

Monitors

The monitoring organization will require procedures on planning, conducting, reporting, and following up on monitoring visits. The monitors usually follow a trial-specific monitoring plan which documents how much monitoring will be done and the extent of the monitoring. This document is usually developed by the Sponsor but could be delegated.

Document Management Systems

As the reader can see, the requirements for documents are substantial, and it is beneficial to develop a system for creation, maintenance, and storage of these documents.

The Sponsor and all other parties involved in the conduct of the trial (e.g., site, coordinating center, ISC, and monitors) should aim to maintain an inspection ready TMF at all times. In other words, a regulatory inspector should be able to reconstruct the conduct of the trial using only the documents and metadata present in the TMF. While the concept of an inspection-ready TMF sounds simple, it is not easily achieved, and the quality of the TMF is a growing area of risk for the clinical research industry. There are many aspects to maintenance of the TMF, and some aspects are more challenging than others, such as managing electronic correspondence including emails in the TMF.

TMF quality is determined by both the quality of the individual records held therein and the quality of the systems and processes in place to maintain the TMF. The following section gives some suggestions for such a system.

Document Creation

Having a standard template for the development of a plan or an SOP simplifies the process when a new one needs to be developed. When a standard format is used for all documents, it also makes it easier for users to find something within the document as they are familiar with the layout of the sections. Figure 2 shows a sample layout for an SOP template. The document is normally prepared by someone with knowledge of the particular process (a subject matter expert). Once drafted, the document should be routed for appropriate review and, once all changes have been incorporated, final approval. This entire process should be documented. Signature is usually with wet ink, but there is a growing trend to use of digital signatures to approve essential documents. The implementation of electronic signatures should comply with international electronic signature requirements. Once approved, the document should be circulated to all individuals who are required to follow the process. Training in the contents should be documented in each individual training record.

Maintenance and Storage

There is a requirement for SOPs and other procedural documents to be routinely reviewed and updated when relevant. Part of the document management process is therefore to build in a timeline for re-review at a regular interval. This can be anything from 1 year to 3 years depending on the policy of the organization developing the SOP. Updated versions should be version-controlled with a clear record of what changes were made at what time. All approved versions of an SOP should be held in the TMF.

In general, the TMF held by the investigator (at sites) must be stored and archived separately from other documents that are part of the central TMF (e.g., from Sponsor, coordinating center, monitors). Confidential documents such as those held by the ISC and IDMC are usually transferred to the Sponsor once the primary analysis is completed. While site files are part of the TMF, they may continue to be maintained at the site rather than submitted to a central TMF. This is due partly to subject

[Document Number]

[Document Title]

Version:

Date of Approval:

Effective Date:

Next Review Date:

Security Level:

	Name	Role	Signature	Date
Approver				

	Name	Role
Author/Subject Matter Expert		
Reviewer		
Reviewer		
Reviewer		
Reviewer		

[Document Title /Document ID]   Version No.

VERSION HISTORY

Version	Effective Date (previous versions)	Issue Description	Summary of Changes Made

TABLE OF CONTENTS

1. PURPOSE
2. SCOPE
3. INTENDED USERS
4. PRE-REQUISITES
5. ROLES AND RESPONSIBILITIES
6. PROCEDURES
7. REFERENCES

LIST OF TABLES

LIST OF FIGURES

Template Version No.   Page 2 of X

Fig. 2 Sample SOP template

confidentiality issues and partly to the requirement that the investigator must maintain control of the source documentation held at site.

TMFs will usually be a combination of both paper and electronic files. It should be noted that the main requirements for storage and archival are the same for both.

The TMF itself should be well structured with records filed in an organized and timely manner. This enables ease of identification and retrieval of both the documents and the associated metadata – a key requirement for regulatory inspections. Metadata attributes give context and meaning to the records. An audit trail is a form of metadata, providing information on actions relating to the documents and records. Access to the TMF must be appropriately controlled to ensure no authorized disclosure of information, and the TMF itself protected from damage, unauthorized changes, and records loss. TMF documents are subject to review at audit/inspection, and any party involved in the trial could expect requests for direct access to the TMF during an audit/inspection.

Individual documents within the TMF must be version controlled, with an audit trail for changes made. Finally, the contents of the TMF must be clearly indexed with "signposts" to the relevant TMF repositories and systems.

Using a specialized eTMF system can greatly assist with the challenge of meeting the above requirements and streamline the processes of managing the active eTMF and of archiving the eTMF at study close-out. An eTMF system can also solve some of the issues faced by the Sponsor when the TMF documentation is being generated by a number of collaborating partners.

Quality Control of the TMF

The TMF should be monitored throughout the course of the trial for quality in terms of completeness, timeliness, document quality, and ease of retrieval.

Document Archiving

The Sponsor is responsible for archiving the TMF at the end of the study. An archive is a physical facility or an electronic system designated for the secure long-term retention and maintenance of archived materials. In the UK, such a system must be under the control of one or more named archivists, with access limited to those individuals.

Responsibilities for archiving the TMF should be agreed between the Sponsor, the sites and all other parties involved in the trial such as the coordinating center, ISC, and monitors. The Sponsor should ensure that all parties involved are capable of archiving their TMFs in a manner that meets GCP requirements. If files are transferred from one entity to another, then the transfer process should be tested and validated to ensure that all files are transferred completely and correctly.

The required retention period for archiving the TMF will depend on the applicable regulatory requirements. The principles for archiving paper and electronic TMFs are the same:

(a) All archived materials must be stored in a way that ensures their integrity and continued access throughout the required period of retention.
(b) Procedures should be established for making archived materials available for inspection, e.g., by regulatory authorities.
(c) Any alteration to archived records shall be traceable.
(d) Any transfer of materials within the archive from one location, media, or file format to another must be documented and validated if appropriate.
(e) The Sponsor shall maintain contact with any external organization that archives its materials throughout the period of retention.

The challenge of meeting requirement (a) above, for an electronic archive retained over a period of many years, can be significant due to the fast-changing nature of computer software and hardware. Archived digital files can become irretrievable unless consistent effort is made to maintain digital continuity throughout the retention period.

Destruction of Essential Documents

The requirements for long-term storage of essential trial-related documents vary in different regulatory jurisdictions. For example, in the EU the retention period is about to become 25 years. In the USA, it is often defined as "until two years after the last filing of data with regulatory authorities." As this is obviously vague and hard to define, it is recommended that documents be stored until the Sponsor gives approval for their destruction. Given the huge volumes of information that must be stored, it is easy to see why electronic archives are becoming the preferred way of storing documents.

Summary

This chapter has provided information on the documentation requirements for clinical trials. Clinical trials are increasingly governed by stringent rules and regulations which require development and maintenance of standardized ways of doing things and detailed documentation of those actions. While some of the regulations and requirements apply specifically to trials of medicinal products, it is recommended that clinical trialists use the same procedures for all types of clinical research. First of all, it is easier to have one set of rules for all trials, and secondly, it ensures that all clinical research is done to the same standards. However, it is acknowledged that compliance with all the requirements adds a considerable administrative overhead to clinical trials conduct. This overhead is not always recognized by those funding the trials – yet it is a requirement that all the standards be met. This is another reason to try to streamline procedures so that SOPs cover all clinical trial activity within an organization and that study-specific documentation is kept to a minimum.

The requirement to be able to "reproduce" the conduct of a trial from the TMF leads to an increasing volume of documentation required for each trial, particularly if it is to be used in a regulatory submission. While there are agreed international standards for trial conduct defined by the International Conference on Harmonization, there are national variations on these around the world. It is important for the Sponsor of the trial to ensure that all parties involved in the trial are fully aware of their responsibilities in terms of documentation and that all national requirements are met.

Use of standard templates and document management systems and following ALCOA+ principles will make it easier to develop, maintain, and implement essential documents and SOPs.

Key Facts

- Accurate and complete documentation is essential
- Conduct and results should be reproducable
- All parties have responsibility for compliance with procedures, for documenting key decisions and contributing to a complete and accurate TMF
- TMF must be retrievable throughout the active phase of a trial and the archiving/ retention period

Cross-References

- ▶ Data Capture, Data Management, and Quality Control; Single Versus Multicenter Trials
- ▶ Design and Development of the Study Data System
- ▶ Good Clinical Practice
- ▶ International Trials
- ▶ Responsibilities and Management of the Clinical Coordinating Center
- ▶ Trial Organization and Governance

References

Ben-Yehuda N, Oliver-Lumerman A (2017) Fraud and misconduct in clinical research: detection, investigation and organizational response. University of Michigan Press. ISBN – 0472130552, 9780472130559

DIA TMF (2018) Reference Model. Retrieved from: https://tmfrefmodel.com/resources/

Ellenburg S, Fleming T, De Mets D (2003) Data monitoring committees in clinical trials. Wiley, New York

Good Clinical Practice Guidelines, E6 (R2) (2016). Retrieved from: http://www.ich.org/products/guidelines/efficacy/efficacy-single/article/integrated-addendum-good-clinical-practice.htmlICH GCP Guidelines/

McFadden E et al (2015) The impact of registration of clinical trials units: the UK experience. Clin Trials 12(2):166–173

Weiss RB (1998) Systems of Protocol Review, quality assurance and data audit. Cancer Chemother Pharmacol 42(Suppl 1):S88

Consent Forms and Procedures

21

Ann-Margret Ervin and Joan B. Cobb Pettit

Contents

A.-M. Ervin (✉)
Johns Hopkins Bloomberg School of Public Health, Baltimore, MD, USA

The Johns Hopkins Center for Clinical Trials and Evidence Synthesis, Johns Hopkins University, Baltimore, MD, USA
e-mail: aervin@jhu.edu

J. B. Cobb Pettit
Johns Hopkins Bloomberg School of Public Health, Baltimore, MD, USA
e-mail: jpettit@jhu.edu

Abstract

Obtaining the informed consent of a participant is a prerequisite for enrollment in a clinical trial. In the United States, federal regulations provide the framework for establishing informed consent with additional protections for persons considered vulnerable due to incarceration, illiteracy, or other condition. Investigators are tasked with providing sufficient information about the research to satisfy the ethical and regulatory requirements while communicating it in a manner that maximizes the participant's ability to make an informed decision regarding study enrollment. There are clinical trial design features that are essential to include in the consent form with care to describe topics such as randomization, allocation ratio, and masking in a manner understood by the lay public. The informed consent discussion should continue throughout the course of the trial as informally reaffirming the participant's willingness to continue participation and reconsenting them when there are significant changes to the study protocol are important considerations for providing truly informed consent.

Keywords

Informed consent · Assent · Consent forms · Institutional review board

Introduction

The guidance in this chapter primarily pertains to clinical trials conducted in the United States, but the general principles may apply more broadly to trials conducted elsewhere.

Before enrolling a potential participant in a clinical trial, investigators must obtain the individual's informed consent. While people may think they know what "informed consent" is, there is no set formula as to how to best achieve it. Informed consent is a conversation between the participant and investigator that begins at recruitment and ends with study exit. Presenting information about the trial to the target population, taking into consideration the common characteristics of that population, e.g., age, sex, common disease, or condition, can be challenging. The ethical, legal, and procedural components of informed consent are intertwined; and while the ethical objective is static, regulatory/legal authorities will modify requirements over time, causing changes to procedural mechanisms. Investigators must have operational systems in place to ensure compliance with regulatory changes that may affect their studies.

The Office of Human Research Protections (OHRP), the US government entity that oversees federally funded human subjects research for the Department of Health and Human Services (DHHS), describes the investigator's obligation in the Code of Federal Regulations, Title 45, Part 46 (45 CFR 46.116):

Except as provided elsewhere in this policy, before involving a human subject in research covered by this policy, an investigator shall obtain the legally effective informed consent of the subject or the subject's legally authorized representative. An investigator shall seek informed consent only under circumstances that provide the prospective subject or the legally authorized representative sufficient opportunity to discuss and consider whether or not to participate and that minimize the possibility of coercion or undue influence. The information that is given to the subject or the legally authorized representative shall be in language understandable to the subject or the legally authorized representative. The prospective subject or the legally authorized representative must be provided with the information that a reasonable person would want to have in order to make an informed decision about whether to participate, and an opportunity to discuss that information Department of Health and Human Services, Office for Human Research Protections (n.d.).

This chapter summarizes the components that contribute to a successful informed consent process.

Who May Obtain Informed Consent?

Under guidance from the OHRP, obtaining informed consent is a study procedure that, alone, is enough to establish that a research institution is engaged in human subjects research and must have oversight by an Institutional Review Board (IRB) (also known as Ethics Committee or Research Ethics Committee (REC) in many parts of the world) (Department of Health and Human Services, Office for Human Research Protections 2008). The IRB has the obligation of ensuring that the investigators performing research activities are qualified and trained to so. Thus, the consent designees for a trial must be identified, and their qualifications and training submitted to the IRB for review and approval. The investigator must identify consent designees who are appropriately credentialed to obtain consent for clinical procedures. Qualified study team members may also work with the investigators and consent designees to support the informed consent process.

If the person who obtains informed consent has a clinical care relationship with the potential participant, the issue of "therapeutic misconception" arises (Sisk and Kodish 2018). Thus, when the clinician introduces a research study, the patient may interpret that introduction as a recommendation from the clinician, and may improperly attribute the possibility of direct personal benefit to study participation. The clinician must clearly explain that the trial is separate from clinical care and the patient's decision about participation will not affect the care that the clinician provides.

Who May Provide Informed Consent or Assent?

Participants, or their legal agents, must provide their voluntary informed consent in order to enroll in a research study. Adults, as defined by the locale's law on the age of majority, may provide informed consent for themselves unless they lack capacity to do so.

Lack of Capacity

If an adult lacks capacity to provide informed consent, a legally authorized representative (LAR), as defined by local law, may provide consent on their behalf. Lacking the capacity to provide informed consent is not the same as being cognitively impaired. The Alzheimer's Association (2004) defines the capacity to consent as "the ability to comprehend a research protocol, the meaning of personal participation in this protocol, including risks and benefits, as well as the ability to make and communicate a choice about participation." If a trial is likely to include adults who lack capacity to provide consent, the protocol must explain how study personnel will assess capacity. Studies that enroll adults who may lose capacity during the study may ask participants to identify an individual (a Research Agent) who may provide continuing consent on their behalf. A participant with limited capacity should provide assent, if able, and the study team should respect their dissent from participation.

Other Vulnerabilities

Some adults may not lack capacity to consent, but may be otherwise vulnerable due to incarceration, immigrant status, pregnancy, illiteracy, or another similar situation. Each participant must be considered as a unique individual, and investigators must consider and address any personal characteristics that may obstruct the possibility of obtaining legally effective informed consent.

Nonnative Speaker

If the target population is anticipated to be non-English speaking, the investigators should provide translations of the English consent document by qualified translators. If an unexpected non-English speaker who is otherwise eligible for the study is interested in participating and there is no time to fully prepare a translated consent form, both the Food and Drug Administration (FDA) and OHRP permit the use of generic short-form consents, translated into the potential participant's language, in conjunction with an oral translation of the official English version of the form by someone fluent in the participant's language. The process involves several components, including the participation of a nonstudy affiliated witness who is fluent in both English and the participant's language, and the procedures must receive IRB approval prior to implementation (Department of Health and Human Services, U.S. Food and Drug Administration 2014).

Parental Permission

Parents (biological or adoptive parents) and legal guardians must provide parental permission for minors (under the age of majority) to participate unless the study falls under a specific exception to this rule. The exceptions are:

- The study addresses a topic that is protected by a statute that allows minors to provide consent for themselves.
- The study meets the standards for waiver of informed consent and the IRB agrees to waive parental permission.
- The study includes a population of children for whom requiring parental/guardian permission is not appropriate given the study topic or the special characteristics of their relationship, and the regulations governing the study permit the IRB to approve a substituted mechanism to protect the minor participants. The DHHS provides this exception at 21 CFR 46.408(c), with the example being a population of neglected or abused children.

Depending upon the risk associated with the trial and the prospect of direct personal benefit, permission may be required from one or both parents. In the Randomized Trial of Peanut Consumption in Infants at Risk for Peanut Allergy (LEAP Study), infants as young as 4 months old at high risk for a peanut allergy were randomly assigned to avoid or consume peanuts in their diet until 5 years of age. Because the IRB determined that the study offered the possibility of direct personal benefit to the minor participants consent was obtained from one parent or guardian (Du Toit et al. 2015).

Assent

Minors must have the opportunity to provide assent to study participation. Assent means "a child's affirmative agreement to participate in research. Mere failure to object should not, absent affirmative agreement, be construed as assent" (45 CFR 46.402(b)). The IRB must determine whether children have the capacity to assent to trial participation. The IRB must consider the "ages, maturity, and psychological state of the children involved" (21 CFR 50.55(b), 45 CFR 46.408(a)). This determination may be for all children participating, for subgroups, or for individual minors. Assent may be waived for certain minimal risk studies, and for an FDA-regulated study which "holds out a prospect of direct benefit that is important to the health or well-being of the children and is available only in the context of the clinical investigation" (21 CFR 50.55(c)(2)).

Community Approval

For clinical trials that occur in community settings and in some international locations, investigators may obtain the consent or approval from local leaders. Community acceptance of the proposed trial may be important to successful recruitment and enrollment of study participants. It is also important to establish a communication mechanism with the community to facilitate the dissemination of results once the trial is completed. The Surveillance and Azithromycin Treatment for Newcomers and Travelers Evaluation (ASANTE) Trial recruited 52 communities in the Kongwa district, Tanzania, to receive annual mass drug administration (MDA) or annual MDA plus a surveillance and treatment program for newcomers and travelers to determine if the surveillance program would reduce infection with *Chlamydia trachomatis* (Ervin et al. 2016). In the ASANTE Trial, community leaders provided verbal consent for the participation of the community. Guardians provided consent to enroll children, and children aged 7 years and older provided assent to participate.

What Must the Documentation of Informed Consent Include?

The consent form for a clinical trial must include specific regulatory elements that may change over time, as well as provisions required by the institution where the research will take place. The US regulations governing federally funded human subjects research from 1991 until the 2018 revisions required eight basic elements and provided six "additional elements" to be added to consent documents when appropriate (Department of Health and Human Services, Office for Human Research Protections n.d.). The revised regulations, effective January 21, 2019, include new basic and additional elements and new format requirements. Some of these changes increase the focus on the collection and use of identifiable data and biospecimens.

While the consent form is the primary documentary evidence that a study interaction with a participant occurred, other notes that the study team records contemporaneously about that interaction may help record the context of the discussion. The consent form may also reference other IRB-approved tools, such as brochures, videos, and patient information sheets that the study team may use to help explain the study. Table 1 presents the current US regulatory requirements for informed consent. HIPAA Authorization is also included as many clinical trials in the United States must also comply with the HIPAA mandate.

Consent forms for clinical trials will also include a description of the study arms, including the use of placebos and sham procedures. The method of assigning participants to different study arms should be discussed along with a lay description of the allocation ratio. Additional important elements include:

- Persons masked/blinded during the course of the trial
- How and when study products (drugs, devices, etc.) are administered with detailed descriptions of all testing, procedures, and medications
- Details about the follow-up period, including the time points and methods of contact with participants
- Indications for discontinuing the study product during the course of the trial
- Description of the examinations, surveys or other assessments conducted at each study visit and any interim telephone (or other) contacts
- The availability of study products to all participants (or those receiving the placebo or other control treatment) once the trial has concluded

Table 1 US federal regulatory requirements for informed consent

Requirement	Description
Common rule consent elements	**Informed consent required elements 45 CFR 46.116 (1991)**
	1. A statement that the study involves research, an explanation of the purposes of the research and the expected duration of the subject's participation, a description of the procedures to be followed, and identification of any procedures which are experimental;
	2. A description of any reasonably foreseeable risks or discomforts to the subject;
	3. A description of any benefits to the subject or to others which may reasonably be expected from the research;
	4. A disclosure of appropriate alternative procedures or courses of treatment, if any, that might be advantageous to the subject;
	5. A statement describing the extent, if any, to which confidentiality of records identifying the subject will be maintained; if the study is FDA regulated, *noting the possibility that the Food and Drug Administration may inspect the records (21 CFR 50.25(a)(5));*
	6. For research involving more than minimal risk, an explanation as to whether any compensation and an explanation as to whether any medical treatments are available if injury occurs and, if so, what they consist of, or where further information may be obtained;
	7. An explanation of whom to contact for answers to pertinent questions about the research and research subjects' rights, and whom to contact in the event of a research-related injury to the subject; and
	8. A statement that participation is voluntary, refusal to participate will involve no penalty or loss of benefits to which the subject is otherwise entitled, and the subject may discontinue participation at any time without penalty or loss of benefits to which the subject is otherwise entitled.
	Additional elements
	1. A statement that the particular treatment or procedure may involve risks to the subject (or to the embryo or fetus, if the subject is or may become pregnant) which are currently unforeseeable;
	2. Anticipated circumstances under which the subject's participation may be terminated by the investigator without regard to the subject's consent;
	3. Any additional costs to the subject that may

(continued)

Table 1 (continued)

Requirement	Description
	result from participation in the research; 4. The consequences of a subject's decision to withdraw from the research and procedures for orderly termination of participation by the subject; 5. A statement that significant new findings developed during the course of the research which may relate to the subject's willingness to continue participation will be provided to the subject; and 6. The approximate number of subjects involved in the study.
January 2018 revisions to 45 CFR 46.116; effective January 21, 2019	**Expanded general requirements; 46.116(a)** (1) Before involving a human subject in research covered by this policy, an investigator shall obtain the legally effective informed consent of the subject or the subject's legally authorized representative. (2) An investigator shall seek informed consent only under circumstances that provide the prospective subject or the legally authorized representative sufficient opportunity to discuss and consider whether or not to participate and that minimize the possibility of coercion or undue influence. (3) The information that is given to the subject or the legally authorized representative shall be in language understandable to the subject or the legally authorized representative. (4) The prospective subject or the legally authorized representative must be provided with the information that a reasonable person would want to have in order to make an informed decision about whether to participate and an opportunity to discuss that information. (5) Except for broad consent obtained in accordance with paragraph (d) of this section: 　(i) Informed consent must begin with a concise and focused presentation of the key information that is most likely to assist a prospective subject or legally authorized representative in understanding the reasons why one might or might not want to participate in the research. This part of the informed consent must be organized and presented in a way that facilitates comprehension. 　(ii) Informed consent as a whole must present information in sufficient detail relating to the research, and must be organized and presented in a way that does not merely

(continued)

Table 1 (continued)

Requirement	Description
	provide lists of isolated facts, but rather facilitates the prospective subject's or legally authorized representative's understanding of the reasons why one might or might not want to participate.
	(6) No informed consent may include any exculpatory language through which the subject or the legally authorized representative is made to waive or appear to waive any of the subject's legal rights, or releases or appears to release the investigator, the sponsor, the institution, or its agents from liability for negligence
	New basic elements: 46.116(b)
	(b)(9)
	(i) A statement that identifiers might be removed from the identifiable private information or identifiable biospecimens and that, after such removal, the information or biospecimens could be used for future research studies or distributed to another investigator for future research studies without additional informed consent from the subject or the legally authorized representative, if this might be a possibility; or
	(ii) A statement that the subject's information or biospecimens collected as part of the research, even if identifiers are removed, will not be used or distributed for future research studies.
	New Additional Elements: 46.116(c)
	These require that a subject be informed of the following, when appropriate:
	(7) That the subject's biospecimens (even if identifiers are removed) may be used for commercial profit and whether the subject will or will not share in this commercial profit;
	(8) Whether clinically relevant research results, including individual research results, will be disclosed to subjects, and if so, under what conditions.
	(9) For research involving biospecimens, whether the research will (if known) or might include whole genome sequencing (i.e., sequencing of a human germline or somatic specimen with the intent to generate the genome or exome sequence of that specimen. For the purposes of this Chapter, the concept of "…broad consent for the storage, maintenance, and secondary research use of

Table 1 (continued)

Requirement	Description
	identifiable private information or identifiable biospecimens" introduced by the DHHS in the 2018 revisions to the Common Rule, will not be addressed.
HIPAA authorization requirements if the study involves using or disclosing protected health information (PHI) from a U.S. covered entity	**HIPAA authorization core elements** (see Privacy Rule, *45 C.F.R.* §164.508(c)(1)) Description of protected health information (PHI) to be used or disclosed (identifying the information in a specific and meaningful manner). The name(s) or other specific identification of person(s) or class of persons authorized to make the requested use or disclosure. The name(s) or other specific identification of the person(s) or class of persons who may use the PHI or to whom the covered entity may make the requested disclosure. Description of each purpose of the requested use or disclosure. Researchers should note that this element must be research study specific, not for future unspecified research. Authorization expiration date or event that relates to the individual or to the purpose of the use or disclosure (the terms "end of the research study" or "none" may be used for research, including for the creation and maintenance of a research database or repository). Signature of the individual and date. If the Authorization is signed by an individual's personal representative, a description of the representative's authority to act for the individual. **Authorization required statements** (see Privacy Rule, *45 C.F.R.* § 164.508(c)(2)) The individual's right to revoke his/her Authorization in writing and either (1) the exceptions to the right to revoke and a description of how the individual may revoke Authorization or (2) reference to the corresponding section(s) of the covered entity's Notice of Privacy Practices. Notice of the covered entity's ability or inability to condition treatment, payment, enrollment, or eligibility for benefits on the Authorization, including research-related treatment, and, if applicable, consequences of refusing to sign the Authorization. The potential for the PHI to be re-disclosed by the recipient and no longer protected by the

(continued)

Table 1 (continued)

Requirement	Description
	Privacy Rule. This statement does not require an analysis of risk for re-disclosure but may be a general statement that the rivacy Rule may no longer protect health information
NIH certificate of confidentiality (suggested language)	"This research is covered by a Certificate of Confidentiality from the National Institutes of Health. The researchers with this Certificate may not disclose or use information, documents, or biospecimens that may identify you in any federal, state, or local civil, criminal, administrative, legislative, or other action, suit, or proceeding, or be used as evidence, for example, if there is a court subpoena, unless you have consented for this use. Information, documents, or biospecimens protected by this Certificate cannot be disclosed to anyone else who is not connected with the research except, if there is a federal, state, or local law that requires disclosure (such as to report child abuse or communicable diseases but not for federal, state, or local civil, criminal, administrative, legislative, or other proceedings, see below); if you have consented to the disclosure, including for your medical treatment; or if it is used for other scientific research, as allowed by federal regulations protecting research subjects."
NIH guidance on consent for future research use and broad sharing of human genomic and phenotypic data subject to the NIH genomic data sharing policy 2015	In order to meet the expectations for future research use and broad sharing under the GDS Policy, the consent should capture and convey in language understandable to prospective participants information along the following lines: Genomic and phenotypic data, and any other data relevant for the study (such as exposure or disease status), will be generated and may be used for future research on any topic and shared broadly in a manner consistent with the consent and all applicable federal and state laws and regulations. Prior to submitting the data to an NIH-designated data repository, data will be stripped of identifiers such as name, address, account, and other identification numbers and will be de-identified by standards consistent with the Common Rule. Safeguards to protect the data according to Federal standards for information protection will be implemented. Access to de-identified participant data will be controlled, unless participants explicitly

(continued)

Table 1 (continued)

Requirement	Description
	consent to allow unrestricted access to and use of their data for any purpose.
	Because it may be possible to re-identify de-identified genomic data, even if access to data is controlled and data security standards are met, confidentiality cannot be guaranteed, and re-identified data could potentially be used to discriminate against or stigmatize participants, their families, or groups. In addition, there may be unknown risks.
	No direct benefits to participants are expected from any secondary research that may be conducted.
	Participants may withdraw consent for research use of genomic or phenotypic data at any time without penalty or loss of benefits to which the participant is otherwise entitled. In this event, data will be withdrawn from any repository, if possible, but data already distributed for research use will not be retrieved.
	The name and contact information of an individual who is affiliated with the institution and familiar with the research and will be available to address participant questions.
GINA (if appropriate)	"A Federal law, called the Genetic Information Nondiscrimination Act (GINA), generally makes it illegal for health insurance companies, group health plans, and most employers to discriminate against you based on your genetic information. This law generally will protect you in the following ways: Health insurance companies and group health plans may not request your genetic information that we get from this research. Health insurance companies and group health plans may not use your genetic information when making decisions regarding your eligibility or premiums. Employers with 15 or more employees may not use your genetic information that we get from this research when making a decision to hire, promote, or fire you or when setting the terms of your employment."
Conflict of interest	A statement that one or more investigators have a financial or other conflict of interest with the study and how it has been managed.

(continued)

Table 1 (continued)

Requirement	Description
FDA "applicable clinical trials"	Under 21 CFR 50.25(c), the following statement must be reproduced word-for-word in informed consent documents for applicable clinical trials: "A description of this clinical trial will be available on http://www.ClinicalTrials.gov, as required by U.S. Law. This Web site will not include information that can identify you. At most, the Web site will include a summary of the results. You can search this Web site at any time."

Consent Materials

The consent process begins as soon as an informational exchange between the investigator and potential participant about the trial yields personal information from the participant; and it continues throughout study participation. Recruitment materials are used as part of the consent process and must be IRB approved. No materials should overstate the potential benefits of the study using persuasive words like, "exciting" or "important" to describe the research. The traditional model of obtaining informed consent involves the use of an IRB-approved consent document that includes all the required elements of consent, potentially the elements of a HIPAA Authorization, plus any institutional provisions required by the local site. While the informed consent document is the standard mechanism for introducing a study and explaining its purpose, procedures, risks, etc., other supplemental tools may also be used. Videos, flipcharts, props, and other media can be very helpful to improve participant access to the study information. IRBs must approve these supplemental materials prior to use, and they must be consistent with the study's informed consent document.

Consent Discussion

The consent process must precede any study-related activities, including screening for eligibility, whether the discussion takes place in-person, by phone, or other remote method. Typically, a study team member approved to obtain informed consent reviews the consent form with the potential participant and answers any questions. The study team member must be cognizant of anything that might interfere with a participant's ability to make an informed decision (e.g., illiterate, language barriers, hearing, visual, or cognitive impairment). The study team member must allow time for the prospective participant to consider whether to participate and to ask questions about the study. In certain circumstances, the initial consent discussion may extend over time to allow the prospective participant to consult with her physician and/or family members. Study team members should not ask for consent when the potential participant feels exposed or vulnerable, for example, when lying on a gurney approaching the operating theater, or when his/her deliberative faculties may be compromised by severe pain, anxiety, or the influence of medication, etc. When the participant is satisfied with the discussion and agrees to participate, the participant, and when applicable, the person obtaining consent, sign and date the consent document. If the study involves clinical procedures for which only credentialed clinicians may obtain consent, the process may be bifurcated such that a trained study team member discusses the consent form with the participant, and then the clinician reviews the consent form with the participant and answers questions. Then, the participant, research staff member, and clinical research staff member all sign and date the consent document. Some trials may include more than one consent form as was utilized in the Randomized Trial of Achieving Healthy Lifestyles in Psychiatric Rehabilitation (ACHIEVE). The aim of ACHIEVE was to assess the efficacy of a behavioral weight loss intervention among persons diagnosed with a serious mental illness who participate in a psychiatric rehabilitation program (Casagrande et al. 2010). Persons at participating rehabilitation centers were orally consented prior to screening for ACHIEVE in order to measure their weight and height. Persons expressing an interest in ACHIEVE were asked to sign a written consent form for procedures related to eligibility screening and a second consent form before randomization.

Understandable Language

The language of the consent document, and discussion, must be understandable to the potential participant. Understandable encompasses many things: the language used in the discussion (English, Spanish, etc.); how well the consent language conveys accurately the information a participant needs to know; and the sophistication of the language, including how well the consent language explains scientific terms to a non-scientist. While IRBs may focus on reading levels and ask investigators to reduce the reading level of consent documents to a certain level (e.g., eighth grade or lower), this effort fails if the result is an oversimplified form that is deficient in conveying the information that a participant needs to know. Translating complex scientific ideas into simpler language accessible to the target population is a challenging task, but is essential to the objective of obtaining legally effective informed consent.

Context

The consent discussion cannot take place under circumstances that introduce a threat that might make prospective participants feel that they must participate (coercion), or that impose undue influence over the decision such that the participants decide to join or remain on a study that they otherwise would not elect to participate in or discontinue participation. These conditions could undermine the voluntary nature of the decision to participate. Investigators must consider the participant's situation and respect their privacy.

Assessing Comprehension

Some studies involve populations for which an assessment of comprehension is appropriate to ensure that the participant really understands what is being agreed to. It also may be appropriate to provide a process for ascertaining comprehension for complex studies. These assessments may take the form of a test following the consent discussion, or could involve the researcher pausing at the end of each section of the consent form to ask the participant questions about the content. It's difficult to know what information each participant absorbs, and it is also difficult to know what information each participant retains. The incorporation of tools such as audio-visual aids during the consent discussion as well as pre-study workshops to improve the communication skills of persons obtaining consent may aid comprehension (Kao et al. 2017). Investigators have considered reducing the complexity of consent forms to improve comprehension. The Strategic Timing of AntiRetroviral Treatment (START) trial compared participant comprehension after receiving a standard versus a concise consent form using a cluster randomized non-inferiority design. The overall comprehension and comprehension of randomization scores did not differ for participants at START trial sites that received the concise consent form when compared to those who received the standard consent form and the investigators concluded that shorter consent forms do not appear to impair the participant's ability to understand the study design and other basic features (Grady et al. 2017). It was however difficult to assess how ancillary information, such as discussions with research team members, might confound the assessment of comprehension among participants.

Re-consent

Re-consent may be required in certain circumstances. For studies that involve multiple interactions over time, additional tools like information sheets or other communications may be advisable to improve the quality of the informed consent. New information that could affect a participant's willingness to continue participation should be communicated to participants, with possible re-consent. Trials that undergo substantive amendments, including stopping or changing the number of arms of the trial, could affect a person's willingness to continue participation and investigators must provide participants an opportunity to re-consent. In the Evaluating the Effectiveness of Prednisone, Azathioprine, and N-acetylcysteine in Patients with Idiopathic Pulmonary Fibrosis (PANTHER-IPF) randomized controlled trial, participants with IPF and lung function impairment were assigned to receive a combination therapy of prednisone, azathioprine, and N-acetylcysteine (triple therapy), N-acetylcysteine (NAC) alone, or placebo (National Institutes of Health, National Heart, Lung, and Blood Institute 2011; The Idiopathic Pulmonary Fibrosis Clinical Research Network 2012). The primary outcome of the trial was change in forced vital capacity (lung function) from baseline to 60 weeks. The Data Safety and Monitoring Board for PANTHER-IPF identified safety concerns among participants enrolled in the triple therapy arm and recommended stopping the administration of the triple therapy and halting further enrollment in the trial while continuing the NAC and placebo arms. Participants in the all three arms were notified of the decision to halt the triple therapy arm and participants in the NAC and placebo arms were re-consented if they chose to continue participation in the study. Studies that enroll minors using parental permission and assent must consent those minors who reach adulthood during study participation. Although a single interaction and a single form may be preferred, legally effective informed consent requires more.

Termination of Consent

A study participant retains the right to leave a study at any time; the consent process must explicitly communicate that right to participants, and if appropriate, the consequences of that decision. It should be clear to the participant whether follow-up is necessary for their own safety and well-being or if there are any other procedures that should occur as a result of that decision.

Regulatory Requirements for Informed Consent in Canada and the United Kingdom

Canada

The Interagency Advisory Panel on Research Ethics developed the Tri-Council Policy Statement: Ethical Conduct for Research Involving Humans (2nd Edition, 2018; TCPS 2). The TCPS 2 is the mandate for the ethical conduct of human participant research in Canada. The TCPS 2 includes the guiding principles and required elements for informed consent (Table 2).

The TCPS 2 includes many of the same informed consent tenets as the US Federal and other policies throughout the world addressing research involving humans. Consent should precede data collection, is voluntary, and can be withdrawn at any time. Information regarding the study procedures and any risks and benefits of participation should be described in detail to facilitate informed decision making. Ensuring a participant's informed consent is a continuous process as events that might alter the risk/benefit ratio during the course of the study should be disclosed and these may affect the participant's willingness to continue participation. Consent

Table 2 Canadian regulatory requirements for informed consent

Requirement	Description
Consent elements	1. A statement that the individual is being asked to participate in a research study;
	2. An explanation of the purpose of the research, study procedures, duration of participation, and participant responsibilities;
	3. Disclosure of the researcher(s) and study sponsor(s);
	4. A description of any reasonably foreseeable risks and benefits to the participants and others;
	5. A statement confirming that participation is voluntary and the participant may withdraw from the research study without penalty or loss of benefits to which the participant is entitled. Information that may affect the participant's decision to continue with the research study will be provided in a timely manner;
	6. A statement that the participant may withdraw access to data or biologic materials with information on the limitations related to the request to withdraw data or materials;
	7. A statement informing the participant of any conflicts of interest (researchers, institutions, sponsors). Participants should also be informed if the research findings will be used for commercial purposes;
	8. A description of the plan for disseminating study results including whether participants will be identified;
	9. Disclosure of the person(s) to contact for research-related queries and unaffiliated person(s) who can discuss ethical concerns with participants;
	10. Disclosure of the types of data that will be collected and the purpose of this data collection;
	11. Notification of the person(s) who will have access to the data collected and how these data will be used including information on confidentiality and requirements to disclose data collected to other entities;
	12. Description of any payments, incentives, reimbursements and compensations for injury that will be provided to participants;
	13. A statement noting that participants do not forfeit their right to legal recourse if the participant experiences a research-related injury;
	14. Clinical trial investigators should also include information on the rules for stopping the trial and the conditions under which participants are removed from the trial.

may be written and a signed consent is required for research regulated under the Heath Canada Food and Drugs Act. The TCPS 2 also acknowledges that oral consent, field notes, exchange of gifts, and other methods may be warranted for documenting consent as cultural norms and research settings vary.

The TCPS 2 addresses the accommodations provided when persons lack the capacity to consent. In this instance the investigator must ensure that the research has a direct benefit to the participant or persons who are similar to the participant. If the investigator is unable to show a direct benefit, then the research must be minimal risk and low burden to the participant. A third party, who is not the investigator or a member of the research staff, will be asked to provide consent on behalf of the participant. If during the course of the trial, the participant regains the capacity to consent, informed consent will be obtained. Assent may be obtained if the participant has some capacity to comprehend the aims of the research. The

TCPS 2 further advises investigators and persons who may be asked to provide consent on behalf of a participant to review research directives for guidance on the participant's preference regarding participation in research activities. A research directive does not, however, modify the Tri-Council's requirements for informed consent.

United Kingdom

Guidance on informed consent for clinical trials in the United Kingdom (UK) is provided in the Medicines for Human Use Clinical Trials Regulations (MHCTR) and Guidelines for Good Clinical Practice (European Medicines Agency International Conference (n.d.); The Medicines for Human Use (Clinical Trials) Amendment (No. 2) Regulations 2006). The underlying ethical principles and general content requirements do not differ from those of the US and Canada. A participant information sheet (PIS) is prepared to support the consent process. The PIS provides a summary of the trial, including the background and objectives, the expectations for volunteers participating in the trial, risks and benefits, what data will be used and who has access to these data, information on withdrawing from the study, and how the results of the trial will be disseminated while maintaining participant confidentiality. The style and length of a PIS are often tailored to inform the persons providing consent or advice on study participation, including children, legal representatives, and relatives.

There are special protections for vulnerable populations, including adults that lack the capacity to consent, children, pregnant women, and patients participating in emergency research. The requirements for the consent for vulnerable populations may depend on the location of the research in the UK (England and Wales, Scotland, or Northern Ireland) and the study type. For clinical trials of investigational drugs or devices a legal representative may provide consent for adults who are unable to consent for themselves in England, Wales, Scotland, and Northern Ireland. For all UK nations the representative may be a person who has a relationship with the adult but is not involved in trial conduct (personal representative) or a professional representative such as a treating physician who is not involved in the study. Scotland regulations further specify that a personal legal representative could be a welfare guardian or attorney and if one is not appointed for the adult, then the closest relative. For greater than minimal risk research in England, Wales, and Northern Ireland that does not include investigational products, a person who cares for or has an interest in the adult's well-being (a personal consultee) or a nominated consultee (a person independent of the study) can provide their opinion on whether the adult would be willing to participate in the study. This opinion is recorded on a Consultee Declaration Form. In Scotland, a legal representative is asked to provide consent for research that does not include investigational products. Specific requirements for children and emergency research in the UK are outlined in Tables 3 and 4.

Table 3 Requirements for the consent of children in the UK

		England, Wales, Northern Ireland, and Scotland
Clinical trials of investigational products	Consent on behalf of a child under 16 years old	1. Parent or person with parental responsibility 2. Personal legal representative (if parent cannot be contacted) 3. Professional legal representative (if personal legal representative is unavailable) Assent of child should be sought when appropriate
	Consent on behalf of a child over 16 years old	Children over 16 may provide consent on their own If the child lacks the capacity to consent, then the regulations for adults that lack capacity to consent for clinical trials of investigational products will apply
Greater than minimal risk research without investigational products		There are no specific legal provisions for a child's consent to participate in research that does not include investigational products

Summary and Conclusion

While there are regulatory and institutional requirements for obtaining consent for clinical trial participation, investigators must also take steps to ensure that the process maximizes the potential participant's ability to make an informed decision. Additional protections are necessary for vulnerable populations. Discussions should occur in the appropriate context and supplemental materials may be important to illustrate specific procedures and expected contacts during the course of the trial. Assessing the potential participant's comprehension of specific elements of the trial should be considered particularly when the methods are complex and participation is expected over an extended period. Informed consent discussions should be continuous and written or other communications should be distributed to update participants during the course of the trial. Re-consent should be considered when modifications may affect the participant's willingness to participate in the trial.

Key Facts

- Voluntary informed consent is an essential prerequisite for clinical trial participation.
- There are additional legal protections for vulnerable persons to facilitate informed consent.

Table 4 Requirements for emergency research consent in the UK

		England, Wales, and Northern Ireland	Scotland
Clinical trials of investigational products	Adults lacking capacity to give consent	May be included without consent if 1) there is an urgency to administer treatment, 2) there is an urgency to administer the investigational drug in the trial setting, 3) obtaining consent from a legal representative is not practical, 4) the trial has been approved by the National Health Service's research ethics committee, and 5) the consent of the legal representative is secured as soon as possible	May be included without consent if 1) there is an urgency to administer treatment, 2) there is an urgency to administer the investigational drug in the trial setting, 3) obtaining consent from a legal representative is not practical, 4) the trial has been approved by the National Health Service's research ethics committee, and 5) the consent of the legal representative is secured as soon as possible
	Children lacking capacity to give consent	Under 16 years old: May be included without consent if 1) there is an urgency to administer treatment, 2) there is an urgency to administer the investigational drug in the trial setting, 3) obtaining consent from a legal representative is not practical, 4) the trial has been approved by the National Health Service's research ethics committee, and 5) the consent of the parent, guardian, or legal representative is secured as soon as possible 16 years and older: Refer to guidance for adults	Under 16 years old: May be included without consent if 1) there is an urgency to administer treatment, 2) there is an urgency to administer the investigational drug in the trial setting, 3) obtaining consent from a legal representative is not practical, 4) the trial has been approved by the National Health Service's research ethics committee, and 5) the consent of the parent, guardian, or legal representative is secured as soon as possible 16 years and older: Refer to guidance for adults
Greater than minimal risk research without investigational products	Adults lacking capacity to give consent	May be included without consent if 1) there is an urgency to administer treatment, 2) obtaining advice from a consultee is not practical, 3) the research has been approved by the National Health Service's research ethics committee, and 4) advice from a consultee is secured as soon as possible.	Consent should be secured from a welfare attorney, welfare guardian, or the nearest relative before the adult is included in the research.

(continued)

Table 4 (continued)

		England, Wales, and Northern Ireland	Scotland
	Children lacking capacity to give consent	May be included without consent if 1) the research has potential benefits to the child, 2) the research has been approved by the National Health Service's research ethics committee, 3) the research cannot be addressed in a nonemergent setting, 4) a parent (or guardian) is notified as soon as possible, 5) Consent and assent when appropriate are obtained as soon as possible, and 6) the child and/or the parent or guardian are informed that the child can withdraw at any time	May be included without consent if 1) the research has potential benefits to the child, 2) the research has been approved by the National Health Service's research ethics committee, 3) the research cannot be addressed in a nonemergent setting, 4) a parent (or guardian) is notified as soon as possible, 5) Consent and assent when appropriate are obtained as soon as possible, and 6) the child and/or the parent or guardian are informed that the child can withdraw at any time

- Consent forms must include specific regulatory elements, institutional language (where applicable), and lay descriptions of study design features that are unique to clinical trials.
- Re-consent should be considered when there are significant changes that may affect the participant's willingness to continue study participation.

Cross-References

▶ Institutional Review Boards and Ethics Committees

References

Alzheimer's Association (2004) Research consent for cognitively impaired adults: recommendations for institutional review boards and investigators. Alzheimer Dis Assoc Disord 18 (3):171–175. https://doi.org/10.1097/01.wad.0000137520.23370.56

Casagrande SS, Jerome GJ, Dalcin AT, Dickerson FB, Anderson CA, Appel LJ, Charleston J, Crum RM, Young DR, Guallar E, Frick KD, Goldberg RW, Oefinger M, Finkelstein J, Gennusa JV, Fred-Omojole O, Campbell LM, Wang N-Y, Daumit GL (2010) Randomized trial of achieving health lifestyles in psychiatric rehabilitation: the ACHIEVE trial. BMC Psychiatry 10:108. https://doi.org/10.1186/1471-244X-10-108

Department of Health and Human Services, Office for Human Research Protections (2008) Engagement of institutions in human subjects research. Available at https://www.hhs.gov/ohrp/regulations-and-policy/guidance/guidance-on-engagement-of-institutions/index.html. Accessed 23 June 2020

Department of Health and Human Services, Office for Human Research Protections (n.d.) Protection of Human Subjects 45 CFR §46.116 (a) and (b). Available at https://www.hhs.gov/ohrp/regulations-and-policy/regulations/45-cfr-46/index.html. Accessed 23 June 2020

Department of Health and Human Services, US Food and Drug Administration (2014) Informed consent information sheet: guidance for IRBs, clinical investigators, and sponsors. Available at https://www.fda.gov/RegulatoryInformation/Guidances/ucm404975.htm#genrequirments Accessed 23 June 2020

Du Toit G, Roberts G, Sayre PH, Bahnson HT, Radulovic S, Santos AF, Brough HA, Phippard D, Basting M, Feeney M, Turcanu V, Sever ML, Lorenzo MG, Plaut M, Lack G for the LEAP Study Team (2015) Randomized trial of peanut consumption in infants at risk for peanut allergy. N Engl J Med 372:803–813

Ervin AM, Mkocha H, Munoz B, Dreger K, Dize L, Gaydos C, Quinn TC, West SK (2016) Surveillance and azithromycin treatment for newcomers and travelers evaluation (ASANTE) trial: design and baseline characteristics. Ophthalmic Epidemiol 23(6):347–353. https://doi.org/10.1080/09286586.2016.1238947

European Medicines Agency International Conference on Harmonisation Guideline for Good Clinical Practice ICH GCP E6(R2) Step 5. Available at https://www.ema.europa.eu/en/documents/scientific-guideline/ich-e-6-r2-guideline-good-clinical-practice-step-5_en.pdf. Accessed 23 June 2020

Grady C, Toulomi G, Walker AS, Smolskis M, Sharma S, Babiker AG, Pantazis N, Tavel J, Florence E, Sanchez A, Hudson F, Papadopoulos A, Emanuel E, Clewett M, Munroe D, Denning E, The INSIGHT START Informed Consent Substudy Group (2017) A randomized trial comparing concise and standard consent forms in the START trial. PLoS One 12(4): e0172607

Kao CY, Aranda S, Krishnasamy M, Hamilton B (2017) Interventions to improve patient understanding of cancer clinical trial participation: a systematic review. Eur J Cancer Care 26: e124124. https://doi.org/10.1111/ecc.12424

National Institutes of Health, National Heart, Lung, and Blood Institute (2011) Questions and answers: PANTHER-IPF study. Available at https://www.nhlbi.nih.gov/node-general/questions-and-answers-panther-ipf-study. Accessed 23 June 2020

Sisk BA, Kodish E (2018) Therapeutic misperceptions in early-phase cancer trials: from categorical to continuous. IRB Ethics Hum Res 40(4):13–20

The Idiopathic Pulmonary Fibrosis Clinical Research Network (2012) Prednisone, azathioprine, and N-acetylcysteine for pulmonary fibrosis. N Engl J Med 366:1968–1977

The Medicines for Human Use (Clinical Trials) Amendment (No. 2) Regulations (2006). Available at http://www.legislation.gov.uk/uksi/2006/2984/pdfs/uksi_20062984_en.pdf. Accessed 23 June 2020

Tri-Council Policy Statement: Ethical Conduct for Research Involving Humans – TCPS2 (2018). Available at http://www.ethics.gc.ca/eng/policy-politique_tcps2-eptc2_2018.html. Accessed 23 June 2020

Contracts and Budgets

22

Eric Riley and Eleanor McFadden

Contents

E. Riley (✉) · E. McFadden
Frontier Science (Scotland) Ltd., Kincraig, Scotland, UK
e-mail: eric.riley@frontier-science.co.uk; eleanor.mcfadden@frontier-science.co.uk

© Springer Nature Switzerland AG 2022
S. Piantadosi, C. L. Meinert (eds.), *Principles and Practice of Clinical Trials*,
https://doi.org/10.1007/978-3-319-52636-2_47

Abstract

The clinical research landscape in the twenty-first century continues to evolve. Over the last three decades, the clinical trials landscape has changed dramatically with increased regulations, worldwide standards (ICH E6 Guidelines), and intense scrutiny. Most recently, there has been substantial impact from changes to legislation on data protection (US Health Insurance Portability and Accountability Act, EU General Data Protection Regulations) rather than legislation directed specifically at clinical trials. There is an increase in large multicenter clinical trials, many of them international in scope. Trials are increasingly becoming more automated and complex in their design, management, and implementation.

The complexity of the clinical trials environment and the increase in regulations requires all those involved, whatever their level of contribution, to adapt to the changes and to be very clear on the costs associated with carrying out research (Mashatole, Conducting clinical trials in the 21st century- adapting to new ways and new methods. Retrieved from https://www.clinicaltrialsarena.com/news/conducting-clinical-trials-in-the-21st-century-adapting-to-new-wasy-and-new-methods-4835722-2/, 2016). Equally important, the terms of agreement and division of responsibility between relevant parties involved in a trial, including the Sponsor and/or funder, must be clearly specified in advance in the form of a legally binding agreement.

This chapter provides guidelines for preparing Clinical Trial Agreements/Contracts and for developing budgets/funding requests for the work involved, both essential activities during the start-up phase of a trial.

Keywords

Contract · Clinical Trial Agreement · Data Transfer Agreement · Budget · Sponsor

Introduction

A "Signed Agreement between Involved Parties" and "Financial Aspects of the Trial" are listed as essential documents in ICH E6 Good Clinical Practice Guidelines (ICH 2016). This chapter will consider key considerations in preparation of these documents. For clarity, the "Signed Agreement" is referred to as a contract in this document, and the "Financial Aspects" as a budget. The budget is usually an appendix to the contract. In this chapter, the term Sponsor can mean the legal Sponsor of the trial or it can be the funder. Sometimes they are both the same entity, but not always, and, for the purpose of this text, are effectively interchangeable.

In broad terms, the steps usually followed to develop partnerships and a structure for a new clinical trial are typically as follows:

1. Request for proposal from Sponsor/funder/research organization/investigator, including specifications for the conduct of the trial
2. Preparation of submissions, including costs estimates

3. Selection of relevant partners
4. Negotiation of contract terms, including finalization of budget
5. Signature of contract
6. Activation of trial activities covered by the contract

In the chapter, the focus is primarily on steps 2 and 4 in the above list, but the other steps will be touched on briefly. Firstly, it is important to provide an overview of the funding landscape of clinical research and a background to the key issues, which ultimately inform the budget development process and more specifically the steps above.

Funding Landscape

There have been many changes in the approaches, regulations, and funding models of clinical research in the past 30 years ultimately affecting the source and level of investment. In 1991, 80% of US clinical trials were funded by government or philanthropic organizations, including by one of largest sponsors of biomedical research in the world, the US federal government. However, this number has been steadily in decline as the pharmaceutical industry's contributions continue to grow. By 2005, industry funded an estimated 70% of US clinical trials. Given the fact that commercial research is now assuming a larger share of the market, academic research that was once mainly funded through public grants is having to rely more on industry funding. As a result, these academic research groups are needing to adjust how they operate in order to align with the goals of industry, which is to bring drugs to the market in a timely and efficient manner (Pfeiffer and Russo 2016).

Much of the reason for the increased cost of doing research is the need for compliance with legal and regulatory requirements. For example, the initial EU Directive on Clinical Trials (Directive 2001/20/EC) stipulated that the same standard of conduct had to be maintained for all drug trials, regardless of whether there was an investigational agent involved or not. These regulations have been relaxed slightly, but there are still extensive standards to follow.

In several countries, private nonprofit organizations and state/local governments have been increasing their stake in research and now compete with the traditional key stakeholders. As all parties battle the increasing costs and complexities of clinical trials, which has been accelerated by global recessions and fluctuations in funding, research organizations in every sector have to strategically position themselves and find ways to work with each other for sustainability and advancement of their missions (Hind et al. 2017).

Types of Clinical Research

The contract and budget process is connected to the funding model for a particular trial, which from a high-level perspective is dependent on the various types of research. By having an understanding of the type of research being conducted, one can better appreciate the key elements that define these processes. Regardless of the type however, the information generated by any clinical research ultimately leads to the commercialization of a new drug or device, advancement of scientific knowledge, and/or changes in health policy and legislation (Camps et al. 2017).

Broadly speaking, there are two types of clinical research, noncommercial and commercial. In noncommercial research, the aim of the research project is to generate knowledge that benefits the good of the wider public. It usually involves government or nonprofit organizations such as academic institutions or foundations, but it can also involve financial support from commercial entities such as a pharmaceutical or a biotech company, often in the form of an educational grant.

Commercial research is mainly sponsored by private industry. While there is a genuine interest in advancing the development of scientific knowledge, there are inevitably financial interests in this type of research specifically related to bringing a new product to market or expanding the use of an existing product. This type of research typically involves one organization which funds, designs, and carries out a clinical trial either entirely under one roof or with delegated tasks outsourced to other organizations which provide research services, such a Clinical Research Organisation (CRO). CROs can provide a range of services from project management, database design and build, clinical trial data management, statistical analysis, and administration of Independent Data Monitoring Committees (IDMC)/Data Safety Monitoring Boards (DSMB). Due to this diversity and scope, they are becoming a major force in drug development and clinical trial recruitment (Carroll 2005). Other organizations such as AROs (Academic Research Organisations) and CCOs (Contract Commercial Organisations) can also be involved in providing a range of specialist services to support clinical research such as recruitment support, clinical knowledge and expertise, marketing and regulatory filing support, and drug launch.

Key Funding Sources

Within each type of research, there are various funding sources and mechanisms. As part of their drug development programs, private industry is naturally a major funder of clinical research. Another significant source of investment is the US federal government, namely, through the National Institutes of Health (NIH). NIH is considered the largest funder among the world's top public and philanthropic organizations in the world investing $26.1 billion in health research. The European Commission and the UK Medical Research Council follow in second and third places for research investment with recent contributions investments of $3.7 billion and $1.3 billion, respectively (Viergever and Hendriks 2016).

Charities like Cancer Research UK and the Wellcome Trust make significant investment to research and development in the UK and worldwide (Cooksey 2006). Private donors or foundations such as the Bill and Melinda Gates Foundation and The Michael J. Fox Foundation for Parkinson's Research also fund clinical research. Additionally, there are global philanthropic groups such as The European Organisation for Research and Treatment of Cancer (EORTC) or the

Breast International Group (BIG) who support and fund research in specific disease areas. An organization such as BIG has expansive global reach and influence. As a key stakeholder in breast cancer research, BIG represents a network of collaborative groups connecting over 59 academic research groups on over 30 clinical trials or research programs at a given time and affecting over 95,000 patients since its inception (BIG 2018).

Key Differences in Funding Models

Overall, the motivation and incentives for each funding model vary. Often the motivation for noncommercial research does not align with the current needs of the pharmaceutical industry. In these cases where industry is sponsoring the research, there is a need to ensure independence and impartiality to address the scientific hypothesis. This has implications for budgeting given that there could be extra costs involved in ensuring the scientific integrity of the trial, such as the need for Data Safety Monitoring Boards (DSMBs) or in other ways like ensuring the proper firewalls are in place between the relevant partners.

There are other potential differences between commercial and noncommercial models, which relate to timelines and trial procedures. In academic settings, time-lines are typically more relaxed than for industry trials. The rigor of trial procedures can also vary. In commercial research, or any trial involving investigational drugs, the infrastructure and standards are usually more resource intensive and to a very high standard. This rigor is necessary to satisfy regulatory bodies as results of these trials are used to ensure products can make it to the consumer market safely and effectively.

Distribution of Funds

The distribution of funds will vary depending on the individual trial, the main stakeholder(s), and how the contracts are written. As stated, there may be several parties involved in ensuring a trial is carried out successfully (e.g., research sites, CRO, data management services, drug distribution services, sample processing labs), and the main funder (which may be the Sponsor) is responsible for paying the partners either directly or indirectly.

In academic trials the Sponsor/funder, which could be a government body, nonprofit organization, or a commercial partner, typically pays a participating university or affiliated medical center directly. In another model, the Sponsor pays the Coordinating Center, which subcontracts to each participating site. Usually at major academic centers, research groups are able to access the necessary support resources through the institution's research infrastructure sometimes called a CTU or clinical trial unit. This may include central personnel, laboratory resources, additional medical services like imaging or equipment, bio sample storage, and Institution Review Boards (IRBs)/Ethics Committees (ECs).

In contrast, a large global trial being sponsored by a major pharmaceutical company may have a multitude of partners and individual contracts with each party or possibly even a setup with a main CRO and only a few select partners. Another model is a large collaborative group, which manages and handles all contracts and payments across services. In these cases, the collaborative group would likely have access to a network of global organizations who would pool their resources to identify the best sites to recruit the required study population.

Overall, the distribution of funds for a clinical trial is dependent upon the type of clinical research being implemented, the source of the funds, and the funding model being applied. Prior to these steps though, the clinical trial process starts with a request for proposal.

Request for Proposal

A clinical trial originates with a scientific concept for testing one or more treatments for a particular condition. This concept can then follow one of many different pathways. It could, for example, be an investigator-initiated concept, a concept from a pharmaceutical company, or a concept from a funding agency. At a high-level description, the idea is built in to a draft protocol and a trial Sponsor and funder is agreed. The Sponsor and the funder can be the same entity or two separate entities. The next step is to decide how the trial will be conducted and by whom. Quite often, a formal request for proposal (RFP) is developed and circulated to any interested party to allow them to submit a proposal outlining their plan for the specific role that they would play in the trial. This RFP is usually particularly relevant for the Clinical Trials Coordinating Center, and both this model and the Coordinating Center role are the primary focus of this chapter.

Sometimes it is predetermined that a specific Coordinating Center will be responsible for the conduct of the trial, perhaps because of a direct association with an investigator, expertise in the specific condition being tested, or existing contractual relationships. For other trials, there is a competitive process where any interested parties (or sometimes-selected parties) are invited to participate.

Regardless of the model, this step is when certain details of the trial conduct are first defined so that those responding (or those preselected) can develop a proposal for their role in the conduct of the trial. The proposal will include logistical details about proposed procedures and scope of work but will also include a preliminary budget. Examples of things, which may be defined, and impact on required resources (and therefore the budget) are:

1. Required accrual
2. Number of participating sites
3. Number of countries
4. Volume of data
5. Method of data collection (paper/electronic)
6. Any specific software requirements

7. Requirements for central reviews
8. Expected dropout/ineligibility rate
9. Extent of on-site monitoring required
10. Whether the trial involves investigational product
11. Whether there is intent to file with regulatory authorities
12. Any other criteria which could impact the scope of work and budget

The detail included in the request for proposal can vary in detail. In some instances, all of the above will be well defined making it more straightforward to develop a budget and proposal. In other instances, the specifications can be vague and poorly defined, and some interaction will be required with the party requesting proposals so that a reasonable estimate can be made.

Preparation of Proposal and Budget

This step is the first opportunity for a potential applicant to draft a budget to submit as part of the proposal. This step is critical, as there needs to be a balance between being competitive with a proposal and ensuring that the budget is realistic and would cover actual costs of doing the trial.

The escalating and complex costs of clinical research are forcing the main funders including the pharmaceutical and biotechnology companies, CROs, and government to tightly manage and control the financial particulars of their trials. This is having a large impact on organizations and is requiring them to better understand the sponsor's position and the wider funding landscape in order to create a proposal that will stand out. Rising costs are also forcing them to adapt their budget models so they can remain competitive and to be able to deliver high quality and on target work.

All clinical research studies require a budget, regardless of the funding sources, size of research project, or parties involved in the research activities (Fine and Albertson 2006). The budget can be seen as a planning document, which covers the financial life of the study and supports the functions necessary for its success (Floore 2019). Along with other key trial documentation such as the protocol, schedule of events, or informed consent, the budget is important and should be designed to be the best attempt at evaluating and planning for the resources and costs needed to implement the study in order to achieve the scientific goals for the study.

Budget Considerations

There are several things to consider when developing a research budget. The primary financial consideration is ensuring that the research can be effectively carried out with the available funds. Planning inefficiency and insufficient budget forecasting are notable areas where many organizations are failing, which often jeopardizes the financial sustainability of a clinical trial (Grygiel 2016).

Another challenging area for the bottom line of a clinical trial is the therapeutic area being studied and the protocol design. There is evidence to suggest that the complexity of the trial protocol is associated with higher study costs, lower levels of data quality, and longer study durations (Friedman et al. 2010). The protocol defines much of how the study will be implemented and what components are required. Additional specifications as defined above will also factor into budget calculations, such as how many research sites are needed, estimated duration of the trial, relevant regulations, and scope of responsibilities. All of these areas have a significant impact on a research budget and should be carefully examined to ensure the costs are properly considered.

The costs of increasing and complex regulations and compliance are becoming a more common part of research budgets (Matula 2012). This refers to both the personnel responsible for fulfilling these obligations and the costs associated with fulfilling IRB/ethics requirements, local, national, or even international regulations including General Data Protection Regulation (GDPR), a European Union regulation that has a global reach and impact on data protection. There are also the costs attached in ensuring research personnel are adequately trained in the appropriate areas of clinical research such as Good Clinical Practice (GCP). While these costs may not be directly listed as budget line items, the costs may be reflected in travel or training costs or by specific compliance roles such as a Quality Assurance Officer.

Rising costs in running clinical trials are also stemming from the fact that per patient costs are increasing at astronomical rates. In the USA, the average cost per patient in a clinical trial increased 88% between 2008 and 2011 (Hargreaves 2016). Some reasons include poor patient recruitment and retention, which is resulting in massive cost overruns, missed deadlines, and in some cases premature closure of the study.

Budget Format

Any party involved in a trial will have to develop a budget relevant to their roles and responsibilities and will have different formats to use. The parties involved could include a Coordinating Center, participating sites, Contract Research Organisations, central laboratories, and drug distribution centers.

The format of a budget submission for a specific proposal is usually predefined by the Sponsor/funder for the trial and can be in many different forms. It is important to prepare and submit the budget proposal in the required format. Some budget requests are based on providing estimates of effort over time for relevant personnel, some are hourly rates and estimated total number of hours per position, or some could be a fixed rate per task. It is important to ensure that any relevant overhead (add-on/indirect) costs are incorporated into the budget proposal.

The process of developing the research budget can be streamlined by having standard tools available for the initial costing process. Research institutions could have a "budget toolbox" in place to use when developing a draft budget, regardless of the required format for a submission (Appelman-Eszczuk 2016). The diversity of these tools depends upon the funding portfolios and overall experience with previous applications or bids. All toolboxes should contain the ability to understand and analyze several key areas including the funding model being applied, the funding source, the therapeutic area being researched, the essential components of an effective trial budget, and, of course, an understanding of the tasks which will be the responsibility of the applicant. An organization with this type of "budget toolbox" in place when responding to a request for proposal will be able to develop and submit a budget more quickly and more effectively than those who do not have these tools at hand.

Preparing the Response to a Request for Proposal

The previous sections show the complexity of budget preparation and the importance of knowing the relevant factors, which contribute to the drafting of a budget proposal. The budget should be prepared in the required format and according to specifications provided by those making the proposal request. The proposal also needs to demonstrate an understanding of the regulatory requirements for the specific project under consideration. If any assumptions are made in the preparation of the draft budget, they should be well documented so that if those assumptions are incorrect, the budget can be adjusted accordingly. Adequate justification for all budget line items should also be provided.

In addition to the budget, there will be text to be added to the proposal, and it is important to follow all instructions in preparing the proposal. There may be a questionnaire to complete or free text to write to summarize the plan to meet the requirements for the trial and to justify the budget request. The written component of the proposal should be clear and concise and cover all relevant information. It should be clear from the text which responsibilities are being included in the proposal and the budget and text should match. Finally, it is important to submit the proposal by any stipulated deadline and to include all information that was requested. Late or incomplete proposals may be rejected.

Selection of Relevant Partners

Once the party who requests submissions has received proposals from all interested parties, there is a process of selection. There may be a requirement for the applicant to give a presentation to the requester or to answer some additional questions. A final selection will be made, and the successful applicant will then move on to negotiating a legal contract with the Sponsor/funder.

Negotiation of Contract Terms

Once a proposal has been accepted, the two (or more) parties involved have to negotiate a legal agreement outlining the terms under which the work will be done and incorporating the final accepted budget, which may differ from the budget in the proposal as more details of the project are fully defined. It is important to ensure that appropriate legal cover is in place prior to starting to work on a project and to understand that the contract negotiations can be a lengthy process, especially for a complex trial.

Contract Content

There are standard sections, which would routinely be incorporated into a contract for the conduct of a clinical trial, often referred to as a Clinical Trial Agreement or CTA. These sections include:

1. Names and addresses of parties involved in the contract
2. Definitions of any key terms
3. Period/duration covered by the contract
4. Description of responsibilities of each of the parties (may be detailed in an Appendix)
5. Financial provisions including details of how and when payments will be made and the agreed budget (usually in an Appendix)
6. Contract termination/early termination conditions/rules
7. Governance structure for the trial and responsibilities of those involved (e.g., a Trial Steering Committee may have the ultimate decision-making power)
8. Ownership of study data and materials
9. Intellectual property rights
10. Liability and indemnity
11. Data protection
12. Rules for future amendments to contract terms

Other sections, which may be relevant depending on the trial and the roles and responsibilities of the contracting parties, could include:

1. Access to data while trial ongoing (or restrictions to access)
2. Collection of biological samples
3. Drug/device distribution system
4. Rules for publication and presentation of data once results are available
5. Interactions with regulatory agencies
6. Conflict of interest
7. Entities excluded by debarment
8. Assignment of responsibilities
9. Ability to subcontract
10. Governing law and procedures for any disputes
11. Commitment to accrual (for site contracts)
12. Permission for monitoring/audits/inspections

As the contract is a legally binding document and would hold any party to account, it is essential that this document has detailed legal input by representatives of each party prior to agreement and signature. Quite often, the legal counsel for involved parties will negotiate terms among themselves once the assignment of responsibilities and general structure have been agreed. While legal advice can be expensive, it is much less costly than the alternative, which is finding out that you are not covered if something goes wrong.

Clinical Trial Agreement Guidance

There are templates online, which provide a starting point for a Clinical Trial Agreement document. In the UK, the UK Clinical Research Collaboration (UKCRC) has developed model agreements in several areas. Their website has links to several model templates, including ones relevant to clinical investigation, CROs, primary care and commercial trials, and one for site agreements (UKCRC website – https://www.ukcrc.org/regulation-governance/model-agreements/). These nationally approved model agreements have been developed and published to help to speed up the trial development process and simplify negotiations. National Health Service Trusts in England and the devolved nations (Scotland, Wales, and Northern Ireland) are expected to use them for relevant contracts.

Other guidance can be found in the NIHR Clinical Trials Toolkit, "an interactive color-coded route map to help navigate through the legal and good practice arrangements surrounding setting up and managing a Clinical Trial of an Investigational Medicinal Product (CTIMP) (www.ct-toolkit.ac.uk)."

A clinical trial podcast (Kunal 2017) details nine essential components of a CTA and provides insight into pitfalls in their formulation.

Scope of Work

As mentioned above, one of the key components of the contract should be a detailed summary of roles and responsibilities for each party. It is essential that this is well documented and understood so that there are no misunderstandings or omissions once the trial gets under way. The list of tasks can be extensive and may be best included as a detailed Appendix to the contract.

Table 1 shows a sample list of high-level topics for a scope of work to be considered in a contract between a Sponsor and a Coordinating Center. Each of these high-level topics can be broken down into activities that are more detailed. For example, under the Statistics header, it can be documented which party is responsible for preparing the statistical analysis plan development; under Interactions with Authorities and IRBs/ECs, it can be documented which party interacts with regulatory authorities and which is responsible for ensuring materials are prepared for, submitted to, and approved by Institution Review Boards and Ethics Committees; under Clinical Data Management, it can be defined which party is to hold the clinical database, which does quality control and interacts with sites. These are just examples, but it is recommended that each high-level category be broken down into these

Table 1 High-level scope of work topics

#	Trial activities	Sponsor	CTU	Trial sites
1	Trial protocol and Informed Consent Form (ICF) development			
2	Selection of trial sites			
3	Interaction with authorities and IRB/ECs			
4	Other trial documents preparation, printing, and distribution			
5	Management of trial drug and supplies			
6	Management of central patient randomization			
7	Management of investigator/team meetings			
8	Project management and administration including committees, contracts, and budget			
9	Monitoring (coordination and execution)			
10	Drug safety/SAE reporting			
11	Clinical data management (including systems setup)			
12	Clinical data review			
13	Statistics (development, programming, and analyses)			
14	Clinical study report writing			
15	Quality control and assurance			
16	Protocol-defined sample management			

Instructions: Enter L in column for party taking the lead; X for party involved but not in lead

detailed subcategories so that the division of responsibility for each task is predefined.

This example is for the division of responsibilities between a Sponsor and a Coordinating Center, but similar lists can be created for other kinds of contracts, for example, between a Sponsor and a drug distribution center or between a Coordinating Center and a randomization provider. Similarly, there needs to be a legal agreement between all related parties in the conduct of a trial.

Budget Evaluation

At this stage in the start-up process and before the contract is signed, there should be a thorough evaluation of the initial budget proposal which was submitted as part of the response to the proposal request. It is highly likely that additional detail about the trial and its conduct has become evident during the intervening period between the initial submission and the contract signature. There may be additional responsibilities that have been added to the scope of work since the RFP was issued, and any additional tasks or increase in responsibility can impact the initial budget.

All assumptions made in preparing the initial budget should be reexamined to see if they are still relevant, and revised budget calculations made and negotiated with the funder. It is also advisable to add language to the contract saying that there will be new negotiations if the scope of the contract changes and that no such changes can be made without agreement of both parties.

Signature of Contract

Once the terms of the contract, budget, and scope of work have been agreed, legal representatives of each party should sign the document. Someone senior within an organization would normally do this. The primary researcher would not normally be authorized to sign such documents on behalf of an organization. Signatures can be wet-ink, with a document being circulated to all parties to add their signature(s). Sometimes multiple copies are signed so that each party receives a fully signed/ executed copy with original wet-ink signatures, and sometimes each party retains their own wet-ink signature on site, and a scanned copy is sent to other parties. More recently, electronic signatures have become more common with document signature software that is compliant with relevant regulations. Often the method is dependent on the laws within the relevant countries involved.

Activation of Trial

Once the contract is signed, the study can be activated and work commence. It is not advisable to start work on the trial until such a contract is in place, as an organization would have no legal basis for doing work before the document is signed.

Other Legal Documents/Contracts/Contract Amendments

There are other legal agreements, which may be needed for a specific trial. Some examples of these are as follows.

Confidentiality Agreements/Nondisclosure Agreements
These agreements are usually issued at the beginning of the proposal process to protect any proprietary information about a study or company before being released to a tendering site or organization.

Data Transfer/Data Use/Data Specification Agreement
This agreement would cover transfer of data between parties. For example, if there are two parties each contracted directly by the Sponsor but with no contract between the other for statistical analysis, a Data Transfer Agreement would be needed. This agreement should clearly specify which data is being transferred, the mechanism for transfer (e.g., secure portal), the timing of transfers, how the data can be used once transferred, and specifications of file formats for the transfer. The two parties involved should sign this agreement.

Vendor Agreements

If specific software/services are contracted by a party involved in the trial and used for fulfilling their responsibilities in the trial, there should be agreements signed with each vendor. Examples of these would be software support, software provider, and database/electronic data capture (EDC) host.

Contract Amendments and Budget Review

During the course of the trial, if work scope changes are made to the operation of the trial, it is essential that these changes be reflected in an updated contract and budget amendment. Examples of changes are:

1. Modified accrual goals
2. Change in study design
3. Additional recruitment sites
4. Changes to scope of monitoring requirements

These are some examples, but any of these changes would impact the work scope and the budget, and an updated contract should be negotiated.

Summary and Conclusion

The preparation of contracts and budgets to cover activities in a clinical trial is essential and critical. While it is important to submit a competitive budget if responding to an RFP, it is also important to ensure that the budget request covers all relevant costs particularly given the escalating costs and complexities to running a clinical trial today. Review of all available documents about the study will help to ensure that items are not missed. Budgets can be formulated in many different ways and each funder will have their own rules for submission. Guidelines should be followed, and questions asked if these are unclear, and there should be a good understanding of the roles and responsibilities of each party involved.

The negotiation of contracts and budgets is usually a lengthy process and this should be factored into study planning. A key part of this planning is ensuring the organization's contract and budget development process is regularly reviewed in order to streamline its efficiency and effectiveness. Additionally it is essential for an organization to make sure the budgets, which are being developed, are accurately reflecting the work being carried out. These reviews can be a result of contract amendments, which can take several forms including changes in accrual goals or study design or as part of an organization's regular improvement process.

Key Facts

- Rules provided by the funder should be followed in preparing a budget.
- Ensure that the budget meets the requirements of the party doing the work.

- Allow scope for budget amendments in the contract.
- Ensure that all contracts have had appropriate legal review before signing.
- Ensure contracts are signed before work starts on the project.

Cross-References

▶ Documentation: Essential Documents and Standard Operating Procedures
▶ Funding Models and Proposals
▶ Multicenter and Network Trials
▶ Responsibilities and Management of the Clinical Coordinating Center

References

Appelman-Eszczuk S (2016) Clinical research site budgeting for clinical trials. J Clin Res Excell 87:15–21

BIG (2018) Annual Report 2018 Spreading hope- advancing breast cancer research. Belgium. [Last accessed: 24 November 2020] Available at: https://www.bigagainstbreastcancer.org/news/annual-report-2018

Camps I, Rodriguez A, Agusti A (2017) Non-commercial vs. commercial clinical trials: a retrospective study of the applications submitted to a research ethics committee. Br J Clin Pharmacol 84:1384–1388

Carroll J (2005) CRO crowing about their growth. Biotechnol Healthc 2(6):46–50. https://www.ncbi.nlm.nih.gov/pmc/articles/PMC3571008

Cooksey D (2006) A review of UK health research funding. HM Treasury, Norwich

Fine and Albertson P.C (2006) Budget development and staffing. In: Penson DF, Wei JT (eds) Clinical research methods for surgeons. Humana Press, Totowa

Floore T (2019) Balancing the clinical trial budget. J Clin Res Excell 101:16–21

Friedman L, Furberg C, DeMets D (2010) Data collection and quality control in the fundamentals for clinical trials, chapter 11. Springer Science and Business Media, Dordrecht, pp 199–214

Grygiel A (2016) The struggles with clinical study budgeting. Contract Pharma. http://www.contractpharma.com/issues/2011-10/view_features/the-struggle-with-clinical-study-budgeting/

Hargreaves B (2016) Clinical trials and their patients: the rising costs and how to stem the loss. Pharmafile (Online). Available at: http://www.pharmafile.com/news/511225/clinical-trials-and-their-patients-rising-costs-and-how-stem-loss

Hind D et al (2017) Comparative costs and activity from a sample of UK clinical trials units. Trials 18:1–11. 203

International Council of Harmonization E6 (R2) (2016) Good Clinical Practice [Last accessed on 2020 November 24]. Available from https://www.ema.europa.eu/en/ich-e6-r2-good-clinical-practice

Kunal S (2017) Clinical Trials Arena 9 Essential Components of a Clinical Trials Agreement. https://www.clinicaltrialsarena.com/news/9-essential-components-of-a-clinical-trial-agreement-5885280-2/

Matula M (2012) Evaluating a protocol budget. In: Gallin J, Ognibene F (eds) Principles and practices of clinical research, 3rd edn. Elsevier/Academic, Amsterdam/Boston, pp 491–500

Pfeiffer J, Russo H (2016) Academic institutions and industry funding: is there hope? J Clin Res Excell 90:23–27

Viergever R, Hendriks T (2016) The 10 largest public and philanthropic funders of health research in the world: what they fund and how the distribute their funds. Health Res Policy Syst 14:1

Long-Term Management of Data and Secondary Use

23

Steve Canham

Contents

Abstract

The reasons for retaining data after a study is finished are reviewed. The nature and implications of the legal obligations to keep data are explored, with a brief discussion around each of the main questions that need to be considered. The increased pressure to make individual-level data available to others is then examined. Some of the barriers to such secondary use, or "data sharing," are described as well as some of the ways data re-use can be anticipated and thus facilitated. Practical issues such as data de-identification and data use agreements are discussed. The importance of promoting data inter-operability using standards and common vocabularies is stressed, followed by a brief discussion about data repositories and the selection of a suitable long-term home for data. Processes and systems to support the secondary re-use of data, from the point of view of a trials

S. Canham (✉)
European Clinical Research Infrastructure Network (ECRIN), Paris, France
e-mail: steve.canham@ecrin.org

© Springer Nature Switzerland AG 2022
S. Piantadosi, C. L. Meinert (eds.), *Principles and Practice of Clinical Trials*,
https://doi.org/10.1007/978-3-319-52636-2_286

427

unit, are suggested. A recurrent theme is the need to consider and plan the long-term management of data from the very beginning of the study, because plans to store and, especially, to share data may have profound implications for data design and study costs.

Keywords

Data retention · Good clinical practice · Metadata · Secondary use · Data sharing · HIPAA · Data standards · Data repositories · Data use agreements

Introduction

Trials eventually reach a point when all data entry is complete, all the analyses have been performed, and all the associated papers and result summaries are written. Direct access to the trial data for its primary research purpose is either no longer required or limited to occasional read-only access. The data cannot, however, be destroyed – there is a regulatory and legal obligation to retain it, at least for a defined minimum period. In addition, there is increasing recognition that the data has potential scientific value to others and that – suitably de-identified and usually with controlled access – it could and should be made available for possible re-use. For both of these reasons, therefore, the data will require management in the long term.

Regulatory Obligations for Data Retention

The regulatory requirement for data retention stems from the possible need to re-examine data, in the context of assessing, or re-assessing, either the safety of a product or the general conduct and regulatory compliance of the study. There may be a suspicion that the data has been interpreted wrongly, or that a particular safety-related signal was missed, or even deliberately suppressed or mis-classified in the original trial summaries. There may be a need – fortunately rare – to investigate alleged fraud by individual investigators, or there may be actions for compensation from individual participants. For all these reasons, the sponsor is responsible for ensuring that the data is retained, enabling it, if necessary, to be examined within legal or regulatory processes or institutional or professional disciplinary procedures.

Data retention also allows the completion of analyses originally abandoned at an early stage and thus never published, as well as the re-analysis of results where misreporting is suspected. Promoting such analyses was the aim of the RIAT (restoring invisible and abandoned trials) initiative (Doshi et al. 2013; RIAT Support Center 2020). GSK's "study 329," which looked at the effects of paroxetine (Paxil or Seroxat) and imipramine (Tofranil) in the treatment of depression in adolescence, is an example of a high-profile trial that was re-published as part of RIAT.

This study had been originally published in 2001 (Keller et al. 2001) and had claimed that the drugs were "generally well tolerated and effective" in the target population. During litigation, brought by New York State against GSK in 2004 after it appeared that paroxetine in fact *increased* suicidal behavior among adolescents, it emerged that the underlying data had never really supported the 2001 assertion. The study had never been republished with a corrected analysis, however, and the original paper had never been retracted (in 2020 it is still not retracted) so it was re-examined within RIAT. The re-analysis (Le Noury et al. 2015) confirmed that the drugs were not "statistically or clinically significantly different from placebo for any prespecified primary or secondary efficacy outcome" but that there were "clinically significant increases in harms, including suicidal ideation and behavior and other serious adverse events in the paroxetine group and cardiovascular problems in the imipramine group."

Le Noury and colleagues had used not only the clinical study report (CSR) for their analysis but also individual patient data (as SAS datasets) and about 77,000 pages of de-identified individual CRFs. Importantly, the authors noted that "Our analysis indicates that although CSRs are useful, and in this case all that was needed to reanalyze efficacy, analysis of adverse events requires access to individual patient level data in case report forms."

The principle of data retention is set out in the Good Clinical Practice Regulations or GCP (ICH 2016). Although strictly speaking these only apply to investigations involving medicinal products, the *principles* of GCP are usually seen as applicable to, and are followed by, all types of trials. GCP uses the concept of "Essential Documents" which are defined (section 8.1) as "those documents which individually and collectively permit evaluation of the conduct of a trial and the quality of the data produced." The "Essential Documents," often collectively referred to as the "Trial Master File" or TMF, include:

8.3.14 SIGNED, DATED AND COMPLETED CASE REPORT FORMS (CRF) To document that the investigator or authorized member of the investigator's staff confirms the observations recorded Investigator/ Institution.
   8.3.15 DOCUMENTATION OF CRF CORRECTIONS To document all changes/additions or corrections made to CRF after initial data were recorded.

Essential documents therefore include the data, specifically in the form in which it was collected and including amendments to that data, reflecting the fact that the purpose of data retention is essentially to provide an audit trail for possible later inspection. The retention period is given by section 5.5.11 of the GCP guidance:

The sponsor specific essential documents should be retained until at least 2 years after the last approval of a marketing application in an ICH region and until there are no pending or contemplated marketing applications in an ICH region or at least 2 years have elapsed since the formal discontinuation of clinical development of the investigational product. These documents should be retained for a longer period however if required by the applicable regulatory requirement(s) or if needed by the sponsor.

The final sentence is important. The relatively short retention period demanded by GCP may be extended by other regulations, applied at international, national, state, or institutional level, and those regulations are subject to change. In the USA, the retention period specified in CFR 21 (1) broadly follows the GCP requirement (US Code of Federal Regulations 2020), but in Europe the period has been considerably longer. The Clinical Trials Directive amendment of 2003 required:

> ... at least 15 years after completion or discontinuation of the trial,
> — or for at least two years after the granting of the last marketing authorization in the European Community ... (European Commission 2003),

but the Clinical Trials Regulation of 2014 extended this period to 25 years:

> Unless other Union law requires archiving for a longer period, the sponsor and the investigator shall archive the content of the clinical trial master file for at least 25 years after the end of the clinical trial. However, the medical files of subjects shall be archived in accordance with national law. (European Commission 2014, Article 58)

To complicate things further, the required retention period may also depend on the type of trial and the population under study. For pediatric studies (because any statute of limitation on claims may not come into effect until the child is 18, and then last for a further period, e.g., 4 years), retention may be necessary until the youngest participant reaches a certain age, e.g., 23 or 25. Similar considerations may need to apply to studies that allow pregnant women, or the partners of pregnant women, to participate. In such cases the retention period will depend on the relevant law within the applicable legal jurisdiction. Some treatment types – especially if they are relatively new and untested – may also demand longer retention periods.

A further aspect of the GCP guidance on data retention is that it requires data to be kept both centrally by the sponsor, and/or the trial's operational managers (i.e., a trials unit or CRO) on the sponsor's behalf, *and* at each clinical site. Useful detailed guidance on what records should be kept where, for the TMF as a whole, is provided by the European GCP Inspectors Working Group (EMA 2018). Although originally written for a European context, the points made in this document should be relevant to most other environments.

For data, GCP makes it clear that the sponsor should retain the original CRFs while each clinical site should keep a copy of the data that they generated. In the days of three-part carbon paper CRFs, this was automatic; the sites simply retained a copy of whatever data they sent to the sponsor's central facility. Nowadays, with almost universal use of electronic remote data capture, this means a copy of the site's data, as collected by a clinical data management system (CDMS) and usually incorporating the investigator's signature in electronic form, is returned back to the site in a human readable form at the end of the trial.

A potential complication was introduced into this process with the advent of the latest version of GCP (E6(R2)). Here an addendum to section 8.1 makes the point explicitly that:

> The sponsor should ensure that the investigator has control of and continuous access to the CRF data reported to the sponsor. The sponsor should not have exclusive control of those data. . . . . . .
>   The investigator/institution should have control of all essential documents and records generated by the investigator/institution before, during, and after the trial.

This seems reasonable – if a sponsor has exclusive control of the data, it could, in theory, make unaudited changes to the data before it was returned to the site. Unless the investigator had the time and inclination to check the returned data (e.g., against the source documents), he or she would likely be unaware of any changes made. But what this addendum means in practice is unclear. Does the use of a CRO, as a third party managing the data, ensure that the sponsor does not have exclusive control? Probably, though some have suggested a CRO, paid by the sponsor, may not be independent enough. Academic- or hospital-based trials units rarely use CROs, though increasingly they use hosted CDMS solutions. But if they directly control and can access the CDMS, and thus the data, and are also the sponsor, how can they show that the site, rather than themselves, has "control of all essential documents and records generated by the investigator/institution"? If they cannot, are they then in breach of this addendum to GCP? Further discussion would seem to be necessary to clarify exactly how this addendum should be interpreted.

Regulatory Obligations and Long-Term Management

Organizing the long-term retention of the data equates to answering a set of questions:

- What material needs to be retained?
- Who should keep the data and where?
- What format(s) should be used?
- What metadata is also required?
- How long should the data be retained for?
- What data should the sites retain?
- How should final data destruction (if it ever occurs) be managed?

The increasingly common additional question, of how data could also be made available for possible re-use by others, is discussed in a later section. The final responsibility for resolving the questions listed above rests with the sponsor, but they will normally be discussed with investigators and the trial's operational managers, i. e., a CRO or trials unit. That discussion will usually encompass all the essential documents, i.e., the whole of the TMF, although here only the data is considered.

It is clearly better to consider these questions as *part of the initial study planning*, so that everyone is clear about what will happen to the data and essential documents at the end of the study, and what their role and responsibilities will be, from the very beginning. It also allows necessary resources to be identified and costed (and included in bids for funding). The issues will probably be revisited when the end of the study arrives, but in truth the focus and energy of those involved are usually elsewhere by that point. This is especially the case if the trial was managed by a collaboration of some kind, which may have dissolved by study end. There is therefore a danger that data (or some parts or versions of the data) are simply left where they are, with little active management, unless arrangements for the long term have already been settled. The issues that need to be discussed are considered in more detail below.

What material needs to be retained? The essential documents include all the data *as collected*, i.e., as in the (e)CRFs. But should it be in *exactly* the same format as when it was collected, i.e., as a database file? Or in the format in which it was extracted from the clinical data management system (CDMS) for analysis, which will usually be as a collection of flat files, e.g., CSV or SAS transport files? Or in some form of read-only archive format (e.g., as pdf files)? The latter two may not include all the data amendments, but would normally be easier to access.

How should additional data that was never in the CDMS (e.g., treatment allocation lists or image or lab data) be retained? What about the analysis datasets themselves – which again might not be exactly the same as the data as extracted (they might be MedDRA coded, for instance, or include reconciled SAE data). And data for analysis may also exist in different versions – interim datasets taken at different times, subsets representing sub-studies, and datasets for different populations (e.g., for intent-to-treat versus safety analysis). Which of these should be retained?

Who should keep the data and where? In some cases a sponsor and the CRO or trials unit that is managing the data have a close, long-term relationship (or may be the same organization). In this scenario, it is usually easier to retain the data within the infrastructure in which it was collected. Given that storage capacity is so cheap, and the datasets from a clinical trial are not, in terms of modern storage devices, very large, it is quite possible to keep *all* the different versions of the data, but they will need careful organization into a clearly labelled set of folders and files, including a "read me" file explaining the contents.

If the sponsor has a more temporary, contractual relationship with the CRO or trials unit, they will normally want the data as collected returned at the end of the study, often to carry out the analysis themselves as well to meet their obligation to retain the data. But what should happen to the copy of the data that remains on the servers which collected it? This question becomes more acute when the servers are not directly managed by the CRO/trials unit but are part of a remote SaaS (software as a service) clinical data management system, which may in turn use a separate "cloud" infrastructure. If the decision is taken that the data, once extracted, should be removed from the data collection infrastructure (for a combination of security, commercial, and financial reasons), then some thought will be required as to how that can be managed. An absolute guarantee of data destruction, when an infrastructure is outside an organization's direct control, is very difficult (Ramokapane et al. 2016), but some form of assurance that the data has been removed should be sought. This should also cover the scenario when a virtual machine or a collection of data is restored onto an infrastructure from a backup – in such a case data marked as deleted will need to be re-deleted.

What format(s) should be used? The proprietary structures used by many clinical data management systems, both for database storage and for a "data export," do not lend themselves to long-term storage. Even if systems remain in existence, they will evolve, and a file created by one version may soon become unusable by later versions. Twenty-five years is a very long time in technology. On the other hand, such files often provide the most complete picture of the data as collected, with previous values and audit trails included. Data is much easier to re-access if it is stored in simpler non-proprietary formats, e.g., CSV (comma separated values), or using a global XML schema, although such schemas are also likely to evolve over time. But it may take additional work to ensure that the full set of data required, including previous values, is included when using such formats.

The best answer is probably to use *both* format types. The lifetime of proprietary files can be extended by using a virtual machine (VM) or, increasingly these days, a server "Container" to preserve not just the data but also the context, e.g., the CDMS, database, and operating system, in which it was housed. When a CDMS is updated or replaced, old studies could be transferred to the new system, but it may be simpler to split off the old system and the studies completed on it as a separate VM or Container and "freeze" that in long-term storage. This has resource implications, however, hence the need to consider this option at an early stage.

Complementing the data retained in this "native" format are the datasets in a non-proprietary flat file format, i.e., the data as extracted and the data as analyzed, if different. These should already exist because they have been required for the analysis process. Organizing and retaining them should therefore be a relatively straightforward exercise.

What metadata is also required? Data in any format quickly becomes useless unless its meaning is clear, which means that metadata, for all types of retained data, is essential. This should include, for each data item, its code, name, type, description, and possible values. Most CDMSs can generate metadata for each study they support, so including the metadata for data in its original format should be straightforward. Flat files created from the data may require additional, specific data dictionaries, however, although again these should have already been created to support the analysis process. Care needs to be taken that this descriptive metadata is present or generated for all the data files, and included in the final data package.

As well as the descriptive metadata, the read me or "contents" file should include – along with a general listing of the files included and the provenance and purpose of each – any technical details about the files, e.g., the versions of systems used to generate them. Text-based files like CSVs can all look the same to humans, but machines can get confused by the different coding schemes used to generate them (e.g., UTF-8 versus UTF-16) or the presence of technical marks in the file (e.g., byte order marks). These may be unimportant at the time the data is generated because all systems are set up to work with a specific configuration, but a few years later they could cause problems if restoration is attempted. These details should therefore be documented.

How long should the data be retained for? As indicated in the previous section, there may not always be a simple answer to this question. Most sponsors, trials units, and CROs become familiar with a particular regulatory regime and its data retention guidelines, but it is worth checking to see if any exceptions apply or if the regulations seem likely to change soon. For relatively new trialists (e.g., a new biotech startup or an inexperienced investigator), it may be worth obtaining professional advice from a CRO or trials unit, to ensure the regulations are well understood.

Some sponsors will stipulate a longer period for data retention than the strict minimum (e.g., 30 years), often making it a blanket rule for all types of studies, interventional and observational, to keep everything relatively simple. Exceptions may still occur, but they should be less common. Some sponsors may even decide to simply "keep everything" indefinitely. This is easy to say for a relatively new sponsor with little if any data in long-term management, but decisions about how and where the data needs to be stored still need to be resolved. It also raises an ethical issue – if data is relatively identifiable, the longer it sits in an IT infrastructure, the longer it risks being lost or hacked. Once the period required by regulation is over therefore (admittedly a long time in Europe), there is a good argument that says such data should be destroyed (or anonymized) and not simply left indefinitely in its original state.

What data should the sites retain? The sites should end up with a copy of the data they provided as input to the study. They are unlikely to have the systems to read the data in the way it is stored centrally, so a database file is not appropriate. The data will therefore need conversion to some more readable format – e.g., pdf, csv files, and spreadsheets. This may need to be negotiated at the beginning of the study, and it certainly needs to be planned as – especially for a large study with many sites – it could be a time-consuming and costly exercise. Different CDMS have different capabilities in this respect – some have an 'archive' function which will generate the required data in a suitable format, while for others it will be more of a manual exercise. The use of optical storage is a common way of transferring the data, i.e., sending the site a CD-ROM. If not copied to local systems, however, the disk may not be accessible after several years – CD-ROMs have a finite lifetime – so arrangements should be in place to ensure that the copying takes place, even though this is the site's responsibility.

How should final data destruction (if it ever occurs) be managed? If and when some or all of the data is to be destroyed, then this should be explicitly authorized and then documented. This can be quite difficult if the infrastructure where the data sits is not under the direct control of the sponsor or the sponsor's agents, but some form of certification or assurance should be sought to show that the sponsor has done their best to ensure full destruction.

A related issue is that elements of the underlying infrastructure will be periodically replaced. Machines and storage devices have a finite lifetime – indeed the physics of solid-state storage devices (SSDs) means that they can only be written to so many (million) times. There will therefore inevitably come a time when these devices need replacing, with their data being transferred to new systems. It is important that the infrastructure's users are aware of this and are satisfied that device removal also renders the data on that device completely inaccessible, usually through physical destruction of the device. If the IT infrastructure is "in-house," this is relatively straightforward – procedures can be established to ensure it happens. When the infrastructure is external, it becomes more difficult, requiring explicit recognition of this issue with suitable assurances sought and provided.

To ensure that all the questions listed above are considered, even if only in the form of a checklist that needs to be worked through, it is important that both the sponsor and the operational managers of a trial, the CRO or trials unit, have a standard operational procedure (SOP) in place covering long-term data management. It should be integrated with the other SOPs covering trial setup and design, and the decisions taken as a result of working through it should be documented in the trial's data management plan (DMP). Much later, when the study ends, the same DMP can be used to document the actions taken as a result of the plan.

Data for Secondary Use

Over and beyond simply keeping the data because it is a regulatory requirement, which at base is a rather passive and defensive exercise, there is a growing recognition that the data from a clinical trial has potential scientific value to other researchers and through them to society as a whole. Over recent decades therefore, there has been a steadily growing acceptance that a study's individual participant data (IPD) should be *actively* prepared for possible secondary use (so called because it is outside the primary use of the original research study) and then be openly advertised as available, albeit usually under controlled access.

The Push for Secondary Data Use

Making data available in this way has been driven by the convergence of a number of different arguments and trends. Among the arguments advanced in favor of data re-use are:

- It allows the conclusions from trials to be re-examined and verified or corrected, although naturally enough it is the corrections that tend to generate the most coverage. The example of GSK's study 329 has already been quoted. Another controversial case (where researchers were compelled to give up their data under a Freedom of Information Act) was the re-analysis of the PACE trial on treatments for myalgic encephalomyelitis (White et al. 2011; Geraghty 2016; Torjesen 2018).
- IPD re-analysis can trigger a debate over methodology and analytic methods that may stimulate further work, as well as clarifying the value of the original research. The re-analysis of an influential de-worming trial in Kenya, where the researchers made their data available voluntarily, provides one example (Miguel and Kremer 2004; Davey et al. 2015; Özler 2015), as does the re-analysis of the FEAST trial,

looking at fluid resuscitation in African children with shock and severe infection (Maitland et al. 2011; Levin et al. 2019; Maitland et al. 2019).

- In times of global pandemics like Ebola or COVID-19, the availability of IPD can be critical in allowing investigators to properly evaluate the often hastily prepared reports, as well as allowing the possible pooling of data from different sources. In this context, calls for data sharing have been issued by the WHO (2015), the Wellcome Trust (2020), and the Research Data Alliance (2020).

- Data availability makes it possible to compare or combine the data from different studies. An example is the cross-study "data platforms" that have been established in some specialist disease areas, for example, the Ebola Data Platform (IDDO 2020). It also allows data aggregation for participant-level meta-analysis, where, despite the potential advantages of such analyses, data has often been difficult to obtain (Riley et al. 2010).

- Secondary use can reduce unnecessary duplication of work and make it easier to build upon a trial with additional ancillary studies. An early example was the Diabetes Control and Complications Trial (DCCT) of 1993 that made their data available to other investigators. By 2015 over 220 ancillary studies had been carried out using or building upon DCCT data, i.e., with the same cohort of participants (Henry and Fitzpatrick 2015; EDIC 2020).

- Secondary use can lead to novel analyses and/or tool generation. In an experiment in 2016, the *New England Journal of Medicine* hosted the SPRINT data analysis challenge. People were invited to analyze the IPD from the NIH-sponsored SPRINT trial (SPRINT Research Group 2015), "to identify a novel or scientific or clinical finding that advances medical science." A total of 143 different applications were received, each representing a new application of the data (NEJM 2016).

- Economically, because data sharing can increase the quality and efficiency of clinical trials through the mechanisms described above, it can help to reduce the wastage in research (Chan et al. 2014). Not surprisingly, funders are often strong supporters of data sharing and mandate it in the studies they support. The Wellcome Trust, the UK's Medical Research Council, Cancer Research UK, and the Bill and Melinda Gates Foundation all require that data be made available for re-use. In a joint declaration, they concluded "It is simply unacceptable that the data from published clinical trials are not made available to researchers and used to their fullest potential to improve health" (Kiley et al. 2017).

- Ethically, IPD sharing has been framed as a way of better respecting the generosity of clinical trial participants, as it increases the utility of the data they provide and thus the value of their contribution. It has also been argued that, if access to health and healthcare is a basic human right, access to data that can improve health is similarly a fundamental right (Lemmens 2013). Those involved in research therefore have an obligation to respect and promote that right by making their data available (Lemmens and Telfer 2012).

- Socially, the substantial public investment in science, including clinical research, demands a similarly public response: "publicly funded research data are a public good, produced in the public interest, which should be made openly available with as few restrictions as possible in a timely and responsible manner" (UKRI 2020). Because clinical research has a key role in promoting and maintaining health, and in determining regulatory and safety decisions, it has been further argued that clinical trial data should be shared and treated as a public good whoever generates it, i.e., whether it is created by publicly funded or commercial research (Reichman 2009).

- Culturally, making IPD from clinical research available is part of a wider shift in science as a whole, toward making data FAIR (findable, accessible, interoperable, and reusable), itself part of a more general move toward "open" science (Wilkinson et al. 2016). Clinical research is increasingly aligning itself with the more open data sharing already practiced in many disciplines, including basic biological sciences as well as physics, astronomy, geology, etc. The fact that clinical research IPD is sensitive personal data certainly makes data sharing more complex, but not impossible.

For all of the reasons listed above, the *idea* of data sharing in clinical research has become much more acceptable, to the extent that Vickers was able to claim a "tectonic shift in attitudes" over 10 years (Vickers 2016). In addition, many trial registries now include sections for trialists to describe their plans for data sharing, and there is strong encouragement from many journals for authors to indicate how they will make the underlying data for a paper available to others. *BMJ journals*, for example, for most of its major titles, stipulate the following (BMJ 2020):

- "We strongly encourage that data generated by your research that supports your article be made available as soon as possible, wherever legally and ethically possible.
- We require data from clinical trials to be made available upon reasonable request.
- We require that a data sharing plan must be included with trial registration for clinical trials that begin enrolling participants on or after 1 January 2019. . . ."

The last requirement is in line with the data sharing recommendations of the influential International Committee of Medical Journal Editors, which also stipulate that clinical trials must include a data sharing plan in the trial's registration, from 2019 onward. The ICMJE currently stop short, however, of *requiring* the availability of data for secondary use. *Not* making data or documents available is still listed as an example of a valid data sharing plan (ICMJE 2020). This may be a recognition that, despite the various "top-down" pressures to make data available, e.g., from publishers and funders, and the growing cultural acceptance of data sharing, from a "bottom-up" perspective there are several potential risks that can make it less appealing.

Barriers and Issues with Secondary Use of Data

Some investigators fear that others could "mine" their data for insights and results that would otherwise be available only to them. The critical value of published papers for career progression can make this concern, that others might pre-empt "their" papers using "their" data, a critical factor in deciding *when* data should be made more generally available. It also influences the debate about whether the whole dataset produced by a study should be made available, or just the data used to support the conclusions of published papers, which may be subsets of the whole. There have also been claims that researchers in low- and middle-income countries could be particularly disadvantaged if their data is made available to those with more developed capacities for analysis (Tangcharoensathien et al. 2010), a case of FAIR being potentially unfair. The call has therefore been made for data sharing in such contexts to be considered as a partnership, and more of a mutual learning exercise, than the simple appropriation of one group's data by another.

There is also a reticence of some authors to allow their data and analyses to be examined and possibly misunderstood, misused, or simply criticized, with a consequent need to enter into a public debate that could endanger their reputation, as well as demanding time and effort. This was one of the major reasons quoted by researchers as a barrier to data sharing in a survey conducted by the Wellcome Trust (Van den Eyndon et al. 2016) across a range of researchers in the biological, medical, and social sciences. The same survey, however, also found that in reality – despite some of the high-profile cases reported above – very few researchers reported these types of negative experiences from data sharing. In fact side effects when they did occur were almost always positive, including more collaboration opportunities and an increase in citations.

The lack of conventional academic reward for "simply" sharing data has also been recognized as a barrier to data sharing. At the technical level, there needs to be consensus on the best ways in which re-used data should be cited to ensure that the original data generators are properly recognized (including tackling the issue of different versions of data being available), but more importantly those citations then need to be included in the evaluation of a researcher's work, for example, when considering grant applications or career progression. One scheme (Bierer et al. 2017) proposes the use of the term "data author" in the literature, to clearly distinguish the contribution of the data generators to the research, in not only initially collecting but also managing, cleaning, curating, and preparing the data for re-use.

It seems likely that over time experience will show that there is less to fear from data sharing than some researchers believe. Greater clarity should emerge from publishers and others about their expectations for making data available, and the time periods when that should occur; and systems will evolve to give greater recognition to the researchers who provided the data. There will remain, however, some very practical issues that contribute to the complexities and costs of supporting secondary data use, which are often a cause of concern to researchers. An overview of some of the main issues is provided below.

Appropriate Preparation of Data for Re-use

To preserve participant privacy, as well as the reputation of the investigators and their institutions or companies, data must almost always be modified before it can be released for secondary use, and it must conform to the relevant data protection and privacy regulations. The difficulty is that those regulations will vary across both space and time. For example, currently (mid-2020) there appears to be a contrast between a relatively pragmatic approach to secondary use of IPD in the USA, based on de-identification of the data, and the more complex situation in the EU, where the General Data Protection Regulation (GDPR) has brought several contentious issues to the fore, including the exact characterization of pseudonymous data and the potential role of consent (Peloquin et al. 2020). In addition, while the GDPR was supposed to harmonize regulations relating to personal data use across the EU, it returned some of the powers to regulate personal research data back to the member states, so that a simple, single European regime has not been realized. The result is that the regulations around secondary use of IPD in the EU continue to evolve.

No attempt is made here to try and survey the different and developing privacy and data protection requirements that apply around the world. It will always be necessary for sponsors and investigators to familiarize themselves with those requirements and comply with them, which for multi-national trials may involve multiple jurisdictions. There are, however, some common components to data preparation that will need to be considered.

The Need for De-identification

The expectation is that data will need to be de-identified before it can be shared. The de-identification should be sufficient to render the dataset anonymous in practical terms – i.e., the amount of effort required to identify individuals, for instance, the collection and collation of additional information from external sources like social media, should outweigh any potential benefit to anyone trying to identify individuals.

De-identification techniques described in the literature. For instance, Appendix B of the Institute of Medicine's (2015) paper on data sharing, "Concepts and Methods for De-identifying Clinical Trial Data," provides an overview of both the assessment of risks and strategies to mitigate them, focused on but not restricted to the US context. Also in the USA, the Health Insurance Portability and Accountability Act (HIPAA) Privacy Rule gives detailed explicit guidance on de-identification techniques. One option is to use a documented "expert determination" that a dataset does not contain personally identifiable information, but the other (the "safe harbor method") is to remove all of a checklist of direct identifiers. The main identifiers are listed below, but the HHS website should be consulted for details of the full compliance required (HHS 2020).

- Names
- Geographic locations smaller than a state, including street address, city, county, post code
- All elements of dates (except year) for dates that are directly related to an individual, including birth date, admission date, discharge date, and death date
- All ages over 89 and all elements of dates (including year) indicative of such age, aggregated into a single category of age $>= 90$
- Fax numbers, telephone numbers

- Device identifiers and serial numbers
- Email addresses, Web Universal Resource Locators (URLs), and IP addresses
- Social security numbers, medical record numbers, and health plan beneficiary numbers
- Vehicle identifiers and serial numbers, including license plate numbers
- Full-face photographs and comparable images; biometric identifiers
- Account numbers, certificate/license numbers
- Any other unique identifying number, characteristic, or code

In the USA at least, following the fairly straightforward and public rules should normally allow secondary use. The loss of dates (apart from the year element) is something that could seriously impact the scientific usefulness of a study dataset, given the central importance of the timing of events. One way around this is to "rebase" dates to numbers of days after a fixed point (e.g., randomization), so that they become integers with no relationship to the calendar.

Other de-identification techniques take the obfuscation of data further. One approach ensures that no collection of data values is unique to a single individual, instead being shared by at least k individuals ("k-anonymization"). This can include techniques such as:

- Aggregating categories to reduce unique combinations (for instance, birth years become age ranges)
- Data perturbation, where the distribution of data is preserved but the actual values are changed
- Removal of detailed text fields, such as reports of serious adverse events

The problem with de-identification is that if pursued too enthusiastically, the scientific usefulness of the data may decline. Data perturbation, for example, may make sense in the context of an epidemiological study with many thousands of subjects, but unless done with great care, it may distort the statistical analysis in a clinical trial with just a few hundred participants.

Ideally therefore, the documentation of the de-identification process (which should always be available with the de-identified data) should indicate if the primary analyses can be re-run and give the same results as with the original data. A useful example of a de-identification process being applied in practice is provided by Keerie et al. (2018), who used guidance provided by the UK's Medical Research Council (MRC 2015). The de-identification process included explicit confirmation that the original analysis could be replicated.

De-identification is almost always a necessary part of data preparation for re-use and applies to data classified as either pseudonymized or anonymized – the need to prevent re-identification from the data itself is the same in each case. Nor does it matter if the term lacks any formal significance within the jurisdiction's legal framework (for instance, the term is not defined in the GDPR), the process will still be required to protect study participants.

Anonymized Versus Pseudonymized Data

One of the problems of any discussion around data sharing and re-use is that the terms "anonymized data" and "pseudonymized data" are subject to a range of interpretations, both in common use and more formally within legal frameworks. It is therefore usually necessary to preface any discussion of secondary IPD re-use by setting out the definitions used in any particular case (e.g., as in Ohmann et al. (2017)).

From the point of view of preparing data, it is necessary to be clear about the legal implications, if any, of labelling data either pseudonymized or anonymized, and then to be clear how the various datasets in question are categorized along this dimension. In some cases it will also be necessary to clarify how data can be moved from a pseudonymized to an anonymized state, to take advantage of what are usually lesser restrictions around anonymized data.

Both anonymized and pseudonymized data prepared for re-use should be de-identified, and the datasets themselves are likely to be identical. The difference is only that with pseudonymized data there is additional information, kept separately, that can be used to link the data back to the individual participants.

All clinical trial data starts off as pseudonymized – it can always be linked back to the participants at the source clinical sites. During data collection it remains pseudonymized, and the linkage must remain during the legal retention period, which as described above may be decades. But the fact that a pseudonymized version of the data exists does not necessarily mean that data released for secondary use is also pseudonymized (although, inevitably, it depends how those terms are defined). Some have argued that if a dataset is de-identified and released without the pseudonymizing linkage data, with the recipients having no (legal) means of obtaining that linking data, it is "effectively anonymized." Whether this distinction is applicable within any particular legal jurisdiction would need to be clarified.

It has also been proposed that for extra security the participant identifiers attached to an "effectively anonymized" data should also be regenerated as a separate, independent set with no links to those used in the primary study. The difficulties with that is that (a) it does not stop the data theoretically being matched back to the pseudonymized data, using the full sets of data values linked to each participant, and (b) if a new signal is detected in secondary analysis that may be relevant to the treatment of some of the participants, it makes it much more difficult to make that information known to the participant and/or their clinician.

The Role of Consent

Data classified as pseudonymized generally requires consent from the data donors, the study participants, for any particular usage. This may, however, depend on the legal basis claimed for the data processing, with the options available being dependent, as always, on the local legal framework. If the legal basis is something other than consent (e.g., is "public interest"), then the presence or not of an associated consent is likely to be irrelevant. This is particularly important in a public health emergency such as the COVID-19 pandemic. Many states retain the right to process individual health and research data in the interests of public health, with suitable safeguards but irrespective of the presence or not of explicit consent. Secondary re-use of data may therefore be allowed under such regulations.

Even when consent is the basis of processing pseudonymized data, as it often is with the primary study, the difficulty with consent for secondary use is that it cannot be fully informed. By definition, at the time of the primary study, the nature of any secondary usage is unknown. Attempts have been made to promote the use of a "general consent" for secondary use for research purposes, linked to assurances about data de-identification and data location (as has been proposed for bio-bank materials), but it is not clear if such a consent would be acceptable in all jurisdictions.

Consent therefore remains a tricky issue whose relevance urgently needs clarification in circumstances where data remains classified as pseudonymized. Having said that, whether consent is deemed relevant from a legal standpoint or not, there remains an *ethical* imperative to inform the study participant of any plans to make the data they provide available for data sharing. Such information should be provided as part of the information sheets given to participants when they enter a study, and include relevant details such as the de-identification measures that will be applied, the location of data storage, and restrictions that will be placed on any secondary users (in turn meaning that establishing these details is a necessary part of initial study planning).

The question then arises as to whether a participant should be able to object to their data being re-used beyond the primary study, and be able to withdraw their data from such re-use, either at the beginning of the study or at any time afterwards, even after data collection has ceased. Again, different legal jurisdictions may have something to say about whether this is possible or desirable, and what mechanisms might be necessary to put in place to support it.

The Role of Data Use Agreements

Although it is possible that anonymized and heavily de-identified IPD may simply be released into the public domain, the difficulties with guaranteeing full anonymization while retaining scientific utility mean that in many cases investigators and sponsors will prefer to control access to the data, wrapping that access within a formal "data use agreement" (or "data sharing agreement"). This allows them, for example, to insist that applicants for access to the data provide a full explanation of their reasons, e.g., in a research protocol, and possibly also provide evidence of ethical approval of that protocol. It also allows them to insist, within a contractual agreement, that the data applicants will not misuse the data, e.g., by trying to identify participants or by passing it on to third parties. The agreement can also clarify the nature of the data access – which might be by on-screen access only, perhaps even in a specified location, rather than by a simple file download.

Data use agreements can therefore provide a powerful and flexible mechanism for reducing risks associated with data re-use. Whether or not they can modify the legal position in respect of allowing data re-use in any particular case will depend, as usual, on the local legal framework – on whether, for example, it demands that proportionate risk management measures are put in place. Even if not strictly required, however, a data use agreement is evidence of good intent and can help to protect sponsors from reputational damage. It is noteworthy that two major data repositories managing secondary re-use of data from the pharmaceutical industry – ClinicalStudyDataRequest.com and the Yale University Open Data Access project – both insist on data use agreements being in place before data is released (CSDR 2020; Yoda 2020).

Maximizing Scientific Value with Data Standards

Traditionally clinical studies have been designed in relative isolation, and study datasets have therefore also tended to be idiosyncratic, each with a distinct set of differently defined and coded data points, often categorized in different ways. Unfortunately this can be a huge problem when trying to compare and/or aggregate data from different studies, making those processes error prone, time-consuming, and costly, as well as constraining what comparisons are possible.

The use of standards and conventions for data definitions, however, allows data to be compared and/or aggregated much more easily across studies (and also, as described in the chapter on the study data system, allows studies to be designed more quickly and efficiently). As secondary re-use of data increases, it is vital that investigators and study designers maximize the inter-operability, and thus the potential scientific value, of the data they generate, by increasing the use of data standards.

Data standardization operates at various levels:

- The data points selected
- The detailed definition of those data points
- How the data is categorized – the "controlled vocabularies" used in categorized questions
- How the data is structured and coded in the database
- How the data is described (i.e., associated metadata)

The data points selected will depend upon the outcomes and safety signals to be measured, as specified in the protocol. The nature of clinical trials means that sometimes a study will have novel end points and safety signals, but a high proportion of the data points collected will be very similar across studies. This applies not just to the common variables found in most studies (e.g., demographics, medical history, vital signs, adverse events, concomitant medications) but often also to more disease-specific measures. One aid to selecting outcome measures is the COMET (Core Outcome Measures in Effectiveness Trials) initiative, designed to identify and support the generation of core outcome sets (COS) in trials, with a core outcome set being defined as "an agreed standardised set of outcomes that should be measured and reported, as a minimum, in all clinical trials in specific areas of health or health care." COMET maintains a database of papers that describe the generation and content of over 400 core outcome sets (Comet 2020).

Professional, national, and international bodies may also develop outcome measures and measuring schemes for particular disease areas, such as cancer staging (e.g., TMN) and tumor measurement (e.g., RECIST) or, as an example of a response to a specific disease threat, the set of data points developed by ISARIC for COVID-related trials (ISARIC 2020). A further source of standardized data items is published and validated questionnaires, e.g., those dealing with aspects of the quality of life of participants or for assessing cognition or mood. Care must be taken that the instrument is valid for the population under study (and translations in a multi-national/multi-lingual context must also be validated), but in general using a pre-existing questionnaire or rating scale will be more useful, less expensive, and more generalizable than trying to develop a study-specific instrument.

Ensuring detailed definition of data points is critical for meaningful comparison, within as well as between studies, and underlines the need for good descriptive metadata that makes such definitions explicit. Although many data points are relatively unambiguous (date of surgery, weight, blood biochemistry, etc.), some are not. A notorious example is "blood pressure," which for consistency should be further characterized by position (lying, sitting, standing) but rarely is, or perhaps for timing (e.g., before or after a procedure). Time points for events, despite their importance for analysis, can also be ill-defined. Is a recurrence of a tumor dated from the date the patient first reported the associated symptoms, the date of the scan that confirmed disease progression (possibly one of several scans and tests), or the date of the multi-disciplinary meeting that formally confirmed the recurrence diagnosis? There may be several weeks between these dates, so some consistent rules need to be developed, applied, and described.

The use of different categorization schemes can also be a headache when comparing data, though it is sometimes possible to find mapping schemes between the major controlled vocabularies. MedDRA is widely used for adverse event reporting (and is mandated for such use within the EU) and is a *de facto* international standard for that purpose. But medical history, for example, might be gathered using MedDRA, ICD, SNOMED CT, or MESH terminology, among others. Unfortunately there are few formal requirements or guidelines regarding the use of one controlled vocabulary scheme over another – the choice may come down to such factors as previous training and/or exposure to different systems, the existence or cost of licenses, the practicalities of use, and the required levels of granularity and compatibility with other systems. Whatever controlled vocabularies are selected, however, they will almost certainly be more informative and easier to analyze than free text.

The most comprehensive and established framework for using data standards in clinical research, one that is both global in scope and internationally recognized, is that provided by CDISC, the Clinical Data Interchange Standards Consortium. Beginning in 1997, CDISC has provided a broad range of standards and related tools, covering all phases of the clinical study life cycle, including schema for structuring pre-clinical data, for study protocols, for data collection, for data transport, and for data submission and analysis. It also provides lists of questionnaires and controlled vocabularies (CDISC 2020).

The key CDISC resources, in terms of study design and data re-use, are the Clinical Data Acquisition Standards Harmonization (CDASH) standards and the Therapeutic Area (TA) user guides. Taken together, these provide a means of structuring, coding, and defining the data in a consistent fashion, especially those relating to the data domains commonly found across studies – demographics, adverse events, subject characteristics, vital signs, treatment exposure, etc.

CDASH and the TA guides are currently used much more within the pharmaceutical industry than the non-commercial sector. The FDA, in the USA, and the PMDA, in Japan (though not yet the EMA in the EU) have stipulated that data submitted in pursuance of a marketing authorization must use CDISC's Study Data Tabulation Model (SDTM), a standard designed to provide a consistent structure to submission datasets. Creating SDTM structured data is far easier if the original data has been collected using CDASH, which is designed to support and map across to the submission standard.

The CDASH system is relatively simple conceptually, but it is comprehensive, and it does require an initial investment of time to appreciate the full breadth of data items that are available and how they can be used. It provides standardized terms for common study and demographic variables (e.g., SUBJID, SITEID, BRTHDAT, AGE) and then uses a prefix-suffix system to define further variables in various domains – 24 such domains are listed in CDASH 2.0. The prefix is a two-letter code for the domain (AE = adverse events, MH = medical history, CM = concomitant mediation, EX = Exposure (to the drug under investigation, PR = Procedures, etc.). The suffix indicates the type of data value, so, for instance:

- The start date of an AE event = AESTDAT
- The name of the adverse event = AETERM
- Whether the AE is still ongoing = AEONGO
- The outcome of the AE = AEOUT
- The start date for a concomitant medication = CMSTDAT
- Whether the concomitant medication is ongoing = CMONGO
- The name of the concomitant medication = CMTRT
- The individual dose of the concomitant medication = CMDSTXT
- The start of the investigative treatment = EXSTDAT
- The individual dose of the treatment = EXDSTXT
- The units of the treatment dose = EXDSU
- The route of the treatment dose = EXROUTE
    etc., etc.

The Therapeutic Area (TA) user guides supplement both the CDASH and the SDTM standards, providing a steadily growing list of therapeutic or disease area specific terminology and detailed explanations of how SDTM and CDASH definitions can be applied. The list of therapeutic area standards already developed, or being developed, is available on the CDISC website. In August 2020 there were 44 areas listed (from acute kidney injury, Alzheimer's, and asthma through to tuberculosis, vaccines, and virology).

An evaluation of CDASH and any relevant TA standards is highly recommended because they represent a relatively complete system for standardizing data collection. Readers are referred to the CDISC website (CDISC 2020), which provides comprehensive implementation guides for each standard. While trials units in the non-commercial sector have not been forced into preparing CDASH and SDTM datasets, many have already experimented with using parts of the system. Ultimately, wide use of the CDISC standards could enable an SDTM-based archiving and data sharing model that could be used across all sectors of clinical research, allowing a huge pool of more inter-operable data to become available.

One caveat is that using CDASH can have consequences for the structure of the data that is exported from a CDMS, i.e., the nature of the analysis datasets, and it is therefore important that statisticians are happy about the data being presented to them in this way. Traditionally, CDMS systems generate a series of tables, each corresponding to an eCRF, with the data arranged as a row/subject visit within that table. Because the CDASH approach tends to make greater use of small repeating groups of questions, it creates many "ribbon"-shaped tables instead, each focused on a particular domain, with relatively few data fields in each but often with many rows. These tables are organized as one row/event, where the "event" is represented by a cluster of related data points. Some statisticians may be wary of accepting data in this form, preferring to transform it to a more traditional structure, or face modifying their normal approach to analysis and the library of tools they have established. In other words, making use of the CDISC standards requires the full understanding and cooperation of the statisticians tasked with analyzing the exported data.

The final aspect of standardization to consider is the generation of descriptive metadata for the study data – the characterization of the data points: their codes, names, descriptions, types, ranges, possible values, etc. This has traditionally been done using a variety of methods, from simple "data dictionaries" in spreadsheets through to XML schemas, for example, using the CDISC Operational Data Model (ODM). To make this metadata more useful, and in particular more easily searched and processed by machines, it would be useful to have such metadata in a standard format, the most appropriate – because it exists specifically for this purpose – being CDISC's "Define.xml" standard.

Unfortunately, current use of Define.xml seems very limited outside of the pharmaceutical industry. There is a need for CDMS developers to incorporate Define.xml exports in their systems, for tools to help statisticians and others read or search Define.xml files more easily, for tools to allow machines to search and/or describe Define.xml content, and for funders, trials units, sponsors, and investigators to push for greater consistency in generating metadata using this single standard rather than the variety of approaches that currently exist. The first part of re-using data is to understand what is in it, and without a consistent approach to metadata, that is going to be more time-consuming and costly than it should be.

Managing Data and Data Repositories

Currently, much of the clinical research data objects made available for sharing are simply retained by the research team that produced them, somewhere on the disk storage allocated to their department. The alternative, and other things being equal the preferred option in the longer term, would be to make a conscious decision to move the whole data package (i.e., datasets and related documents) to a dedicated data repository. This might be the institution's or the company's own data repository, specifically set up for storing the research outputs of its staff, or it might be a third-party repository – perhaps a general one storing all types of scientific data, or one specializing in clinical research data, or even one specializing in a particular disease area.

Note that putting a copy of the data in a repository does *not* mean granting public access to it; it simply means preparing the data for possible sharing and then advertising that it is available. Those wishing to use it would still have to meet any conditions that the researchers stipulated, e.g., provide a rationale for their usage and/or adhere to a data use agreement. The data in the repository could be pseudonymous (i.e., could be linked if required to the pseudonymous data held securely by the researchers) or anonymous (could not be practically linked to that data) depending on legal requirements.

The advantages of using a separate, dedicated data repository (including one set up by the researchers' own institution) include:

- Long-term data management. The original research team (or collaboration) will change its composition, or may even cease to exist, and it may then become difficult or impossible for data to be managed and requests for it to be properly considered.
- Transfer of data to a repository helps to ensure that preparation of the data for sharing (e.g., de-identification, provision of metadata) occurs and that the data and related documents are properly described.
- Advertising the data and metadata in a repository's catalog can help to make that data and related documents more easily discoverable.
- It can, depending on the arrangements made with the repository, relieve the original research team/sponsor of the need to review requests and even of the need to make the decisions about agreeing to such requests.
- Anticipating transfer to a repository aids in explicitly identifying data preparation and sharing costs at an early stage of the trial.

The problem is that most existing data repositories are not, yet, well organized to manage the sensitive personal data generated by clinical research and have only limited facilities for controlled access. The default for data repositories in most scientific domains is open public access, with the only control a possible embargo period on data release, so controlled access to sensitive data presents a challenge.

A recent study (Banzi et al. 2019) looked at data repositories that were potentially available to non-commercial researchers for clinical research data. Twenty-five such repositories were identified and assessed against eight key criteria (filtered down from an initial list of 34), seen as particularly relevant to clinical researchers and their data storage needs. The criteria were that the repository should have:

- Guidelines for data upload and storage
- Support for data de-identification

- Data quality controls
- Contracts for upload and storage
- Exposure of metadata
- Application of identifiers
- Flexibility of access
- Plans for long-term preservation

None of the repositories fully demonstrated all of the eight items included in the indicator set, although three were judged as demonstrating or partially demonstrating all of them. Other repositories appeared less suitable in a variety of ways, although this may have been because in many cases the relevant information was not available publicly on the repository's website – many repositories do not do a good job of advertising their services.

This situation may improve but at the moment it is clear that the full potential for data re-use for clinical research data is hampered by the lack of suitable places to store that data in the long term. This problem also underscores the need for robust and public assessments of data repositories, so that potential users can make an informed decision. Various general schemes have been proposed for this (e.g., see CoreTrustSeal 2020), but they have not yet been expanded to include specialist certification schemes for groups with particular requirements. Such a development will be necessary, however, in order that clinical researchers can make informed decisions about the storage of their data.

Trials Unit Systems for Managing Secondary Re-use of Individual Participant Data

Managing the secondary use of clinical study IPD is complex, with a range of technical, resource, and legal issues to consider. In many cases decisions will be required as part of study planning – for example, deciding how to integrate data standards in the study's database design and what to include about potential data re-use in the information sheets prepared for participants. Even when decisions and activities could be postponed until the end of the study (e.g., deciding where data should be stored in the long term, de-identifying the data), they should be anticipated at the beginning of the study in order to estimate the resources required for those activities and include the associated costs in bids for funds (not least because the impetus for data sharing often comes from funders).

Managing the potential re-use of data is also a relatively new activity – one more aspect of running a trial to add to all the other responsibilities and requirements faced by investigators and operational managers. So how should a trials unit (using that term in the most general sense, i.e., the trial management department in a pharmaceutical company, CRO, university, or hospital) integrate managing data re-use with the other services it offers to investigators and sponsors? It seems clear that two broad types of activity are necessary:

- A general preparation, of systems and staff, to understand and be prepared for the various aspects of data re-use
- Study-specific activity, to manage the details of data re-use in the context of a particular study. The latter will be split into two time points:
  - That required during study planning, and
  - That required at study end

As a brief practical guide to supporting data re-use, but also to summarize many of the points made earlier in this chapter, suggestions for the main elements of each of these activities are listed below:

General Preparation
- Clarify the legal regulations and requirements for data sharing in the relevant legal jurisdiction(s). "Relevant" usually means those in which any study participants live, and not just the jurisdiction of the trials unit itself. Among the things to be clarified are the legal basis, or bases, under which data re-use is justified, the role of consent (if any), the definitions and relevance of anonymized and pseudonymized data, the need for data de-identification, and the need to demonstrate risk assessment and/or risk management.
- Clarify any existing policies and procedures relevant to data sharing of the parent organization (if there is one, e.g., a hospital, university, or company), and incorporate them as necessary into the trials unit's own procedures.
- For external sponsors or funders involved with a lot of studies, clarify their policies and procedures relevant to data sharing (and data retention), with a view to incorporating them, as necessary, into the trials unit's own procedures.
- Ensure sufficient staff are familiar with regulations and policies relating to data re-use, as described above, for study-specific work in this area to be carried out effectively. Consider giving one or two roles operational oversight of the preparation for data re-use.
- Ensure sufficient staff are familiar with data standards and their application in local systems for systems such as CDASH to be applied – perhaps at relatively low levels initially but increasing over time. (Application of data standards may require separate SOPs).
- Explore the options available for long-term data storage and data management, within the department, within the larger parent organization, and within external third-party repositories.
- Develop an SOP for preparing data for re-use, to be applied in the context of any particular trial (unless all the decisions relating to data re-use in that trial are taken entirely by an external sponsor). Integrate it into more general SOPs on study preparation so that the data re-use is considered, planned, and costed at the outset of the trial's setup. The elements of the SOP are described in more detail in the study-specific section below.
- Develop an SOP on responding to requests for data, to be applied in the context of any particular trial (unless all such requests in that trial are managed entirely by an external sponsor).

Study-Specific Activity (within study planning):

- Any IPD sharing policies/procedures of the study sponsor (or other data controller) and/or the study funder should be checked and the implications of these for IPD sharing identified (if not already known from the more general review described above).
- The IPD sharing policies and expectations of any collaborating groups should also be checked and incorporated into the proposed plan for IPD secondary use.
- The sponsor as the data controller should normally take overall responsibility for making decisions about possible data re-use, though may delegate this in practice to a Trial Management Group (TMG). The TMG may in turn delegate the function to a smaller group.
- The datasets to be made available for sharing should be identified, together with an estimate of the time points when they will become available (e.g., in months after the primary paper has been published).
- The documents to be made available for sharing should be identified (e.g., protocols, results summary) together with an estimate of the time points when they will become available. Times are likely to differ between different documents.
- Depending on the legal requirements, the need for a specific consent to enable data re-use needs to be considered. If such a consent is deemed necessary, it and associated information will need to be written and incorporated into the consent forms and other participant documents.
- Likely de-identification steps need to be identified to aid in estimating the work that will be involved.
- The pros and cons of transferring data and documents to a dedicated data repository, in the same or an external organization, should be considered. At this stage this might only be a "decision in principle," but it may have a cost implication and therefore needs to be considered.
- The extent and type of the use of data standards in the study should be decided, planned, and documented.
- The type of access to be offered needs to be decided, at least in principle. For example, access might be public, or by prior request to the investigator, with a reasoned scientific justification, or it might be initially to an expert review panel who could screen requests and recommend appropriate action.
- The likely costs of preparing data for sharing and then storing it in the long term should be estimated. These may include the costs required for (a) de-identification, (b) checking the impact of de-identification on scientific utility, (c) preparing metadata, (d) identifying a suitable repository and negotiating with it, and (e) long-term storage costs, if any. Costs should be included in bids for funds.
- Text needs to be prepared so that the data sharing plan can be summarized (a) within the protocol, (b) within the trial registration entry (or entries) and (c) within patient information sheets.

Study-Specific Activity (at study end)

- The plans for data re-use should be reviewed, in the light of available resources, possible changes in legislation (or the interpretation of that legislation), changed scientific expectations about data sharing, etc.
- The data preparation required to support IPD sharing should be carried out according to the agreed strategy. This will include (a) application of de-identification techniques and (b) checking of the impact of de-identification on the analyses carried out on the data.
- If and as required by local regulation, risk assessment and risk management documents may have to be prepared. The latter may need to include descriptions of the data use agreements to be employed.
- Additional metadata for the dataset(s) and documents should be prepared. This includes (a) descriptive metadata for the de-identified dataset(s), e.g., using CDISC's Define.xml, and (b) provenance/discovery metadata, for use in "advertising" the data and documents, e.g., in the context of a data repository. Both these steps may need to be repeated multiple times, as different datasets and documents become available.
- If a dedicated external repository is to be used, datasets and documents should be transferred to that repository. The transfer should be subject to formal agreements that stipulate the responsibilities of each party.

Conclusion

Study data management does not end with the end of the study. Data must be retained for a set period to allow re-analysis if necessary, and, increasingly, data – or a de-identified subset of it – is expected to be made accessible to others, if they can justify the reasons for that access.

The simple retention of data is not difficult and has long been a requirement, but it does require clear planning and resourcing, and it needs to be comprehensive – all forms of the data need to be considered and archived or destroyed as necessary. Because interest in the data may have waned at study end, it is important that all decisions relating to data retention are taken at the beginning of the study, by the sponsor but usually in collaboration with the study's operational managers, and that all activities are properly resourced.

Making data available for secondary re-use is a more complex, active process that is relatively new for most trialists and trials units, but it is increasingly becoming an expectation. The details of the processing required will inevitably depend on the legal framework that applies, but as a minimum data will need to be de-identified. To make the shared data more useful, it will also be important to ensure that the data is as inter-operable as possible, by incorporating data standards into the study design from the outset (applying such standards retrospectively can be done in theory, but in practice is a very difficult and costly process). Finally, to make the data and associated documents available in the long term, it will often be necessary to transfer them to a dedicated data repository.

Again, the only way this end of study activity can be delivered efficiently is by planning and resourcing it from the beginning of the study planning process. That means setting up systems (including adequately trained staff as well as relevant SOPs) that allow preparation for data re-use to be integrated into the rest of study management.

Key Facts

1. Clinical trial data must be retained, for potential re-analysis and investigation, for periods determined by the relevant legal jurisdiction(s).
2. Data retention is also required for compliance with Good Clinical Practice (GCP).
3. Data should be retained both centrally and at each clinical site.
4. The sponsor has the final decisions with regard to the details (files, format, location, etc.) of retained data.
5. Arrangements for retaining data in the long term should be established by the sponsor, in collaboration with the trial's operational managers (e.g., CRO or trials unit) as part of study planning.
6. In recent years there has been increasing pressure on sponsors and investigators to make de-identified individual participant data and study documents available to others, for secondary research purposes.
7. Funders and publishers in particular have been keen to encourage secondary re-use, as a mechanism for raising both the cost-effectiveness and the quality of research.
8. The regulations governing secondary re-use will vary from one legal jurisdiction to another and over time.
9. Almost all data will need to undergo de-identification before it is suitable for secondary re-use. A variety of techniques have been published, but the stronger the de-identification applied, the greater the risk to the scientific utility of the data.
10. Data use agreements offer an additional level of risk management around secondary use and are an important reason why access to the data should often be controlled rather than freely available.
11. To maximize the value of secondary use, it is important to make data as inter-operable as possible, by the use of data standards – e.g., with common outcome sets, consistent data definitions and categorizations, standardized data structures and codes, and a standardized metadata scheme.
12. In the longer term, data is best transferred to a dedicated data repository. Unfortunately, at the moment, few existing repositories are well adapted to managing sensitive personal data available under controlled access.
13. Sponsors and study operational managers need to develop systems and processes to support the preparation of data for re-use. This includes adequate training of staff as well as SOPs and other quality documents.

14. Although much of the activity related to data re-use occurs at the end of the study, much of the planning for it needs to take place at the beginning, as part of the general study planning process.

Cross-References

► Archiving Records and Materials
► De-identifying Clinical Trial Data
► Design and Development of the Study Data System
► Documentation: Essential Documents and Standard Operating Procedures
► Responsibilities and Management of the Clinical Coordinating Center

References

Banzi R, Canham S, Kuchinke W et al (2019) Evaluation of repositories for sharing individual-participant data from clinical studies. Trials 20:169. https://doi.org/10.1186/s13063-019-3253-3. Available at https://trialsjournal.biomedcentral.com/articles/10.1186/s13063-019-3253-3. Accessed 13 Aug 2020

Bierer B, Crosas M, Pierce H (2017) Data authorship as an incentive to data sharing. N Engl J Med 376:1684–1687. https://doi.org/10.1056/NEJMsb1616595. Available at https://www.nejm.org/doi/10.1056/NEJMsb1616595. Accessed 14 June 2020

BMJ (2020) BMJ author Hub: data sharing. Available at https://authors.bmj.com/policies/data-sharing/. Accessed 8 June 2020

CDISC (2020) CDISC standards in the clinical research process. Available at https://www.cdisc.org/standards. Accessed 13 Aug 2020

Chan A, Song F, Vickers A et al (2014) Increasing value and reducing waste: addressing inaccessible research. Lancet 383:257–266. https://doi.org/10.1016/S0140-6736(13)62296-5

COMET (2020) Core outcome measures in effectiveness trials. Available at http://www.comet-initiative.org/. Accessed 13 Aug 2020

CoreTrustSeal (2020) CoreTrustSeal certification. Available at https://www.coretrustseal.org/. Accessed 13 Aug 2020

CSDR (2020) ClinicalStudyDataRequest.com: data sharing agreement. Available at https://clinicalstudydatarequest.com/Help/Help-Data-Sharing-Agreement.aspx. Accessed 13 Aug 2020

Davey C, Aiken A, Hayes R, Hargreaves J (2015) Re-analysis of health and educational impacts of a school-based deworming programme in western Kenya: a statistical replication of a cluster quasi-randomized stepped-wedge trial. Int J Epidemiol 44:1581–1592. https://doi.org/10.1093/ije/dyv128

Doshi P, Dickersin K, Healy D et al (2013) Restoring invisible and abandoned trials: a call for people to publish the findings. BMJ 346. https://doi.org/10.1136/bmj.f2865. Available at https://www.bmj.com/content/346/bmj.f2865. Accessed 5 June 2020

EDIC (2020) The epidemiology of diabetes interventions and complications. Available at https://edic.bsc.gwu.edu/. Accessed 7 June 2020

EMA (2018) Guideline on the content, management and archiving of the clinical trial master file (paper and/or electronic). EMA/INS/GCP/856758/2018 Good Clinical Practice Inspectors Working Group (GCP IWG). Available at https://www.ema.europa.eu/en/documents/scientific-guideline/guideline-content-management-archiving-clinical-trial-master-file-paper/electronic_en.pdf. Accessed 5 June 2020

European Commission (2003) Directive 2003/63/EC, amending Directive 2001/83/EC relating to medicinal products for human use. Available at https://ec.europa.eu/health/sites/health/files/files/eudralex/vol-1/dir_2003_63/dir_2003_63_en.pdf. Accessed 5 June 2020

European Commission (2014) Regulation 536/2014 of the European Parliament and of the Council of 16 April 2014 on clinical trials on medicinal products for human use. Available at https://ec.europa.eu/health/sites/health/files/files/eudralex/vol-1/reg_2014_536/reg_2014_536_en.pdf. Accessed 5 June 2020

Geraghty K (2016) 'PACE-Gate': when clinical trial evidence meets open data access (Editorial). J Health Psychol. https://doi.org/10.1177/1359105316675213. Available at https://journals.sagepub.com/doi/10.1177/1359105316675213. Accessed 8 June 2020

Henry D, Fitzpatrick T (2015) Liberating the data from clinical trials (editorial). BMJ 351:h4601. https://doi.org/10.1136/bmj.h4601

HHS.Gov (2020) Guidance regarding methods for de-identification of protected health information in accordance with the Health Insurance Portability and Accountability Act (HIPAA) privacy rule. Available at https://www.hhs.gov/hipaa/for-professionals/privacy/special-topics/de-identification/index.html#standard

ICH (2016) International council for harmonisation of technical requirements for pharmaceuticals for human use (ICH) guidelines for good clinical practice E6(R2). Available at https://database.ich.org/sites/default/files/E6_R2_Addendum.pdf. Accessed 5 June 2020

ICMJE (2020) International Committee of Medical Journal Editors: data sharing. Available at http://icmje.org/recommendations/browse/publishing-and-editorial-issues/clinical-trial-registration.html#two. Accessed 13 Aug 2020

IDDO (2020) Infectious diseases data observatory: Ebola. Available at https://www.iddo.org/ebola/data-sharing/accessing-data. Accessed 7 June 2020

Institute of Medicine (2015) Sharing clinical trial data, maximizing benefits, minimizing risk. Appendix B. Concepts and methods for de-identifying clinical trial data. National Academies Press, Washington, DC. Available at https://www.nap.edu/read/18998/chapter/10. Accessed 12 Aug 2020

ISARIC (2020) Clinical data collection – the COVID-19 case report forms (CRFs). Available at https://isaric.tghn.org/COVID-19-CRF/. Accessed 13 Aug 2020

Keerie C, Tuck C, Milne G et al (2018) Data sharing in clinical trials – practical guidance on anonymising trial datasets. Trials 19:25. https://doi.org/10.1186/s13063-017-2382-9. Available at https://trialsjournal.biomedcentral.com/articles/10.1186/s13063-017-2382-9. Accessed 12 Aug 2020

Keller et al (2001) Efficacy of paroxetine in the treatment of adolescent major depression: a randomized, controlled trial. Am Acad Child Adolesc Psychiatry 40(7):762–772. https://doi.org/10.1097/00004583-200107000-00010. Available at http://www.dcscience.net/keller-2001-paroxetine.pdf. Accessed 5 June 2020

Kiley R, Peatfield T, Hansen J, Reddington F (2017) Data sharing from clinical trials – a research funder's perspective. N Engl J Med 377:1990–1992. https://doi.org/10.1056/NEJMsb1708278. Available at https://www.nejm.org/doi/full/10.1056/NEJMsb1708278. Accessed 8 June 2020

Le Noury J, Nardo J, Healy D et al (2015) Restoring study 329: efficacy and harms of paroxetine and imipramine in treatment of major depression in adolescence. BMJ 351. https://doi.org/10.1136/bmj.h4320. Available at https://www.bmj.com/content/351/bmj.h4320. Accessed 5 June 2020

Lemmens T (2013) Pharmaceutical knowledge governance: a human rights perspective. J Law Med Ethics 41(1):163–184

Lemmens T, Telfer C (2012) Access to information and the right to health: the human rights case for clinical trials transparency. Am J Law Med 31(1):63–112

Levin M, Cunnington AJ, Wilson C et al (2019) Effects of saline or albumin fluid bolus in resuscitation: evidence from re-analysis of the FEAST trial. Lancet Respir Med 7:581–593. https://doi.org/10.1016/S2213-2600(19)30114-6. Available at https://www.thelancet.com/journals/lanres/article/PIIS2213-2600(19)30114-6/fulltext. Accessed 8 June 2020

Maitland K, Kiguli S, Opoka R et al (2011) Mortality after fluid bolus in African children with severe infection. N Engl J Med 364(26):2483–2495. https://doi.org/10.1056/NEJMoa1101549. Epub 2011 May 26. Available at https://www.nejm.org/doi/10.1056/NEJMoa1101549?url_ver=Z39.88-2003&rfr_id=ori:rid:crossref.org&rfr_dat=cr_pub%20%200www.ncbi.nlm.nih.gov. Accessed 8 June 2020

Maitland K, Gibb D, Babiker A et al (2019) Secondary re-analysis of the FEAST trial (correspondence). Lancet Respir Med 7(10):E29. https://doi.org/10.1016/S2213-2600(19)30272-3

Miguel E, Kremer M (2004) Worms: identifying impacts on education and health in the presence of treatment externalities. Econometrica 72(1):159–217. https://doi.org/10.1111/j.1468-0262.2004.00481.x.

MRC (2015) Good practice principles for sharing individual participant data from publicly funded clinical trials. MRC Hub for Trials methodology research, UKCRC, Cancer Research UK, Wellcome Trust. Available at https://www.methodologyhubs.mrc.ac.uk/files/7114/3682/3831/Datasharingguidance2015.pdf. Accessed 12 Aug 2020

NEJM (2016) The SPRINT data analysis challenge. Available at https://challenge.nejm.org/pages/about. Accessed 8 June 2020

Ohmann C, Banzi R, Canham S et al (2017) Sharing and reuse of individual participant data from clinical trials: principles and recommendations. BMJ Open 7:e018647. https://doi.org/10.1136/bmjopen-2017-018647. Available at https://bmjopen.bmj.com/content/bmjopen/7/12/e018647.full.pdf. Accessed 12 Aug 2020

Özler B (2015) Worm wars: a review of the reanalysis of Miguel and Kremer's deworming study. World Bank Blogs. Available at https://blogs.worldbank.org/impactevaluations/worm-wars-review-reanalysis-miguel-and-kremer-s-deworming-study. Accessed 8 June 2020

Peloquin D, DiMalo M, Bierer B, Barnes M (2020) Disruptive and avoidable: GDPR challenges to secondary research uses of data. Eur J Hum Genet 28:697–705. https://doi.org/10.1038/s41431-020-0596-x. Available at https://www.nature.com/articles/s41431-020-0596-x. Accessed 12 Aug 2020

Ramokapane K, Rashid A, Such J (2016) Assured deletion in the cloud: requirements, challenges and future directions. Conference paper at ACM, October 2016. https://doi.org/10.1145/2996429.2996434. Available at http://eprints.lancs.ac.uk/81611/1/Assured_deletion_Final_version.pdf. Accessed 7 June 2020

Reichman J (2009) Rethinking the role of clinical trial data in international intellectual property law: the case for a public goods approach. Marquette Intellect Prop Law Rev 13(1):1–68

Research Data Alliance (2020) RDA COVID-19 recommendations and guidelines (5th Release). Available at https://www.rd-alliance.org/system/files/RDA%20COVID-19%3B%20recommendations%20and%20guidelines%2C%205th%20release%20%28final%20draft%29%2028%20May%202020.pdf. Accessed 7 June 2020

RIAT Support Center (2020) Restoring invisible and abandoned trials. Available at https://restoringtrials.org/. Accessed 5 June 2020

Riley R, Lambert P, AboZaid G (2010) Meta-analysis of individual participant data: rationale, conduct, and reporting. 340:c221. https://doi.org/10.1136/bmj.c221. Available at https://www.bmj.com/content/340/bmj.c221. Accessed 7 June 2020

SPRINT Research Group (2015) A randomized trial of intensive versus standard blood-pressure control. N Engl J Med 373:2103–2116. https://doi.org/10.1056/NEJMoa1511939. Available at https://www.nejm.org/doi/full/10.1056/NEJMoa1511939. Accessed 8 June 2020

Tangcharoensathien V, Boonperm, Jongudomsuk P (2010) Sharing health data: developing country perspectives. Bull World Health Organ 88(6):468–469. https://doi.org/10.2471/BLT.10.079129. Available at https://www.ncbi.nlm.nih.gov/pmc/articles/PMC2878166/. Accessed 14 June 2020

Torjesen I (2018) Pressure grows on Lancet to review "flawed" PACE trial (News article). BMJ 362: k3621. https://doi.org/10.1136/bmj.k3621

UKRI (2020) Common principles on data policy. Available at https://www.ukri.org/funding/information-for-award-holders/data-policy/common-principles-on-data-policy/. Accessed 7 June 2020

US Code of Federal Regulations (2020) Title 21, Chapter I, 312 D – responsibilities of sponsors and investigators, section 312.62 investigator recordkeeping and record retention. Available at https://www.govregs.com/regulations/expand/title21_chapterI_part312_subpartD_section312.61#title21_chapterI_part312_subpartD_section312.62. Accessed 5 June 2020

Van den Eyndon, V, Knight G, Vlad A et al (2016) Towards open research, practices, experiences, barriers and opportunities. Wellcome Trust. https://doi.org/10.6084/m9.figshare.4055448

Vickers A (2016) Sharing raw data from clinical trials: what progress since we first asked, "whose data set is it anyway?". Trials 17:227. Available at https://www.ncbi.nlm.nih.gov/pmc/articles/PMC4855346/. Accessed 8 June 2020

Wellcome Trust (2020) Sharing research data and findings relevant to the novel coronavirus (COVID-19) outbreak. Available at https://wellcome.ac.uk/coronavirus-covid-19/open-data. Accessed 7 June 2020

White P, Goldsmith K et al (2011) Comparison of adaptive pacing therapy, cognitive behaviour therapy, graded exercise therapy, and specialist medical care for chronic fatigue syndrome (PACE): a randomised trial. Lancet 377(9768):5–11, 823–836. https://doi.org/10.1016/S0140-6736(11)60096-2. Available at https://www.sciencedirect.com/science/article/pii/S0140673611600962. Accessed 8 June 2020

WHO (2015) Developing global norms for sharing data and results during public health emergencies. Available at https://www.who.int/medicines/ebola-treatment/data-sharing_phe/en/. Accessed 7 June 2020

Wilkinson MD, Dumontier M et al (2016) The FAIR guiding principles for scientific data management and stewardship. Sci Data 3:160018. https://doi.org/10.1038/sdata.2016.18

Yoda (2020) Yale open data access project: data use agreement training. Available at https://yalesurvey.ca1.qualtrics.com/jfe/form/SV_0P7Kl30x4aAZDRX?Q_JFE=qdg. Accessed 13 Aug 2020

Part III

Regulation and Oversight

Regulatory Requirements in Clinical Trials

24

Michelle Pernice and Alan Colley

Contents

M. Pernice (✉)
Dynavax Technologies Corporation, Emeryville, CA, USA
e-mail: mpernice@dynavax.com

A. Colley
Amgen, Ltd, Cambridge, UK
e-mail: acolley@amgen.com

© Springer Nature Switzerland AG 2022
S. Piantadosi, C. L. Meinert (eds.), *Principles and Practice of Clinical Trials*,
https://doi.org/10.1007/978-3-319-52636-2_51

Abstract

Understanding the regulatory requirements for initiating and conducting clinical trials is a crucial starting point and success factor in any plan to advance drug development in humans. Regulatory requirements go beyond what is considered compliance with good clinical practice (GCP) and other standards. Regulations provide the guardrails and opportunities for safe, efficient, and purposeful drug development. While regulations provide the groundwork of what is to be considered "right" and "wrong" in drug development, there is a level of uncertainty that is intentionally left for sponsor interpretation in order to provide flexibility. Further, regulators usually represent the views of the country or region within their specific purview, a structure which lends itself to dissonance between different regulations/guidelines, furthering the need for sponsor interpretation. Such interpretation is conveyed in the finished clinical trial application (CTA) or investigational new drug (IND) application and then subject to the regulators' review and approval. As important as it is to understand the written requirements, it's equally important to understand how and when to engage with the regulators to expedite drug development. If done well, the combination of understanding the regulations, implementing sponsor interpretation, and utilizing opportunities for engagement with regulatory agencies can lead to ultimately deliver useful treatments to patients.

In this chapter, global, regional, and national clinical trial regulatory considerations will be described to enable the reader to understand the principles and practice of conceptualizing, submitting, initiating, and completing clinical trials in the regulated environment of drug development.

Keywords

Regulatory · FDA · EMA · Marketing authorization · BLA/NDA · MAA · IND · CTA · Approval · Sponsor

Introduction

When a patient goes to see a doctor and walks out with a prescription, the ability for that treatment to be prescribed is the result of regulatory approval or "marketing authorization." Marketing authorization is only granted once sufficient clinical trial data are generated to prove that the benefits of the treatment outweigh the risks. As explained in the US Code of Federal Regulations (CFR), the purpose of conducting clinical trials is to distinguish the effect of a drug from other influences (e.g., rule out "placebo effect"). The Food and Drug Administration (FDA) considers adequate and well-controlled studies to be the primary basis for determining whether there is "substantial evidence" to support the claims of effectiveness for new drugs. Substantial evidence is defined in Section 505(d) of the Food, Drug, and Cosmetic (FD&C) Act[2] as, "evidence consisting of adequate and well controlled investigations, including clinical investigations, by [qualified experts who could fairly and responsibly conclude that the drug will have the effect it purports or is represented to have in the labeling]." The clinical trial data which serve to comprise substantial evidence as the basis of such an approval are submitted to the regulator in a marketing authorization application (MAA) or, in the USA, a new drug application (NDA)/biologics licensing application (BLA). Standardly, the MAA or BLA/NDA will contain the data from Phase 1, Phase 2, and Phase 3 clinical trials. However, there are exceptions to this standard where development may be expedited (e.g., Phase 2 data being considered sufficient for approval under FDA's Accelerated Approval program) based on unmet need and other factors.

As the name denotes, Phase 1 trials are the starting point to understand how the drug candidate will perform in humans from a safety perspective, including identification of the appropriate dose(s) to be studied further. Phase 2 trials are meant to develop information on the potential efficacy and to generate more safety data in the larger population. Phase 3 trials are intended to provide sufficient data to prove that the benefits outweigh the risks of the experimental treatment, using a clinically meaningful endpoint (e.g., survival or mortality). Typically, the Phase 3 trial(s) are referred to as the "registrational" or "pivotal" trials. However, in situations where there is a high unmet medical need and new treatment options are urgently needed, an earlier-phase trial (e.g., Phase 2 trial) can serve as the "registrational" or "pivotal" trial. This would usually occur under a specific regulatory designation (e.g., "Accelerated Approval" in the USA and "Conditional Approval" in the EU), which is sought by the manufacturer of the product (referred to as the "sponsor") and granted by the regulator (e.g., the FDA in the USA, European Medicines Agency [EMA] in the EU).

There are regulatory requirements that apply across all phases of clinical trials. As an example, all clinical trials must comprehensively disclose the risks of the trial to the people volunteering to be enrolled and receive the volunteers' consent to be treated and have the results used as data. There are also regulations and regulatory guidance that apply to specific trial phases. For example, in a Phase 3 study where the investigational treatment is compared against an approved therapy, the design will be required to control for possible bias between treatment arms (e.g., the protocol procedures must employ blinding) in order to generate a reliable, clinically meaningful conclusion (e.g., proven superiority or non-inferiority).

In addition to Phase 1–3 data intended for inclusion in the submission of an MAA, NDA, or BLA, there are also clinical trials which may be conducted after the product's approval, referred to as Phase 4 clinical trials or post-marketing studies. Phase 4 trials may be required by the regulator to answer remaining questions about the efficacy or safety of the now-approved product or could be initiated voluntarily by the sponsor company. Either way, Phase 4 trials usually seek to generate more information on the treatment over a longer duration of time, in a larger population or in specific patient populations not sufficiently represented in the original Phase 1–3 trials. Phase 4 trials aren't the only trials that can be conducted after a product approval, however. As the approved product continues to be explored in other disease areas and/or patient populations, additional Phase 1–3 trials with that product may be conducted (e.g., a product approved for the treatment of adult patients with melanoma may then be included in a new Phase 1 trial to assess the product's safety in pediatrics with a different malignancy).

Clinical trials are often conducted in more than one country. This is partly due to the intent for the product to ultimately be approved in multiple countries, and therefore data that is representative of each country's population and local medical practice is likely to be required by that country's regulator. This is also due to the need to expeditiously accrue patients to a trial, necessitating the ability to recruit study volunteers from a larger population than what would be feasible in a single country. While conducting clinical trials globally should lead to data that are more representative of the real-world patient population, this also opens the sponsor up to inconsistencies between requirements and advice received from different national and regional regulators. As an example, the approval to conduct a clinical trial in the USA is the subject of FDA review of the Investigational New Drug (IND) application, which includes a multitude of detailed documents (e.g., information on the manufacturing of the product, the preclinical data on the product). Thereafter, when a subsequent trial is proposed (e.g., after the completion of the Phase 1 trial, a Phase 2 trial will be proposed), that individual trial's clinical protocol will be submitted "to the IND." The clinical trial protocol is just one document usually less than 200 pages, whereas there are typically 30 or more documents amounting to thousands of pages in the original IND. To conduct the same Phase 2 trial in the EU, a new clinical trial application (CTA) must be submitted to the regulators of those countries within the EU where the clinical trial will be conducted, even though a CTA was submitted for the original Phase 1 trial. There are some documents that may be prepared to support both an IND and CTA filing, whereas there are a number of other documents that only serve to support one or the other. Unlike in the USA, where after the FDA review of the original IND subsequent studies require less documentation, in the EU, CTAs are submitted each time a new study is proposed. While certain initial CTA documents can be referenced or resubmitted for subsequent CTAs, the submission package still tends to be much larger than what is required for such subsequent studies in the USA.

As exemplified above, in order to be successful in developing a new treatment for patients, it is important for the sponsor to have capabilities to understand not only basic global regulatory requirements but also the details of individual country regulations.

Fundamentals of Global Regulatory Affairs

Unlike the IND and CTA differences described, some regulations are consistent globally, or have been harmonized between regions, and comprise the bedrock of initial clinical development inception and planning. Developed by regulators around the world, good manufacturing practice (GMP) and good clinical practice (GCP) form the fundamental basis of what is required throughout global clinical development. Adhering to the standards set forth in these practices is a requirement for clinical trials to be conducted safely and ethically. Various bodies globally have published what comprise the principles of GMP and GCP, including the World Health Organization (WHO) and the International Council of Harmonization (ICH). ICH was founded in 1990 with the mission to achieve greater harmonization worldwide to ensure that safe, effective, and high-quality medicines are developed and registered in the most resource-efficient manner. Since then, ICH has developed guidelines across the various pillars of a drug development program, which include the development of the experimental product's quality attributes (referred to as the "Q" category; e.g., stability and shelf life), the generation of preclinical toxicology data ("S" category) and clinical efficacy and safety ("E" category) data, and multi-disciplinary topics which apply across categories ("M" category; e.g., standardized medical terminology). Such foundational globally relevant guidance was developed based on core principals often reflected in individual country regulations and in turn also influence future evolution of those individual country regulations.

Regulatory Strategy: "Black and White" vs. "Gray Zone"

Within the practice of regulatory affairs, there are clear-cut regulations that need to be understood and adhered to, provided through the rules and regulations written in "black and white," meaning there is intentionally little room for interpretation considering the criticality of the concept (e.g., regulations that govern patient safety and adverse event reporting). As regulators and sponsors consider the adherence of these rules as more than just "regulatory affairs," this practice is more often termed "compliance."

The "Black and White"

In the USA, written regulations are laid out in the CFR. The CFR documents all actions that are required under the applicable federal law which, in this case, is the Federal Food, Drug, and Cosmetic Act (FD&C Act, codified into Title 21 Chap. 9 of the US Code) (The CFR is organized into a hierarchical series which will be exemplified hereon consistent with the subject focus of this book chapter. The hierarchy begins with Titles, and Title 21 of the CFR contains 'Food and Drugs' regulations. Next, are Chapters classified by regulatory entity, and Chap. 1 covers the 'FDA Department of Health and Human Services'. Chapters are broken down into Subparts, where Subpart D describes 'Drugs for Human Use'. Within Subpart D there are a number of Parts, including Part 312 which describes 'Investigational New Drug Applications'. Collectively, this example selection within the CFR would be referred to as "21 CFR Part 312," "Chap. 1" and "Subpart D" are assumed by "Part 312" as Chap. 1, Subpart D is the only component of 21 CFR that contains a "Part 312."). Among other topics, the CFR contains the central principals of safely and ethically conducting a clinical trial. For a regulatory affairs professional with a purview that includes the USA, the CFR is often the first pillar of decision-making and considered a necessity to achieve "compliance." This section considers the CFR, and comparable written regulations globally, as "The Black and White" seeing as the rules and regulations set forth in the CFR are most often standard requirements in order to achieve regulatory approval to conduct a clinical trial and the subsequent approval of an MAA/BLA/NDA based on data from the conducted clinical trials. These regulations tend to avoid overprescriptive details and instead issue broadly impactful rules. An example can be found in 21 CFR Part 312.20 (a) which states, "A sponsor shall submit an IND to FDA if the sponsor intends to conduct a clinical investigation with an investigational new drug that is subject to §312.2 (a)" (where §312.2(a) refers to 21 CFR Part 312.2(a) which addresses the products within scope of the overall 21 CFR Part 312 regulations). The concept that a sponsor must submit an IND to FDA prior to conducting a clinical investigation with an investigational new drug within the scope referred to is not a subject that should typically be considered negotiable. This requirement is necessary to enable the appropriate oversight of the investigational clinical trial by the regulator, a critical component of safe and ethical drug development.

The "Gray Zone"

The next pillar of decision-making for a regulatory affairs professional is found in written regulatory guidance or guidelines. Written guidance elaborates on the written regulation text, offering more detailed description of the intent of the regulation based on the regulator's current thinking. Most often, guidance documents will begin with reference to the statutory and regulatory requirements that comprise the basis of the topic being presented for guidance (e.g., text from the CFR). Meaning, written guidance introduces a combination of the "black and white" and the "gray zone." The "gray zone" can be interpreted as regulator-issued considerations that could be the subject of further discussion and alignment, even negotiation, between the sponsor, regulator, and other stakeholders (e.g., healthcare professionals, patients, and patient advocates). Most written guidance will contain introductory text to this effect, as an example FDA guidance text includes:

> In general, FDA's guidance documents do not establish legally enforceable responsibilities. Instead, guidances describe the Agency's current thinking on a topic and should be viewed only as recommendations, unless specific regulatory or statutory requirements are cited. The use of the word 'should' in Agency guidances means that something is suggested or recommended, but not required.

This flexibility is often evident in the guidance text itself being inconclusive or situation-dependent, leaving the "door open" for the sponsor to consider what is the most appropriate proposal for the particular investigational drug, specific patient population, and disease landscape. Diseases that are life-threatening or otherwise remain a high unmet medical need are of particular relevance for further consideration, discussion, and even negotiation with the regulator. With the betterment of public health as a shared common goal between all stakeholders (regulators, sponsors, healthcare professionals, and patients themselves), circumstances which challenge the chances of a patient's success are replete with opportunity to be open, collaborative, and communicative between stakeholders, namely, between the sponsor and regulator.

Another helpful component to guide decisions to meet the regulators' expectations is regulatory precedents (e.g., examples of past agreements between a sponsor and a regulator). Every approved product is issued a public document describing the product's core information. In the USA, this document is called the US Prescribing Information (USPI), and in the EU, it is called the Summary of Product Characteristics (SmPC). Documents of this type will reflect a multitude of information, including the pivotal clinical trials conducted in order to achieve the marketing authorization. Further, regulators often publish documents publicly which stipulate the rationale behind the decision to approve the product. In the USA, this document is called the Summary Basis of Approval (SBA), and in the EU, this document is called the European Public Assessment Report (EPAR). Within these documents, a description of the registrational pivotal trials will be described, often including the primary endpoint, selected secondary endpoints, sample size, demographics, specific safety assessments, and results. Such precedents are helpful to understand circumstances when products were successfully developed and approved in addition to what is provided in official labeling.

Once the plans for a particular clinical trial's design are formed, a sponsor can choose to seek regulatory agency advice. This represents the final major pillar of decision-making for a regulatory affairs professional and where the opportunity to really explore the "gray zone" comes into action. Some regulator advice procedures are described in the CFR, denoting how common and how strongly encouraged they tend to be. Of note, 21 CFR 312.47, entitled "Meetings," presents the below alongside additional information:

> Meetings between a sponsor and the agency [FDA] are frequently useful in resolving questions and issues raised during the course of a clinical investigation. FDA encourages such meetings to the extent that they aid in the evaluation of the drug and in the solution of scientific problems concerning the drug, to the extent that FDA's resources permit. The general principle underlying the conduct of such meetings is that there should be free, full, and open communication about any scientific or medical question that may arise during the clinical investigation.

Such engagement constitutes the third pillar of regulatory wherewithal to guide drug development in an ethical, safe, and productive manner. The ability to combine information and learning from each of the pillars outlined into a plan that suits the aim of all stakeholders is what constitutes a regulatory strategy. Regulatory strategies are developed by regulatory affairs professionals for each critical decision within a drug candidate's development plan. Such critical decisions span across the life of the drug's development and touch on topics both with immediate need and with long-term impact, such as the optimal timing for an initial IND submission, whether or not to develop in pediatric populations, and choosing a marketing authorization pathway to aim toward throughout the drug's development.

Hypothetical Case Study

A hypothetical case study can be found within the requirements surrounding clinical trial endpoint selection in potentially registrational clinical trials for patients with a disease of high unmet need, using certain cancers as an example of such disease. When designing a clinical trial, the regulatory affairs professional is often tasked with selecting and confirming the appropriate endpoint of a given clinical trial. In this case study, consider that the team has requested the regulatory affairs professional to advise on whether there are any other endpoints that can be acceptable by regulators for a marketing authorization, as a mortality endpoint may take too long to reach in the clinical trial setting, considering the present-day unmet need of this population.

Knowing that the clinical trial being designed is intended to study a patient population of high unmet need, and aims to pursue a pathway that is as expedited as possible toward marketing authorization, the regulatory affairs professional could start with comprehending the "black and white" around the clinical trial results and data requirements to support such an application in the USA. Accordingly, in searching first through the CFR, the regulatory affairs professional will find 21 CFR part 314, subpart H entitled, "Accelerated Approval of New Drugs for Serious or Life-Threatening Illnesses," including 21 CFR part 314.510, "Approval based on a surrogate endpoint or on an effect on a clinical endpoint other than survival or irreversible morbidity," which states:

> FDA may grant marketing approval for a new drug product on the basis of adequate and well-controlled clinical trials establishing that the drug product has an effect on a surrogate endpoint that is reasonably likely, based on epidemiologic, therapeutic, pathophysiologic, or other evidence, to predict clinical benefit or on the basis of an effect on a clinical endpoint other than survival or irreversible morbidity. Approval under this section will be subject to the requirement that the applicant study the drug further, to verify and describe its clinical benefit, where there is uncertainty as to the relation of the surrogate endpoint to clinical benefit, or of the observed clinical benefit to ultimate outcome. Postmarketing studies would usually be studies already underway. When required to be conducted, such studies must also be adequate and well-controlled. The applicant shall carry out any such studies with due diligence.

Based on this, the regulatory affairs professional can advise the team that a clinical trial should be proposed to FDA containing an endpoint that acts as a "surrogate" that is "reasonably likely" to predict what a traditional, clear clinical benefit endpoint would assess (e.g., mortality). Acknowledging that there are currently no approved therapies in the malignancy being studied, and therefore nothing to design a comparative, head-to-head trial against, the regulatory affairs professional may consider whether a Phase 2 study would be sufficient for initial marketing authorization. Along with guiding the team in planning such a clinical trial, the team will also need to be advised to plan for a post-marketing study including a certain clinical benefit endpoint. As this is written in "black and white," it is pertinent information for the drug development team. Next, the regulatory affairs professional knows to seek information beyond the CFR and identifies written FDA guidance titled, "Clinical Trial Endpoints for the Approval of Cancer Drugs and Biologics" which advises, among other content:

> Surrogate endpoints for accelerated approval must be reasonably likely to predict clinical benefit (FD&C Act § 506(c)(1)(A); 21 CFR part 314, subpart H; and 21 CFR part 601, subpart E). While durable objective response rate (ORR) has been used as a traditional approval endpoint in some circumstances, ORR has also been the most commonly used surrogate endpoint in support of accelerated approval. Tumor response is widely accepted by oncologists in guiding cancer treatments. Because ORR is directly attributable to drug effect, single-arm trials conducted in patients with refractory tumors where no available therapy exists provide an accurate assessment of ORR. Whether tumor measures such as ORR or PFS are used as an accelerated approval or traditional approval endpoint will depend on the disease context and the magnitude of the effect, among other factors.

With this, the regulatory affairs professional is empowered to advise the team of regulation- and guidance-supported suggestions of possible endpoints for the team to consider within the context of this particular malignancy and patient population. Further, the regulatory affairs professional perceives an element of regulatory precedents that plays heavily into the FDA written guidance. In searching through the USPIs and SBAs of approved treatments for other forms of cancer that previously represented a high unmet need, a number of surrogate endpoints can be identified and noted as successful in serving as pivotal evidence to support the marketing authorization of that particular product.

Culminating the rules, regulations, guidance, and precedents, the team will generate a proposed clinical trial design, including a selected surrogate endpoint, to seek advice from major regulators. Such advice will generate a collaboration between the regulator and sponsor to meet the common goal: the betterment of public health.

With the refined clinical trial design, the sponsor will seek approval from the regulators to conduct the study. This will entail multiple country- and region-specific processes. In order to maximize the efficiency of the sponsor's preparation, the regulator's review, and the applicability across countries, regulators worldwide (FDA, EMA, and Japan's Ministry of Health, Labor and Welfare (MHLW)) developed a set of specifications for applications to be submitted regulators, entitled the Common Technical Document (CTD) which is broken into five parts or "modules." Module 1 is a region-specific part that contains documents required by the regulator in that specific country or region. Module 2 through Module 5 are constant internationally, shown in Fig. 1.

The electronic version of the CTD (eCTD) was developed by ICH, enabling electronic submissions in lieu of the previous paper-based submissions. This structure is employed for marketing authorization applications (MAA, BLA, NDA) in all participating countries (referred to as "ICH countries"), including but not limited to the USA, EU, Japan, Canada, Switzerland, and Australia. It is also employed for IND submissions in the USA to FDA but is not uniformly employed for CTA submissions to regulators within the EU.

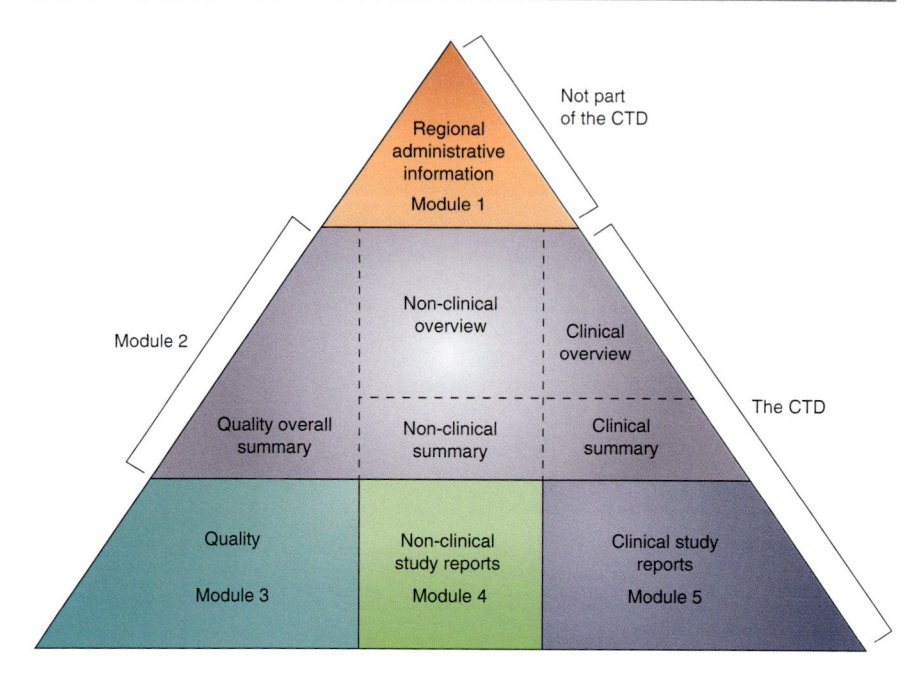

Fig. 1 The CTD triangle

Regulatory Affairs Considerations for Clinical Trials in the USA

Submitting an IND to FDA

The submission of an IND to FDA requires that the details of the investigational product's development be explained across many documents. These documents are organized within the eCTD structure when an IND is being submitted to FDA.

Module 1 contains a cover letter, administrative forms, table of IND contents, the investigators brochure, and an introductory statement including a brief summary of what the clinical development plan is foreseen to include. Module 2 contains the summaries of all subsequent modules (Modules 3–5).

Module 3 will describe the drug substance and the drug product in terms of ingredients, manufacturing process, name and address of the manufacturer, limits imposed to maintain the manufactured products' integrity, and testing results to show that the products remain stable over time. The drug substance is the manufactured active ingredient before it is prepared in the useable form, the drug product. The drug product is the finished manufactured product prepared in a form ("dosage form") that is able to be used for immediate administration (e.g., a finished tablet or capsule) or for preparation of administration (e.g., a vial containing the drug in a solution to be diluted in a bag of inactive ingredients, like "normal saline," for intravenous infusion).

Module 4 includes the reports containing the results from preclinical studies, meaning testing done in animals and "in vitro." Such testing provides data on safety and toxicology as well as what to expect of the drug in humans in terms of how it will be absorbed, distributed, metabolized, and excreted (ADME).

Module 5 includes the clinical proposals in terms of how the investigational drug will be handled in treating the people who have volunteered to participate in the clinical trial. The clinical trial protocol and the informed consent document are of the most important documents in the IND submission, as it contains details of how assessments will be made (e.g., how often the doctor will check the patients' bloodwork, or when an x-ray will be done) and how the investigational drug should be administered (e.g., route of administration, dose, frequency).

Once submitted to FDA, the IND will be reviewed by manufacturing, preclinical, and clinical experts employed by FDA in the "review division." The typical review timeline for a new IND is 30 days, during which time the FDA may ask questions to the sponsor, termed "requests for information." Upon successful review of the IND, the sponsor will receive a letter from FDA entitled "Study May Proceed" which details the FDA acceptance of the proposal set forth by the sponsor in the IND. Alternatively, if the FDA is not comfortable with the sponsor's proposal in the IND, the FDA can issue a "clinical hold" letter detailing what additional information is needed prior to the sponsor being able to initiate the study in the USA. Such a "clinical hold" can also be issued by the FDA during the ongoing conduct of the study, if new information arises that leads the FDA to consider that study participants at undue risk under the current trial protocol.

After the initial IND review has successfully completed, future studies intended for the same or similar patient population can be introduced to the FDA under this now-approved IND, simply with the new protocol and additional new documents supporting the new trial (e.g., toxicology studies for a new patient population). The FDA will review the new documents and will issue questions to the sponsor if necessary. Unlike the original IND, there is no defined formal review timeline. Technically, sponsors can initiate a study in less than 30 days after submitting the new protocol to the IND. However, it is fairly common practice for sponsors to wait an "informal" 30-day period before initiating the study. This practice can be helpful to reduce the risk that the FDA will ask questions or place the study on clinical hold after the study has been initiated; however, the FDA is able to issue "requests for information" at any time, including after the initial 30-day period.

Maintaining the IND

Amendments

As the IND receives initial approval and then stands as the core source of information for an investigational product throughout the product's development, it is common practice for the contents of the IND to change over time. As an example, the IND may've been initially submitted with the drug product in a vial formulation, and over time, the sponsor developed a pre-filled syringe to facilitate ease of preparation and use. Once the sponsor is ready to introduce the drug product utilizing the pre-filled syringe formulation into clinical trials, an amendment to the IND will need to be filed. Such changes can occur in areas that impact the other modules within the IND, also (e. g., additional animal toxicology data become available requiring an amendment to Module 4 of the IND; the clinical trial is changed to also enroll patients with an earlier stage of the disease, requiring an amendment to the protocol in Module 5).

Safety Reporting

One of the most critical aspects of maintaining the IND as the core source of information for the investigational product is safety reporting. Over the course of a clinical trial, the sponsor and the regulator will learn more about the safety of the investigational product. Most of this learning will come from "adverse event reporting." "Adverse event" is defined as any untoward medical occurrence associated with the use of a drug in humans, whether or not considered drug related. Throughout the conduct of the trial, adverse events will be reported based on the study volunteers' experiences while enrolled in the study. These reported events must be promptly reviewed by the sponsor. This is one of the most important regulations stipulated in "black and white" within the CFR and is also a unique exception to regulations presented in the CFR which are typically restricted to conduct in the USA. Safety reporting regulations in the CFR apply to safety reports received from "foreign or domestic sources." Accordingly, sponsors must review safety reports received from every source and assess the reports for their potential reportability to the FDA and impact on continued treatment within the ongoing clinical trials. The CFR is also more prescriptive than usual with regard to the required timeline of safety reporting, outlining which type of reports are mandatory to be submitted no later than 7 calendar days and 15 calendar days.

Annual Reporting

Further to the submission types that occur if and when a qualifying event occurs, as described above, maintaining the IND also comes with a requirement to report certain information annually, within 60 days of the anniversary date of when the FDA review of the original IND came to a successful close. This routine report includes a culmination of what occurred over the reporting period, spanning all topics encompassed in an IND (e.g., manufacturing changes, the status of ongoing preclinical studies, clinical and safety updates, status of the investigational product worldwide).

Regulatory Affairs Considerations for Clinical Trials in the European Union

Evolution of EU Clinical Trials Legislation

A major change to the legislation governing clinical trials in the European Union (EU), the Clinical Trial Regulation (CTReg) EU No. 536/2014[3], currently awaits implementation and could revolutionize the way clinical trials are run in the EU in the next few years. The goal of the CTReg is to create a more favorable environment for conducting clinical trials in the EU by addressing many of the criticisms leveled at the current procedures implemented by the Clinical Trials Directive (CTDir), Directive 2001/20/EC[4], in 2004. It has been widely acknowledged that implementation of the CTDir led to a complexity and lack of harmonization that had direct effects on the cost and feasibility of conducting clinical trials in the EU.

To understand the current procedures for clinical trial authorizations (CTAs) in the EU, and the evolving regulation of clinical trials, it is useful to consider some aspects of the European legislative process in general and the history of clinical trials legislation. Prior to 2004, clinical trials were regulated by the national legislation of each individual member state (MS) of the EU, and significant differences existed between the requirements and procedures in each country. In an attempt to harmonize clinical trial conduct, and the CTA processes, the CTDir was implemented into national legislation of each MS from 2004 onward. The failure of the CTDir to fully harmonize the CTA processes stems largely from the fact that EU directives are legal acts which require each MS to achieve a result without dictating the means of achieving that result in national legislation. This has led to each of the 28 national regulatory agencies (national competent authorities (NCAs)) having differing submission package requirements and/or procedures. In contrast to directives, regulations are legal acts that apply automatically and uniformly to all EU countries as soon as they enter into force, without needing to be transposed into national law. EU regulations are binding in their entirety, on all EU countries, and therefore implementation of the CTReg can be expected to overcome the current lack of harmonization in European CTA procedures.

EudraLex "The Rules Governing Medicinal Products in the European Union"

The body of EU legislation in the pharmaceutical section is compiled into the ten volumes of EudraLex. The basic legislation for medicinal products for human use is contained in Volume 1 and includes the various directives and regulations pertinent to both marketing authorization applications (MAAs) and CTAs. The basic legislation is supported by various guidelines, and Volume 10, "Guidelines for clinical trials," includes guidelines for CTAs approved under the current CTDir and guidelines intended to support the CTReg once it's implemented. Volume 10 includes a chapter on the CTA application, safety reporting, quality of investigational medicinal products (IMPs), inspections, various additional guidelines, and finally links to relevant basic legislation.

Clinical Trials Facilitation and Coordination Group (CTFG)

The Heads of Medicines Agencies (HMA) is a collaborative network of the heads of the NCAs from each EU member state. The CTFG was originally established to coordinate the implementation of the CTDir and has subsequently taken an active role in harmonizing CTA assessment decisions and processes across the NCAs.

In 2009, the CTFG established a process for the assessment of multinational clinical trials (MN-CT) in the EU, the Voluntary Harmonization Procedure (VHP). The VHP was established as a means of achieving a coordinated assessment of MN-CTs within the existing legal framework for clinical trials established by the CTDir. The VHP is discussed in more detail later but can be thought as an intermediate step between the CTDir and the CTReg with the latter being influenced by the experiences of the VHP.

The CTFG publishes guidance relevant to CTAs and the conduct of clinical trials in the EU. With sponsors proposing increasingly complex clinical trial designs, such as basket trials investigating an IMP or multiple IMPs in a variety of populations, or umbrella trials investigating several IMPs in a single population, the CTFG has published a recommendation paper (CTFG, 2019) on initiation and conduct of such trials.

EU Regulatory Agency Advice on Clinical Development and Clinical Trials

The European Medicines Agency (EMA) issues scientific guidelines on most aspects of drug development, and these will influence the design of clinical trials. However, a sponsor may want to seek regulatory advice on the design of a clinical trial prior submitting the CTA, for example, to validate the design will adequately support the regulatory assessment of the benefit and risk during the review of the MAA. In the EU, advice may be sought from the EMA or from individual NCAs. A sponsor may also wish to seek advice from a specific NCA where it is planned to run a clinical trial to facilitate approval of the forthcoming CTA application. In contrast to the situation in the USA where the FDA is responsible for reviewing the IND and the BLA/NDA, in the EU, the review of CTAs is the responsibility of individual NCAs, whereas the EMA is responsible for the review of the MAA submitted through the centralized procedure. If advice is sought, then sponsors should consider whether advice is required at a pan-EU level from the EMA and/or at a country level from one or more NCA. For example, a sponsor might plan to seek advice from an NCA where it is planned to conduct a first-in-human study with the aim of facilitating the review by that authority. Later in the product development, it might be more appropriate to seek advice on the design of a pivotal Phase 3 trial from the EMA especially if there is something novel about the trial design, a lack of guidance, or some planned deviation from EMA guidance. The minutes from scientific advice meetings, whether EMA or national, are required to be included in the CTA application, and any deviation from the advice received may need to be justified either proactively in the application or if questions arise during the review.

Submitting a CTA in the EU

A sponsor planning to conduct a clinical trial in the EU will select one or more European countries for participation by conducting a feasibility assessment that evaluates a wide range of factors including identification of suitable investigators and sites and availability of patients meeting the planned inclusion and exclusion criteria for the trial. Since the access to medicines and standard of care can vary between countries, this can sometimes influence the feasibility assessment.

Once the countries have been selected, a first step is to evaluate the specific document requirements and procedures of the NCA and Ethics Committees (EC) in each MS to plan the CTA submission. As discussed earlier, the exact requirements will vary by MS because the CTDir has not been implemented in a harmonized fashion. In addition to various administrative documents and country-specific required documents, the core package submitted to all NCAs includes the protocol, investigator's brochure (IB), and the Investigational Medicinal Product Dossier (IMPD). The IMPD includes information on the quality of any IMP in the trial as well as relevant nonclinical and clinical data that is available. An overall benefit-risk assessment for the trial should also be included unless already included in the protocol. The possibility also exists to cross-refer to the nonclinical and clinical data summarized in the IB. CTA submissions are not made in eCTD, but sections of the IMPD typically follow a CTD headings with the quality information presented like Module 3 of the CTD.

The CTDir states that assessment of a valid request for clinical trial authorization by the NCA be carried out as rapidly as possible and may not exceed 60 calendar days. The procedure will involve a validation phase to check all the necessary documentation has been provided and is clear. This is followed by the review phase, and usually the NCA will issue a list of questions ("Grounds for Non-Acceptance") requiring adequate responses prior to approval. The exact timelines and procedures vary by MS and are also influenced by the potential for "clock stops" when a sponsor is given additional time to respond to questions.

Typically, the regulatory and ethics procedures run in parallel, and a sponsor may not start the trial in a MS until a favorable opinion is received from both the NCA and the EC.

Voluntary Harmonization Procedure (VHP)

For a MN-CT, the sponsor has a choice of regulatory pathway, either submitting separate CTAs in each MS via the relevant national procedures, as previously described, or requesting assessment via a Voluntary Harmonization Procedure (VHP). The decision to use VHP versus multiple national procedures should be made on a case-by-case basis. The benefits of a single, harmonized procedure may be attractive especially for trials involving many countries where there may be significant operational benefits and the possibility of achieving a harmonized outcome according to a single well-defined timetable. The CTFG particularly rec-ommends use of the VHP for the review of CTAs for MN-CTs with a complex design. However, the VHP is not without its challenges, including very short timelines (10 days) for the response to questions, and overall VHP can be slower than the national procedure in certain countries.

The VHP consists of three phases (not to be confused with clinical trial phases). In Phase 1, the sponsor requests assessment via VHP, and validation of the applica-tion takes place. It is important to remember the "voluntary" nature of the procedure, and individual NCAs can decline to participate, and in that scenario, the sponsor must default to submission via the standard national procedures in that country. If a sponsor requests VHP, then all EU NCAs planned to be involved should be included in the request, and the sponsor should not mix between the national route and VHP, unless advised to do so by the regulators. Sponsors are required to nominate a Reference-NCA (REF-NCA) in the VHP request. The REF-NCA is responsible for leading the scientific assessment in collaboration with the participating-NCA (P-NCA).

Phase 2 of VHP is the assessment step led by the REF-NCA, and it's usual to receive a consolidated list of questions (or "Grounds for Non-Acceptance") on day 32 after the procedure starts. Sponsors have 10 calendar days to respond to ques-tions. Following receipt of the sponsors' response, the REF-NCA continues the assessment with input from the P-NCA. Depending on the acceptability of the response, the Phase 2 will conclude between around 56 and 78 days following the start of the procedure.

Phase 3 of VHP is the "national step" that formally concludes the CTA review according to the requirements of the CTDir. This national step does not include further scientific evaluation of the benefit-risk or quality aspects of investigational medicinal product that were assessed during Phase 2 of VHP. Instead the focus is on national aspects of the CTA, for example, clinical trial labels in national language, ICF, or EC approval letter.

Maintaining the Clinical Trial Authorization

Amendments
The CTDir allows a clinical trial to be amended after it has started, and amendments can be classified as non-substantial or substantial. An amendment to a trial is considered substantial if the changes are likely to have a significant impact on the safety or physical or mental integrity of trial participants or on the scientific value of the trial. Guidance on what is typically considered substantial or not is found in the European Commission communication 2010/C 82/01 (CT-1), and it is the sponsor's responsibility to assess any planned amendment on a case-by-case basis. A substan-tial amendment must be submitted for review and can only be implemented once the necessary NCA and/or EC approvals have been received. Non-substantial amend-ments should be documented internally within the sponsor's records and submitted with the next substantial amendment.

Mechanisms also exist for sponsors to implement urgent safety measures, to protect patients in trials, without the need for approval of a substantial amendment and for a follow-up submission to be made.

Other Maintenance Activities

Sponsors are required to notify NCAs with respect to end of trial and to provide within 1 year (or 6 months for pediatric trials) the results of a trial in a clinical trial report. Usually, this requirement is met providing either clinical study report (CSR) synopsis or the full CSR depending on the MS.

Safety Reporting and Annual Reporting

Safety of patients participating in clinical trials is paramount, and sponsors are required to notify NCAs of life-threatening suspected unexpected serious adverse reactions (SUSARs) as soon as possible and in any case no later than 7 days after becoming aware of the case. Other nonlife- threatening SUSARs can be reported as soon as possible but no later than 15 days after becoming aware of the case.

The requirement for an Annual Safety Report is met by submission of the Development Safety Update Report (DSUR) following adoption in the EU of the ICH guideline E2F on development safety update report. The DSUR is an annual review and evaluation of safety information and describes new issues that may impact the overall development program or specific clinical trials. The DSUR describes known and potential risks and evaluates the impact of new safety information on the clinical development.

Implementation of the Clinical Trials Regulation (CTReg)

When the CTReg becomes applicable, it will replace the CTDir and aspects of the national legislation in each MS that implemented the CTDir. A key benefit of the regulation will be a harmonized electronic submission and assessment process for clinical trials conducted in multiple MS. Submissions to the NCAs and ECs will take place via a new Clinical Trials Information System that includes a submission "portal." The CTA application will be subject to separate parallel scientific (Part I) and ethical reviews (Part I). Part I is led by a reporting member state (RMS) in coordination with the other concerned member states (CMS). Part II is the national ethical assessment conducted independently in each MS, and national laws will still apply for many documents submitted in Part II. It will be up to the individual MS to determine exactly how to involve the NCA and EC in Part I and Part II of the assessments to reach a single decision by country. Timelines will be harmonized, and assuming no validation questions but questions during the review, then the overall assessment time will be 106 days. Some parallels with the VHP are evident although the CTReg takes harmonization and collaboration between MS much further.

The CTReg's full implementation relies entirely on the full functionality of the portal, but due to technical difficulties, testing of the portal was still ongoing as of June 2019, and it seems unlikely that implementation will occur before 2020. The portal will deliver secure workspaces for both sponsors and authorities and will facilitate all interactions between them. The CTReg will become applicable 6 months after the portal is confirmed as achieving full functionality through independent audit. Following implementation, a 3-year transition period will start; during the first year, CTAs can be submitted under the old CTDir or the new CTReg systems. The VHP will no longer be an option for new CTAs immediately once the CTReg is implemented. During years 2 and 3, trials authorized under the CTDir can remain under that system, while new CTAs must be submitted under the CTReg systems. Finally, after 3 years, all trials must switch to the new CTReg system.

Other important aspects of the CTReg will be to simplify safety reporting and to support the continued drive for transparency of clinical trial data in the EU, and increasingly there will be proactive publication of clinical trial information via the clinical trial information system. The implementation of the CTReg will present sponsors, NCAs, and ECs with many challenges and will not entirely remove the complexities associated with conducting a MN-CT in the EU. However, it can be hoped that if the goals of the CTReg are achieved, a more favorable environment for conducting trials in the EU will result and ultimately facilitate the development of new medicines for patients.

Regulatory Affairs Considerations for Clinical Trials in Other Countries

In addition to the detail discussed pertaining to the USA and EU, there are many regulatory considerations regarding the conduct of clinical trials in other countries. Some countries (e.g., China, South Korea, India, Russia) require that, in order to achieve marketing authorization, patients from that country must be included in clinical trials submitted within the marketing authorization application. This requirement can be at least partly due to concerns about ethnic differences in how a drug may be metabolized or a result of notable differences in overall patient care between the studied countries compared to the country with local data requirements. While each country has their own review process and procedures to assess the safety and appropriateness of a proposed new clinical trial, most follow the same basic structure. This basic structure typically starts with the sponsor submitting a clinical trial application containing multifunctional information spanning manufacturing, preclinical, and clinical. Next, the local regulator reviews the submitted application and may issue questions to be answered by the sponsor within a defined period of time. Finally, if successful, the regulator will approve the proposed clinical trial to be conducted in that country.

There are additions and exceptions to this basic structure, which a global sponsor needs to develop the capabilities to understand and anticipate. An example can be found in Japan, where the Pharmaceuticals and Medical Devices Agency (PMDA) is the regulator with purview over clinical trial applications and marketing authorization applications. In Japan, the sponsor typically plans to meet with PMDA prior to submitting the clinical trial application for a consultation with PMDA to advise on the overall acceptability of the basic proposal for the new clinical trial (e.g., checks whether a proposed clinical trial complies with the requirements for regulatory submission).

During the clinical trial planning, the regulations for all countries selected by the sponsor to be included in the recruitment for study volunteers must be taken into account to enable timely approval and initiation of the trial in the given country. In particular, if a country with local data requirements for marketing authorization is not included in the clinical development of the product, it is likely that additional, dedicated studies may need to be conducted if the sponsor aims to have marketing authorization in that country. Unfortunately, it is not uncommon that the conduct of these additional, dedicated studies can lead to years-long delays in access to the new treatment in that country. Therefore, up-front planning leveraging regulatory acumen and guidance is critical to the success of enabling global approval and access to new medicines.

Summary

Regardless of country or region, the need for sophisticated regulatory strategy is a critical component of the development of any drug candidate. While some rules and regulations seem clear and simply the subject of wrought memorization or ability to research and reference, most drug development decisions span beyond what is written in "black and white." Beyond coming to an agreement with a particular regulatory authority on a complex topic, sponsors are often also tasked with integrating differing advice and procedures from regulators globally. This frequently proves to be very challenging and can even slow the development of a promising new drug candidate. However, this divergence can also be a motivator behind what can result in some of the best examples of innovation. Regardless of how divergent the views of individual regulators and sponsors may be, the betterment of patients' health is always the shared goal. Accordingly, the regulatory affairs professional's ability to maintain focus on the patient as the end goal is what will ultimately drive innovative solutions to complex drug development challenges.

Cross-References

- ► ClinicalTrials.gov
- ► Cluster Randomized Trials
- ► Consent forms and Procedures
- ► Data and Safety Monitoring and Reporting
- ► Data Capture, Data Management, and Quality Control; Single Versus Multicenter Trials
- ► End of Trial and Close Out of Data Collection
- ► Evolution of Clinical Trials Science
- ► Good Clinical Practice
- ► Implementing the Trial Protocol

► International Trials
► Investigator Responsibilities
► Multicenter and Network Trials
► Participant Recruitment, Screening, and Enrollment
► Post-approval Regulatory Requirements
► Reporting Biases

References

Clinical Trial Regulation (CTReg) EU No. 536/2014. Available via European Commission. https://ec.europa.eu/health/sites/health/files/files/eudralex/vol-1/reg_2014_536/reg_2014_536_en.pdf. Accessed 02 Sept 2019

Clinical Trials Directive (CTDir), Directive 2001/20/EC. Available via European Commission. https://ec.europa.eu/health/sites/health/files/files/eudralex/vol-1/dir_2001_20/dir_2001_20_en.pdf. Accessed 02 Sept 2019

Code of Federal Regulations. Available via Electronic Code of Federal Regulations (e-CFR). https://www.ecfr.gov/cgi-bin/ECFR?page=browse. Accessed 02 Sept 2019

European Commission communication 2010/C 82/01 (CT-1). Available via European Commission. https://eur-lex.europa.eu/LexUriServ/LexUriServ.do?uri=OJ:C:2010:082:0001:0019:EN:PDF. Accessed 02 Sept 2019

Sect. 505(d) of the Food, Drug and Cosmetic (FD&C) Act. Available via FDA webpage on FD&C Act Chap. V: Drugs and Devices. https://www.fda.gov/regulatory-information/federal-food-drug-and-cosmetic-act-fdc-act/fdc-act-chapter-v-drugs-and-devices#Part_A. Accessed 02 Sept 2019

ClinicalTrials.gov

25

Gillian Gresham

Contents

Abstract

ClinicalTrials.gov is a federally supported, web-based clinical trials registry maintained by the United States (US) National Library of Medicine (NLM) at the National Institutes of Health (NIH). It is available to health care professionals, researchers, patients, and the public. Since its launch in 2000, over 325,000 clinical research studies have been registered in ClinicalTrials.gov. Unlike other clinical trial registries and databases, clinical trials registration for certain types of clinical trials is mandated by law under Section 801 of the US Food and Drug Administration Amendments Act (FDAAA 801). There are several components that make up the ClinicalTrials.gov registration process, including trial registration itself, results reporting, and the download and analysis of the ClinicalTrials.gov content.

G. Gresham (✉)
Samuel Oschin Comprehensive Cancer Institute, Cedars-Sinai Medical Center, Los Angeles, CA, USA
e-mail: gillian.gresham@cshs.org

© Springer Nature Switzerland AG 2022   479
S. Piantadosi, C. L. Meinert (eds.), *Principles and Practice of Clinical Trials*,
https://doi.org/10.1007/978-3-319-52636-2_266

While the previous chapter focuses on clinical trials registration in general, this chapter pertains to clinical trials registered in ClinicalTrials.gov. This chapter provides an overview of the history of ClinicalTrials.gov, a description of the trials currently registered in ClinicalTrials.gov, and a review of the Federal Requirements for Registration in the United States. A summary of the registration process, trial reporting, and data analysis procedures follows. The chapter concludes with an overview of the limitations associated with the analysis and reporting of ClinicalTrials.gov registration data.

Keywords

Clinical trials registration · ClinicalTrials.gov · Clinical trial · Interventional study · Clinical trials database · Results reporting

ClinicalTrials.gov: History

Trial registration and its regulation in the United States, as we know it today, has evolved and expanded over the last 30 years. Key events and policies related to the ClinicalTrials.gov are illustrated in the historical timeline (Fig. 1). ClinicalTrials.gov definitions are consistent with those provided by the NIH and are listed in an online glossary as part of the ClinicalTrials.gov website: https://clinicaltrials.gov/ct2/about-studies/glossary. Some key definitions from the glossary are transcribed in Table 1.

International calls for trial registration first emerged in the late 1980s in response to increasing awareness of publication and reporting biases (Dickersin 1990; Simes 1986). In 1986, Simes demonstrated the value of an international registry for clinical trials using two case examples in ovarian cancer and multiple myeloma (Simes 1986). Simultaneous calls for registration were published at the turn of the twenty-first century, providing additional examples of reporting biases and arguments for the need for a comprehensive, prospective trial registry (Dickersin 1990; Dickersin and Rennie 2003; Piantadosi 2017).

In 1997, the first Federal law to require trial registration was passed under Section 113 of the Food and Drugs Administration Modernization Act (FDAMA) related to data bank containing information on privately or federally funded trials being conducted under investigational new drug applications for serious or life-threating disease and conditions:

"A registry of clinical trials (whether federally or privately funded) of experimental treatments for serious or life-threatening diseases and conditions under regulations promulgated pursuant to section 505(i) of the Federal Food, Drug, and Cosmetic Act, which provides a description of the purpose of each experimental drug, either with the consent of the protocol sponsor, or when a trial to test effectiveness begins. Information provided shall consist of eligibility criteria for participation in the clinical trials, a description of the location of trial sites, and a point of contact for those wanting to enroll in the trial, and shall be in a form that can be readily understood by members of the public. Such information shall be forwarded to the data bank by the sponsor of the trial not later than 21 days after the approval of the protocol."

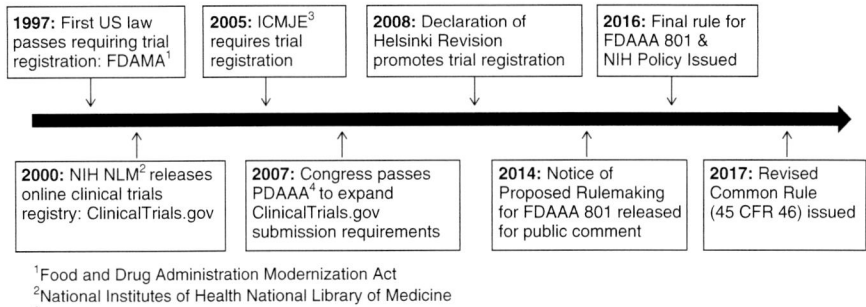

[1]Food and Drug Administration Modernization Act
[2]National Institutes of Health National Library of Medicine
[3]International Committee of Journal Editors
[4]Food and Drug Administration Amendments Act

Fig. 1 ClinicalTrials.gov timeline

Table 1 Selected terms and definitions used on ClinicalTrials.gov

Term	ClinicalTrials.gov definition
Clinical study	*A research study involving human volunteers (also called participants) that is intended to add to medical knowledge. There are two types of clinical studies: interventional studies (also called clinical trials) and observational studies*
Interventional study (clinical trial)	*A type of clinical study in which participants are assigned to groups that receive one or more intervention/treatment (or no intervention) so that researchers can evaluate the effects of the interventions on biomedical or health-related outcomes. The assignments are determined by the study's protocol. Participants may receive diagnostic, therapeutic, or other types of interventions*
Observational study	*A type of clinical study in which participants are identified as belonging to study groups and are assessed for biomedical or health outcomes. Participants may receive diagnostic, therapeutic, or other types of interventions, but the investigator does not assign participants to a specific interventions/treatment*
Expanded access	*A way for patients with serious diseases or conditions who cannot participate in a clinical trial to gain access to a medical product that has not been approved by the US Food and Drug Administration (FDA). Also called compassionate use. There are different expanded access types*
ClinicalTrials.gov identifier (NCT number)	*The unique identification code given to each clinical study upon registration at ClinicalTrials.gov. The format is "NCT" followed by an 8-digit number (e.g., NCT00000419)*
Funder type	*Describes the organization that provides funding or support for a clinical study. This support may include activities related to funding, design, implementation, data analysis, or reporting. Organizations listed as sponsors and collaborators for a study are considered the funders of the study*
Sponsor	*The organization or person who initiates the study and who has authority and control over the study*

(continued)

Table 1 (continued)

Term	ClinicalTrials.gov definition
Collaborator	*An organization other than the sponsor that provides support for a clinical study. This support may include activities related to funding, design, implementation, data analysis, or reporting*
Phase	*The stage of a clinical trial studying a drug or biological product, based on definitions developed by the US Food and Drug Administration (FDA). The phase is based on the study's objective, the number of participants, and other characteristics. There are five phases: early phase 1 (formerly listed as phase 0), phase 1, phase 2, phase 3, and phase 4. Not applicable is used to describe trials without FDA-defined phases, including trials of devices or behavioral interventions*
Phase 1	*A phase of research to describe clinical trials that focus on the safety of a drug. They are usually conducted with healthy volunteers, and the goal is to determine the drug's most frequent and serious adverse events and, often, how the drug is broken down and excreted by the body. These trials usually involve a small number of participants*
Phase 2	*A phase of research to describe clinical trials that gather preliminary data on whether a drug works in people who have a certain condition/disease (i.e., the drug's effectiveness). For example, participants receiving the drug may be compared to similar participants receiving a different treatment, usually an inactive substance (called a placebo) or a different drug. Safety continues to be evaluated, and short-term adverse events are studied*
Phase 3	*A phase of research to describe clinical trials that gather more information about a drug's safety and effectiveness by studying different populations and different dosages and by using the drug in combination with other drugs. These studies typically involve more participants*
Phase 4	*A phase of research to describe clinical trials occurring after FDA has approved a drug for marketing. They include postmarket requirement and commitment studies that are required of or agreed to by the study sponsor. These trials gather additional information about a drug's safety, efficacy, or optimal use*
Phase not applicable	*Describes trials without FDA-defined phases, including trials of devices or behavioral interventions*

All definitions transcribed from the ClinicalTrials.gov glossary available at: https://clinicaltrials.gov/ct2/about-studies/glossary

The 1997 FDAMA law resulted in the subsequent release of ClinicalTrials.gov in 2000 by the National Institutes of Health NLM as the primary registry for federally and privately funded trials conducted in the United States. At the time of its launch, ClincialTrials.gov included information on over 4000 medical studies in over 47,000 locations across the United States (Zarin et al. 2017a). The launch of ClinicalTrials.

gov was followed by FDA guidance for Industry, issued in 2002 and withdrawn by the FDA in September 2017 (US guidance for industry 2002).

In 2004, the International Committee of Medical Journal Editors (ICMJE) implemented a policy that required registration of all clinical trials as a condition of consideration for publication (De Angelis et al. 2004). The policy applies to any trial that started enrollment after July 1, 2005, where registration must occur before patient enrollment and requires registration of trials by September 13, 2005, for those that began enrollment before July 1, 2005. The ICMJE registration policy represents an important landmark for trial registration, where a significant increase in trial registration occurred after its implementation (Zarin et al. 2017a).

The World Health Organization (WHO) established a trial registration policy shortly after, in 2006, releasing a minimum trial registration dataset of 20 items (Appendix 10.12.) Additional information regarding the history of the development of the WHO International Clinical Trials Registry Platform (ICTRP) is described in the previous Chapter on "Trial Registration" Chap. 3.2. Additional international efforts by the World Medical Association (WMA) to encourage trial registration were made in 2008 at the 59th WMA General Assembly in Seoul, Republic of Korea. At this time, the Declaration of Helsinki was amended to include trial registration requirements initially outlined in Sections 19 and 30 (World Medical Association 2013). These principles were again modified and re-ordered in 2013 at the 64th WMA General Assembly, now corresponding to Sections 35 and 36 (World Medical Association 2013). Section 35 indicates that every research study involving human subjects should be registered in a public database, while Section 36 raises the ethical obligation to publish and disseminate the results of research regardless of whether the findings are statistically significant or "negative or inconclusive" (Appendix 10.3). While not legally binding, the Declaration of Helsinki has increased recognition and awareness of the importance and ethical obligations of trial registration, especially among physicians conducting research in human subjects.

The Food and Drug Administration Amendments Act (FDAAA) of 2007 became one of the most important and influential policies for trial registration in the United States. The FDAAA Public Law 110-85 was passed by Congress on September 27, 2007, and expanded registration and reporting requirements for ClinicalTrials.gov. Such requirements, as detailed in Section 801 of FDAA, included expanding the clinical trial registration information for applicable clinical trials and adding a results database (FDAAA 801). The law also mandated submission of results for applicable clinical trials of drug, biologics, and devices that were approved, cleared, or licensed by the FDA. The law includes the requirement that the responsible party of an applicable clinical trial must submit results within 1 year of data collection including summary results of the demographic and baseline characteristics, primary and secondary outcomes, points of contact, and agreements. Submission of adverse events, including frequent and serious adverse events, was not required by law until 2009 (FDA 801). Finally, the FDAAA law of 2007 introduced civil penalties of "not more than $10,000 for each day of the violation after such period until the violation is corrected" (FDAAA 801).

The FDAAA Section 801 was modified and released in September 2016, expanding on definition of the clinical trial and providing additional requirements regarding trial registration and reporting (Zarin et al. 2016). The NIH simultaneously issued a policy, requiring that all NIH-funded trials should be registered regardless of whether they are covered under FDAAA 801 requirements.

ClinicalTrials.gov: Content and Features

Characteristics of Trials Registered in ClinicalTrials.gov

A summary of the registration process itself, trial reporting, and data analysis will then be provided.

ClinicalTrials.gov includes clinical trials being conducted in 207 countries, with over a third being conducted in the United States only, half outside of the United States, and the rest in both the United States and non-US countries. Study locations were not specified in 12% of the registered trials. ClinicalTrials.gov is a living database that is constantly being updated with new studies as well as undergoing modifications and revisions to the study records as well as to the site itself. Therefore, counts will vary with time, and the following summary of characteristics of trials registered reflects trial counts completed as of December 31, 2019. Overall, there were 325,860 studies registered in ClinicalTrials.gov of which 256,924 (79%) were interventional, 67,486 (19%) were observational, and 601 were expanded access. Types of interventions include drugs or biologics (59%), behavioral interventions (31%), surgical procedures (10.5%), and devices (12.5%). Among the registered trials, 175,691 were completed to date (December 31, 2019). Trials can also be characterized by lead sponsor, where industry was lead sponsor for 106,775 trials as of December 31, 2019, the US Federal Government including NIH was lead sponsor for 37,706 trials, and all other funding sources were lead sponsor for 184,040 trials. While industry tends to fund larger, randomized drug intervention trials, the NIH focuses on smaller, early development studies (Gresham et al. 2018; Ehrhardt et al. 2015). An increasing number of behavioral trials funded by NIH have also been observed in the last 10 years, which may include exercise and nutritional studies.

ClinicalTrials.gov Website Content

ClinicalTrials.gov is an online resource maintained by the NLM with a target audience of health-care professionals, researchers, patients, and the general public. Information and resources for different users are integrated throughout the website links. The home page includes a search bar for users to find trials by recruitment status, condition or disease, other terms (e.g., NCT identification number, investigator, drug name), and country. An advanced search allows users to further filter their search by trial type, intervention, outcome measure, eligibility criteria, location, phase, funder type, and recruitment status. The menu at the top of the page includes five tabs: "Find Studies," "About Studies," "Submit Studies," "Resources," and "About Site." Within the "Find studies" menu, users can access a map of the studies and information on how to search for studies as well as how to use, find, and read a study record. The "About Studies" tab provides information about the studies, a list of additional websites about studies, and the glossary of common terms. Resources for administrators including registration guidelines help with registering the studies; support and training materials as well as FAQs can be found under the "Submit Studies" tab. A "Resources" tab includes a list of selected publications, clinical trials alerts, RSS feeds, the metadata for ClinicalTrials.gov, and information on downloading ClinicalTrials.gov content for analysis. Finally, the top menu includes additional information about the site where readers can learn more about the history of ClinicalTrials.gov; the history, policy, and laws surrounding trials registration; and the terms and conditions of the site. An additional link to the Protocol Registration and Results System (PRS) site is available for administrators and study sponsors/investigators to access and register their trials. To access the PRS site, users must have a PRS account linked to their organization name, username, and password. More information on this will be provided in a later section.

Clinical trials are organized by the ClinicalTrials.gov study identification number (NCT number) which is unique to each trial registered. Every study record includes the NCT number, which is listed at the top of the record along with the study title, key dates (e.g., First posted, Results first posted, Last update), and names of the sponsors, collaborators, and responsible party. Every record also includes a disclaimer that states the following:

> The safety and scientific validity of this study is the responsibility of the study sponsor and investigators. Listing a study does not mean it has been evaluated by the U.S. Federal Government. Read our disclaimer for details.

Each trial record includes the ICMJE/WHO minimum 20-item Trial Data Set (Appendix 10.12). Trial information is organized by tabs including "Study Details," "Tabular View," and "Study Results." Additional links to the disclaimer and resources for patients on how to read and interpret a study record are also available. The "Study Details" divides trial information by section: study description, study design, arms and interventions, outcome measures, eligibility criteria, contacts and locations, and more information (e.g., publications). Related citations are automatically identified from the NLM and added to the publication tab using the study identification number (NCT number) and updated directly to the publications field.

The tabular view provides the same information as listed in the "Study Details" page with some additional features and links. Links to study documents (e.g., protocol, consent forms) can be accessed and downloaded, if available. A "Change History" link also exists, where a complete list of historical versions for the specific study is available and posted to the ClinicalTrials.gov archive site. When applicable, study results are posted under the results tab and organized by baseline table, primary outcome measures, secondary outcome measures, and adverse events by treatment group (Section 5.3).

ClinicalTrials.gov: Registration and Results Reporting

Registering a Trial in ClinicalTrials.gov

Trial registration is required by law if it fits the definition of an "applicable clinical trial," as defined in the Final Rule (42 CFR Part 11) and under the FDAAA Act of 2007, Section 801. A checklist for determining whether a trial is considered an "applicable trial" is available online at https://prsinfo.clinicaltrials.gov/Voluntary SubmissionFlowchartChecklist.pdf.

To register a clinical trial, a ClinicalTrials.gov PRS account must first be requested if one does not already exist for the organization from which the trial is being registered. One PRS account per organization is established, for which investigators and administrators from that organization can subsequently be added. Once a PRS account has been created, the responsible party for the trial, defined as the "sponsor of the trial unless and until a principal investigator has been designated the responsible party in accordance with 42 CFR 11.4(c) (2)," can register their trial. Only one record per trial should be created. Trial registration must occur within 21 days after enrollment of the first trial participant and posted to the public within 30 days after initial submission (Zarin et al. 2016).

Initial registration of the trial in ClinicalTrials.gov involves provision of the study title, description, study type (interventional, observational, or expanded access), and status (e.g., recruiting, completed, withdrawn, etc.). Specification of the study start date, primary completion, and study completion dates must also be provided. These dates may be actual or anticipated, depending on the study status. Details on the sponsors and collaborators follow in addition information regarding the study oversight, such as details on the US FDA-regulated drug and IND number (if applicable), the name and information of the human subjects review board, and the corresponding human subjects review board's approval number.

A brief and detailed summary of the study that includes the purpose and general information of the study is included along with a selection of MeSH terms for conditions and keywords. Details on the study design (type, phase, number of arms, masking, allocation, and enrollment) and a description of the study arms and interventions follow. Eligibility criteria for the trial must be provided, with separate fields for age, sex, and acceptance of healthy volunteers included.

One of the most important data elements to be registered is the study outcomes and secondary outcomes. ClinicalTrials.gov requires detailed specification of the outcome title, description, and timeframe or the specific timepoint at which the study participant is assessed for that measure (Zarin et al. 2016). Some general data entry tips for each data entry element, as obtained from the PRS information pages, have been summarized in Table 2.

Table 2 Data entry tips for common data elements entered in ClinicalTrials.gov

Data element	Definition	Data entry tips
Study status	**Overall recruitment status:** *the recruitment status for the clinical study as a whole, based upon the status of the individual sites* **Study start date:** *the estimated date on which the clinical study will be open for recruitment of participants, or the actual date on which the first participant was enrolled* **Primary completion date:** *the date that the final participant was examined or received an intervention for the purposes of final collection of data for the primary outcome, whether the clinical study concluded according to the pre-specified protocol or was terminated* **Study completion date:** *the date the final participant was examined or received an intervention for purposes of final collection of data for the primary and secondary outcome measures and adverse events (e.g., last participant's last visit), whether the clinical study concluded according to the pre-specified protocol or was terminated*	Study status can alternate between the following: *Not yet recruiting: participants are not yet being recruited* *Recruiting: participants are currently being recruited, whether or not any participants have yet been enrolled* *Enrolling by invitation: participants are being (or will be) selected from a predetermined population* *Active, not recruiting: study is continuing, meaning participants are receiving an intervention or being examined, but new participants are not currently being recruited or enrolled* *Completed: the study has concluded normally; participants are no longer receiving an intervention or being examined* *Suspended: study halted prematurely but potentially will resume* *Terminated: study halted prematurely and will not resume; participants are no longer being examined or receiving intervention* *Withdrawn: study halted prematurely, prior to enrollment of first participant* If the trial registered is multisite and one of the individual sites is recruiting, then the overall recruitment status for the study must also be "recruiting" Once the first patient is enrolled, the study start date should be updated to include the actual date Once the study has reached the study completion date, the study completion date should be updated to reflect the actual study completion date
Study description	***Brief summary:*** *a short description of the clinical study, including a brief statement of the clinical study's hypothesis, written in language intended for the lay public.* ***Detailed description:*** *extended*	The brief summary should be brief and written for a lay audience (limit 5000 characters) The detailed description can include more technical information The detailed description should not

(continued)

Table 2 (continued)

Data element	Definition	Data entry tips
	description of the protocol, including more technical information compared to the brief description	include the entire protocol nor should it duplicate information that is already recorded in other data elements (limit 32,000 characters)
Study design	*Study design: a description of the manner in which the clinical trial will be conducted, including the following information: primary purpose*	Primary purpose can be selected from drop-down menu and includes treatment, prevention, diagnostic, supportive care, screening, health services research, basic science, and device feasibility The study phase should be selected based on the NIH definitions (Table 1) The interventional study model may include single group, parallel, crossover, factorial, or sequential All the roles that are masked should be indicated including participant, care provider, investigator, outcomes assessor, or open-label (no masking) Study allocation can be randomized or non-randomized. Note that quasi-randomized is not a true form of randomization Anticipated enrollment should be specified based on the primary outcome power calculation. Once the study is complete, the actual enrollment should be updated
Arms and interventions	*Arm: a pre-specified group or subgroup of participants in a clinical trial assigned to receive specific interventions (or no intervention)* *Intervention: a process or action that is the focus of a clinical study*	The arm title should be concise, but allow for easy distinction from one arm to another The arm definition is selected from a drop-down menu and includes experimental; active comparator; placebo comparator; sham comparator; no intervention; other If the intervention is a drug, the generic name should be used as well as the dosage form, dose, frequency, and duration Intervention type is selected from a drop-down menu and can include drug, device, biological/vaccine, procedure/surgery, radiation, behavioral, genetic, dietary supplement, combination product, diagnostic test, or other If conducting an observational study, intervention name can be used to identify the intervention or exposure of interest

(continued)

Table 2 (continued)

Data element	Definition	Data entry tips
Eligibility criteria	*The eligibility module specifies the criteria for determining which people are (or are not) eligible to participate in the study*	Enter age limits, if applicable. Otherwise, enter "N/A (no limit)" from a drop-down menu Sex refers to the classification of male or female based on biological distinctions, with drop-down of "all," "male only," and "female only" Gender refers to the person's self-representation of gender identity. If applicable, a user can indicate that eligibility is based on gender in addition to descriptive information about gender criteria When entering eligibility criteria, include headings for the inclusion and exclusion criteria followed by a bulleted list under each heading
Outcome measures	***Primary outcome****: the outcome measure(s) of greatest importance specified in the protocol, usually the one(s) used in the power calculation. Most clinical studies have one primary outcome measure, but a clinical study may have more than one*	When specifying an outcome, include the specific domain, method of aggregation, specific metric, and timepoint Do not use acronyms Each outcome measure should be presented separately, regardless of whether they share the same metric If using a scale or questionnaire, specify the number of items, how they are scored, the minimum and maximum ranges, and how the scores are interpreted

Definitions and information obtained from: https://register.clinicaltrials.gov/prs/html/definitions. html

It is the responsibility of the record owner to maintain and update the clinical trial information within the required timepoints in accordance with Section 801 of FDAAA and 42 CFR 11.64. Records for active studies are required to be updated at least once a year with some data elements requiring more frequent updates. Once the record has been reviewed for accuracy and modified as necessary, the verification date will be updated, and the responsible party/PRS administrator can approve and release the record.

Reporting Results in ClinicalTrials.gov

The ClinicalTrials.gov registry provides access to study results, regardless of whether they have been published. While all registered trials may submit their study results to ClinicalTrials.gov, results for applicable clinical trials, as previously defined, are required by the FDAAA to be submitted within 1 year after the trial's primary completion date (date that the final subject was examined or received the intervention for the purposes of final data collection for the primary outcome). Trials that are not considered "applicable clinical trials" (Non-ACT) are not required to submit results, such as Phase 1 trials, feasibility, or observational studies. However, under the NIH Policy, any trial that meets the NIH definition for clinical trial and is funded in whole or in part by the NIH must provide summary results.

As of December 31, 2019, a search of the ClinicalTrials.gov registry identified 41,074 studies (interventional or observational) with posted results. This has increased dramatically from the 2,178 records with results identified in September 2010 and 23,000 in 2016, probably as a result of the expanded FDAAA reporting requirements (Zarin et al. 2011, 2016). It is anticipated that this number will continue to grow as more applicable trials are completed after the January 18, 2017 implementation date. Understanding and training in the results submission process will become more important to ensure timely and accurate data entry.

Results Submission Process

Results are entered and submitted using the PRS results page in a similar fashion to the registration process. Results can be entered directly into the interactive tables provided on the results tab or uploaded using XML files. Unlike journal publications, they are not accompanied with detailed narrative text to explain the results (Zarin et al. 2017a). Results are displayed by study arm or comparison group, where applicable, as well as combined totals. In addition to tabulations, statistical comparisons and summary results can be provided for the corresponding outcome data (e.g., within and between group differences). During the preparation of results for submission, it is important that the responsible party works with the study statistician and other investigators to ensure complete and accurate information being entered into the results system.

Results are organized into the following sections: participant flow, baseline characteristics, outcome measures and statistical analyses, and adverse events. The participant flow chart includes a summary of the progress of trial participants, by comparison group, if applicable. The purpose of the flow chart is similar to that of a CONSORT flow diagram, where it displays the number of participants at each stage or study time interval (e.g., screening, randomization, treatment, study completion, follow-up, etc.) (Appendix 10.5). The second results section to enter is the baseline characteristics, which includes a table of demographic and baseline measures by each comparison group and combined totals. All results will include the total number of participants and the number of participants analyzed for each result at the specified timepoint.

Baseline measures include age (continuous, categorical, or customized), sex or gender, race, and ethnicity, as defined by the NIH Office of Management and Budget (OMB), region of enrollment (e.g., United States, Canada), and study-specific measures. The study-specific measures are customized to the study population and protocol and may include baseline anthropometric measures, clinical and diagnostic characteristics, or other factors specific to the disease or condition under study.

Baseline measures may be summarized as counts, means, median, least squares means, geometric means, numbers, or other. Measures of dispersion should also be included, if applicable, where a standard deviation, standard error, interquartile range, or full range may be provided. The system provides space to add the unit of measure (e.g., lbs., mmHg, participants) and explanation if a particular entry is not applicable.

Results for both primary and secondary outcomes, as defined and pre-specified in study the protocol and registration record, are entered by group along with the result from the statistical analysis for that particular outcome. Each outcome should include the type (mean, median, count, etc.), measure of dispersion/precision (e.g., standard deviation, confidence interval, interquartile range), and number of participants analyzed. Additionally, a description of the statistical test (e.g., superiority, non-inferiority), hypothesis (e.g., p-value), method to calculate p-value (e.g., log rank, ANOVA, regression), estimation parameter (e.g., hazard ratio, mean difference, odds ratio, etc.), and its corresponding dispersion/precision parameter should be included.

The last component of the results reporting system is the adverse events section, which includes a tabular summary of all anticipated or unanticipated serious adverse events, as well as other adverse events that exceed a specific frequency threshold. This information is categorized into three tables including all-cause mortality, serious adverse events, and other adverse events. A checklist and adverse event reporting template are available on the ClinicalTrials.gov Administrative Information Page to assist with the preparation and submission of adverse event results: https://clinicaltrials.gov/ct2/manage-recs/how-report#AdministrativeInformation

Adverse event reporting elements include the description of the adverse event reporting system along with source vocabulary (e.g., MedDRA 10.0, CTCAE 5.0), the collection method (systematic or non-systematic), the title, and description of the adverse event. In the all-cause mortality table, the number of participants that died from any cause and the number of participants that were assessed for death should be included by group. For the serious adverse event table, the number of participants who experienced each AE by adverse event term and organ system must be provided including the number of participants affected, the number at risk (denominator), and the number of events. The time frame, arm description, adverse event collection approach, and all-cause mortality table are required for trials that had primary completion dates after January 18, 2017, as per the updated Final Rule.

A third table for other adverse events can be included for all adverse events (not including serious adverse events) and may be reported based on a frequency threshold of occurrence that the adverse event must exceed. This number must be less than or equal to the allowed maximum of 5% within at least one of the comparison groups.

Once results have been entered, they can be released by the sponsor. They will undergo verification by a PRS administrator, similar to the registration process, and all queries and errors will be identified and addressed, prior to releasing the record to the public.

Quality Control Review of ClinicalTrials.gov Records

All submitted trial records undergo a quality review prior to being released to the public. Quality control review of ClinicalTrials.gov records includes both automated validation rules incorporated within each item for entry and review by PRS staff. Once the responsible party/PRS administrator has released and submitted the initial record, PRS staff reviews the record for completeness and any additional errors, deficiencies, or inconsistencies (ClinicalTrials.gov 2019). Implementation of standard quality control review criteria, standardized review comments, and similar trainer programs across PRS staff ensures consistency of the reviews. Reviews are also audited by other review staff members to ensure proper review of the records. Specific quality control review criteria and accompanying documents are publicly available and can be found under "Support Materials" at the PRS User's Guide and Review material link: https://clinicaltrials.gov/ct2/manage-recs/resources#ReviewCriteria. Review criteria are organized by data entry element, which are categorized within 13 different modules for describing the study protocol. PRS review of the trial registration record is estimated to take between 3 and 5 days for registration and within 30 days for results. Reviewers provide comments throughout the record that address general issues, formatting, and specific notes on the completeness and appropriateness of each data element or result. Comments may be identified as "major" which are required to be corrected or addressed within 15 calendar days or "advisory" which are meant to improve the clarity of the record and can be addressed within 25 days from when the PRS Staff sent notification (ClinicalTrials.gov 2019). While they are able to identify errors in the entry of information, the reviewers are not responsible for ensuring the scientific validity and merit of the trial and cannot confirm that the information is compliant with policy or legal requirements (Tse et al. 2018).

The most common problem identified upon quality review of registration information is incomplete or insufficient information for the primary and secondary outcomes. Common issues encountered when reviewing results include invalid or inconsistent units of measure, insufficient information about scales, internal inconsistencies between different sections in the record, the inclusion of written results or conclusions, and unclear baseline or outcome measure (Tse et al. 2018).

Once PRS comments have been received and addressed, the record owner will resubmit the information for further review and comment. At this point, reviewers may respond with additional comments and suggestions or release the record to the public along with the assigned NCT identification number.

Downloading and Analyzing Content from ClinicalTrials.gov

Downloading Content for Analysis

There are two primary methods for downloading clinical trials content from ClinicalTrials.gov. The first is directly from the ClinicalTrials.gov database, where some search results are available for download. For instance, a search of studies within a particular disease site may be conducted, and the total records or a selection of records from the search can be exported and downloaded to different formats (.csv, XML, plain text, tab-separated values, and PDF). The record for an individual trial can also be downloaded directly from the study record page. The downloaded content includes 20 fields in long format with trials listed by study ID. Exported data types include NCT ID, title, study status, whether results are available, conditions, interventions, outcome measures, phases, sponsors, gender/age, enrollment (sample size), funders, study type (interventional or observational), design, and key dates (start date, completion date, date last updated, etc.). While downloading content directly from ClinicalTrials.gov can be a simple and efficient method to access up to date study information, it is limited to 10,000 records at a time and does not include all registration fields and study results.

The second method for downloading ClinicalTrials.gov content for analysis is through the Clinical Trials Transformation Initiative (CTTI) Aggregate Analysis of ClinicalTrials.Gov (AACT): https://www.ctti-clinicaltrials.org/aact-database. The AACT database contains restructured and aggregated information on Clinical Trials registered in ClinicalTrials.gov that is refreshed daily and available in different formats (e.g., Oracle dmp, Pipe delimited text output, and SAS CPORT transport). It also includes static versions of the databases that are updated monthly and available for download. Access to the cloud-based platform can be accessed upon free registration and download of the required programs: https://aact.ctti-clinicaltrials.org/download. The AACT database is a relational database linked by NCT ID and organized by trial registration fields and categories. A comprehensive data dictionary and schema are available on the website at the following link: https://aact.ctti-clinicaltrials.org/schema. Data in the AACT database have been cleaned, sorted, and created with additional calculated fields generated to facilitate and improve the analysis of trials. The AACT CTTI database has also integrated the MeSH thesaurus, thus improving search and indexing capabilities. Regardless of the method used to obtain and analyze clinical trials data, it is important to take the limitations of the registries into consideration when interpreting and reporting the results.

Limitations of Analyzing Data from ClinicalTrials.gov

There are several limitations associated with the use and analysis of data from ClinicalTrials.gov. First of all, the analysis is based on the assumption that all trials are registered (Zarin et al. 2017b; Gresham et al. 2018). Although registration has significantly improved over time, especially during the last decade, one cannot assume that the studies registered in ClinicalTrials.gov are unbiased representation of the clinical research enterprise (Tse et al. 2018). A recent paper published by Tse et al. (2018) identifies and describes ten common problems encountered when using ClinicalTrials.gov for research (Tse et al. 2018). Some of the key issues raised include the fact that ClinicalTrials.gov includes more than just interventional studies, with approximately 20% of the registered studies being observational and 450 with expanded access records (Tse et al. 2018). Thus an understanding of the definitions and specific registration elements and requirements for each study type is essential.

Trial records may also be incomplete or incorrect, thus leading to potentially inaccurate reports and interpretations of the trial data. For example, missing registration fields, especially for optional data elements, or misclassification of data elements can occur, make it difficult to estimate and compare trends in clinical trials. Incomplete records may also be a result of the changing database elements over time, where the ClinicalTrials.gov structure has evolved since its establishment in 2000 (Zarin et al. 2017b). Mandatory data elements have also been added and modified over time, such as the primary outcome measure data elements and sub-elements (Tse et al. 2018). Data entered in the trial record can also be modified at any time, making it difficult to determine which information is most appropriate for analysis. While the change history of modifications can be accessed, it is difficult to obtain and download previous versions of the trial record for analysis. Furthermore, while review of the quality review of the trial record and results is performed, it does not include verification of the scientific merit and validity of the information (Zarin et al. 2007).

Finally, an increasing problem includes duplicate registrations of clinical trials, which can occur within ClinicalTrials.gov or across different trial registries (e.g., ICTRP). Duplicates within the ClinicalTrials.gov database are often a result of follow-on or expansion studies being registered as separate records (Tse et al. 2018). There is currently no automated way to identify duplicates, although searches of the trial titles and acronyms, summaries, and eligibility can be used to identify similar records. As a result of a growing number of international trial registries, there are also duplicate registrations across multiple registries, where almost 45% of duplicates go unobserved or undetected (van Valkenhoef et al. 2016). There are currently no methods for identifying identical trials across registries, thus distorting and overestimating the number of trials registered. Prevention of duplicates across registries would require coordination and potential linkage using one universal registration number within a single platform such as the World Health Organization (Zarin et al. 2007).

Conclusion

ClinicalTrials.gov is an important resource for researchers, policy makers, providers, and the general public that provides access to information that, prior to registration, difficult to obtain. As a result of key regulatory events and policies, registration is now widely accepted as standard practice. ClinicalTrials.gov continues to evolve and incorporate new methods and policies to further improve its overall quality and function such as recent efforts to import study documents (e.g., protocols, consent forms) into the registration record (Zarin et al. 2017a) or the incorporation of individual participant data (IPD) to in ClinicalTrials.gov to increase the accountability and transparency of clinical trial data. Researchers are also beginning to use ClinicalTrials.gov as a more efficient method for conducting systematic reviews using automatic extraction of the quantitative data (Pradhan et al. 2019). While the use and analysis of ClinicalTrials.gov registration data can provide valuable information about a particular intervention, it is complex and requires an in-depth understanding and knowledge of the registration and reporting requirements. Thus, it is the responsibility of the lead sponsors as well as study investigators, staff, and responsible parties to provide complete and accurate registration information in order to contribute to scientific advancement and improve the clinical trials research enterprise.

References

De Angelis C, Drazen JM, Frizelle FA, Haug C, Hoey J, Horton R, Kotzin S, Laine C, Marusic A, Overbeke AJPM, Schroeder TV, Sox HC, Van Der Weyden MB, E. International Committee of Medical Journal (2004) Clinical trial registration: a statement from the International Committee of Medical Journal Editors. CMAJ: Can Med Assoc J 171(6):606–607

Dickersin K (1990) The existence of publication bias and risk factors for its occurrence. JAMA 263(10):1385–9. PubMed PMID: 2406472

Dickersin K, Rennie D (2003) Registering clinical trials. JAMA 290(4):516–23. PubMed PMID: 12876095

Ehrhardt S, Appel LJ, Meinert CL (2015) Trends in National Institutes of Health funding for clinical trials registered in ClinicalTrials.gov. JAMA 314(23):2566–2567

Gresham GK, Ehrhardt S, Meinert JL, Appel LJ, Meinert CL (2018) Characteristics and trends of clinical trials funded by the National Institutes of Health between 2005 and 2015. Clin Trials 15(1):65–74

Piantadosi S (2017) Clinical trials: a methodologic perspective. John Wiley & Sons

Pradhan R, Hoaglin DC, Cornell M, Liu W, Wang V, Yu H (2019) Automatic extraction of quantitative data from ClinicalTrials.gov to conduct meta-analyses. J Clin Epidemiol 105:92–100

Simes RJ (1986) Publication bias: the case for an international registry of clinical trials. J Clin Oncol 4(10):1529–41. PubMed PMID: 3760920

Tse T, Fain KM, Zarin DA (2018) How to avoid common problems when using ClinicalTrials.gov in research: 10 issues to consider. BMJ (Clinical Research Ed) 361:k1452

van Valkenhoef G, Loane RF, Zarin DA (2016) Previously unidentified duplicate registrations of clinical trials: an exploratory analysis of registry data worldwide. Syst Rev 5(1):116

World Medical Association (2013) World medical association declaration of Helsinki: ethical principles for medical research involving human SubjectsWorld medical association declaration of HelsinkiSpecial communication. JAMA 310(20):2191–2194

Zarin DA, Ide NC, Tse T, Harlan WR, West JC, Lindberg DA (2007) Issues in the registration of clinical trials. JAMA 297(19):2112–2120

Zarin DA, Tse T, Williams RJ, Califf RM, Ide NC (2011) The ClinicalTrials.gov results database–update and key issues. N Engl J Med 364(9):852–860

Zarin DA, Tse T, Williams RJ, Carr S (2016) Trial reporting in ClinicalTrials.gov—the final rule. N Engl J Med 375(20):1998–2004

Zarin DA, Williams RJ, Tse T, Ide NC (2017a) The role and importance of clinical trial registries and results databases. In: Gallin JI OF, Johnson LL (eds) Principles and practice of clinical research. Academic, London, pp 111–125

Zarin DA, Tse T, Williams RJ, Rajakannan T (2017b) Update on trial registration 11 years after the ICMJE policy was established. N Engl J Med 376(4):383–391

Funding Models and Proposals

26

Matthew Westmore and Katie Meadmore

Contents

Abstract

Clinical trials require funding – often a lot. Funders of clinical trials are not just sources of funding however. They are actors in their wider research systems, have their own philosophies, values, and objectives, and operate within different

M. Westmore (✉) · K. Meadmore
University of Southampton, Southampton, UK
e-mail: m.j.westmore@soton.ac.uk; k.meadmore@soton.ac.uk

© Springer Nature Switzerland AG 2022
S. Piantadosi, C. L. Meinert (eds.), *Principles and Practice of Clinical Trials*,
https://doi.org/10.1007/978-3-319-52636-2_55

political, social, and economic environments. While there are commonalities, differences in their context and culture shape their approaches to funding decisions, what they are looking for from the research community, and therefore how to successfully engage with them. By understanding the commonalities and differences between funding agencies, the types of funding models they may use, what they are trying to achieve, and what the decision-making process looks like may help increase the success of proposals.

This chapter summarizes the similarities and differences of clinical trial funding agencies around the world and the implications for funding models and proposals. It is primarily aimed at trialists seeking to understand and ultimately succeed in applying and funding; it will also be of interest to research funding agencies (RFAs) and regulators.

Keywords

Research funding agency · Funders · Funding model · Decision-making · Funding decision · Sources of funding · Proposals and applications

---

Introduction

This chapter summarizes the similarities and differences of clinical trial funding agencies around the world and the implications for funding models and proposals. It is primarily aimed at trialists seeking to understand and ultimately succeed in applying and funding; it will also be of interest to research funding agencies (RFAs) and regulators.

Funders of clinical trials are not just sources of funding. They are actors in their wider research systems, have their own philosophies, values, and objectives, and operate within different political, social, and economic environments. While there are commonalities, differences in their context and culture shape their approaches to funding decisions, what they are looking for from the research community, and therefore how to successfully engage with them.

Figure 1 shows a hierarchy of factors from the wider environment, through to the internal organizational setting that ultimately affects how funding schemes are designed and what is expected of applicants.

Types of Research Funding Agencies and Their Societal, Political, and Organizational Context

Clinical trial funding agencies are not all alike. Broadly, they share the ultimate aim of improving human health through research but the way they operate and the way they measure success differ. These differences depend on the societal, political, economic, research system and organizational context in which they operate. With

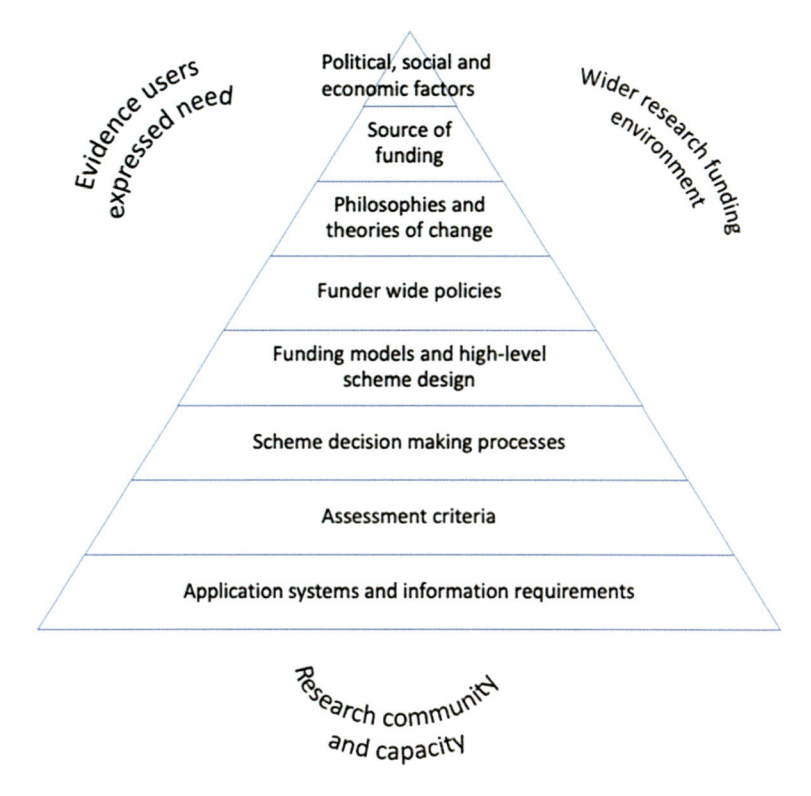

Fig. 1 Hierarchy of factors that influence research funding agency policies and procedures and ultimately what applicants have to address

many commonalities, these differences lead to different aims and theories of change of how to achieve those aims. This section outlines some of those differences.

The information presented in this chapter is solely meant to provide an overview of the different types of contexts in which funding organizations operate and are molded by. To do this, we have necessarily caricatured different types of organizations and generalized their objectives, values, and approaches. We have done this in best faith to inform readers in a simple way rather than suggest any actual funding agency neatly fits the character.

Political Context for Public Research Funding Agencies

The allocation of funding for research is not just a technical process but is a political one as well; this is especially true for publicly funded research. At what level and how influential politicians should be is a controversial topic and beyond the scope of this work. What is important to understand is how the political context flows through the hierarchy of factors, Fig. 1, through to the expectations placed on researchers.

Politics (and therefore policy makers) can influence the research that is funded across a spectrum of ways. From direct involvement into individual decision-making, for example, in the prioritization of individual calls for research as the primary customer of the eventual evidence, to setting the wider policy context in which research funding agencies interpret their role; for example, in how some countries national policy for economic growth has been internalized in funding agencies into a desire to demonstrate potential impact at the application stage.

When done well, this connects researchers with policy makers and ensures research reflects the needs and desires of those that fund it through taxation; when done badly, this represents an unacceptable imposition on academic freedom and allows political bias to cast a shadow across research.

Politicians who take little interest in research is perhaps no less worrying than those that take too much; a survey of Canadian members of parliament and/or senior aids found that 32% knew nothing about the role of the Canadian Institutes of Health Research (CIHR) despite it being the primary federal funder of research (Clark et al. 2007).

US President Barack Obama summed up the tension:

> Obama pledged in a speech to protect "our rigorous peer-review system" to ensure that research "does not fall victim to political manoeuvres or agendas" that could damage "the integrity of the scientific process." However, he added that it was important that "we only fund proposals that promise the biggest bang for taxpayer dollars". (Obama 2013)

Sources of Funding

One of the most influential characteristics of funding agencies on funding models is the source of their funding.

Public RFAs funded through public finance (e.g., taxation, public borrowing) are accountable to society more broadly and therefore tend to operate in ways that promote societal values such as inclusivity, democracy, fairness, and transparency. Different public RFAs will operate in different areas of research depending on the prevailing theory of change. An important characteristic is the sponsoring government department or legislation. Research councils in the UK, for example, are sponsored by the government department responsible for business, energy, and industrial strategy, whereas the National Institute for Health Research (NIHR) is sponsored by the department responsible for the UK's health, public health, and social care services. What they each look for from the research community only makes sense within that context.

Until relatively recently, the last 10–20 years, public funding has valued long-term incremental advances to societal value and shorter term scientific breakthroughs. Public RFAs tend to be broad in their remits but may set strategic areas of focus. Where they differ more markedly is in the domains of science in which they operate. For example, the UK Clinical Research Collaboration assesses public and philanthropic funding (UK Health Research Analysis – http://www.ukcrc.org).

It categorizes funding into disease categories and in research activity categories: underpinning etiology, prevention, diagnosis and detection, treatment development, treatment evaluation, disease management, and health services. The analysis shows different RFAs focusing on different categories.

Philanthropic RFAs, funded by high net worth individuals or fundraising led by the founders, may have objectives significantly influenced by their founders. This may be because of direct lived experience, such as trusts established in someone's name, say a child of the founder who died from a particular disease, or because of wider interests in helping humanity benefit from their "excess" wealth, or as is sometimes termed "giving back to society." These organizations are also influenced by the founders in the way they operate. For example, founders whose background is in venture capital may employ venture capital thinking and ways of working, so-called philanthropic venture capital. They tend to focus more on portfolios of research, value overall return on investment, and are often characterized (or perhaps caricatured) as seeking rapid and transformative change to health outcomes. Funding is often not limited to specific countries or specific disciplines. They may be more utilitarian and tangible in their metrics of success compared to other types of funders.

Medical research charities are philanthropic in their outlook but are heavily influenced by their constituents and donor communities. Medical charities broadly operate in four main domains: fund raising, lobbying, service provision, and research funding. Different charities will have different profiles across these domains, with some being predominantly active in one domain and having less or have no role in others. This can lead to differences in the way they operate within the research funding domain. For example, charities whose primary interest is lobbying and service provision may see research funding as a powerful tool to drive fundraising. They will therefore prioritize newsworthy and high-profile research, working with esteemed institutions. Given that the overall organization culture and expertise within the charity is focused on other areas, these charities' research agendas are driven predominantly by the research communities with whom they work and may be more science driven, focusing on more headline grabbing exploratory and discovery phases of research. Charities whose primary interest is in medical research itself may be more driven by the immediate needs and perspectives of their current patient communities. They are perhaps more likely to support a more balanced research portfolio across prevention, cure, and symptom management and are more likely to more actively steer the research agenda themselves.

Commercial RFAs clinical trials are dominated by the pharmaceutical sector followed by medical devices. These studies could be completely funded by the company or collaborative research with funding coming from other partners – other companies, charities, or public RFAs. Commercial funding (or investigator-sponsored trials or studies as they are also referred to) focuses on developing approaches to health problems for the benefit of people but that obviously have a commercial emphasis and application. As this research is often for commercial gain, the research outputs are not always open and accessible to all. In addition, to attract private funding researchers might require a good understanding of market context and awareness of potential conflicts of interest around intellectual property, especially ownership of the research and freedom to disseminate knowledge.

Many organizations will fund so-called *own account research*. The original funding into the organization comes from a variety of sources but there is very little link between the original source of those funds and what research it goes to fund. The research will be carried out by the employees of the organization itself. The important characteristics in terms of what research would be prioritized, the processes, and oversight are defined by the organization itself. Organizations will tend to have a wide variety of different mechanisms and schemes aimed at supporting the aims of the organization (rather than source funder). Commercial organizations fund large amounts of research in this way and this will form the spine of their in-house research and development pipelines; public institutions tend to fund small projects (e.g., developmental, pilot, and feasibility studies in the context of this book) aimed at developing opportunities and capacity for future external proposals to other RFAs.

A new *democratized* model of research funding is now also emerging that will change the nature of the relationship between the source of funding and the recipient researcher. Crowd funding approaches are being used directly by researchers to raise funding for research projects from the public at large through (typically) online platforms. Traditionally, research is funded by collecting a large number of small contributions, such as through taxation or donations, but there is an intermediary institution between the person making the contribution and the researcher who receives it. Crowd funding removes that intermediary. On the assumption that the intermediary is not just a source of funds, it influences priorities and the conduct of research, a quality assurance role, and acts on behalf of other stakeholders, these new approaches will ultimately have a significant impact on what research happens and how it is delivered.

A final category to explore is that of the *transnational* RFA; funders that have a role to play in funding across national boundaries. The nature of these RFAs expectations differs depending on whether their funding comes from a single national entity, such as a philanthropic trust with an interest in funding global health research such as the UK's Wellcome Trust or The Bill and Melinda Gates Foundation, or multinational collaboration with an interest in the collective advantage of the member states, such as the European Union Horizon 2020 program. These different factors can again lead to aims, expectations, policies, and procedures that are markedly different compared to other RFAs. For example, the European Union's Horizon 2020 values, indeed mandates, multinational collaborative research involving member states with high and low national incomes. Its aims are not just around scientific or health benefits but to reduce inequality across member states and to promote overall cohesiveness of the European Union – these are political, not scientific or clinical aims.

Philosophies and Theories of Change of Funding Agencies

What funders are trying to achieve and how they believe they will achieve them also significantly influences their policies and procedures. These could loosely be called philosophies and theories of change. Some funders will be quite explicit about this and others will be influenced by a wider set of norms, culture, and tacit knowledge. There are philosophies and theories that apply very generally to research and those that are very focused on clinical trials.

Starting generally, the oldest and most influential concept is the Haldane principle. This is the idea that politicians may set the overarching strategic allocation of funding (e.g., what to spend on research into the liberal arts, what to spend on engineering, what to spend on health-related research); these are political questions. Beyond that, decisions about what to spend research funds on should be made by researchers rather than politicians; these are technical questions. This principle has underpinned the entire peer review process since the Haldane report was published in 1918 (HMSO 1918) and has been influential in subsequent funding policy not just in the UK but around the world. Haldane in its purest sense gives primacy to academic freedom in deciding on the direction of research. This has been highly successful and has led to many modern economies being based on the advances in knowledge, culture, and technology that has resulted from it. Haldane has its limitations however.

The research community may well be the best experts to decide on highly scientific technical questions but which research to support and how it should be delivered are often subjective, value-laden issues. This is particularly the case when the intended purpose of research is more utilitarian than enlightenment or non-specific advances in knowledge; when the intended user of the research is not another researcher (but, for example, a policy maker, clinician, or patient). This requires a wider range of opinions, experiences, and expertise.

The first major challenge to the Haldane principle also originated in the UK. In 1971, the Rothschild Report (HMSO 1971) raised the issue, and proposed solutions to it, that the research community and commercial funders while undoubtedly successful in some fields were failing to deliver in others. Most notably in applied research areas where parts of society needed more immediate answers to more specific questions; in the context of this work, questions like is treatment A better than treatment B? Rothschild developed the concept that applied R&D must have a customer and that customer should be influential in deciding which research should be carried out. Rothschild was and in some ways remains highly controversial. It has nonetheless changed the nature of research and research funding.

Rothschild also led to the concept of market failure research funding. Whereby public funders should not be supporting research that would happen anyway – research that would be funded by commercial funders or philanthropic funders. Doing so is not only unnecessary, and therefore a poor use of limited public funding that could be spent on other areas but can also lead to crowding out. Those that would have funded in that area now do not either because they do not need to or because it now does not make commercial sense; for example, public funding results in public knowledge that cannot be protected for commercial gain. This has the result that the additional public funding actually reduces the over-investment in an area rather than increases it.

Influenced by the work of Mariana Mazzucato in The Entrepreneurial State (Mazzucato 2018), an alternative view has also developed. In certain circumstances, public funding can indeed have the opposite effect whereby the injection of funding in an area causes other private and philanthropic funders to also fund in that area: this concept is called crowding-in (as opposed to crowding-out). The public funder must of course choose the area and nature of its investment carefully – this in turn will again change the ways in which it makes its funding decisions.

More specifically relating to clinical trials. A common narrative in the development of new treatments is the *translational pathway*. The US NIH defines translational research as:

> Translational research includes two areas of translation. One is the process of applying discoveries generated during research in the laboratory, and in preclinical studies, to the development of trials and studies in humans. The second area of translation concerns research aimed at enhancing the adoption of best practices in the community. Cost-effectiveness of prevention and treatment strategies is also an important part of translational science. (Rubio et al. 2010)

How strongly the funder subscribes to this model, and sees their role in facilitating ideas move along the pathway, will have significant impact on not only the methodology expected but also who is setting research priorities and what outcomes would be of greatest interest.

Whose Priority Is It Anyway?

A critical aspect of a research funder's philosophy is to whom do they feel accountable and who therefore should define its priorities. A research funder who sees their role in supporting the research community develop and deliver to their full potential will pay greatest attention to that community in priority setting (c.f. Haldane principle); a funder who sees their role in delivering direct patient benefit will look to clinical and patient communities to set priorities (c.f. Rothschild). This is important because when different stakeholders are consulted on research priorities, they provide different answers – patient priorities don't completely align with clinician priorities, nor completely align with researchers; a further list might be generated when asking policy makers. When you coproduce priorities with people from each of these communities you end up with another different list. Understanding that will inform applicants on how to set their own priorities, who to work with to do that, and ultimately how to succeed in obtaining funding.

Of growing importance to funders of health-related research in general, and clinical trials in particular, is the role of the patient, carer, consumer, lay representative, or member of the public above and beyond as participants recruited into trials. Different terminology is used across the world and across funders – for the sake of clarity, we will use *patient and public*. Funders are increasingly expecting patients and the public to play a number of varied and more active roles. Again different terminology is used such as involvement, advocacy, engagement; we will use involvement. The UK's INVOLVE (http://www.invo.org.uk) defines consumer involvement in research as research being carried out "**with**" or "**by**" members of the public rather than "**to**," "**about**," or "**for**" them. This includes, for example, working with research funders to priorities research, offering advice as members of a project steering group, commenting on and developing research materials, and undertaking interviews with research participants. More on this topic can be found in section 3 ▸ Chap. 30, "Advocacy and Patient Involvement in Clinical Trials."

Impact

Research impact is the effect research has beyond academia. There is no single definition nor approach to measuring it, but it is often described as research that has wider benefits and influences on society, culture, and the economy. It remains a contentious and complex subject and also depends on the individual funder's context and where they sit in the translational pathway; one funder's impact is another funder's input. What is universal, however, is every funder wants it. It speaks to the funder's fundamental purpose and it forms an important part of how the funder is held to account by those providing the funding. A public funder has to justify its overall impact to government, a philanthropic to its donors, and a commercial to its shareholders. A discussion of the nature and role of research impact is beyond the scope of this work but it is important to underline its importance to the relationship between research funder, funded researcher, and wider stakeholders.

Funder Policies

Funders encode all of the above into policies and procedures that guide their own actions and the expectations placed on the research community. These will cover all areas relating to the research over which the funder either has responsibility (such as legislative requirements or financial rules ensuring good use of funds) or wish to have influence (such as research integrity or transparency).

Different funders with different contexts will of course have different sets of rules, policies, and procedures that must be understood and complied with.

The Importance of Remit

All funders will have limitations on the nature of research they will support. This flows from the fundamental purpose of the organization through the intended purpose of the scheme being applied to. Remits will operate at different levels – the whole funder, a funding program, or a specific call. Different funders will specify their remits differently; some might be methodologically driven (e.g., by clinical trial phase), others by clinical area or health need. It cannot be overstated how important it is to understand the remit of a call or program being applied to. Preparing applications can be an enormous piece of work, yet up to 20% of applications (for example, see the NIHR Health Technology Assessment success rates https://www. nihr.ac.uk/documents/hta-programme-success-rates/23178) can be deemed out of remit and will not be considered for funding.

The Impact of Funder Policies on Research Culture

While the majority of the focus of RFAs is on the relevance, quality, and impact of the research they support, funders are increasingly paying attention to how their policies and procedures have a wider influence on research delivery and culture. RFAs sit in a highly influential position and are increasingly using that position to improve research. For example, the move from a Haldane denominated view of the world to Rothschild; the rise of the impact agenda, insistence on open access publication, and wider clinical trial transparency.

Of particular importance is the global movement toward quality improvement in research is the Research Waste and Rewarding Diligence Alliance (REWARD). The REWARD Alliance was launched at the REWARD/EQUATOR Conference, 28–30 September 2015, stimulated by the seminal work of Iain Chalmers and Paul Glasziou on avoidable research waste in 2009 (Chalmers and Glasziou 2009) and a series of articles in the Lancet in 2014 (Lancet Series Research: increasing value, reducing waste 2014), detailing expert consensus recommendations for all sectors of the research ecosystem. The Alliance's purpose is to facilitate efforts to maximize the potential for research contributions by addressing five cross-cutting ideals: (1) The "right" research priorities are set, with input from the users of research, including patients and clinicians; (2) Studies are appropriately designed by building on what is already known and are robustly conducted and analyzed through using up to date methods to minimize bias; (3) Research regulation and management requirements are proportionate to risks; (4) All information on research methods and study findings are accessible; (5) Study reports are complete and usable. Both the REWARD Alliance and the 2014 Lancet series noted that progress would require action independently and collaboratively by different stakeholders, namely researchers, funders, regulators, and publishers, with the inclusion of patients and the public embedded in the activities of each of these stakeholder groups. An international group of RFAs called *Ensuring Value in Research* (http://www. ensuringvalueinresearch.org) has formed and developed a conceptual model and ten guiding principles to address these issues. These are now beginning to inform RFA policies globally (Fig. 2).

A second initiative particularly relevant to this work is the World Health Organizations' Joint statement on public disclosure of results from clinical trials (World Health Organization 2017). This sets out a number of expectations regarding clinical trial transparency namely:

- Clinical trials must be registered in design specific registries
- Clinical trial protocols must be made publicly available at the start of studies
- Registry information must be kept up to date

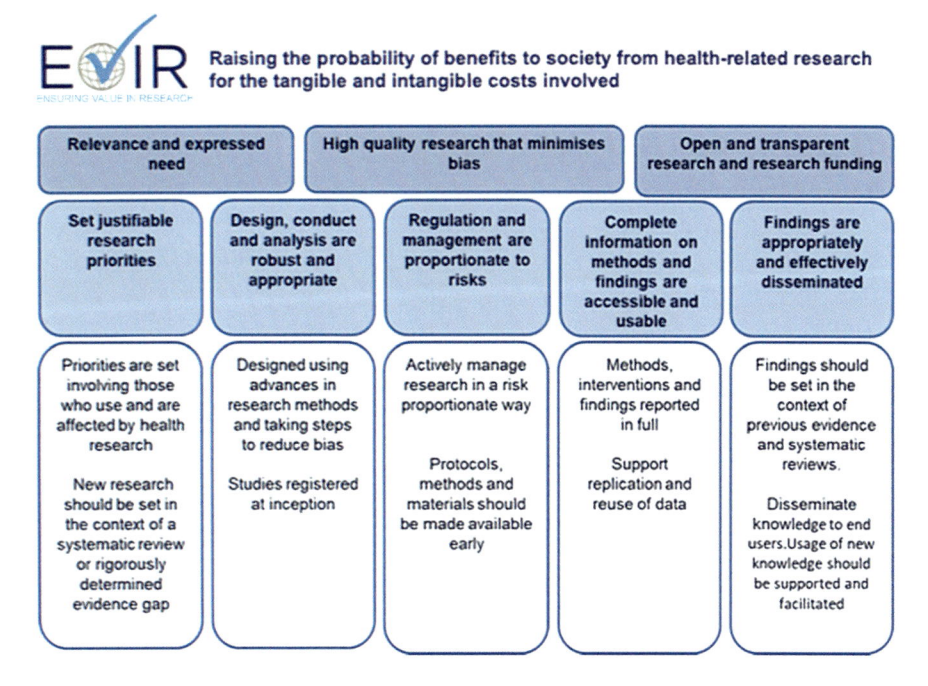

Fig. 2 Ensuring value in research conceptual model and guiding principles

- Summary findings must be made publicly available within 12 months of the completion of the primary study
- Full results must be made publicly available within 24 months of the completion of the primary study
- Past registration and publication performance should be taken into account when applying for new funding
- Individual patient level data should be shared

At the time of writing, 21 RFAs had signed up and are now implementing policies to deliver on this. Even where RFAs are not formal signatories, however, the importance of transparency policies is growing and are likely to be part of the requirements for funded researchers.

Funding Models

Given the different contexts, environments, aims, and objectives of funders, different models of funding have been developed. Each will follow a different process of decision-making and place different expectations on the research community during the application and delivery phases of research. Fundamentally, however, all are attempting to achieve the same aim. The delivery of relevant, high quality, usable, and accessible answers to specific research questions. Where they differ is how and who crafts the research question.

Open Versus Commissioned Calls

The two most common funding models used are open call (or researcher-led or response mode) and commissioned call (or targeted or contract research). In open call, researcher-led or response mode funding models, the RFA sets a high level remit and the research community develops the research question and methodology. In contrast in commissioned call funding models the RFA, working with stakeholders, fully specifies the research question and the research community compete to be the best team to deliver it. Typically, in these cases applicants will be provided with a specific brief or vignette and the program of research in the application must address this. Researcher-led calls or responsive mode funding is where the researchers drive the research questions and topics and can propose research questions on any topic (so long as they are within the organization's remit).

Sitting between open and commissioned calls are thematic calls. Some funding organizations also issue themed calls for research in areas that have been identified as health challenges, scientific, clinical, or community priorities. These are specified more tightly than open calls but more broadly than commissioned calls.

Across all of these models, the importance of remit should be restated. Applicants must ensure they are not only within the remit of the funder or program but also the call in question. Deviations from the call specification may be tolerated but this would be a high-risk strategy and would have to be robustly defended by the applicant.

Common Funding Models

Table 1 summarizes some common funding models.

Proposal Assessment Processes

Regardless of which RFA is applied to and where the funds are sourced (public, philanthropic, commercial, etc.), all RFAs have to make decisions regarding which research applications they should invest in. Good decision-making processes are seen as integral and essential to the research process (Nurse 2015). This is no easy challenge as the number of applications received by funding organizations is often large and the amount requested by the applicants typically outweighs the amount of resource available (Guthrie et al. 2018). As such, funding organizations have rigorous processes in place to facilitate decision-making in order to whittle down the number of competitive applications and ensure that funds are awarded to the best applications. However "best" does not have just one definition, and instead depends

Table 1 Common funding models used by different types of funder

Funding model	Description	Purpose	Typically used by
Response mode (a.k.a. grant rounds, researcher-led, open call)	Funder specifies a broad remit to the program. Researchers develop and submit applications or proposals	Allows the research community to flexibility propose any project (within remit). Allows the funder to decide on a project-by-project basis	Public Philanthropic
Commissioned call (a.k.a. targeted)	Funder specifies a specific piece of research (e.g., may advertise a PICO) that applicants apply to deliver	Allows the funder to fully specify the research project. This would normally be in response to an identified need. For public philanthropic, evidence users' expressed need (e.g., patient community, policy maker, clinical community). For commercial, an internal R&D pipeline is needed	Public Philanthropic Commercial
Challenge areas (a.k.a. moon shots)	Funder sets out a major challenge facing society needing a coordinated and concerted response across a range of projects and disciplines	A way of focusing a wide (possibly transdisciplinary) community to work over a longer period of time	Public Philanthropic
Strategic or thematic calls	Funder sets out a strategic or thematic area needing number of projects to be funded	Useful where there are a number of uncertainties needing addressing, where the funder wants to guide the research community but not fully specify	Public Philanthropic
Call-off contracts	Funder enters into a contract for future research where the individual projects are not known at the point of award	Funder is able to initiate research very rapidly from a team that is established and expert	Public Commercial
Contract or grant funding	Public funder enters into a contract for research or issues a grant	Grant funding typically comes with limited oversight from the funder. Grants are efficient and useful instruments when academic freedom is paramount. Where the funder wants greater control over the delivery of the research project a contract of research would be used	Public Commercial

(continued)

Table 1 (continued)

Funding model	Description	Purpose	Typically used by
Project funding	Funding of a single project. The project may have multiple subprojects that collectively address a narrow need	Where a single or small number of interconnected subprojects are required	Public Philanthropic Commercial
Block funding	Research institution is awarded substantial funding with limited direction from the funder on what to use it for	Provides long-term sustaining and capacity-building funding. Allows for the highest levels of academic freedom and creativity	Public Philanthropic Commercial
Infrastructure funding	Funding to provide infrastructure to support research projects funded by other means	Provides long-term sustaining and capacity building to support a wider research community	Public Philanthropic Commercial
Sandpits and other variants	Prefunding workshops	To bring research communities together to collaborate in ways that would not otherwise happen, e.g., where highly creative or radical approaches or transdisciplinary research is required	Public Philanthropic

on the organizational context and priorities. RFAs also need to balance academic freedom and creativity with accountability and value for money. This balance will again vary depending on the nature of the funder and nature of the research.

Typical Application Route and Decision-Making Processes

There are many types of approaches and processes involved in allocating research funding (see Table 2).

The overarching processes for allocating funding are largely similar across public and philanthropic funders (Nurse 2015). Commercial, own account, self-funded, and crowd-funded research follow a vast heterogeneity of processes that cannot be usefully summarized here. This section therefore focuses on public and philanthropic funders.

In the current landscape, the use of triage, face-to-face committee meetings, and external peer review comprise a typical approach by funders to decide which applications to fund (see Fig. 3). This standard route has been developed over many years to embed the Haldane Principle and principles of openness and fairness. Typically, once an application has been submitted, it goes through an internal triage

Table 2 Stages for research fund allocation

Stage	Brief description	Pros (not exhaustive)	Cons (not exhaustive)
Remit and competitiveness checking	Usually a gate-keeper for initial submissions. It is a type of internal triage in which applications are shortlisted into those that are believed to be within the program remit and are competitive (e.g., reasonable costs, methodology)	Reduces the number of applications that go to the next round or are sent out to review by excluding those that are weaker or not in remit	Sometimes seen as a hidden review process that is not transparent and could filter out potentially good applications or let through bad applications. Increased burden to funder – another process and staff need appropriate training
One-stage application	One-stage applications require submission of a full application upfront	Reduce time to make a decision process	Increased burden to funder as potentially more full applications to review. Limits opportunity for feedback to applicants
Two-stage applications	Require an expression of interest or a reduced application form at stage one. If the applicant is successful, then they are invited to submit a full application at stage two	Reduces the number of applications that go to the next round or are sent out to review by excluding those that are weaker	Increase time for decision-making process. Could filter out potentially good applications or let through bad applications. Ability to give feedback to applicants between stages
External peer review	Applications are sent to experts in the field for comments and recommendations. External peer reviewers do not sit on the research programs funding committee	Funders are gaining expert opinion on the application	Biases exist (e.g., age, gender, stage of career); unreliable as scores and comments can vary; high burden for funders to find reviewers, reliant on quality and timely reviews
Face-to-face committee meetings	Applications are reviewed by a range of experts in different fields in a face-to-face meeting	Provides opportunity for thorough discussion and clarification	Biases exist, certain members of a committee may be better at arguing a case (and so more likely to get applications they like funded), high time, and cost burden
Virtual committee meetings	Applications are reviewed by a range of experts in different fields in a virtual	Provides opportunity for thorough discussion and clarification; more	Biases exist, certain members of a committee may be better at arguing a case

(continued)

Table 2 (continued)

Stage	Brief description	Pros (not exhaustive)	Cons (not exhaustive)
	environment (e.g., telephone conference or online such as Skype)	inclusive than face-to-face as reduces travel, time, and geographic constraints	(and so more likely to get applications they like funded), reliant on technology
Inclusion of stakeholder perspectives	Applications are reviewed by lay people, patients/carers of people with a specific health condition, or people from a specific population	Funders are gaining lay, patient, and/or population perspective	Biases exist (toward own health condition/population); can be difficult to find PPI for narrow criteria
Sandpits and other variants	A sandpit model aims to bring together researchers, funders, and reviewers to interactively discuss and revise proposals at a workshop	Provides a forum for brainstorming to foster creativity and generate research proposals quickly; shorter timeframe for proposal review and revision	Relies on appropriate selection of participants; may not be inclusive as involves 3–5 day workshops
Random allocation for applications above a certain threshold	There are many different ways that this could be done. Sorting applications into three groups through peer review according to a certain threshold (e.g., not fundable, probably fundable, definitely fundable). Not fundable are declined and definitely fundable are accepted. Decisions in the middle tier are made through random allocation up to the amount of resource available	Eliminates biases, transparent	Uncertainty around outcome, may not capture very good applications, still needs reviewers and/or a committee for initial ranking process Even if statistically fair the use of random chance to decide funding is not welcome by the research community

system. Applications which are considered competitive are then sent to peer reviewers. Different RFAs approach peer review differently; some will rely on sending applications singularly or in small numbers to individual external and independent experts; others will send all applications in a call to a face-to-face committee of experts; other funders do both.

If both external and committee peer review are used, external reviewers comments and recommendations on the proposal are considered at a funding committee meeting (also referred to as panels or boards). Applications considered fundable may then be ranked and a final list of funded applications is drawn. Before applicants are

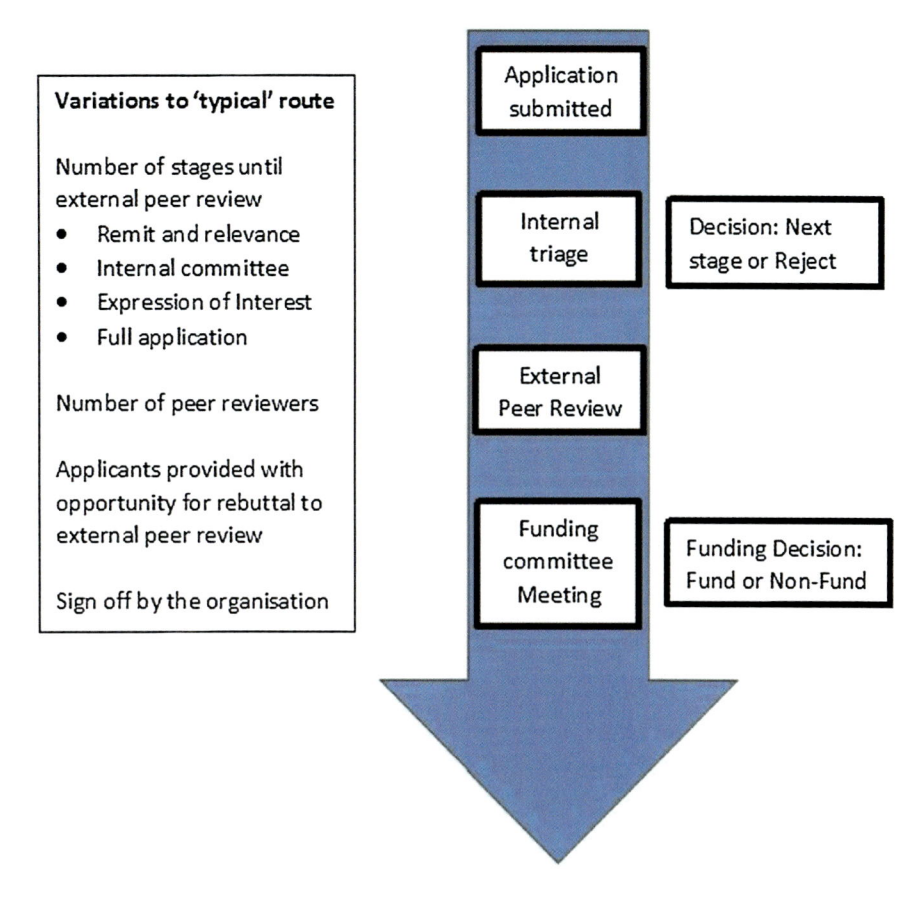

Fig. 3 Illustration of the common elements involved in an application route and potential areas for differences

informed, the outcome may first need to have formal sign off from the RFAs governance structures and/or external sponsoring agency (such as government department for a public funder).

Different funders will operate variations on the process steps included in this model. For example, the Canadian Institutes for Health Research (CIHR) and the Australian National Health and Medical Research Council do not send proposals out to external peer review. Other funders will not hold face-to-face meetings; instead making their decision via electronic panels, scoring, and discussion.

Differences in the way different process steps are carried out may also include the assessment criteria to which applications are judged (see Table 3), whether the application is in response to a commissioned call or researcher-led, whether applicants can make revisions and rebuttals following feedback from reviewers, the number of internal triage stages, and the scoring system used for rating the application (Guthrie et al. 2018).

Table 3 Common assessment criteria used by funding organizations

Common assessment criteria	Examples of how the criteria may be defined
Remit and relevance	Does it fit the funder objectives and research strategy? Does it fit the research program objectives, e.g., global health initiatives expect to see plans in the application to work collaboratively with partners in low- and middle-income countries? Does it fit the specific call?
A need to generate evidence	Is the question of importance and has it been tested before? Is it based on a systematic review? Is there equipoise?
Scientific rigor	Is an appropriate methodology used? Will the outcome measures answer the research question? For example, is the sample size big enough and are there adequate recruitment strategies in place?
Innovation/originality of proposal	Has the study previously been conducted? Is it investigating a topic using novel methods? Is it studying a novel topic?
Patient and public involvement	Is there meaningful and sufficiently resourced patient and public involvement throughout the research project?
Team	Are the team multidisciplinary? Do the team engage appropriate stakeholders? Does the team have an excellent track record or have adequate mentoring and support been put in place? Is the team balanced and credible? What is the track record?
Stakeholder perspectives	Different funders expect to see this at different levels to stakeholders reading materials, to stakeholder steering groups involvement throughout the project, to coproduction
Value for money	Does the application generate value for money given the importance of the question? Has the study been adequately and sufficiently costed?
Potential societal impact	Who will benefit from this research? Will the research make a change in policy or practice? Is that credible? Is that value for money?
Potential research impact	What is the pathway for academic impact? Will a paper be published? Who else will benefit from the results of this study? Will the research have potential for implementation in practice?
Intellectual property and commercialization review	Do the outcomes from the study have the potential for IP or commercialization? How will that be managed? How will the IP be exploited? Is that appropriate given the nature of the funder? For example, a public funder will have a different view of commercialization to a commercial funder
Conflicts of interest	What are the actual or perceived conflicts of interest? How are they being managed? Do any residual conflicts threaten scientific integrity (bias) or confidence in the eventual results?

Although these processes are widely used, there is also much criticism surrounding them. For example, it is suggested that peer review (both external and internal funding committees) is heavily biased and not reliable (Guthrie et al. 2017). Opinions on what is fundable can be very subjective and vary widely. Largely these issues, real or perceived, come from the long-term trend of research funding becoming a professionalized, largely technical, and bureaucratic process. These trends are in turn due to the desire for funders to operate fair, transparent and efficient processes.

Over the last decade, funders have begun to explore variations to this typical approach as well as alternative processes for funding, such as sandpits. However, these approaches (alternative and more traditional) still have limited evidence on how efficient and effective they are. Future work needs to explore in which circumstances different approaches work best, how, and for whom.

Who Reviews the Applications?

The application is therefore reviewed by a large number of people. Under the Haldane principles, it is suggested that scientists should assess other scientific work as they are best placed to make a judgment on the excellence of the proposal. Funders have since gone beyond these principles and it is recognized by many that expertise encompasses a wide range of reviewer expertise. Accordingly, many funding organizations seek external peer reviews and committees/panels that comprise a mix of experts. For example, academics, clinicians, health economists, methodologists, patients, and public. Some funding organizations will ask each reviewer to read the whole application and others will ask them to focus on their areas of expertise. For example, a methodologist will look at the methodology of the proposed research studies and a patient representative may look at the aspects of the proposal relating to PPI. Each will then be asked to score the application based on specific assessment criteria. Applicants need to understand the nature of the decision makers in order to understand how to ensure their application is compelling and addresses the expectations of a wide range of experts; for example, an application that is a tour de force methodologically will make a compelling case to methodologists but may fall flat when read by the clinical or patient experts.

Assessment Criteria

To assess applications, each organization will have a set of specific assessment criteria that are applied to each application (see Table 2). These assessment criteria may change from organization to organization and from research program to research program (Guthrie et al. 2018). They will incorporate the funding organizations' strategic research plans, as well as the aims and objectives of specific research programs. Therefore, there is not a one size fits all and applicants are advised to check the remit of the organization and the research program/call they are submitting to before writing on writing the application begins.

General or higher level assessment criteria usually consist of a few core values that are important to a funder. For example, the UK's NIHR states three general assessment criteria: (1) need for the evidence; (2) value for money; (3) scientific rigor. In a review of the UK research councils, Nurse (2015) suggests that there are three key factors that should be considered when funding decisions for scientific research: (1) who the researcher(s) are; (2) content of the research program; and (3) the context within which the research being undertaken. In practice, more criteria that focus on more specific questions under these headings are used during review.

Common assessment criteria include scientific rigor, remit, and relevance (to fit the funder and research programs objectives and research strategy), potential research impact, innovation/originality of proposal, value for money, a need to generate evidence, and potential societal impact (see Table 3). Funding organizations may use a combination of these criteria and may weigh the criteria according to their values. For example, a funder of late phase pragmatic trials will weight meaningful and sufficiently resourced patient and public involvement throughout the research project more highly than a funder of early phase efficacy study.

Success Rates

Not all submitted applications will get funded. Given the effort involved in developing and submitting an application, applicants have careful decisions to make regarding where to submit their research proposals to enhance their chances of success. In addition to checking the funding organizations remit and objectives, applicants may also want to consider the success rates associated with a funding organization or a particular research program. More interesting than the numeric value of the success rate may well be the reasons behind it being high or low and what the applicant can learn from that.

Success rates provide information about the percentage of applications that receive funding from the total number of applications that are reviewed. Note that there are also a number of applications (generally about 10–20%) which will not make it past the first internal triage stage (i.e., remit and relevance). This is sometimes a stage which is forgotten about and success rates often do not include these application numbers in their calculations; i.e., the true success rate could be lower than stated.

At each decision stage of the review process, some applications are rejected. These figures are fairly consistent across funders internationally and are reported by the funding organizations (usually found on their website). In general the overall success rate of funding organizations is between 15% and 25% (for example, see https://www.timeshighereducation.com/news/uk-research-grant-success-rates-rise-first-time-five-years for UK examples and https://report.nih.gov/success_rates/ for NIH data). For those funding organizations that have a two-stage review process, for example, the UK's NIHR and the Welcome Trust, about 50% of applications are rejected at each stage.

Tips for Success

Taking all these considerations together, all the layers of Fig. 1 hierarchy of factors, there are a number of practical tips for success that seem simple yet are not always followed. Doing these things can have a big impact on success rates:

- Choose your funder and program carefully. Squeezing an ill-fitting idea into the wrong funder or scheme is unlikely to work.
- Make sure it is in remit and has a chance of being competitive. Look at the funder's past portfolio to get an idea of the type and quality of projects previously funded.
- Write your application specifically for the funder and scheme of choice.
- Consider the broader expectations of the funder, scheme, or expert reviewers. Don't just focus on one element such as methodology. Different funders will have different criteria and will weight them differently.
- You need to convince the peer review experts, external or committee, that the question is important. This will be highly dependent on the nature of the funder and the makeup of the expert and peer reviewers. Consider who it is important to and why. Challenge yourself – is it important or just interesting – the question may be important but the proposed study might not.
- Cut and paste high level prevalence or incidence figures are not convincing on their own. Funders will want to know what difference the proposed trial will actually make to those that use, deliver, or plan health services and treatments.
- Remember you will need to convince those outside of your specialty. That will include trialists and clinicians working in other areas, methodologists and statisticians, patients, and the public.
- Make sure there is a real research gap that the proposed trial will add to what is already known and that what you are proposing is plausible given the existing evidence base. The best way of doing this is to base the new proposal on a systematic review of the existing evidence. If there isn't one, do one.
- You need to convince the RFA that you have the right approach to delivering the trial. This will include methodology but will also be much broader. How feasible is it? Who are you partnering with? Do you have the right multidisciplinary team? (clinicians, statisticians, patients, etc.).
- Make sure your sample size is credible and meaningful. Will it be achievable? Will it change the meta-analysis?
- Consider wider issues around how you will do the research. Consider issues of transparency, integrity, and openness.

- Consider value for money. Is the answer to the question worth the investment? How much is the trial costing per participant? The more expensive studies will be expected to make a bigger difference to society.

Summary and Conclusions

Funders of clinical trials are not just sources of funding, they are actors in their wider research systems, have their own philosophies, values, and objectives, and operate within different politi cal, social, and economic environments. These will all affect their policies and practice and ultimately what applicants need to work successfully with them. Different funding agencies will use a range of funding models depending on what they are trying to achieve. The decision-making process will vary by funder and by scheme. It is likely to be based on multiple criteria; all must be considered (see Table 3). Applications will be reviewed by a range of experts and usually beyond the field of expertise of the applicant.

Key Facts

- Not all funders of clinical trials are alike; they have their own sources of funding, stakeholders, philosophies, values, and objectives, and operate within different political, social, and economic environments. These will all affect their policies and practice, and ultimately what applicants need to do to work successfully with them.
- Different funding agencies will use a range of funding models depending on what they are trying to achieve; from open calls for proposals limited only by broad remit statements through to commissioned calls where the funder specifies the full research question.
- With nuanced variations, many funders make decisions following a standard procedure involving internal review, external expert and peer review, and funding committee review.
- Understanding the political, philosophical, and contextual issues of funding agencies is important, but there are also some simple practical tips for success for applicants that are useful across all funders.

Cross-References

▶ Advocacy and Patient Involvement in Clinical Trials

References

Chalmers I, Glasziou P (2009) Avoidable waste in the production and reporting of research evidence. Lancet 374(9683):86–89. https://doi.org/10.1016/S0140-6736(09)60329-9

Clark DR, McGrath PJ, MacDonald N (2007) Members' of parliament knowledge of and attitudes toward health research and funding. CMAJ 177(9):1045–1051. https://doi.org/10.1503/cmaj.070320

Guthrie S, Ghiga I, Wooding S (2017) What do we know about grant peer review in the health sciences? F1000Res 6:1335. https://doi.org/10.12688/f1000research.11917.2

Guthrie S, Ghiga I, Wooding S (2018) What do we know about grant peer review in the health sciences? An updated review of the literature and six case studies. RAND Corporation, Santa Monica. https://www.rand.org/pubs/research_reports/RR1822.html

HMSO (1971) A framework for Government research and development. HMSO, London

HMSO (1918) Report of the Machinery of Government Committee under the chairmanship of Viscount Haldane of Cloan. HMSO, London. https://www.civilservant.org.uk/library/1918_Haldane_Report.pdf. Accessed 10 June 2020

Mazzucato M (2018) The entrepreneurial state, 1st edn. Penguin, London

Nurse P (2015) Nurse review of research councils. GOV.UK. Available at: https://www.gov.uk/government/collections/nurse-review-of-research-councils. Accessed 27 June 2019

Obama B (2013) Public papers of the Presidents of the United States: Barack Obama, Book I, p 345. https://www.govinfo.gov/app/details/PPP-2013-book1/PPP-2013-book1-doc-pg342. Accessed 10 June 2020

Rubio D, Schoenbaum E, Lee L, Schteingart D, Marantz P, Anderson K, Platt L, Baez A, Esposito K (2010) Defining translational research: implications for training. Acad Med 85(3):470–475. https://doi.org/10.1097/ACM.0b013e3181ccd618

Series. Research: increasing value and reduce waste when research priorities are set. (2014) The Lancet 383(9912):156–185 e3–e4. https://doi.org/10.1016/S0140-6736(13)62229-1

World Health Organization (2017) Joint statement on public disclosure of results from clinical trials. Available at: https://www.who.int/ictrp/results/jointstatement/en/. Accessed 28 June 2019

Financial Compliance in Clinical Trials

27

Barbara K. Martin

Contents

B. K. Martin (✉)
Administrative Director, Research Institute, Penn Medicine Lancaster General Health,
Lancaster, PA, USA
e-mail: barbara.martin@pennmedicine.upenn.edu

© Springer Nature Switzerland AG 2022
S. Piantadosi, C. L. Meinert (eds.), *Principles and Practice of Clinical Trials*,
https://doi.org/10.1007/978-3-319-52636-2_267

Abstract

Financial compliance considerations are an important aspect of the design and funding of clinical trials. Such research often involves a mixture of sponsor funding and insurance billing for the clinical services provided in the trial. In the United States, what can be billed to insurance and what must be paid by a sponsor are in general determined by the Centers for Medicare & Medicaid Services (CMS). Other third-party payer policies largely mimic those of CMS.

Medicare reimbursement for clinical trials is determined by the interagency agreement between the Food and Drug Administration and CMS regarding investigational devices, the clinical trials policy, and CMS guidance on coverage with evidence development. Non-compliance in research billing carries risk of monetary penalty. To ensure compliance, providers and institutions must conduct coverage analyses to determine if a trial qualifies for CMS coverage and, if it does, which clinical items and services can be billed to CMS. Claims with items and services being billed to CMS must be identified with research codes and modifiers. While these policies and procedures have brought some clarity to research billing, there are still murky waters that providers and institutions need to navigate.

The risk from non-compliance is not theoretical. Several cases of large fines to major research institutions have been well publicized. The imperative for having a comprehensive program for billing compliance continues to mount, and the cost of this necessary infrastructure must be part of the calculation of institutional overhead for clinical research.

Keywords

Billing compliance · Coverage analysis · Clinical Trial Policy · Coverage with evidence development · Qualifying clinical trials · Waiving of co-pays · Subject remuneration · Subject injury

Introduction

The design and conduct of an appropriate, informative, and successful clinical trial of course is multifaceted. The trial must be based on a scientific question worth answering. It must be ethically sound. The design must give the trial a reasonable chance to actually answer the question that it is intended to answer. It must be conducted with rigor and integrity. Also importantly, it must be adequately and appropriately funded.

The funding of clinical trials differs from and is more complex than the funding of other research studies. That is, studies that involve clinical services of any type, from diagnostic testing or monitoring to surgery to administration of drugs, biologics, or devices, could be funded entirely by a sponsor, but they are more likely to involve a mixture of sponsor funding and billing to insurance for some or all of the clinical services provided as part of the trial. In the United States, what can be billed to insurance and what must be paid by a sponsor in general are determined by policy of the Centers for Medicare & Medicaid Services (CMS). Many third-party payers have policies and practices that largely mimic those of CMS. However, with CMS policy come consequences for non-compliance that involve monetary and even criminal penalties. Therefore, the issue of financial – particularly billing – compliance is now an important concern in the conduct of clinical trials. This chapter explores the history of current US policy and the resulting financial compliance considerations that are now necessary. Acronyms frequently used in this chapter are explained in Table 1.

CMS Policy Regarding Reimbursement of Costs in Clinical Trials

The standard for CMS reimbursement has always been anchored to the phrase "reasonable and necessary" from the Social Security Act, which established the Medicare program. More specifically, Medicare is intended to reimburse for clinical services and products that are "reasonable and necessary for the diagnosis and treatment of an illness or injury, or to improve the functioning of a malformed body member" (42 US Code § 1395y). Experimental treatments generally have not met this standard for reimbursement, as it has been interpreted to mean that the service or product must be demonstrated to be safe and effective. However, confusion has long existed around the "routine" testing and treatment that individuals might receive as part of a clinical trial that they would also receive if they were not enrolled in a clinical trial.

Categorization of Devices

The first classification of CMS reimbursement policy came in 1995, with an interagency agreement (FDA 1995) between what was then the Health Care Finance Administration (HCFA) – the precursor to what became CMS in 2001 – and the US Food and Drug Administration (FDA). In the years preceding the agreement, the Office of the Inspector General (OIG) was investigating whether hospitals and providers improperly billed Medicare for the facility and professional fees associated with the implantation of cardiac devices being tested under investigational device exemptions (IDEs) and was indeed finding this to be the case (Aaron and Gelband 2000). Device manufacturers claimed that they could not feasibly pay for all the costs associated with the clinical research necessary to advance the development of medical devices. Furthermore, FDA recognized that some "experimental" devices represented refinements of existing technologies, and treatment of patients with existing technologies would have resulted in similar charges outside of the clinical trials. Concern that hospitals and providers might discontinue participation in device trials out of fear of the OIG investigation and potential fines and penalties led to

Table 1 Frequently used acronyms

Acronym	Full form	Description
CED	Coverage with evidence development	The mechanism by which the Centers for Medicare & Medicaid Services agrees to cover an item or service not otherwise covered, due to a shortage of adequate evidence that the item or service is reasonable and necessary, with the condition that data are collected on utilization and impact of the item or service as part of a protocol that the agency has reviewed and approved; the data generated are intended to be used to inform future coverage decisions; the agreement to provide coverage is published in a national coverage determination
CMS	Centers for Medicare & Medicaid Services	The federal agency within the US Department of Health and Human Services that oversees and administers the Medicare, Medicaid, and Children's Health Insurance programs; among other things, it determines what items and services these programs cover for their beneficiaries
CSP	Coverage with study participation	A type of coverage with evidence development; the mechanism by which the Centers for Medicare & Medicaid Services agrees to cover an item or service not otherwise covered if beneficiaries are receiving the item or service in the context of clinical studies that the agency has reviewed and approved as specifying the process for gathering data and as providing protections and safety measures for beneficiaries
CTP	Clinical trials policy	The commonly used name for the national coverage determination that states that the Centers for Medicare & Medicaid Services provides coverage for the costs of routine items or services delivered in the context of qualifying clinical trials
FDA	Food and Drug Administration	The agency within the US Department of Health and Human Services that, among other things, regulates the sale, labeling, and shipment of drugs, biologics, and medical devices
HCFA	Health Care Financing Administration	The former name for the federal agency within the US government department then known as Health, Education, and Welfare; it oversaw and administered the Medicare and Medicaid programs
IDE	Investigational device exemption	The means by which a device manufacturer obtains permission from the Food and Drug Administration to conduct human clinical studies to collect safety and effectiveness data for a new or modified medical device before the device is approved for marketing
IND	Investigational new drug [application]	The means by which a pharmaceutical company obtains permission from the Food and Drug Administration to conduct human clinical trials (1) with an experimental new drug before it can be approved for marketing or (2) with an existing (approved) drug being testing for a new indication before a labeling change can be approved

(continued)

Table 1 (continued)

Acronym	Full form	Description
NCD	National coverage determination	A determination by the Centers for Medicare & Medicaid Services as to whether Medicare will pay for an item or service; in the absence of a national coverage determination, an item or service is covered at the discretion of the local Medical Area Contractor
OIG	Office of the Inspector General	Specifically, the Office of the Inspector General of the US Department of Health and Human Services (HHS) dedicated to protecting the integrity of HHS programs, combating fraud, waste and abuse, and improving program efficiency; the majority of resources go toward oversight of Medicare and Medicaid

consideration by the FDA and HCFA of a means to determine whether some devices might legitimately be covered by Medicare.

In the interagency agreement between FDA and HCFA regarding reimbursement of investigational devices, FDA agreed to categorize the clinical investigation of medical devices to aid HCFA in its reimbursement decisions. Specifically, FDA would label as Category A those investigations of Class III devices (requiring pre-market approval) that are innovative and for which the safety and effectiveness of the device has not been established (i.e., they are experimental). Category B investigations, on the other hand, would be those that involve devices where the incremental risk of the device is the primary risk in question (i.e., the underlying questions of safety and effectiveness have already been resolved). Therefore, devices in Category B investigations were able to meet the criteria of "reasonable and necessary," and the devices and the associated hospital and professional charges could qualify for reimbursement by HCFA.

The Clinical Trial Policy

Reimbursement for care in non-device trials remained unclear until 2000. Early in that year, the Institute of Medicine of the National Academy of Sciences released the report, "Extending Medicare Reimbursement in Clinical Trials" (Aaron and Gelband 2000). The report summarized the state of reimbursement at that time, suggesting that although Medicare did not have a policy to reimburse for care in clinical trials, and many private insurers had policies that excluded coverage, a significant proportion of costs of patient care in clinical trials were indeed paid for by insurers. This was because providers bill for the services, and without any obvious identification of a beneficiary's participation in a clinical trial, the insurers were none the wiser. That current state, though not untenable, left patients and providers with uncertainty regarding whether costs would be covered. The IOM report recommended an explicit policy that "Medicare should reimburse routine care for patients in clinical trials in the same way it reimburses routine care for patients not in clinical trials." (Aaron and Gelband 2000).

As a result of the IOM report, President Clinton on June 7, 2000, issued an executive order directing Medicare to create explicit policy and to immediately begin to reimburse for the costs of routine services provided to participants in clinical trials (The White House 2000). In response to the executive order, HCFA issued the national coverage determination (NCD) for Routine Costs in Clinical Trials on September 19, 2000 (CMS 2000). This NCD is widely referred to as the Clinical Trial Policy and exists in much the same form today. To state first what the policy excludes, it does not allow for coverage of investigational items or services themselves, unless an item or service is "otherwise covered outside the trial." Additionally, "items and services provided solely to satisfy data collection and analysis needs and that are not used in the direct clinical management of the patient" are not covered. What the policy does require is the coverage of routine costs from "qualifying" clinical trials. Qualifying clinical trials must have therapeutic intent for patients with a diagnosed disease, or intent to diagnose a clinical disease. The policy also outlines seven desirable characteristics of a qualifying clinical trial. HCFA, or now CMS, has never instituted a method for investigators to certify that their research meets the seven desirable characteristics. Instead, clinical trials are deemed as qualifying if they are federally funded, are conducted under an investigational new drug (IND) application, or meet criteria to be exempt from having an IND. The policy also provides that if Medicare is billed for a study that is not qualifying, the providers are liable for the costs and could be investigated for fraud.

Coverage with Evidence Development

The IOM in its report, in addition to advocating for coverage of costs of routine care in clinical trials, urged HCFA "to use its existing authority to support selected trials and to assist in the development of new trials" (Aaron and Gelband 2000). That is, the agency should identify research that is of particular significance to the care of its beneficiaries and provide reimbursement for more than just routine care. The Committee pointed to the example of the National Emphysema Treatment Trial, in which HCFA agreed to pay for lung volume reduction surgery (LVRS) only when the procedure was performed as part of the trial, which was a randomized comparison between LVRS and standard medical management of emphysema.

Response to this recommendation of the IOM report took longer. On July 12, 2006, CMS published guidance on "National Coverage Determinations with Data Collection as a Condition of Coverage" (CMS 2006). The so-called coverage with evidence development (CED) allows for coverage of a service under specific conditions. One such condition, more specifically labeled "coverage with study participation" (CSP), provides for reimbursement of the item or service "only when provided within a setting in which there is a pre-specified process for gathering additional data, and in which that process provides additional protections and safety measures for beneficiaries, such as those present in certain clinical trials."

The intention is to allow coverage of items and services for which CMS does not find there to be enough evidence to support their use as "reasonable and necessary" but for which additional data could help clarify the value of the service. The decision to allow coverage under the CED mechanism is made as part of the CMS coverage determination process, and as such, it is open to public comment (CMS 2014b).

When CMS revised the Clinical Trial Policy in July of 2007, it added reference to coverage of items and services "when provided in a clinical trial that meets the requirements defined in [a specific] national coverage determination" (CMS 2007). This version of the CTP has remained unrevised for the subsequent decade and more.

Billing Compliance in Clinical Trials

CMS policies that began to be put in place a couple decades ago have provided much needed clarity to reimbursement for services provided in the context of clinical trials. However, with this clarity has come the requirement for compliance, and the possibility of penalty for non-compliance. This is a big concern to providers and institutions that bill CMS and/or receive federal grant funds. This section will discuss what is entailed in billing compliance in clinical trials.

Coverage Analysis

In the 2000 IOM report, the Committee discussed the status quo in reimbursement and concluded that much of routine care in clinical trials was indeed already billed to, and paid for, by insurance, mostly without the payers knowing when their beneficiaries were in trials. However, because of the lack of clarity in policy, the possibility remained that either providers or patients could be left holding the bill after a denial of coverage or when sponsor support did not adequately cover services. Providers and institutions differed in their billing practices. According to the Committee, only General Clinical Research Centers (GCRCs), typically funded by the National Institutes of Health and located within major academic hospitals, seemed to have a rigorous and consistent approach to billing for tests and services provided in the context of their clinical trials (Aaron and Gelband 2000). These centers reviewed all the charges for participants in their studies, often early phase research with intensive treatment and monitoring, and determined which charges were for unproven therapies or for tests and services that the participants would not have had outside the clinical trial. These costs were not billed to CMS or other payers, while routine charges were. At the time of the IOM report, this practice was uncommon and mostly confined to GCRCs, which were able to devote substantial resources to their clinical trial billing.

Today, this practice is considered imperative to a comprehensive system for billing compliance. Such a system starts first with coverage analysis, the term that has come to refer to the process of (1) determining if a trial qualifies for coverage under the CTP, under CED, or as a Category A or B IDE study approved by CMS and (2) analyzing all activities required by the study and whether they will be supported by study funds or billed to insurance. Then, as was modeled by GCRCs, all clinical trial charges must be reviewed and triaged for payment according to the coverage analysis.

Determining coverage for a study is the first challenge in billing compliance, as discussed below.

Qualifying for Medicare Coverage Under CTP

The interagency agreement and the CTP have done much to clear up uncertainty regarding clinical trial billing. However, a couple issues remain unclear, and institutions and providers are still left to make their own determinations of the appropriateness of billing or to consult with their local Medicare area contractors (MACs).

One area that has generated much discussion, particularly in the oncology field, is that of early phase clinical trials. As mentioned above, to qualify for coverage under the CTP, a trial must have therapeutic intent for patients with a diagnosed disease or intent to diagnose a clinical disease. Many phase I trials are designed with safety and toxicity measures as the primary outcomes of interest. Can such trials be considered therapeutic in nature, as required under the CTP? Many oncology researchers argue that these trials do have therapeutic intent; if the drugs under study were not thought to have the potential to be therapeutic, they would not be under study. Nonetheless, if the measure of therapeutic intent is the primary outcome of the study for which it is designed and powered, then phase I studies arguably might not meet this criterion.

A second murky area is that of research on a device, such as diagnostic tool, that did not require an IDE, or research on a procedure or technique, such as the use of surgical intervention instead of medical management. Because these interventional studies do not involve an IDE, IND, or IND exemption, the rules for covered devices and qualifying trials do not apply. If the trial has federal sponsorship, it qualifies under the default of the CTP, but if it does not, the trial can be caught in a dead zone of no clarity on coverage. Federal sponsorship or CED coverage for a procedure and technique gaining foothold in practice may be more likely for later phase studies. However, non-sponsored early phase development may be hampered by virtue of the lack of ability to bill for an innovative procedure or technique in the context of a clinical trial.

Device Classification and Medicare Coverage

In the two decades following the interagency agreement that established the categorization of devices by the FDA, this process in and of itself was not enough to establish Medicare coverage. That is, mere classification by the FDA did not guarantee that Medicare would cover routine costs or that it would cover the costs for a Category B device. Local MACs had to be consulted and pre-authorization sought, often for each patient enrolled. CMS, with FDA concurrence, subsequently made changes to its regulations regarding coverage of devices and routine costs as part of IDE studies, with the intent to streamline its coverage determinations. Effective on January 1, 2015, Medicare coverage determinations for IDE studies were centralized (CMS 2014a). That is, sponsors are now required to submit IDE protocols to CMS for a central review process. Studies that are approved for coverage of the investigational device (Category B only) and routine costs are published on the CMS website.

CMS and FDA further collaborated to revise the definitions of Category A and B devices, to support CMS's centralized decision-making on coverage (FDA 2017). Each category has three similar sub-categories of devices, and whether or not there are data to support the questions of safety and effectiveness determines the classification of the device as Category A or B. That is, a new device with no marketing approvals will be considered Category A if "data on the proposed device or similar devices do not resolve initial questions of safety and effectiveness" and Category B if there is available information on the proposed device or similar devices that supports the proposed device's safety and effectiveness. If an approved device is being studied for a new indication, it will be classified as Category A if the information from the proposed or similar devices related to the previous indication does not resolve questions of safety and effectiveness for the new indication and Category B if it does. Finally, a proposed device that has "different technological characteristics compared to a legally marketed device," such that the information from the marketed device can't resolve the questions of safety and effectiveness, will be considered Category A, while a device that has similar technological characteristics would be classified as Category B if the information on the approved device provides applicable data on safety and effectiveness. The amendment to rules on device categorization further allows for changes in the categorization – most likely from A to B but in some instances from B to A – as research on the device progresses. FDA will categorize a device at the start of an IDE study but can consider changes to the categorization with amendments or supplements to the study or at the request of the sponsor.

As a consequence of device categorization by FDA and centralized review by CMS, billing in the device research space may seem more focused and defined. However, questions about coverage may arise from non-significant risk (NSR) device studies (FDA 2006) or studies that can be conducted without an IDE (21 CFR § 812.2(c)), as these studies are not reviewed by FDA or approved by CMS. Rather, one or more IRBs serve as the surrogate for the FDA in reviewing and approving the study. Such studies may involve, for example, investigations related to the clinical use of a new imaging approach, or optimal clinical use of an approved monitoring device. Providers and institutions may need to negotiate with sponsors and local MACs over payment for approved items and services that are being used outside of common practice. For monitoring devices, it is not just the cost of the devices themselves that may be in question but also coverage for medical review of the data being reported by those devices. Providers and institutions may need to determine their risk tolerance for practices for which the "reasonable and necessary" standard could perhaps be challenged.

Qualifying for Medicare Coverage with Evidence Development

When CMS issues a national coverage determination for a specific item or service, the NCD may limit coverage to certain indications, populations, or providers and centers with demonstrated expertise in delivery of the item or service. It also may allow for reimbursement only when the item or service is provided in the context of a research study, under the coverage with evidence development mechanism. For a trial to qualify for reimbursement of the item or service under the CED mechanism, CMS must review and approve the protocol. The items and services that may be covered under CED are listed on the CMS webpage. The CMS webpage typically references the NCD for the item or service it is covering under CED. The NCD then lists the research questions that CMS is interested in having answered and the research studies that are currently approved by CMS.

It is worth noting that the CED mechanism for coverage pertains only to items and services that are covered under Medicare parts A and B. The CED mechanism of coverage could not be applied to self-administered drugs that fall under Medicare part D.

Identifying Research Charges Billed to CMS

Charges that are billed to CMS as routine care provided in the context of clinical trials are to be labeled as such in the claims. This requirement by CMS also has its roots in the events surrounding the advent of the CTP. President Clinton's executive order directed HCFA to establish a tracking system for the charges billed to and reimbursed by Medicare that were generated in clinical research (The White House 2000).

First, an International Classification of Diseases (ICD) code is required. The ICD10 code Z00.6 identifies a charge as part of an "encounter for examination for normal comparison and control in [a] clinical research program." Second, the National Clinical Trials (NCT) number assigned by the clinicaltrials. gov registry is required. Conveniently, this registry had already been established by the Food and Drug Administration Modernization Act of 1997 (FDAMA), developed in conjunction with the National Institutes of Health, and made publicly accessible in 2000 (National Library of Medicine). Initially, federally and privately funded clinical trials conducted under investigational new drug applications were required to be registered and to provide this information to the public, healthcare professionals, and researchers. In 2005, the International Committee of Medical Journal Editors (ICMJE) began to require that authors seeking to publish clinical trial results provide evidence of registration of the clinical trial. The ICMJE's interest was to promote clinical trial registration as a means of addressing the well-documented bias in the publication and reporting of clinical trial results. The requirement for registration of clinical trials has since been expanded by the FDA Amendments Act of 2007 (FDAAA). As a result, this registry provides a comprehensive mechanism for identifying clinical trials when billing for items and services provided in these trials.

CMS additionally requires modifiers on charges for outpatient or professional clinical services that are billed to Medicare for a clinical trial (CMS 2008). The modifier Q0 designates an experimental item or service. Experimental items and services are not reimbursable under the CTP, so the use of this modifier is essentially limited to charges for Category B devices and for items and services allowed under CED. The Q1 modifier is used to designate all other charges for routine items and services.

It is not clear if and how Medicare has used this tracking data. However, it is also apparent that the labeling of claims could allow CMS "to undertake significant data-mining to compare different institutions' billing practices for the same research study" and provides a "powerful mechanism for the government's billing compliance enforcement" (Meade & Roach LLP 2008).

Medicare Advantage Plans

Medicare Advantage plans pose another challenge to billing in clinical trials. When Medicare Advantage plans came into being, the interagency agreement between FDA and CMS regarding coverage of investigational devices was already in place, so the cost of this benefit was calculated into the capitated payments made by CMS to the Medicare Advantage plans. Therefore, Medicare Advantage plans are required to cover costs from device trials that have been approved by CMS for Medicare billing. Drug studies, on the other hand, get complicated. After the CTP went into effect in 2000, "CMS determined that the cost of covering these new benefits was not included" in the capitated payments to Advantage plans (CMS 2014c). Therefore, it was decided that CMS should pay for the covered clinical trial services outside of the capitated payment rate. This means that, for a Medicare Advantage beneficiary, routine costs in trials subject to the CTP need to be billed to Medicare Fee-for-Service rather than to the beneficiary's Advantage plan. Providers need to have a mechanism to redirect claims appropriately. Then, the Medicare Advantage plan is required to cover the difference between its beneficiary's out-of-pocket costs and those incurred under Medicare Fee-for-Service (CMS 2013). The capitated payment rates have yet to be adjusted, so this band-aid solution has remained in place for a couple decades.

Issues in Non-compliance

This section is not intended to be a comprehensive review of laws and regulations, their interpretation, or their enforcement. However, it is intended to highlight issues that require careful consideration when determining the financial arrangements for covering the costs of clinical care provided in the context of clinical trials.

Subject Remuneration

Subject remuneration in clinical trials is a generally accepted practice, though some institutional review boards (IRBs) do not allow it and those that do typically want to review the reason for the remuneration, the amount, and the schedule of payment. This chapter will not cover the larger discussion on the appropriateness of subject remuneration but will only address the billing compliance issues that are raised in some circumstances.

Subject remuneration in clinical trials, like any form of gift or payment, is viewed by the OIG as an inducement to Medicare beneficiaries that could influence their selection of a particular provider of healthcare services. The OIG, in its Special Advisory Bulletin dated August 2002, stated that a person who offers remuneration to Medicare beneficiaries "could be liable for civil money penalties (CMPs) for up to $10,000 for each wrongful act" (HHS OIG 2002). However, the Advisory Bulletin allows that providers may offer gifts and remuneration that fit within five statutory exceptions; subject remuneration in clinical trials is potentially applicable to only one of these, which are practices allowed in the "safe harbor" provisions of the federal anti-kickback statute. Payments related to clinical trials (i.e., payments of industry sponsors to providers, payments of providers to research subjects) are typically judged against the requirements of the "personal services and management contracts" safe harbor of the anti-kickback statute (42 CFR § 1001.952(d)). This safe harbor category requires that the payments occur under a written and signed agreement that details the services to be provided and the schedule and term of the agreement (which cannot be for less than a year). It also requires that the compensation for the clinical trial activities is set in advance, is consistent with fair market value, and doesn't exceed what is reasonably necessary for the performance of the activities. Finally, the activities performed under the agreement cannot involve business promotion, and the compensation for the activities cannot be determined by the volume of referrals for services paid by federal healthcare programs. If a clinical trial agreement is so constituted and executed, providers should not incur liability for penalty for subject remuneration set out in such an agreement. That said, it is prudent, when determining subject remuneration, to have standard practices in place for the amount of compensation for specific things such as extra time, travel, parking, or other expenses incurred by subjects by virtue of being in the study. Stated in the converse, it is prudent to avoid paying subjects when their research participation is not requiring much in the way of time and expenses over and above what they would be investing for standard care. For example, when a study is merely abstracting data on the results of routine services, subjects are not incurring additional expenses by virtue of being in the study, and providing them with remuneration could arguably constitute inducement to receive those routine services as a research subject, and from the research provider.

Waiving of Co-pays

As providers are likely well aware, CMS considers the waiving of co-pays by providers to be in violation of the beneficiary inducements statute and the anti-kickback statute. That is, such waivers are seen as inducements to use services paid for by Medicare or inducement to receive services from a specific provider. Waiving of co-pays in clinical trials is largely seen in the same light, with the additional concern that it may sway beneficiaries to forego available proven therapies in favor of an experimental one (HHS OIG 2008). However, leaving subjects with out-of-pocket expenses that they would not have incurred, but for their participation in a clinical trial, are also not satisfactory. The IOM Committee, in its 2000 report, put forth the recommendation that subjects should not incur expenses for participation, over and above what might be expected for standard care, but recognized that, while this may be a guiding principle, it is not enforceable (Aaron and Gelband 2000). Indeed, not only is it unenforceable but in some instances is very difficult to achieve within the confines of current laws and their interpretations.

The OIG has issued a series of opinions in specific cases in which it has declined to impose sanctions for the payment of co-pays. The OIG is clear that these opinions are relevant to the specific cases only, but they are informative on the thinking of the Department of Health and Human Services. For example, in one case of a trial of oxygen therapy supported by the National Heart, Lung, and Blood Institute, investigators made the assertion that cost-sharing would result in the intervention group having more expenses than the control group and could decrease compliance. The OIG decided that the trial did not present risk of fraud and abuse, at least in part because it was co-sponsored by CMS and was not a commercial, product-oriented study (HHS OIG 2008). The OIG explicitly stated that "commercial or private studies pose significantly different risks under the fraud and abuse authorities." In another opinion, the OIG declined to impose sanctions when the payment of co-pays by Medicare beneficiaries would have unblinded the research subjects in a CED study as to whether they were in the active treatment or sham procedure group (HHS OIG 2015). In a third case, a trial sponsored by the National Cancer Institute, the OIG concurred that payment of co-pays by subjects could create an economic barrier to participation in a cancer prevention trial in people with HIV and could skew the research population toward a higher and less representative, socioeconomic status (HHS OIG 2016). These instances are all good examples in which the requirement for subjects to pay co-pays for care received as part of a clinical trial could affect the feasibility and/or scientific validity of the study, but it is clear that unless the OIG issues an opinion in a particular case, waiving of co-pays in clinical trials creates risk for the investigators.

Reimbursement for Subject Injury

Subject injury is a somewhat sticky issue in clinical research. Let us first consider clinical trials covered under the CTP. The CTP allows for billing of services related to monitoring for, preventing, and treating adverse effects related to the investigational therapy. So, for example, in an oncology chemotherapy trial, treatment of nausea and laboratory tests to monitor blood counts are billable. This seems quite reasonable when medical monitoring and management of adverse effects are to be expected with most therapies. It also is quite reasonable when it may be difficult to determine whether a clinical event is related to an investigational therapy or to the patient's larger clinical circumstances. However, there may be instances in which patients clearly suffer significant subject injury from an investigational therapy. The CTP provision for coverage of adverse effects was not intended to release industry sponsors from liability for their products or to transfer catastrophic costs to insurers. Additionally, it again is important to remember that when insurers are billed, in this case for adverse effects of therapy, subjects frequently may share in those costs through co-pays or deductibles. Therefore, it is important to carefully think through subject injury costs and who should be responsible for them. Industry sponsors historically have pledged to cover costs not covered by insurers, but this has proven problematic in a couple of regards.

Again, co-pays are at issue. Even in the case of treatment of adverse effects resulting from the study intervention, the waiving of co-pays could generate risk of penalty. A second issue is that of Medicare Secondary Payer (MSP) rule, which defines the circumstances under which Medicare is not obligated to pay until a primary insurer has paid, or because a primary insurer can reasonably be expected to pay for a covered item or service (42 US Code § 1395y). It is long been debated whether the MSP is invoked in so-called conditional payment clauses in clinical trial agreements; that is, does it violate MSP rules if a sponsor, in a clinical trial contract, agrees to pay for subject injury costs in the event that such costs are not covered by insurers? CMS in 2010 announced a policy for sponsor payments in clinical trials that stopped short of answering this question. The policy states that when sponsors pay for subject injury, they are acting as a liability insurer. It also states that such payments must be reported to CMS, which allows CMS to ensure that it has not paid for the same items and services. The naming of sponsors as liability insurers in clinical trials has generated discomfort by providers with contractual provisions to bill Medicare when there is a possibility of payment by the sponsor, i.e., another insurer. In the absence of definitive policy by Medicare, sponsors are seeming to recognize that to help providers mitigate compliance risk, they may need to accept financial obligations for subject injury. Some sponsors have attempted to limit the financial obligations by carving out subject injury payment for beneficiaries of federal programs only, as there are no potential legal implications for billing private insurers when there is a possibility of sponsor payment. However, such an approach puts additional compliance burden on providers to modify their clinical trial billing practices based on patients' source of insurance, but perhaps more ethically unsatisfactory is the creation of a situation in which the sponsor pays in whole for some patients' medical costs, while other patients experience cost-sharing with their insurers. In recognition of the above, it is the current recommendation of Model Agreements & Guidelines International (MAGI), an organization of industry players with the mission to standardize best practices for clinical operations, business, and regulatory compliance, to avoid such carve-outs in the contract and to provide for sponsor payment for subject injury. As pointed out by Meade & Roach, LLP, a leading law firm offering advisement in the research billing compliance space, "This arguably defers to the clinical trial agreement to define when – and presumably under what myriad of circumstances – the sponsor will pay for complications and injury related to the clinical trial. In essence, it becomes a matter of contract law as to what…the sponsor will consider to be complications." (Meade & Roach LLP 2010).

In a return to where we started in this section, it is important to note that the above issues relate to clinical trials falling under the CTP. For non-qualifying studies, device studies, and CED studies, there is no clear guidance on the billing of services related to monitoring for, preventing, and treating adverse effects related to the investigational therapy. Sponsors and providers are left to negotiate this space.

Billing Non-compliance

By far the issue that has gotten institutions in the most trouble has been the inappropriate or double billing of Medicare and Medicaid for services provided in the context of clinical research. There are a few well-known cases of penalties imposed on major medical centers for research billing found to be in violation of the False Claims Act (31 US Code § 3729). An early case is that of the University of Alabama at Birmingham. The US Department of Justice announced in April of 2005 that it had reached an agreement with the university to pay $3.39 million to settle allegations related to its research billing practices (DOJ 2005). The investigation of the institution resulted from two lawsuits brought by whistleblowers – a former physician and a former compliance officer at the medical school. It was alleged that the university "unlawfully billed Medicare for clinical research trials that were also billed to the sponsor of research grants." In December of that same year, Rush University Medical Center announced that it had voluntarily disclosed billing errors to the federal government (RUMC 2005). Under the False Claims Act, the government can impose fines up to three times the amount of the false claims. Rush, because of its self-disclosure and cooperation with the investigation, was only fined 50% of the amount of the false claims. With these penalties and restitution of the claims, the fine paid by Rush reportedly totaled about $1 million, substantially less than that paid by the University of Alabama at Birmingham.

Five years later, the Tenet HealthSystem/USC Norris Cancer Center agreed to pay $1.9 million (HHS OIG 2010). The health system was already operating under a 5-year corporate integrity agreement with the OIG as part of the resolution of a wide range of investigated fraudulent activities. Under the disclosure requirements of the agreement, the health system revealed that it submitted improper claims for "(1) items or services that were paid for by clinical research sponsors or grants under which the clinical research was conducted; (2) items or services intended to be free of charge in the research informed consent; (3) items or services that were for research purposes only and not for the clinical management of the patient; and/or (4) items or services that were otherwise not covered under the Centers for Medicare & Medicaid Services (CMS) Clinical Trial Policy." The fine for its research billing practices paled in comparison to the more than $900 million paid by the health system in 2006 to settle its other billing liabilities.

In 2013, Emory University admitted to overbilling Medicare and Medicaid in clinical trials conducted at its Winship Cancer Institute (DOJ 2013). The case was brought to light by a former research finance manager at the university. Emory University agreed to pay $1.5 million to settle its claims related to billing for services for which clinical trial sponsors either had paid or had agreed to pay.

To put these cases into perspective, one can compare them to the overall recoveries by the federal government under the False Claims Act. In 2018, the federal government collected $2.5 billion in such settlements from the larger healthcare sector, the ninth consecutive year that this amount exceeded $2 billion (DOJ 2018). In this light, non-compliance in clinical trial billing is a small fraction of the cases pursued by the Department of Justice. However, for premier research institutions, it is not only their clinical revenue but also their research grant revenue that could be put in jeopardy by research billing non-compliance. As these institutions have increasingly joined forces with community healthcare systems and are expanding their research bases, the imperative for billing compliance continues to mount.

Summary: Best Practices for Billing Compliance

In summary, this chapter has discussed the evolution of the rules regarding financial compliance in clinical trials. The Institute of Medicine report set the stage for the clinical trials policy, and the GCRCs referenced in the report were leaders in establishing best billing compliance practices.

Today, a comprehensive program for financial compliance must include the below elements.

- *Determination of Qualification*: Every research study that involves interaction of a healthcare provider with a patient must be examined to determine if the study meets the criteria of a qualifying clinical trial.
- *Coverage Analysis*: Every item, service, and activity that is required by the clinical trial protocol must be analyzed to determine if it is billable or not. This determination should be documented and referenced for billing review.
- *Review and Comparison of Contract and Consent*: The contract should be examined carefully for what the sponsor is obligated to cover, especially regarding subject injury. Any language that could invoke the Medicare as Secondary Payer rule is best avoided. The consent must be reviewed for any promises of coverage to subjects and should be consistent with the terms of the contract.
- *Billing Review*: Charges that are incurred by participants in clinical research studies should be reviewed in a systematic fashion to ensure that they are being triaged correctly. There are a number of philosophies and mechanisms to achieve this that run the gamut from a manual, charge-by-charge comparison against the coverage analysis of 100% of participants' items and services while enrolled in a study to sophisticated, automated methods to find research charges and label them with the appropriate codes and modifiers. Whatever the mechanism for billing

review, documentation that a charge was reviewed is necessary for quality control and auditing of the process.
- *Auditing*: The loop is closed by audit of at least a subset of study subjects to ensure that all expected research charges were identified and billed as appropriate to the sponsor or the subject's insurer. It can lead to further auditing if errors are detected that could be more widespread or systemic.

Such a comprehensive program requires infrastructure and resources to support it. The costs of the software to track research finances, the IT resources to customize, implement, and integrate research-specific tools, and the personnel to conduct coverage analyses, billing reviews, and audits are not insignificant. These costs typically do not generate a return on investment; they are the costs of doing business and of being compliant while doing so. If not covered as a direct cost in research budgets, these costs need to be part of the calculation of institutional overhead, as they are a necessary component of research infrastructure.

Key Facts

- In the United States, what can be billed to insurance and what must be paid by a sponsor are largely determined by CMS.
- Medicare reimbursement for device trials is governed by an interagency agreement between FDA and CMS, which has been in place since 1995.
- Medicare reimbursement for drug trials is governed by the Clinical Trial Policy, which went into effect in 2000.
- CMS uses the mechanism of Coverage with Evidence Development to allow coverage of items and services for which CMS does not find there to be enough evidence to support their use as "reasonable and necessary" but for which additional data could help clarify the value of the service.
- Research institutions need to have processes for determining at the start of a trial if it qualifies for CMS coverage and for conducing coverage analyses to determine which clinical items and services are to be paid by the research study and which can be billed to CMS.
- Charges that are billed to CMS as routine care provided in the context of clinical trials are to be labeled as such through the use of modifiers and codes on the claim.
- Subject remuneration, payment of co-pays, and reimbursement for subject injury are three complicated issues for which special care must be taken to avoid noncompliance.
- Noncompliance in research billing carries risk of monetary penalty, as set forth in the False Claims Act.
- There have been four cases of large fines to research institutions for billing noncompliance.
- A comprehensive program to ensure financial compliance in clinical trials requires investment in research infrastructure by institutions.

References

Aaron HJ, Gelband H (eds) (2000) Committee on routine patient care costs in clinical trials for medicare beneficiaries, Institute of medicine. Extending medicare reimbursement in clinical trials. National Academy Press, Washington, DC

Centers for Medicare and Medicaid Services. National coverage determination (NCD) for routine costs in clinical trials (310.1). Publication 100-3, Version 1. Effective date September 19, 2000

Centers for Medicare and Medicaid Services. Guidance for the public industry, and CMS staff: national coverage determinations with data collection as a condition of coverage: coverage with evidence development. Issued July 12, 2006

Centers for Medicare and Medicaid Services. National coverage determination (NCD) for routine costs in clinical trials (310.1). Publication 100-3, Version 2. Effective date July 9, 2007

Centers for Medicare and Medicaid Services. CMS manual system: medicare claims processing. New HCPCS Modifiers when Billing for Patient Care in Clinical Research Studies Publication 100-04. Effective date January 1, 2008

Centers for Medicare and Medicaid Services. CMS manual system: medicare managed care. Chapter 4, Benefits and beneficiary protections. Publication 100-16. Effective date August 23, 2013

Centers for Medicare and Medicaid Services. CMS manual system: medicare benefit policy. Publication 100-02. November 6, 2014a

Centers for Medicare and Medicaid Services. Guidance for the public industry, and CMS staff: coverage with evidence development. Issued November 20, 2014b

Centers for Medicare and Medicaid Services. Medicare managed care manual. Chapter 8, Payments to medicare advantage organizations. Revision 118. September 19, 2014c

Department of Health and Human Services, Food and Drug Administration, Center for Devices and Radiological Health. Information sheet guidance for IRBs, clinical investigators, and sponsors: significant risk and nonsignificant risk medical device studies. January 2006

Department of Health and Human Services, Food and Drug Administration, Center for Devices and Radiological Health. FDA categorization of investigational device exemption (IDE) devices to assist the centers for medicare and medicaid services (CMS) with coverage decisions: guidance for sponsors, clinical investigators, industry, institutional review boards, and Food and Drug Administration staff. December 5, 2017

Department of Health and Human Services, Food and Drug Administration, Office of Device Evaluation. Implementation of the FDA/HCFA interagency agreement regarding reimbursement categorization of investigational devices. IDE guidance memorandum #95-2. September 15, 1995

Department of Health and Human Services, Office of the Inspector General. Special advisory bulletin. Offering gifts and other inducements to beneficiaries. August 2002

Department of Health and Human Services, Office of the Inspector General. OIG Advisory Opinion 08-11. September 17, 2008

Department of Health and Human Services, Office of the Inspector General. Semiannual report to Congress, Part III: legal and investigative activities related to medicare and medicaid. Fall 2010

Department of Health and Human Services, Office of the Inspector General. OIG Advisory Opinion 15-07. May 28, 2015

Department of Health and Human Services, Office of the Inspector General. OIG Advisory Opinion 16-13. December 13, 2016

Department of Justice. Press release: University of Alabama-Birmingham will pay U.S. $3.39 Million to resolve false billing allegations. April 14, 2005

Department of Justice, Office of Public Affairs. Press release: justice department recovers over $2.8 billion from false claims act cases in fiscal year 2018. December 21, 2018

Department of Justice, U.S. Attorney's Office, Northern District of Georgia. Press release: Emory University to pay $1.5 million to settle false claims act investigation. August 28, 2013

International Committee of Medical Journal Editors. Recommendations: publishing & editorial issues: clinical trials. http://www.icmje.org/recommendations/browse/publishing-and-editorial-issues/clinical-trial-registration.html. Accessed May 29, 2019

Meade & Roach LLP. Compliance advisory: new CMS research modifier rules. http://meaderoach.com/advisory_newsletters.html. April 2008. Accessed 29 May 2019

Meade & Roach LLP. Compliance advisory: CMS issues clinical trials MSP instruction. http://meaderoach.com/advisory_newsletters.html. July 2010. Accessed 29 May 2019

Model Agreements & Guidelines International. Clinical trial agreement template (Annotated). https://www.magiworld.org/Standards?M=1&PK=47. Accessed May 29, 2019

National Library of Medicine. About site: history, policies, and laws. https://clinicaltrials.gov/ct2/about-site/history. Last reviewed September 2018. Accessed 29 May 2019

Rush University Medical Center. News release. Rush settlement with government may help clarify billing requirements for medicare patients in research studies: sets model for provider compliance with national coverage decision on clinical trials. December 8, 2005

The White House, Office of the Press Secretary. President Clinton takes new action to encourage participation in clinical trials: medicare will reimburse for all routine patient care costs for those in clinical trials. June 7, 2000

Statutes and Regulations

29 CFR § 812.2(c)
30 CFR § 1001.952(d)
31 US Code § 3729
42 US Code § 1395y

Financial Conflicts of Interest in Clinical Trials

28

Julie D. Gottlieb

Contents

Abstract

Because clinical trials are the gold standard for evaluating the safety and efficacy of drugs and medical devices, they should be conducted as safely and objectively as possible. Objectivity can be affected by study design and conduct, but additional risks to objectivity – and possible risks to safety – may arise from financial conflicts of interest (FCOIs). The explosion in recent decades of financial relationships between medical researchers and the pharmaceutical and medical device industry means it is very likely that at least some members of most clinical trial study teams will have a financial tie with the sponsor or manufacturer of the study drug or device. Payments of various types are ubiquitous. The data on

J. D. Gottlieb (✉)
Johns Hopkins University School of Medicine, Baltimore, MD, USA
e-mail: jgottlie@jhmi.edu

© Springer Nature Switzerland AG 2022
S. Piantadosi, C. L. Meinert (eds.), *Principles and Practice of Clinical Trials*,
https://doi.org/10.1007/978-3-319-52636-2_275

payments to physicians published by the Center for Medicare and Medicaid Services (CMS) since 2014 offers evidence that approximately half of all physicians have financial ties with industry (Tringale et al. 2017). Social science studies have demonstrated that financial interests can give rise to conscious or unconscious bias in favor of the product being tested or its manufacturer. In addition, when institutions that are clinical trial sites have financial interests related to a clinical trial, the institutional conflicts of interest (institutional COIs) can create risks to the objectivity or safety of the study. So close attention to conflict of interest issues is essential for protecting the integrity of clinical trials. This chapter will examine the nature of the risks at issue, key regulations and standards for addressing FCOIs in research, key elements of FCOI policies, and approaches to evaluating and addressing FCOIs.

Keywords

COI committee · Data safety monitoring board · Disclosures · Financial conflicts of interest · Institutional conflicts of interest · Management plan · Technology licensing

Definition

A common definition of a conflict of interest is "a set of circumstances that creates a risk that professional judgment or actions regarding a primary interest will be unduly influenced by a secondary interest" (Lo and Bero 2017).

Introduction

The primary goals of those who conduct clinical trials must be to carry out safe and objective research that has the potential to advance the science of human health. If the safety of research participants (and future patients) and the objectivity of research are of paramount importance, the potential risks of conflicts of interest must be addressed.

Conflicts of interest (COIs) are ubiquitous in personal and professional life. While there have been calls to consider the risks of intellectual COIs (Ioannidis and Trepanowski 2018), such as strongly held personal beliefs, FCOIs in medical research have received the most attention in large part because of the widespread practice of industry payments to researchers and the incentives associated with inventing, patenting, and licensing new technologies and starting new companies in the biomedical field. And financial interests, unlike potentially competing intellectual interests, can be measured.

Funders and consumers of academic research and the academic research community itself have intensified their focus on FCOIs because of the potential they have to affect research, education, and clinical care. In the wake of various exposés and investigational reporting in the media (Stolberg 2019), scrutiny of the impact of the financial interests of physicians and biomedical researchers increased throughout the early 2000s. National associations have issued recommendations and guidelines for addressing the risks that FCOIs pose in education, clinical care, and to some extent basic and animal research. In academia, most of the attention, including regulation and association standards, has centered on FCOIs in clinical research because the welfare of human research participants is at stake and because research results directly impact medical care and treatment.

This chapter will address FCOIs in clinical trials, including the financial interests of investigators and the institutions where research is often conducted. Not all financial interests create the potential for conflict of interest or the appearance of conflict of interest. If a physician who conducts clinical trials in interventional cardiology owns stock in an energy company, for example, the financial interest is unlikely to create the potential for conscious or unconscious bias related to the value of a particular intervention. However, if the researcher owns stock in a company that sells cardiac stents, that is likely to create an FCOI with her research. So one must define the types of financial interests that have the potential to affect the objectivity and safety of clinical research. Under Public Health Service (PHS) regulation on FCOI, when a grantee institution is conducting research, an investigator must disclose to the institution any financial interest "that reasonably appears to be related to the Investigator's institutional responsibilities." Institutions must review the disclosed interests to identify any "[F]inancial conflict of interest (FCOI)," which is defined as "a significant financial interest that could directly and significantly affect the design, conduct, or reporting of PHS-funded research" (eCFR – Code of Federal Regulations 2019). FCOIs must be addressed with specific management steps. The key roles and responsibilities of the parties involved in clinical research – investigators, institutions, the committees that evaluate potential FCOIs, sponsors, and journals – are set forth in Table 1.

Those conducting or administering clinical trials at hospitals, medical schools, or research organizations that themselves may have financial interests in biomedical research also must deal with institutional COI (Cigarroa et al. 2018). Although there are no US regulations governing institutional COIs in research, many research organizations include institutional COI in their FCOI policies. When the institution where the research is being conducted has a financial interest in the outcome of research, or their senior leaders have ties to companies with financial interests in a study, there may be an actual or apparent institutional COI. For example, an institution that is conducting research on a novel bone harvesting device that it licensed to a start-up company has an institutional COI with the trial testing the device. Of course, it is an institution's agents (deans, department chairs, etc.) who act on behalf of the institution. The risks arise from a concern that in a conscious or unconscious effort to maximize the value of the product or manufacturer in which the institution has a stake, institutional agents may make decisions that conflict with the safety and objectivity of the research project. Another source of concern arises from the personal financial interests of institutional officials when those interests are related to the research they oversee. For instance, even if a research dean or hospital

Table 1 Roles and responsibilities of investigators, institutions, IRB or COI committees, sponsors, and journals in the disclosure, review and management of financial conflicts of interest

Investigator	Institution	IRB and/or COI Committee	Sponsor	Journals
Disclose personal financial interests to institution and/ or IRB as required	Establish, publicize, implement, and enforce FCOI policy	Review disclosures associated with specific clinical trials	For FDA regulated trials, collect disclosures from investigators, manage FCOIs, report FCOIs to FDA	Set policies regarding permissible COIs; require disclosure to journal and in publications
Comply with FCOI management plan	Disclose institutional COIs for review as required	Develop and communicate management plan	If a covered entity, report payments to physicians to Centers for Medicare and Medicaid Services under Physician Payments Sunshine Act	
Follow disclosure requirements of institution (e.g., to patients, study team members, sponsor) and of journals	Monitor compliance with management plans	Identify any failures to comply with management plan		
	Report FCOIs to regulatory bodies as required			
	Make FCOI information related to PHS sponsored studies publicly available per PHS regulations			

president is not directly involved in a particular study but has stock in the manufacturer of the study drug or device, she may – consciously or unconsciously – make decisions affecting the safety and objectivity of the study. Even decisions that are not intended to impact a study may be *viewed* as biased if the decision maker has a related financial interest and that interest is not disclosed or steps are not taken to protect the study.

Risks of Financial Conflicts of Interest: Reality and Appearance

There is a growing body of literature demonstrating strong associations between financial interests and fealty to professional standards, including in medical practice and research (Dana and Loewenstein 2003). Social science research has shown that even modest gifts create an expectation of reciprocity, and studies have demonstrated that there are strong associations between investigators' ties with industry and positive outcomes of related research (Ahn et al. 2017; Lundh and Bero 2017). Research also indicates that many professionals, including physicians, tend to think they are not susceptible to bias and believe they are less vulnerable to the influence of payments and gifts than their colleagues (Cain 2008).

It is important to acknowledge, however, that even the *appearance* of a researcher's or an institution's financial conflict of interest with a study may call into question the integrity of a research project. This is as important as clearly established causation or association. Disclosure of – or, more significantly, the failure to disclose – ties between a researcher or research institution and industry as they relate to clinical research can lead to skepticism on the part of a scientific audience, negative news reports about the research, and doubt on the part of society that medical research is being carried out honestly and is worthy of public support. When patients suffer a bad outcome while participating in a clinical trial, the presence of significant financial interests may strengthen an argument that financial interests played a role in the harm to research participants. There are well-known cases in which plaintiffs' attorneys have linked investigators' (and their institutions') financial interests with the harm suffered by research subjects in clinical trials (Wilson 2009).

Regulations and Other Important Standards

Regulations on conflict of interest in research are varied and inconsistent with one another. There are different standards and recommendations issued by accrediting bodies, journals, professional societies, and national associations (Gottlieb 2015). Institutional officials should be familiar with the array of relevant regulations and standards when developing conflict of interest policies. A brief overview of these standards follows, and additional detail appears elsewhere in this chapter.

Clinical research is subject to the Public Health Service (PHS) regulations on objectivity in research if PHS support is involved. The Food and Drug Administration (FDA) regulation applies (CFR – Code of Federal Regulations Title 21 2019) if the trial data are to be used in marketing applications for FDA approval of a drug, device, or biologic product. Separate standards are maintained by the Association for the Accreditation of Human Research Protection Programs (AAHRPP), which accredits Institutional Review Boards (IRBs), national associations such as the Association of American Medical Colleges (AAMC) and the Association of American Universities (AAU), journals, including those that adhere to the standards set by the International Committee of Medical Journal

Editors (ICMJE), and professional societies such as the American Society of Clinical Oncology (ASCO).

Public Health Service. The 1995 PHS regulation on FCOI (titled "Promoting Objectivity in Research") was substantially revised in 2011, and the revised version went into effect 2012. The regulation covers research supported by PHS agencies (including, among others, the National Institutes of Health, Centers for Disease Control and Prevention, FDA, and the Centers for Medicare and Medicaid Services). It outlines the types of financial interests that investigators must report to a recipient institution that applies for or receives federal research support; how the disclosed interests must be reviewed for potential FCOI with federally funded research projects; and the range of possible approaches to managing FCOIs. While the regulation does not distinguish among different types of research and its focus is on protecting research objectivity rather than research participant safety, it acknowledges that FCOIs in research involving human participants carry the greatest potential risk. Some institutions responded to the 2012 revisions by applying the federal standards to all research regardless of funding source in order to have a single, consistent standard for COI review. Others opted to apply the regulation only to research with federal support, potentially limiting their administrative burden but creating dual standards for federally funded research and research with other sources of support. The 2012 revision lowered the financial "floor" for annual income that must be reported from $10,000 to $5,000 and expanded reporting requirements for reporting of equity ownership. Other reportable interests include royalties from intellectual property, honoraria, consulting fees, and equity in publicly traded and privately held companies. Exceptions to reporting requirements include income from US institutions of higher education and service on certain US federal, state, and local government advisory panels. However, income from non-excluded nonprofit organizations such as foundations and foreign institutions of higher education must be disclosed. There also is a requirement that institutions solicit disclosures of payment or reimbursement for travel. Specified details about FCOIs that institutions have identified and managed must be reported to the awarding agency and must be publicly disclosed on a regularly updated website or upon request.

The PHS FCOI regulation does not require that research support from industry to the recipient institution be disclosed and reviewed for potential FCOI. FDA COI disclosure requirements do not include industry support for the "covered" study (although they do include funds the sponsor may provide the institution that are not directly supporting the covered study). However, there are reasons for institutional policies to consider the role of industry research support, whether financial or in-kind, in the course of their FCOI reviews. Some federally supported research projects also involve support from industry. Many institutions apply their FCOI polices to research that is not federally funded but may be supported by industry (or foundations that are closely tied to a biomedical company with an interest in the research). Journals and professional societies typically require disclosure of research support from industry. Institutions whose FCOI policies do not include research supported by industry take the position that while grants or sponsored research funds awarded to institutions may support a portion of an investigator's salary, the funding is administered by the institution, and it supports a variety of costs of conducting the research. Those that do include industry support tend to view the sources of support for an investigator's salary and the research costs as potential sources of bias. Finally, research grants made directly to investigators who are not part of academic medical centers – for example, those in private medical practices – are more direct personal payments to investigators and may be significant sources of conscious or unconscious bias. In sum, support for the costs of research is treated heterogeneously in the clinical research community.

Food and Drug Administration. The FDA's regulation on conflict of interest for clinical investigators applies to studies being used to support marketing applications for drugs, medical devices, and biologic products. Its purpose is to identify situations in which investigators involved in generating the data have FCOIs exceeding the thresholds set by FDA, address the risk of bias, and thereby enhance the integrity of the approval process for marketing of drugs and medical devices. The sponsor, whether a company or a sponsor-investigator, must collect investigators' financial interest information, apply conflict of interest management measures to mitigate the risks to data associated with FCOIs, and report the information to the FDA. FDA regulation does not prohibit or restrict investigators with FCOIs from participating in research, including as authors of resulting publications. However, in evaluating the potential for bias associated with the data collected by the conflicted investigator, the FDA takes into account the COI management measures applied to the study as well as study design elements such as blinding, objective endpoints, and measurement of endpoints by someone other than a conflicted investigator.

Some institutions have adopted a policy that if an investigator on an FDA-regulated study has financial interests exceeding certain thresholds, that individual may not serve as the sponsor-investigator for the study (and that significant financial interests also disqualify non-investigators from acting as sponsors of FDA-regulated studies).

World Medical Association. The Declaration of Helsinki, which sets forth ethical principles for medical research involving human participants, requires that prospective research participants be informed of any relevant conflicts of interest on the part of investigators (World Medical Association Declaration of Helsinki 2013).

In 2004, the *Office for Human Research Protections* (OHRP) issued a guidance document that governs human subject protection in research conducted under the HHS or FDA regulations. Although it does not have the force of regulation, the document suggests approaches for investigators, institutions, and IRBs to consider in addressing potential FCOIs. The guidance includes IRB operations and cites regulation prohibiting IRB members with conflicting interests in a project from participating in the initial or continuing (HHS.gov 2016).

The *Association for the Accreditation of Human Research Protection Programs* (AAHRPP), which has accredited a substantial majority of human research protection programs (e.g., Institutional Review Boards) in US research-intensive universities and medical schools, includes investigator and institutional conflict of interest as elements in its evaluation process. So organizations seeking this important credential for their human research protection programs need to address COI and institutional COI policies as they prepare for the accreditation process.

The *Association of American Medical Colleges* (AAMC) issued guidance documents for dealing with COIs in human subject research in the early 2000s. The most notable recommendation is that individual FCOIs in human subject research that exceed certain thresholds should be subject to a "rebuttable presumption," i.e., investigators with those interests should not be permitted to participate in the relevant human research project. The AAMC's recommendations challenge institutions to set robust FCOI standards for their human subject research programs.

The *International Committee of Medical Journal Editors* (ICMJE) has issued a series of recommendations, including recommendations for addressing conflicts of interest (ICMJE | Recommendations | Author Responsibilities – Conflicts of Interest 2019) involving authors of journal articles as well as reviewers and editors. The ICMJE developed a detailed COI disclosure form that journals can require authors and those involved in the review of manuscripts to complete so there is transparency about financial interests. The organization recommends that journals publish the disclosure forms (or key FCOI information) with articles as well as a statement about the authors' access to study data. A large number of journals, including many leading biomedical journals, claim to have adopted the ICMJE recommendations.

Developing and Implementing COI Policies for Clinical Trials

Organizations that conduct clinical trials should adopt, publish, and implement a credible FCOI policy. The policy should:

- (i) Outline the financial interests that must be disclosed to the organization as well as when and how they should be disclosed.
- (ii) Describe the process and standards for review of those interests, whether by the IRB or an ancillary committee charged with addressing FCOIs (COI Committee).
- (iii) Require the institution to issue a written management plan designed to manage, reduce, or eliminate risks associated with the FCOI.
- (iv) State that the institution will monitor compliance with the FCOI management plan and address failures to comply.

Disclosure

COI policies should specify who must make disclosures of potential FCOIs, what interests and other information must be disclosed, and the time frame for disclosure.

Policies should detail whether all or a subset of the following must be disclosed: personal income in the form of fees, honoraria, or other payments; patents, patents pending, and trademarks; royalty income or entitlement to royalty under a license agreement; equity interests in publicly traded companies; equity interests in non-publicly traded companies; fiduciary roles, such as service on boards of directors; and the interests of immediate family members. Even organizations that do not receive PHS support should consider adopting an FCOI policy – including disclosure requirements – that complies with the regulation. The regulation applies to sub-recipients, such as sites for clinical trials involving federal funds, and the agreement between the recipient organization and the sub-recipient may require the latter to have a PHS-compliant policy.

Some institutions require disclosure of financial interests in companies that compete with the company that is developing the study product. Defining such interests and evaluating them can be complex and nuanced.

Under PHS regulations, institutions must solicit disclosures of income and payments that, in the aggregate, exceed $5,000 in the 12 months preceding the disclosure; income from intellectual property (e.g., royalties); ownership of equity worth more than $5,000 in publicly traded companies; any equity ownership in privately held companies; and travel payments or reimbursements of over $5,000 in a 12-month period. The disclosure requirements also apply to these interests if they are held by immediate family members.

The policy should specify when and how disclosures should be submitted and updated. (Ideally, there should be an online or other easy-to-use process for submitting and updating financial interest disclosures. There are turn-key systems on the market, and many can be customized.) In the setting of clinical research, disclosures should be made well before the study is approved by the IRB so there can be a complete review of the potential risks of the financial interests. FCOI management may necessitate a change in the protocol or in the roles of investigators. Making changes to study design or personnel too late in the process may be costly and/or inconvenient. The more specific and up-to-date disclosures are, the more robust and effective the review can be. Since investigators' financial interests may change during the course of a clinical trial, FCOI policies need to require that disclosures be updated in a timely way so that new circumstances can be addressed promptly.

Whether FCOIs are reviewed by an IRB or another body, such as a designated COI committee, close integration between the information systems for FCOI disclosure and human subject research is advisable. That, in addition to well-coordinated administrative processes, will maximize the likelihood that FCOIs in clinical trials are identified and addressed in a timely way.

Institutional COIs. Organizations that address institutional COIs need to develop a system for informing the IRB or COI committee of the institution's financial interests as they relate to a particular study. The interests might include income from licensing intellectual property; equity in start-up companies based on inventions made at the institution; or the equity, royalty, consulting income, and board service of senior institutional officials. Aggregating and efficiently communicating the information can be challenging. Many institutional financial interests arise from technology licensing activity, which is often administratively disconnected from research administration and IRBs. Moreover, if an institution has an interest in a drug or device but the inventor is not an investigator on the study, it may be difficult to make the link between study and the institution's financial interest.

So institutions that take institutional COIs into consideration may need manual or custom methods of matching institutional financial information with trial data.

Review for FCOI in Clinical Trials

Substantive review is at the heart of the FCOI process. A robust review should identify the risks that the investigators' and institution's financial interests may generate in the context of a specific clinical trial and within the framework of applicable policy and regulations. There should be a well-defined review process, and the reviewers, whether the IRB members or the members of a COI committee, should have relevant expertise (e.g., experienced clinical trialists, biostatisticians) and independence. If the reviewing body is not the IRB, close coordination with the IRB is essential.

Reviewers should be free of bias. They should disclose any competing personal interests and should recuse themselves from a particular case if they have an interest that may bias or appear to bias their review.

An Initial Consideration: Thresholds for Participation

One threshold question is whether a conflicted investigator should be permitted to have any role in a clinical trial. While there are national guidelines (e.g., AAMC) that recommend limits on the financial interests a clinical investigator may have, neither PHS nor FDA regulations require that investigators whose financial interests exceed certain levels be disqualified from participation. Many leading academic medical centers do, however, set thresholds for permitting a conflicted investigator to participate in a study. These institutions take the position that a researcher who has a "significant" financial interest (however the institution defines it) may not participate in a clinical trial unless the individual completely divests herself of the conflicting financial interests. There are variations among even the most restrictive policies. For instance, some draw the line at allowing conflicted researchers to have any role in a trial; others prohibit conflicted investigators from serving as principal investigators (PIs) but still allow them to be part of a study team.

Social science research has shown that even modest gifts or payments are sources of potential bias (Dana and Loewenstein 2003), but regulators, institutions, and others take into account the nature and size of financial interests. Many policies set thresholds for cash income at a level that may allow for some compensated consulting while, in their judgment, not creating undue bias or an appearance of unacceptable conflict of interest. Equity ownership in a publicly traded company is often treated like cash. If the value of the stock does not exceed a specified limit, the investigator may hold the stock and participate in the study. Equity ownership in a privately held company – especially if the company has licensed the investigator's invention – is widely viewed as disqualifying the researcher from any but the most limited participation in a trial in which the technology is being tested. This is because any trial of the product is likely to directly and significantly impact the value of the equity. Likewise, royalty income and entitlement to future royalty income through inventorship of a study drug or device can create an incentive to demonstrate the safety or efficacy of the product since that can affect regulatory approval, sales, and ultimately personal income. Some institutions allow limited participation for inventors of investigational drugs or devices in an attempt to balance the organization's drive for innovation and translational research with the risks of FCOIs. Finally, service as a board member or officer of a company with an interest in the investigational drug or device is often treated as a bar to participation in trials of the company's products because fiduciary roles require the individual to act in the best interests of the company, a goal that may directly conflict with an investigator's obligation to carry out safe and objective research.

Some institutions set thresholds for the institution's own involvement in a trial. For example, if an institution, through a technology license to a start-up company, holds equity in the manufacturer of an investigational drug and is entitled to royalty on eventual sales of the drug, it may be prudent for trials of safety and efficacy to be conducted at another institution – one that does not have conflicts of interest. Some institutions require that the protocol and/or the institutional COI be reviewed by another institution's IRB or COI Committee, provided that institution does not itself have a conflict of interest with the study. Another approach is to permit the conflicted institution to participate, but not lead the study. That may involve allowing only a small percentage of patients to be enrolled at the institution and ensuring that the institution does not serve as coordinating center or have another other leadership role in the study.

Institutions should clearly outline which FCOIs disqualify an investigator from participating in a trial. To the extent a conflicted individual may be permitted to participate, the institution must undertake a careful, detailed analysis of the study and especially the features that are vulnerable to FCOI risks. Elements of the review are described below. The review should result in a plan to ensure that risks to safety and objectivity are minimized or mitigated and that there is transparency to all key parties about any conflicts of interest.

Study Design and Planning

Clinical trials should be designed to answer scientific questions and not to support a predetermined outcome. Certain study designs can help mitigate the risk that a conflicted investigator will inject bias into the study. One option is to ensure that the investigators are blinded to treatment and control arms. Investigators with FCOIs generate greater risk for unblinded studies, especially Phase I or Phase II studies. For example, in an oncology study comparing standard of care to standard of care combined with an interventional therapy, an investigator with a financial interest in the study drug may be tempted – consciously or unconsciously – to adjust dosages of the standard therapy, as permitted in the protocol, to boost the apparent efficacy of the intervention.

Study designs with objective endpoints that can be recorded, reviewed, and tested by those without FCOIs are likely to be safer from bias than those with subjective endpoints.

Transparency is a powerful tool for protection against bias on the part of a conflicted investigator. Disclosing to all study team members that an investigator has an FCOI builds in a measure of oversight. The study team should also be informed of the measures put in place to address the FCOI, especially since they may be charged with implementing parts of the management plan. For example, a research coordinator who is a consent designee should know if the PI has a conflict of interest so he can clearly inform prospective subjects of the COI (Friedman et al. 2007). Study team members should be advised about how to raise any concerns related to the FCOI and should be protected if they do so.

Expanding a study to more than one center and vesting greater authority in another center, e.g., as coordinating center, especially if the PI and/or her institution have financial interests in the study, can mitigate the risks that any bias in the conduct of the study at the conflicted center will unduly influence the outcome.

Data Safety Monitoring Boards. Establishing independent data safety monitoring boards (DSMBs), especially where the DSMB is informed of the FCOI and formally charged with addressing any FCOI-related risks, can offer powerful protection for trials with conflicts of interest. This is especially true if there is an institutional COI, as long as the DSMB members are independent of the institution. To ensure a DSMB is truly independent, its members should have no conflicting financial interests. Ideally, the DSMB members should not be appointed by the industry sponsor, and if an industry sponsor wants to have a nonvoting representative on a DSMB, that individual may provide information but should not participate in or be present during discussion or voting.

Study Conduct

Recruitment and Consent. FCOIs can inject risk into the recruitment and consenting process. Investigators with FCOIs may be tempted to stretch or expand enrollment criteria to favor a particular outcome. While such behavior may represent noncompliance with a protocol, the risk can be lowered by putting protective measures in place such as prohibiting those with FCOIs from recruiting subjects to trials. Likewise, informed consent should be obtained by individuals other than a conflicted investigator and ideally by individuals who (a) know about the FCOIs and (b) are not supervised by the investigator with an FCOI. Informed consent documents should clearly state if there is an FCOI or an institutional COI and provide contact information for prospective subjects who may have questions.

Intervention. The greatest risk to clinical trial participants may be the investigational intervention. Because administering a drug is fairly straightforward, there is usually no reason a conflicted investigator needs to participate. If the intervention involves an experimental device for which the procedure is novel or very specialized, the conflicted investigator may be able to make a case that his unique expertise is essential for the safety of the procedure. That argument should be tested with independent senior experts in the field. If it is determined that the conflicted investigator has unique expertise, and in particular that his participation is important for subject safety, he may be permitted to implement the procedure as long as other measures are put in place. For example, the investigator may be allowed to carry out a limited number of interventions provided he trains another physician to succeed and replace him in carrying out the procedure. Assigning a non-conflicted investigator responsibility for reporting adverse events and serious adverse events adds a layer of protection if it is judged important for subject safety to allow the conflicted investigator to carry out the intervention.

Data collection is another area of potential vulnerability. Ensuring that endpoints are objective, that non-conflicted investigators collect the data, and that all study team members have access to the study data can help address potential COI risks.

Data Analysis. A conflicted investigator's bias, whether conscious or unconscious, is likely to favor the interventional drug or device. So it is especially important to protect data analysis from any conflict or appearance of conflict. Potential approaches include engaging independent biostatisticians to advise on analytical tools and conduct the analyses; avoiding unacceptable cherry-picking; and avoiding analyses designed to overweight or promote very modest effects of an interventional drug or device.

Publication/Reporting

If a conflicted investigator is allowed to participate in a trial in way that qualifies her for authorship, she must be included as an author on resulting publications. However, steps are needed to protect against bias in the publication and ensure transparency. First, she should not have a role (such as first or senior author) that vests substantial authority over the publication. Her contributions should be reviewed by the first and senior authors for potential bias. If for some reason a conflicted investigator is permitted to serve as first or senior author, the institution should consider having an independent expert with access to study data review the manuscript for potential bias.

Second, whatever role the conflicted investigator is permitted to have, her relevant financial interests should be disclosed (a) to the journal in accordance with its requirements and (b) in the manuscript. Journals have varied disclosure requirements, and the information they publish also varies. But it is the authors' responsibility to understand and follow those requirements. Failure to adhere to journal policies – and the scientific community's expectation of transparency – can lead to corrections, article retractions, being barred from publishing in the journal for a period of time, bad publicity, and even disciplinary action by one's employer (Bauchner et al. 2018; Gottlieb and Bressler 2017).

Documenting and Communicating FCOI Decisions: The Management Plan

The reviewing body should outline a plan for dealing with the FCOIs or institutional COIs associated with the trial. A written management plan should outline clearly the activities in which the conflicted individual (or institution) may participate and under what conditions; which activities the conflicted investigator may not participate in and who will handle them instead; and the disclosures that should be made in various settings. The management plan should be provided to the investigator and others who have a need to know, and there should be infrastructure in place to monitor and help ensure compliance with it. Ideally, there should be a process for the conflicted individual or, in the case of an institutional COI, the responsible individual, to document their agreement to comply with the management plan.

Policies should be flexible enough that in certain circumstances, a reviewing body may determine that an FCOI generates such significant risks for a trial that the individual (or the institution) may have no role in any part of the study. If this determination is made, it should be communicated through a management plan.

Management plans should address, at a minimum, the following items:

- Limitations on the role of the conflicted investigator in areas such as:
  - Recruiting subjects and obtaining consent
  - Carrying out investigational intervention
  - Collecting data
  - Determining adverse events and serious adverse events
  - Analyzing data
  - Authoring publications and making presentations about the study
- If the reviewing organization employs or otherwise has appropriate authority over the investigator, there may be limits imposed on the investigator's relationship with the sponsor or manufacturer of the study drug or device, such as:
  - Limits on annual income and other payments from or interests in the company
  - Limits on the investigator's involvement with the company
  - Prohibition on negotiating terms of the sponsored agreement on behalf of the institution or the company.
- If the conflict involves the institution, the management plan should be communicated to all those with responsibility for and oversight of the study and should outline any conditions being placed on conducting the study at the institution, such as:
  - If a multicenter trial, limit on number or percentage of subjects that may be enrolled at the institution and restrictions on the institution's leadership roles (e.g., as coordinating center)
  - Whether an outside IRB must review the protocol
  - Whether an independent DSMB should be established and details of its composition and charge
- Any changes that need to be made to the study design, such as:
  - Blinding investigators to treatment and control arms

- Ensuring inclusion of objective endpoints
- Adding non-conflicted investigators with special expertise
- Requirements for disclosure of the FCOIs, including details that must be included in the disclosure, to
  - Study team members
  - Prospective research subjects
  - Medical journals and conferences
  - Media and journalists reporting on study outcomes
  - Regulatory bodies (if the conflicted investigator is responsible, e.g., as sponsor-investigator on an FDA-regulated trial).

Once a management plan has been issued, there should be oversight of investigators' compliance with the conditions in the plan. Monitoring may be conducted by the IRB, a COI office, or institutional auditors. The degree of monitoring applied to any particular study may depend on the level of risk associated with the study, its potential impact on drug or device approval and medical practice, and the nature and extent of the financial interests. Failures to adhere to the management plan should be addressed promptly and thoroughly under the institution's policies on research integrity and research compliance. Failures to comply with PHS regulations may result in additional action by the awarding agency.

Summary and Conclusion

FCOIs are ubiquitous and have the potential to create bias and affect the safety of clinical research. Financial relationships between the biomedical industry and those who conduct essential research are likely to be a feature of clinical research well into the future. Regulations and national standards to minimize or mitigate the risks of these relationships will evolve, but investigators and research organizations need to make disclosure, robust review, and careful management of FCOIs a fundamental part of their culture. Adopting policies and procedures that are easy to understand and follow and enforcing policies and procedures consistently will foster a culture of compliance. Institutional leaders should communicate that addressing conflicts of interest is a top priority and is part of a commitment to integrity in research, and they should provide sufficient resources to support robust administration of the FCOI policy. Researchers and institutions that demonstrate a commitment to transparency and to mitigating undue influence of FCOIs in clinical trials will be viewed by the scientific community, the public, and patients as credible and objective.

Key Facts

- Financial conflicts of interest are ubiquitous in clinical research and should be disclosed, reviewed, and managed to ensure the objectivity and safety of clinical trials.

- Management of financial conflicts of interest should be carried out by knowledgeable individuals with the expertise and authority to ensure compliance with and enforcement of management plan conditions.
- Disclosure and transparency regarding financial conflicts of interest are essential.
- Management of financial conflicts of interest may necessitate changes in study design and/or in the roles of investigators with conflicts of interest.
- Some institutions that conduct clinical trials set limits on the conflicting financial interests that investigators may have while leading or participating in clinical trials.
- Financial conflicts of interest in research are regulated by the Public Health Service and the Food and Drug Administration.
- National associations, professional societies, and accrediting bodies maintain standards for addressing financial conflicts of interest.
- Most medical journals require disclosure of authors' financial conflicts of interest.
- Congress and the media have intensified their scrutiny of financial conflicts of interest in recent decades.

Cross-References

▶ Consent Forms and Procedures
▶ Data and Safety Monitoring and Reporting
▶ Data Capture, Data Management, and Quality Control; Single Versus Multicenter Trials
▶ Fraud in Clinical Trials
▶ Implementing the Trial Protocol
▶ Institutional Review Boards and Ethics Committees
▶ Investigator Responsibilities
▶ Paper Writing
▶ Principles of Clinical Trials: Bias and Precision Control
▶ Reporting Biases
▶ Trial Organization and Governance

References

Ahn R, Woodbridge A, Abraham A et al (2017) Financial ties of principal investigators and randomized controlled trial outcomes: cross sectional study. BMJ 356:i6770. https://doi.org/10.1136/bmj.i6770
Bauchner H, Fontanarosa P, Flanagin A (2018) Conflicts of interests, authors, and journals. JAMA 320:2315. https://doi.org/10.1001/jama.2018.17593
Cain D (2008) Everyone's a little bit biased (even physicians). JAMA 299:2893. https://doi.org/10.1001/jama.299.24.2893
CFR – Code of Federal Regulations Title 21 (2019) In: Accessdata.fda.gov. Accessed 28 Jan 2019
Cigarroa F, Masters B, Sharphorn D (2018) Institutional conflicts of interest and public trust. JAMA 320:2305. https://doi.org/10.1001/jama.2018.18482

Dana J, Loewenstein G (2003) A social science perspective on gifts to physicians from industry. JAMA 290:252. https://doi.org/10.1001/jama.290.2.252

eCFR — Code of Federal Regulations (2019) In: Ecfr.gov. https://www.ecfr.gov/cgi-bin/text-idx?c=ecfr&SID=99281785420776721 4895b1fa023755d&rgn=div5&view=text&node=42:1.0.1.4.23&idno=42#sp42.1.50.f. Accessed 28 Jan 2019

Friedman J, Sugarman J, Dhillon J et al (2007) Perspectives of clinical research coordinators on disclosing financial conflicts of interest to potential research participants. Clin Trials 4:272–278. https://doi.org/10.1177/1740774507079239

Gottlieb JD (2015) Financial conflicts of interest in research. In: Suckow M, Yates B (eds) Research regulatory compliance. Elsevier Inc., London, pp 253–276

Gottlieb JD, Bressler NM (2017) How should journals handle the conflict of interest of their editors? JAMA 317:1757. https://doi.org/10.1001/jama.2017.2207

Hhs.gov (2016) Financial conflict of interest: HHS guidance (2004). In: HHS.gov. https://www.hhs.gov/ohrp/regulations-and-policy/guidance/financial-conflict-of-interest/index.html#. Accessed 4 Feb 2019

ICMJE | Recommendations | Author Responsibilities—Conflicts of Interest (2019) In: Icmje.org. http://www.icmje.org/recommendations/browse/roles-and-responsibilities/author-responsibilities%2D%2Dconflicts-of-interest.html. Accessed 28 Jan 2019

Ioannidis J, Trepanowski J (2018) Disclosures in nutrition research. JAMA 319:547. https://doi.org/10.1001/jama.2017.18571. Available at: https://jamanetwork.com/journals/jama/article-abstract/2666008

Lundh A, Bero L (2017) The ties that bind. BMJ 356:j176. https://doi.org/10.1136/bmj.j176

Lo B, Field MJ (eds) (2009) Principles for identifying and assessing conflicts of interests. In: Conflict of interest in medical research, education, and practice, 1st edn. National Academies Press, Washington, DC, pp 44–61. Available at: https://www.nap.edu/read/12598/chapter/4. Accessed 25 Jan 2019

Stolberg S (2019) Youth's death shakes new field of gene experiments on humans. In: Archive.nytimes.com. https://archive.nytimes.com/www.nytimes.com/library/national/science/012700sci-gene-therapy.html. Accessed 28 Jan 2019

Tringale K, Marshall D, Mackey T et al (2017) Types and distribution of payments from industry to physicians in 2015. JAMA 317:1774–1784. https://doi.org/10.1001/jama.2017.3091

Wilson RF (2009) Estate of Gelsinger v. Trustees of University of Pennsylvania: Money, Prestige, and Conflicts of Interest In Human Subjects Research. In: Johnson SH, Krause JH, Saver RS, Wilson RF (eds) Health Law and Bioethics: Cases In Context

World Medical Association (2013) World Medical Association declaration of Helsinki. JAMA 310:2191–2194. https://doi.org/10.1001/jama.2013.281053

Trial Organization and Governance

29

O. Dale Williams and Katrina Epnere

Contents

Abstract

An issue impacting the success of many human efforts is the organizational and management strategy required for their successful completion. This is an important issue for any clinical trial as well. It is always a challenge to match the needs required for a successful trial with the resources available in a management strategy compatible with the experience and personalities of the collection of investigators and staff involved. Clearly the simplest situation is the single-site trial with a single investigator and few or no staff. In this situation, the investigator has only himself or herself to organize and manage. While this is no guarantee of success, it creates much less of a management burden than does a multicenter, long-term trial, especially since such endeavors typically include numerous investigators, central laboratories, reading centers, coordinating center,

O. D. Williams (✉)
Department of Biostatistics, University of North Carolina, Chapel Hill, NC, USA

Department of Medicine, University of Alabama at Birmingham, Birmingham, AL, USA
e-mail: odalewilliams@yahoo.com

K. Epnere
WCG Statistics Collaborative, Washington, DC, USA

© Springer Nature Switzerland AG 2022
S. Piantadosi, C. L. Meinert (eds.), *Principles and Practice of Clinical Trials*,
https://doi.org/10.1007/978-3-319-52636-2_56

and a large number of committees, each with its own purpose, requirements, and personality. The organization and management (OM) issues for this situation are critically important for the overall success of the trial. This chapter highlights issues for such long-term, multicenter studies as these situations encompass all the key, major issues.

Keywords

Organization and management · Organizational structure · Multicenter studies · Steering committee · Executive committee · Coordinating center

Introduction

The number of newly registered trials doubled from 9,321 in 2006 to 18,400 in 2014. The number of industry-funded trials increased by 43%. Concurrently, the number of NIH-funded trials decreased by 24% (Ehrhardt et al. 2015). In a recent communication, Meinert indicated ClinicalTrials.gov included almost 95,000 trials started between 2014 and 2018 (personal communication Meinert 2019). This is a surprising number in many ways and raises the interesting question as to how many are well organized and managed and how many will not meet their stated goals as a consequence of inadequate OM.

It is often said that the inability to recruit adequate numbers of trial participants is the most common cause of the failure of a clinical trial. The root cause of failure in this case, however, is most likely due to an OM strategy that was not up to the task.

This situation was recognized early on in the history of multicenter trials in the USA and was addressed in the Greenberg Report (1967) prepared in 1967 and formally published in *Controlled Clinical Trials* in 1988. This report includes an organization chart that has stood the test of time although the situation has evolved in directions and magnitudes that were perhaps unimaginable in 1967. The key components of this chart are listed in the discussion of committees below.

It is important to point out that it is not uncommon for the OM general issue to receive inadequate attention from the earliest phases of trial planning as these issues, critical as they are, often are much less interesting than the scientific and health-care issues under consideration. The consequence of this lack of appropriate attention can be catastrophic failure. Farrell et al. have repeatedly pointed out that even though eminent trialists have written persuasively and repeatedly of the need for large, randomized, controlled trials, in the scientific literature, little attention has been given to the day-to-day and strategic management of such trials. She emphasizes that the knowledge and expertise gained on running earlier trials are not widely disseminated and new trials often have to begin from scratch. Because randomized trial involves a huge investment of time, money, and people, Farrell suggests it should be managed like any other business (Farrell 1998; Farrell et al. 2010).

Multicenter clinical trials often operate under two separate but related organization charts, one representing the funding structure and its accountability and financial reporting expectations and one representing the committee structure for the overall trial. The funding structure requirements necessarily address issues related to inadequate performance of a trial's individual funded entities. The committee structure performance expectations, while also critical, tend to be less concretely formulated. The remainder of this chapter focuses on the latter.

The overall committee structure typically reflects a balance among the appropriate representation of stakeholders, expertise requirements, and operational efficiency. The first of these may require large committees if there are large numbers of clinical field sites and central units, which may be further augmented should the expertise required not be available from these units. Such large numbers of persons on committees may make it difficult or impossible to proceed with the required efficiency. One strategy used is to create a steering committee, consisting of representatives of all the stakeholders which has overall responsibility for the trial. The role of the steering committee is to provide oversight of the trial on behalf of the sponsor and funder and ensure that the trial is conducted in accordance with the principles of GCP and relevant regulations. The steering committee should focus on the progress of the trial, adherence to the protocol, and participant safety (McDonald et al. 2014). A subcommittee, sometimes called an executive committee, which is much smaller may be more directly responsible for day-to-day issues.

Since the OM strategy for a multicenter, long-term clinical trial typically has a committee structure at its core, it might be worthwhile to reflect on the old adage that a camel is horse designed by a committee. The fact that a key committee exists does not, unfortunately, necessarily mean it will function commendably. Success requires the productive cooperation of all key stakeholders operating in a system that recognizes and takes into account their individual needs as well as those of the overall trial. The WRIST study group wrote a Guide on Organizing a Multicenter Clinical Trial and stated that planning of multicenter clinical trials (MCCTs) is a long and arduous task that requires substantial preparation time. They emphasized an essential asset to planning a MCCT is the fluidity with which all collaborators work together toward a common vision. This would mean a development of a consensus-assisted study protocol and the recruitment of centers and co-investigators who are dedicated, collaborative, and selfless in this team effort to achieve goals that cannot be reached by a single-center effort (Chung et al. 2010).

Key Factors

A list of factors that may be helpful to consider when developing an OM plan for a trial includes the following:

1. Funding source and its relationship to trial operations
2. Individual organizational units, roles, and structure
3. Committees, committee roles, and structure
4. Common threats and failures

A goal for the overall OM scheme can perhaps best be characterized by the simple statement "Who reports to whom about what and when." Which bodies need a report? What types of reports are required? How often are reports required and in what format? What data are required to be included in the report, for example, recruitment data, safety data, and blinded or unblinded data? Who will produce the reports (McDonald et al. 2014)? A scheme that identifies and clarifies roles, responsibilities, and accountability for the entities involved is vitally important.

Funding Source and Its Relationship to Trial Operations

Funding sources for clinical trials include for-profit entities such as pharmaceutical firms; numerous US government agencies and those of other countries and the European Union; various not-for-profit entities including foundations, societies, and others; and international organizations such as the World Health Organization. Each such source has its own expectations as to how trials it funds will be organized and managed in the general sense and what its specific functional role will be for a given trial. It is critically important that these expectations are clearly understood by the investigative team at the very outset of a trial. The expectations and context for pharmaceutical industry-sponsored trials are importantly different from those sponsored by NIH, for example, and the OM scheme to be utilized needs to be fully cognizant of these differences.

It should also be noted that some of the operational units may be funded through subcontracts with other trial organizational units which are funded directly from the funding agency. For example, some laboratories and reading centers may operate under subcontracts to a coordinating center. In this case, the organizational unit offering the subcontract has to have the resources and expertise to select and manage the relationship with the entity under subcontract. Olmstead summarized that several articles and surveys have addressed concerns of pharmaceutical company research staff with the performance of their outside contract researchers. He classified these issues into four categories – credibility, responsiveness, quality of product, and cost. He concluded that strong emphasis on quality control and improved, automated data management are key elements of improvement and added that improved organization and management efforts on the part of contract researchers themselves will go far to reduce the most obvious difficulties (Olmstead 2004).

Individual Organizational Units, Roles, and Structure

A trial may involve 30 or more organizational units. Examples include:

1. Clinical centers. Clinical centers are the core operational unit for a trial. The number of such units is usually based on those required to recruit the required number of trial participants. Clinical centers recruit and interact with trial participants as required for the duration of the trial. They also are responsible for all

local research-related approvals and for collecting and transmitting data, typically to a coordinating center. They also deal with biological samples, sent either to a local laboratory or to a central laboratory, and for the collection and transmission of any images, again, to local readers or to a central reading center. They participate in the trial committee structure as appropriate.

2. Coordinating center. The trial coordinating center is the heart of the trial, whether it is a single-site or multicenter trial. Sometimes the broader function served by this unit is divided into a clinical coordinating center and a data coordinating center. In general, this combined entity is responsible for data-related and study coordinating issues. The data coordinating component typically is responsible for key elements of trial design and for data collection systems, data management, and data analyses. This includes as well the design and testing of data collection forms and data collection quality assessment. The data coordinating center component also would prepare reports for trial overview committees such as Data and Safety Monitoring Boards. The clinical coordinating center component often is responsible for managing and reviewing the adverse and serious adverse events. Responsibility for providing staff support for at least some committees is usual. The data coordinating component team usually consists of chief investigator(s), trial manager, programmer/IT support, database manager and/or data clerks, and trial statistician (McDonald et al. 2014).

3. Central laboratory. Some trials require, in addition to the use of local laboratories, more than one central laboratory. In general, central laboratories are responsible for creating and maintaining shipping procedures for the transmission of samples from the clinical centers to the lab. They are responsible for high-quality laboratory analyses for the parameters under their purview and for transmission of the resulting data to the coordinating center. If abnormal results are considered adverse or serious adverse events, they would be required to transmit appropriate notifications. Importantly, they should participate in the appropriate standardization programs and any quality control activities specific to the trial. They also may serve as an archive for biological materials collected by the trial. Personnel from the central lab also may participate in trial committees.

4. Central reading center. Some trials require the use of central reading centers for images critical to the assessment of patient safety or trial outcomes. These centers typically are responsible for the systems that transmit images from the clinical centers to the reading center and for transmitting the results of assessments they complete to the coordinating center. The center is expected to perform high-quality assessments for the readings they undertake and to participate in quality control activities as appropriate. They, like the central labs, may also serve as an archive for images collected by the trial. Personnel from the center may participate in trial committees.

These individual organizational units also have to be successfully organized and managed for the overall trial's OM to be successful. The individual units report, in many senses, to their home institution and also to the organization structure for the trial of which they are a part. This means that the unit leaders need to have the experience and capability to successfully work with both sets of masters. Keeping in mind that a trial may include more than 30 organization units, it would be ideal if these 30+ units were each led by someone with appropriate OM experience and capability. This doesn't always happen, and a poorly organized and managed unit can jeopardize the overall trial.

Committees, Committee Roles, and Committee Structure

Since the core management strategy for many clinical trials is based on a committee structure, the creation of the committees, selection of their members, and their operational effectiveness and efficiency are of paramount importance. Decisions need to be made up front as to which committees will be needed at least at the outset. Often the first committee created is the steering committee, which includes representatives of all the key stakeholders. Sometimes the chair is designated by the funding agency and sometimes elected from the members. However this is done, this person is key to the overall success of the trial and therefore needs to have the requisite knowledge, experience, and personality for the task. There also needs to be a succession plan that provides backup as needed.

The likelihood of this success may be enhanced by the following considerations:

1. Committee charge: A clear statement as to the role the committee is expected to play is critical.
2. Committee chair: Someone with appropriate knowledge, experience, and personality, possibly along with a designated co-chair, is a fundamental requirement. This person is responsible for organizing and conducting committee meetings and, in general, making sure the committee is satisfactorily addressing its commitments. This likely will include making sure there are appropriate minutes that include action items and assigned tasks. The status of progress on completing these tasks should be addressed at subsequent meetings.
3. Committee members: The critical issue here is the inclusion of appropriate stakeholders and expertise. It may be necessary to go outside the immediate members of the overall team for this expertise. Committee members are responsible for attending and participating fully in the meetings and their deliberations. They also are responsible for completing any assigned tasks in a timely manner.
4. Committee staff: This issue is typically overlooked and is not always needed, but when it is, there needs to be a mechanism for its provision. Staff typically are responsible for arranging the required logistics for meeting and organizing agendas and materials and preparing minutes and action item lists.
5. Scheduling meetings: A clearly delineated meeting schedule, with adjustments as required and available suitably in advance, can be most helpful. One important consequence of such a schedule is the ability of the members to put meetings on their calendars well ahead of time and thus be more likely to be available for meetings.

6. Meeting conduct: Factors that may facilitate the success of the committee meetings include appropriate agendas prepared well ahead of the meeting, accompanied by documents and materials as appropriate; efficiently conducted meetings to include appropriate control of time devoted to individual items and speakers; and clear minutes and follow-up on issues addressed in previous meetings.
7. Committee accountability: Most trial committees are in fact subcommittees to a steering committee or similarly designated committee so that they report to this higher committee. The steering committee should hold the subcommittees accountable for meeting their charge in a high-quality, timely fashion. This typically requires both written reports and presentations at the steering committee meetings.

The trial's committee structure has the responsibility to inform the funding structure component of issues that need to be addressed for specific individual operational entities. This may require special reports and/or special meetings.

The designated committees play key roles, and their successful operation is critical to the success of the overall trial. Examples of committees, which typically operate as subcommittees of and thus report to the steering committee include:

1. Steering committee. Includes representatives of stakeholders and funding entity and may include outside experts. Responsible for the overall management of the trial.
2. Executive committee. Typically, a subcommittee of the steering committee that includes the steering committee chair, the director(s) of the coordinating center, and representatives of the clinical centers. A relatively small committee responsible for the more day-to-day activities.
3. Recruitment and retention committee. Responsible for developing and implementing participant recruitment procedures and also participant retention efforts.
4. Laboratory committee. Responsible for creating list of laboratory tests to be done and monitoring the quality of laboratory performance.
5. Imaging committee. Responsible for creating list of imaging parameters to be included and for monitoring the quality of the reading center performance.
6. Quality control committee. A subcommittee with overarching responsibilities for data quality control. May mandate blind duplicate assessments for some key variables and set standards for acceptable performance.
7. Endpoint committee. For those trials for which a judgment based on several data sources may be required in the assessment of primary outcomes or endpoints, a panel of experts may be required to make this assessment. This panel is required to make this judgment for all such events in the trial.
8. Ancillary studies committee. Some trials include or obtain funds for ancillary studies that add procedures or data to be collected in addition to those for the main trial. This committee would overview that process with careful reference to avoiding conflicts with the main trial.

9. Data form committee. Responsible for the development and testing of data collection forms and sometimes overviews the data collection training and certification procedures.
10. Publication and presentation committee. Responsible for overviewing the publication and presentation process for the trial. This includes efforts to help ensure that trial publications are completed in a timely manner and also deals with authorship conflict issues.
11. Data and safety monitoring board. An independent board of experts in the topic of the trial and biostatistics responsible for trial integrity and participant safety. Typically reports to the funding entity but also may report jointly to the steering committee. Usually operates according to a charter established at the outset of the trial. Reviews adverse and serious events and trial analysis reports.
12. Advisory committee. Some trials may involve an overarching advisory committee which is appointed by and reports to the funding entity. This committee may assist with setting overall directions and with broad overview assessment of trial progress and success.

Common Threats and Failures

As is the case for any endeavor such as a clinical trial, failure can occur. Some key issues are:

1. Participant recruitment. One of the most common causes of a clinical trial failing to be able to operate to completion is failure to recruit adequate numbers of participants to undertake the randomization process. The trial OM process sometimes is too slow to react to this crisis, and when it reacts, it does so with too little too late. It is imperative that the OM process monitor recruitment status from the very outset and react strongly to indications of recruitment problems.
   The assumption should be that the enrollment will be slower than projections and almost every trial should implement proactive measures to foster enrollment. Frequent monitoring of actual vs projected enrollment by site to identify trends gives the opportunity to consider protocol amendment, additional recruitment funds, site closure, etc. (Allen 2015).
   The STEPS study analyzed 114 multicenter trials and showed that 45% failed to reach 80% of the prespecified sample size. Less than one third of the trials recruited their original target number of participants within the time originally specified, and around one third had to be extended in time and resources. Trials that actually recruited successfully shared a common factor – they had employed a dedicated trial manager. The STEPS collaborators suggested that anyone undertaking trials should think about the different needs at different phases in the life of a trial and put greater emphasis on "conduct" (Campbell et al. 2007; Farrell et al. 2010).
2. Clinical center failure. Especially if the trial includes a rather large number of clinical centers, one or more may not perform adequately. Such a situation may

jeopardize the trial. Since this may be a leadership problem at the clinical site, the trial OM system may need to step in quickly and assist or replace as needed.

3. Coordinating center performance. Coordinating centers need to develop data collection, data management, and data analysis systems and operate them in a timely and high-quality fashion. If this does not happen, the consequence can be severe.

   Gathering clean data is among the most important steps to a successful clinical trial. Even if the sites are found and patients recruited, but the data is inaccurate, it will not be of use to the sponsor. Consider doing early and routine review of data – whether remotely or during a monitoring visit. Priority should be given to primary endpoint data. Identifying data quality issues early on, correcting those issues, retraining site personnel, and establishing preventative measures allow for data issues to be addressed and resolved quickly before evolving into significant problems (Allen 2015).

4. Committee failure. If a key committee lags behind and is causing delays in trial development or operation, some corrective action may be needed. Sometimes a new chair should be appointed.

Conclusion and Summary

As described above, numerous entities typically are involved in the organization and management of multicenter long-term trials so that there are numerous opportunities for failure. Clearly, a clear and detailed organization and management strategy needs to be established well before the onset of the trial. The strategy needs to provide an unambiguous answer for the essential question "who reports to whom about what and when." Strong and experienced leadership closely connected with day-to-day operations in a system that provides continuous monitoring and flexibility to adjust to unexpected situations is key to success.

Cross-References

▶ Archiving Records and Materials
▶ ClinicalTrials.gov
▶ Data and Safety Monitoring and Reporting
▶ Data Capture, Data Management, and Quality Control; Single Versus Multicenter Trials
▶ Evolution of Clinical Trials Science
▶ Funding Models and Proposals
▶ Multicenter and Network Trials
▶ Participant Recruitment, Screening, and Enrollment
▶ Publications from Clinical Trials
▶ Responsibilities and Management of the Clinical Coordinating Center

References

Campbell MK, Snowdon C, Francis D, Elbourne D, McDonald AM, Knight R, Entwistle V, Garcia J, Roberts I, Grant A, The STEPS Group (2007) Recruitment to randomised trials: strategies for trial enrolment and participation study. The STEPS study. Health Technol Assess (Winch Eng) 11(48). iii, ix–105

Chung KC, Song JW, WRIST Study Group (2010) A guide to organizing a multicenter clinical trial. Plast Reconstr Surg 126(2):515–523

Ehrhardt S, Appel LJ, Meinert CL (2015) Trends in National Institutes of Health funding for clinical trials registered in ClinicalTrials.gov. JAMA 314(23):2566–2567

Farrell B (1998) Efficient management of randomised controlled trials: nature or nurture. BMJ 317 (7167):1236–1239

Farrell B, Kenyon S, Shakur H (2010) Managing clinical trials. Trials 11(1):78

Greenberg Report (1967) Organization, review, and administration of cooperative studies (Greenberg report): a report from the heart special project committee to the National Advisory Heart Council. Control Clin Trials 1988(9):137–148

Online Documents

Allen S (2015) Best practices for clinical trial operations. https://www.pharmoutsourcing.com/Featured-Articles/180536-Best-Practices-for-Clinical-Trial-Operations/

McDonald A, Lane A, Farrell B, Dunn J, Buckland S, Meredith S, Napp V (2014) Trial managers' network guide to efficient trial management. https://cdn.ymaws.com/www.tmn.ac.uk/resource/collection/77CDC3B6-133F-42E6-9610-F33FF5197D2F/tmn-guidelines-web_[amended_July_2014].pdf

Meinert C (2019) The trend in trials. https://jhuccs1.us/clm/PDFs/NameThatTune.pdf

Olmstead FL (2004) Improved organization and management of clinical trials. http://www.appliedclinicaltrialsonline.com/improved-organization-and-managementclinical-trials

Advocacy and Patient Involvement in Clinical Trials

30

Ellen Sigal, Mark Stewart, and Diana Merino

Contents

Abstract

Patient engagement in research and clinical trials has evolved over time. Patients are no longer simply passive research subjects but are increasingly being integrated into research teams and protocol review teams to help design, implement, and disseminate clinical trial findings. While potential barriers exist for meaningful patient engagement, mechanisms and methods to effectively engage patients and advocacy groups are evolving, and resources and best practices are continually being developed to assist researchers and patients. Additionally, legislation and regulatory guidance are being instituted to promote patient engagement and ensure it is a routine process for clinical trial development. Developing patient-centered clinical trial designs has led to development of innovative clinical trial infrastructures and statistical methods. Patient advocates

E. Sigal (✉) · M. Stewart · D. Merino
Friends of Cancer Research, Washington, DC, USA
e-mail: esigal@focr.org; mstewart@focr.org; dmerino@focr.org

© Springer Nature Switzerland AG 2022
S. Piantadosi, C. L. Meinert (eds.), *Principles and Practice of Clinical Trials*,
https://doi.org/10.1007/978-3-319-52636-2_57

and organizations are also increasingly developing their own data sources and clinical trials, which represent unique opportunities for researchers to partner with patient groups to rapidly advance drug development.

Keywords

Patient advocacy · Drug development · Patient engagement · Patient-Centered clinical trials

Introduction

The role of patients and advocates in clinical research and their involvement in the regulation and oversight of clinical trials have substantially grown over time. In just a few decades, patients have gone from being considered passive human subjects whose clinical measures would contribute to answering research questions to active participants and engaged stakeholders. This growing movement toward a more patient-centered approach aims to provide the best healthcare for each patient, which takes into consideration the patient's own goals, values, and preferences (Manganiello and Anderson 2011). This movement is rooted in early advocacy efforts led by the HIV/AIDS community dating back to 1988 and resulted in fundamental changes to the medical research paradigm.

The path from initial development of a new drug to entry of the new therapy into the patient community relies on clinical trials, which represent the final step in evaluating the safety and efficacy of new therapeutic approaches. Along this developmental path, patients can provide critical input from collecting natural history information; involvement in endpoint selection; protocol design; consent and eligibility; clinical trial recruitment and retention strategies; design of post-market safety studies; and dissemination of trial findings (Fig. 1).

A detailed analysis of several clinical trials indicates that 48% of all sites in a given trial fail to meet their enrollment targets and more than 11% never enroll a

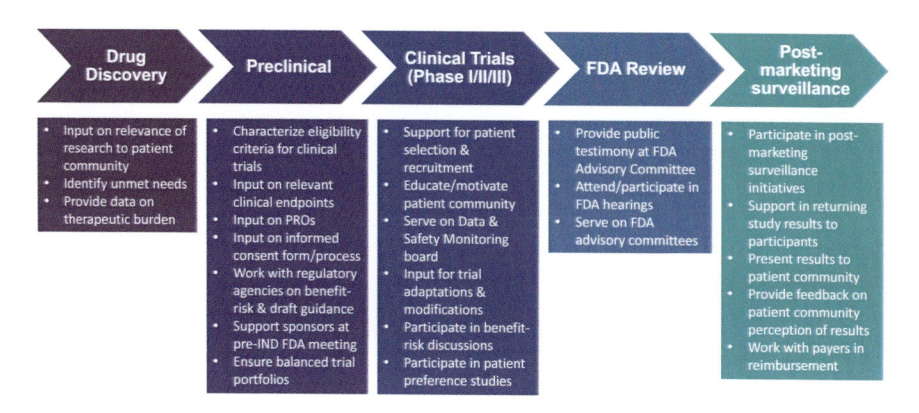

Fig. 1 Opportunities for patient involvement in the drug development process

single patient (Kaitin 2013). It is estimated that less than 5% of adult cancer patients enroll in a clinical trial despite many indicating their desire to participate in clinical trials (Comis et al. 2003; Unger et al. 2016). Thus, significant barriers such as clinical trial access, demographic and socioeconomic challenges, inappropriate or excessive procedures, broad exclusion criteria, lack of patient-centric trial designs, and patient and physician attitudes remain that hinder trial participation. While not every barrier may be readily overcome, engaging patients early and often throughout the entire research and drug development process can help ensure appropriately designed trials that are viewed favorably by patients, answer questions important to the patient community, and ultimately encourage participation.

A growing body of evidence describing the benefits of patient involvement in research and clinical trials is slowly changing scientific, medical, and regulatory practices. In their systematic review, Domecq and colleagues found that patient engagement positively influenced research by increasing study enrollment rates and helping researchers in securing funding, designing study protocols, and choosing relevant outcomes (Domecq et al. 2014). Greater patient engagement in research and clinical trials would help drug developers sponsor trials that are more informed about the needs of the patients, which would translate to more feasible and streamlined trial design generating better outcomes (Hanley et al. 2001; Tinetti and Basch 2013). Increased engagement could also reduce patient accrual time due to improved enrollment, reduce patient attrition, and make findings more applicable and relevant to the target population (Bombak and Hanson 2017), which would significantly decrease trial costs. Implementation of mechanisms for patient engagement can vary.

Patient Engagement in Research and Drug Development

Acknowledging that patients are central to research and drug development, several national and international organizations have invested in clearly defining the role of patient involvement in research practices and the need for the development of innovative infrastructures that will help facilitate the incorporation of the patient voice in all stages of the research process, including design, execution, and translation of research (Domecq et al. 2014). The Patient-Centered Outcomes Research Institute (PCORI) was established in 2010 to improve the quality and relevance of evidence available to help stakeholders make better-informed health decisions and requires that all its funded research projects include patient input throughout the entire research study (www.pcori.org). Patient engagement has been defined by PCORI as "involvement of patients and other stakeholders throughout the planning, conduct, and dissemination of the proposed project" and is becoming institutionalized and incorporated into several funding schemes (PCORI 2018). Patient-driven research activities have ranged from pre-discovery funding for development and acquisition of animal models and cell lines all the way to post-market study design and value discussions.

The US Food and Drug Administration (FDA) recognizes that patients are experts on living with their conditions, and as such, their voice is uniquely positioned to inform stakeholders and provide the right therapeutic context for drug development as well as perspective on the outcome measures that are most relevant to patients and evaluation by regulatory agencies (Anderson and McCleary 2016). Patients may voice their concern or support for the development of certain drugs and provide a firsthand perspective on the proper balance of risk to benefit for a particular disease or patient population. For instance, the patient voice was crucial when reintroducing Tysabri, a monoclonal antibody used to treat multiple sclerosis, which had been previously removed from the market following reports of lethal side effects. After the thorough review of safety information, the FDA convened an advisory committee where patients and caregivers were invited to testify. Weighing all evidence, including the advocates' testimonies, the FDA found enough support to remarket the drug under a special prescription program (Schwartz and Woloshin 2015). Additionally, the FDA has formalized several initiatives to encourage the inclusion of the patient voice in medical product development. Under the fifth authorization of the Prescription Drug User Fee Act (PDUFA V) signed into law in 2012, the FDA began the Patient-Focused Drug Development (PFDD) program with the intent to more systematically incorporate the patient perspective into drug development (FDA 2018). From 2012 to 2017, the FDA organized 24 disease-specific PFDD meetings that have helped capture patients' experiences, perspectives, and priorities and enabled the incorporation of this meaningful information into the drug development process and its evaluation. Duchenne muscular dystrophy advocacy organizations helped to exemplify how patient and advocates can successfully inform regulators, provide meaningful input into benefit and risk assessments, and identify treatment priorities. To build on this success and enable more patient advocacy organizations to shape and influence drug development, the twenty-first Century Cures Act and PDUFA VI have tasked FDA with developing additional guidance to describe approaches to gather patient experience data, quantifying benefit and risks, and using patient-reported outcomes in treatment development. Moreover, the newly formed FDA Oncology Center of Excellence (OCE) has made PFDD a priority and is exploring innovative regulatory strategies that incorporate patient input. Additionally, the National Cancer Institute (NCI) also encourages patient advocates to be involved in the clinical trial process. The SWOG Cancer Research Network, one of five NCI cooperative cancer research groups, has an advocate assigned to every research committee and who is involved in every stage of the process.

Primary Areas of Engagement

A systematic review that searched for reporting of patient engagement on controlled trials and nonrandomized comparative trials conducted from May 2011 to June 2016 reviewed 2777 citations, of which only 23 clinical trials (17 randomized controlled trials and 6 nonrandomized comparative studies) reported patient engagement practices (Fergusson et al. 2018). The methods of engagement most commonly reported involved the development of the research question, selection of outcome, dissemination and implementation of results, and other activities, such as the refinement of the study intervention and protocol review (Fergusson et al. 2018). Thus, there is evidence showing that researchers have engaged patients, especially in trials that reported following the community-based participatory research (CBPR) methods as part of the study design; however, there is still more work needed to get patients meaningfully involved in clinical research. Innovative methodologies, such as CBPR, which aim to have more meaningful relationships with the target population and more effective dissemination and implementation of results are key in improving patient involvement in research (Chhatre et al. 2018).

Another systematic review assessed patient engagement in research including randomized control trials, qualitative studies, single cohort studies, cross-sectional studies, case reports, and systematic reviews (Domecq et al. 2014). This study found that engagement was feasible and most commonly done in the beginning of the research process (agenda setting and protocol development) and less commonly during the execution and translation of research. The study also found no comparative effectiveness research on patient engagement methods. The authors concluded that the lack of this evidence is what may have led to inconsistent and vague reporting of patient engagement research, preventing the incorporation of effective reporting methods.

Using the 2014 Health Information National Trends Survey, one study investigated three aspects of patient engagement: interest, awareness, and participation as research partners in the medical research process to identify different levels of engagement and barriers that prevent engagement (Hearld et al. 2017). The study consisted of a cross-sectional analysis that suggested modest levels of interest in engaging in the research process among respondents. The study also found low levels of awareness of ways in which patients could become involved in research and very low levels of actual participation. Several factors, such as patient health status, attitudes about their health and healthcare, and sociodemographic characteristics, were also examined to provide insights into the types of patients most likely to be engaged in the research process. The study suggested that higher socioeconomic status and positive patient attitudes were associated with increased interest in becoming involved in research but there was no association between respondents with different demographic, socioeconomic, and environmental characteristics to actual participation. The authors concluded that raising awareness of engagement opportunities would improve people's interest in being engaged in research. Moreover, they suggested further research to identify why patients who may be aware of research opportunities are still reluctant to become active participants of the research process.

Challenges Associated with Incorporating Patients into Research and Drug Development

Attitudes toward a more patient-centered or patient-focused approach to care and research are continuing to shift, in part, because of the increasing awareness that active patient participation in research can lead to improvements in the credibility of the study findings and their direct applicability to patients. In addition to the benefits observed for study sponsors and participants, greater patient involvement is also driven by a compelling ethical rationale that lies behind the participation of patients in the democratization of the research process (Domecq et al. 2014). Data shows a compelling relationship between the incidence of clinical trial enrollment and improvement in cancer population survival, and a recent survey indicates the value patient engagement can have on improving patient retention and accelerating trial accrual (Smith et al. 2015; Unger et al. 2016). However, several challenges and concerns remain about the way patient engagement is being conducted (Bombak and Hanson 2017).

Barriers to Patient Engagement

The most commonly described patient engagement barriers were related to logistics and a concern of tokenistic engagement (Domecq et al. 2014). Tokenism refers to involving patients superficially. This can often occur when a small number of participants, who may be involved in the research process minimally, are considered to represent a far larger and diverse patient group. This insincere act of patient inclusion hinders patients from seeking greater involvement in the research process, and it lessens the credibility of the patient voice. Indeed, various research studies have identified that people frequently find that participating in clinical trials is meaningless or disempowering (Mullins et al. 2014), yet people often want to be informed, empowered, and engaged in their medical management (Davis et al. 2005). Some programs may require patients to undergo intense forms of training and involve abundant time, interest, and potentially resources (Bombak and Hanson 2017). These requirements may create preference for observable or quantitative skills over instinct and intuition and may bias the perspectives shared as part of the study. The lack of incentives or payment for a patient's time may also be a barrier for some patients to become engaged in research. Moreover, various erroneous perceptions have been identified as barriers for engagement. Some studies have identified the detrimental perception that patients will not be objective in their decisions and will become a hurdle in the design and development process or that patients and advocates are naïve about the research process and funding problems (Hanley et al. 2001; Bombak and Hanson 2017). These barriers should be assessed in more detail, and greater efforts should be placed on overcoming any perceived drawback that would prevent patients from engaging and getting involved in scientific research.

Historically, few mechanisms existed for systematic engagement of patients in the drug development continuum, and in the very seldom cases in which structures for patient participation exist, they may be disorganized or confusing (Hohman et al. 2015). Efforts to overcome these should be undertaken, and learning modules and information are available to provide best practices. In recognition of these potential barriers, many patient advocacy organizations have research training programs designed specifically for patients to help inform and prepare them to support research studies. They can also provide mechanisms to connect patients with opportunities to participate on advisory boards and research teams to support the development of clinical trials. Most notably, the National Breast Cancer Coalition developed Project LEAD Institute, which provides a series of courses that establish a foundation of scientific knowledge to empower patients to participate actively and collaborate with physicians, industry, and regulatory agencies. In addition, Fight Colorectal Cancer has a Research Advocacy Training and Support (RATS) program, and Susan G. Komen and the American Association for Cancer Research also have programs to train advocates to support research studies. The Clinical Trials Transformation Initiative (CTTI), a public-private partnership, helps develop and drive adoption of practices within physician and patient communities to support patient engagement that will increase the quality and efficiency of clinical trials.

The inclusion of patients as reviewers and on research teams has led to more appropriately designed trials and the development of innovative clinical trial designs and statistical methods. Additionally, studies have demonstrated that patient involvement in the design and development of clinical trials is necessary to improve the efficiency and relevance of drug development and evaluation.

The Contribution of Patient Advocacy to Research and Drug Development

The incorporation of the patient voice has directly impacted the way trials are designed and conducted (Mullins et al. 2014). The way in which clinical trials are designed can transform the evidence generation process to be more patient centered, providing people with an incentive to participate or continue participating in clinical trials. Providing better information to participants and incorporating alternative trial designs will minimize concerns that clinical trials aren't patient centered and will dispel any doubts or concerns that prevent patients from becoming meaningful participants in the planning and design of clinical trials. Addressing the concerns and desires of patients has led to innovative strategies and designs to make trials more patient centric.

Trial Designs and Endpoint Selection

Many new therapies in oncology are molecularly targeted against specific oncogenic driver mutations that may be present in only a fraction of the patient population. Although the advent of targeted therapies holds great promise for patients, it also means that many patients may need to be screened before enough patients harboring the necessary mutation are found. Additionally, patients may not have the mutation of interest and will potentially have to seek out a variety of trials before finding a match. Master protocols are one mechanism to assist with the development and investigation of targeted therapies (Woodcock and LaVange 2017). Perhaps one of the greatest efficiencies of the collaborative clinical trial system is its increased benefit to patients seeking access to genomic screening technologies and experimental therapies. Rather than being forced to undergo multiple screening attempts and to move from trial to trial before ever being matched with a trial and treatment arm, patients who are screened for inclusion in a master protocol study need only be tested once to have a high likelihood of eventually participating in the study. The variety of patient subgroups that are evaluated over the course of a master protocol, as well as the use of non-match substudies, greatly increases patients' chances of receiving a study treatment. Moreover, patients who participate in master protocols are given access to a broad-based screening technology such as next-generation sequencing (NGS), which efficiently screens patients for a multitude of genomic markers and matches them to treatment arms based upon this information. Some select master protocols include the BATTLE program, LUNG-MAP for patients with lung cancer, and NCI-MATCH for patients with solid tumors, lymphomas, and myeloma.

Other patient-centric trial designs include pragmatic trials, adaptive trials, and trials that incorporate Bayesian statistics and allow patient crossover to the experimental treatment (Mullins et al. 2014). Pragmatic clinical trials can produce results that more accurately reflect the outcomes a typical person could expect to experience. Adaptive clinical trial designs allow for modifications to occur partway through the study based on information collected through the trial's progress. The incorporation of Bayesian statistics allows trialists to use prior information learned during the course of the trial and is often employed within adaptive trials. The subsequent Bayesian statistical analysis would describe the probability of a treatment's effect. While these trials provide many advantages for patients, they do have limitations. They can create logistical complications attributable to data management and study design as well as pose risks in the interpretability of the trial results. Trials that allow patients to crossover to the treatment arm, if shown to be superior to the control arm, can attenuate the treatment effect size. Additionally, the specific therapy under study may dictate which trial design is most optimal, particularly if interim results are unattainable to inform an adaptive methodology. The needs of patients and the need to generate solid evidence of efficacy will always need to be balanced.

It is important to engage patients early to understand the endpoints that matter most to them in all settings and stages of a disease. Mortality, for example, is an important outcome measure but is often not the only important outcome to patients. Especially in circumstances when chances of survival can be relatively low, other outcomes such as unnecessary diagnostic procedures or progression-free survival (PFS) are also important to patients. Clinical trials, therefore, must be designed with the patient's needs and preferences in mind within a given disease context. While certain endpoints may be more meaningful to researchers, these endpoints may ultimately not be meaningful to the patient group affected by the clinical trial. With the exception of validated surrogate endpoints, a primary endpoint should generally be a measure of something that is important to the patient (Vroom 2012). These endpoints should measure not only how a patient survives but also how a patient feels and functions.

The ascertainment of certain meaningful clinical endpoints, however, may be burdensome and time-consuming for researchers, hindering potentially lifesaving access for patients to the innovation under investigation. Recognizing this problem, Friends of Cancer Research and the Brookings Institute convened a panel of experts at a 2011 conference to discuss potential methods for streamlining the FDA approval process for drugs that show large treatment effects early in development while still ensuring drug safety and efficacy. The discussion at this conference informed the creation of the "Advancing Breakthrough Therapies for Patients Act" which established the FDA's Breakthrough Therapy Designation (BTD). This designation defines a breakthrough therapy as a drug intended to treat a serious or life-threatening disease or condition and for which preliminary evidence indicates that the drug may demonstrate substantial improvement over existing therapies (FDA Fact Sheet: Breakthrough Therapies). Once BTD is requested by the drug sponsor, the FDA and sponsor work together to determine the most efficient path forward, and if the designation is granted, the FDA will work closely with the sponsor to help expedite the development and review of the drug. Because innovative designation and approval pathways such as BTD take into consideration novel approval endpoints for clinical trials demonstrating higher rates of benefit in carefully selected patients, it is especially critical that patients are involved in identifying and defining the endpoints most important to them.

Given the broad benefits associated with patient involvement in scientific research and clinical trials, it is crucial to focus on greater dissemination and awareness. Strategies for the uptake and implementation of mechanisms for patient involvement should involve patients and patient advocates, health professionals, and drug developers. The creation of more educational resources to support researchers and patients when coordinating the incorporation of the patient voice in clinical trials would also improve the uptake of these mechanisms.

Capturing and Measuring Patient Experience

The patient voice is more commonly being incorporated in regulatory decision-making and has enabled the creation of more modern regulatory pathways. A patient's and their caregiver's experience with the disease and treatment-related symptoms, which may alter their function and health-related quality of life, is important. Capturing this rich experience from both patients and their caregivers helps provide key outcome information to consider in the evaluation of new agents. A recent policy review article written by international regulatory professionals from the USA, Europe, and Canada highlights the need for capturing the patient experience from different sources and focuses on the use of rigorous PRO measures to facilitate the regulatory decision-making process (Kluetz et al. 2018). Among the many advantages that PRO measures provide, these data are critical for supporting the benefit-risk assessment of experimental agents and useful when incorporated into prescribing and product information as descriptive data to inform safety and tolerability (Kim et al. 2018) or as a claim of treatment benefit. This information is particularly important for concerns with quality of life issues that patients and caregivers may have.

All international regulatory agencies acknowledge that robust and accurate data collected from the patient experience can be useful, as it complements existing measurements of safety and efficacy, but warn that poorly defined PRO methodology using heterogeneous analytical methods greatly hinders the incorporation of PRO data in regulatory decision-making (Kluetz et al. 2018; Kuehn 2018; Bottomley et al. 2018). It recommends that sustained international collaboration among regulatory agencies is required to improve patient experience collection and standardize the assessment, analysis, and interpretation of patient data from clinical trials.

The FDA has recognized that a central aspect of PFDD is the use of patient-reported outcomes (PROs) as a way to incorporate the patient voice in drug development and regulatory decisions. PROs are directly reported by the patient and provide a status of the patient's health, quality of life, or functional status (FDA-NIH Biomarker Working Group 2016). PRO measures can provide a better understanding of treatment outcomes and tolerability from a patient perspective and complement current measures of safety and efficacy (Kim et al. 2018). In 2009, the FDA released guidance for industry on the use of PROs in medical product development to support labeling claims and has worked with other advocacy organizations, such as the Critical Path Institute, and industry to form working groups that seek to engage patients and caregivers in the development of robust symptom-measuring tools, such as the PRO Consortium. Although challenges exist when seeking to collect patient and caregiver experience data, such as the need for more personalized and dynamic measuring tools that keep up with the diversity of novel drug classes with wide variety of toxicities, greater efforts to ensure consistency, reliability, and applicability of these data are warranted to support robust use in the drug development space.

Contributors to Data Generation

Patients and advocacy organizations are also actively establishing their own data sources to support clinical drug development and, in some instances, establishing their own clinical trials. These include patient registries, online data-sharing communities, wearable devices, and social media tools for capturing longitudinal data points. Organizations such as the Genetic Alliance, the National Organization for Rare Disorders, and Parent Project Muscular Dystrophy have launched registries to study the natural history of disease, burden of disease, expectations for treatment benefits, and perspectives on tolerable harms and risks. These tools can help inform academia and industry and incentive further study into a particular disease state. Through public-private partnerships, advocacy organizations are also initiating clinical trials within their patient communities. For example, the Leukemia and Lymphoma Society is leading the Beat AML Master Trial, which is a collaborative trial to test targeted therapies in patients with acute myeloid leukemia (AML) (Helwick 2018). Principle investigators should look for opportunities to utilize and integrate these data collection efforts into their research questions and studies in order to develop innovative partnerships that improve research logistics, outreach and communication, funding, and the prioritization of clinical trials.

Future Areas of Innovation and the Evolving Clinical Trial Landscape

There has been great progress in the area of patient engagement in clinical trials and the advancements being made by patient advocacy groups, and additional areas of opportunity continue to be identified. The development of more refined frameworks, models, best practices, and guidelines will help ensure early investigators have foundational knowledge to meaningfully engage patients and advocacy organizations in their research questions and drug development programs. Biopharma is investing heavily to accelerate development timelines. TransCelerate BioPharma Inc., a nonprofit organization that creates collaborations across biopharmaceutical research and development community, has recently launched a new initiative around patient awareness and access (TransCelerate 2018). Toolkits are available to assist research teams in engaging patient advocacy organizations and participants to optimize clinical trial designs. Additionally, some healthcare systems are partnering with cognitive computing platforms to help physicians match, enroll, and support patients (Bakkar et al. 2018).

The incorporation of external data sources to streamline, augment, and support clinical trial development is growing rapidly, due in large part to the advent of technological solutions that include patient collaboration programs, crowdsourcing, and the collection of big data and analytics. The US FDA is currently developing guidance and a framework to describe how real-world evidence can support drug development and regulatory decision-making. These external data sources represent an opportunity to augment clinical trial data and can potentially result in more streamlined drug development with fewer patients. These novel mechanisms of data collection, as well as their use and implementation, will continue to require the involvement of active advocates and consumers, who, through their experience, will contribute greatly to the oversight and eventual success of future clinical trials.

Cross-References

- ▶ Bayesian Adaptive Designs for Phase I Trials
- ▶ Cross-over Trials
- ▶ Implementing the Trial Protocol
- ▶ Orphan Drugs and Rare Diseases
- ▶ Participant Recruitment, Screening, and Enrollment
- ▶ Patient-Reported Outcomes
- ▶ Pragmatic Randomized Trials Using Claims or Electronic Health Record Data
- ▶ Trials in Minority Populations

References

Anderson M, McCleary KK (2016) On the path to a science of patient input. Sci Transl Med 8:1–6. https://doi.org/10.1126/scitranslmed.aaf6730

Bakkar N, Kovalik T, Lorenzini I et al (2018) Artificial intelligence in neurodegenerative disease research: use of IBM Watson to identify additional RNA-binding proteins altered in amyotrophic lateral sclerosis. Acta Neuropathol 135:227–247. https://doi.org/10.1007/s00401-017-1785-8

Bombak AE, Hanson HM (2017) A critical discussion of patient engagement in research. J Patient Cent Res Rev 4:39–41. https://doi.org/10.17294/2330-0698.1273

Bottomley A, Pe M, Sloan J et al (2018) Moving forward toward standardizing analysis of quality of life data in randomized cancer clinical trials. Clin Trials 15:624–630. https://doi.org/10.1177/1740774518795637

Chhatre S, Jefferson A, Cook R et al (2018) Patient-centered recruitment and retention for a randomized controlled study. Trials 19:205. https://doi.org/10.1186/s13063-018-2578-7

Comis RL, Miller JD, Aldigé CR et al (2003) Public attitudes toward participation in cancer clinical trials. J Clin Oncol 21:830–835. https://doi.org/10.1200/JCO.2003.02.105

Davis K, Schoenbaum SC, Audet AM (2005) A 2020 vision of patient-centered primary care. J Gen Intern Med 20:953–957. https://doi.org/10.1111/j.1525-1497.2005.0178.x

Domecq JP, Prutsky G, Elraiyah T et al (2014) Patient engagement in research: a systematic review. BMC Health Serv Res 14:1–9. https://doi.org/10.1016/j.transproceed.2016.08.016

FDA (2018) FDA voices: perspectives from FDA experts. https://www.fda.gov/newsevents/newsroom/fdavoices/default.htm. Accessed 12 Nov 2018

FDA Fact Sheet: Breakthrough Therapies. https://www.fda.gov/regulatoryinformation/lawsenforcedbyfda/significantamendmentstothefdcact/fdasia/ucm329491.htm. Accessed 12 Nov 2018

FDA-NIH Biomarker Working Group (2016) BEST (Biomarkers, EndpointS, and other Tools) Resource [Internet]. Food and Drug Administration (US), Silver Spring; Co-published by National Institutes of Health (US), Bethesda

Fergusson D, Monfaredi Z, Pussegoda K et al (2018) The prevalence of patient engagement in published trials: a systematic review. Res Involv Engagem 4:17. https://doi.org/10.1186/s40900-018-0099-x

Hanley B, Truesdale A, King A et al (2001) Involving consumers in designing, conducting, and interpreting randomised controlled trials: questionnaire survey. BMJ 322:519–523

Hearld KR, Hearld LR, Hall AG (2017) Engaging patients as partners in research: factors associated with awareness, interest, and engagement as research partners. SAGE Open Med 5:205031211668670. https://doi.org/10.1534/genetics.107.072090

Helwick C (2018) Beat AML trial seeking to change treatment paradigm. [Internet] The ASCO Post

Hohman R, Shea M, Kozak M et al (2015) Regulatory decision-making meets the real world. Sci Transl Med 7:313fs46. https://doi.org/10.1126/scitranslmed.aad5233

Kaitin K (2013) 89% of trials meet enrollment, but timelines slip, half of sites under-enroll. Tufts Cent Study Drug Dev Impact Rep 15:1–4

Kim J, Singh H, Ayalew K et al (2018) Use of pro measures to inform tolerability in oncology trials: implications for clinical review, IND safety reporting, and clinical site inspections. Clin Cancer Res 24:1780–1784. https://doi.org/10.1158/1078-0432.CCR-17-2555

Kluetz PG, O'Connor DJ, Soltys K (2018) Incorporating the patient experience into regulatory decision making in the USA, Europe, and Canada. Lancet Oncol 19:e267–e274. https://doi.org/10.1016/S1470-2045(18)30097-4

Kuehn CM (2018) Patient experience data in US Food and Drug Administration (FDA) regulatory decision making: a policy process perspective. Ther Innov Regul Sci 52:661–668. https://doi.org/10.1177/2168479017753390

Manganiello M, Anderson M (2011) Back to basics: HIV/AIDS advocacy as a model for catalyzing change. AIDS 1–29. https://www.fastercures.org/assets/Uploads/PDF/Back2BasicsFinal.pdf

Mullins CD, Vandigo J, Zheng Z, Wicks P (2014) Patient-centeredness in the design of clinical trials. Value Health 17:471–475. https://doi.org/10.1016/j.jval.2014.02.012

PCORI (2018) The value of engagement. https://www.pcori.org/about-us/our-programs/engagement/value-engagement. Accessed 12 Nov 2018

Schwartz L, Woloshin S (2015) FDA and the media: lessons from Tysabri about communicating uncertainty. NAM Perspect 5. https://doi.org/10.31478/201509a

Smith SK, Selig W, Harker M et al (2015) Patient engagement practices in clinical research among patient groups, industry, and academia in the United States: a survey. PLoS One 10:e0140232

Tinetti ME, Basch E (2013) Patients' responsibility to participate in decision making and research. JAMA 309:2331–2332. https://doi.org/10.1001/jama.2013.5592

TransCelerate (2018) Patient experience. http://www.transceleratebiopharmainc.com/initiatives/patient-experience/. Accessed 12 Nov 2018

Unger JM, Cook E, Tai E, Bleyer A (2016) The role of clinical trial participation in cancer research: barriers, evidence, and strategies. Am Soc Clin Oncol Educ Book 35:185–198. https://doi.org/10.14694/EDBK_156686

Vroom E (2012) Is more involvement needed in the clinical trial design & endpoints? Orphanet J Rare Dis 7:A38. https://doi.org/10.1186/1750-1172-7-S2-A38

Woodcock J, LaVange LM (2017) Master protocols to study multiple therapies, multiple diseases, or both. N Engl J Med 377:62–70. https://doi.org/10.1056/NEJMra1510062

Training the Investigatorship

31

Claire Weber

Contents

Abstract

The Investigatorship for clinical trials is a team with specialized experience who are qualified by training and experience to successfully execute clinical trials. The Investigatorship includes the trial sponsor, Good Clinical Practice (GCP) Contract Service Providers (CSPs), and site Investigators, who may also include

C. Weber (✉)
Excellence Consulting, LLC, Moraga, CA, USA
e-mail: cweber@excellence-llc.com

outside experts such as Key Opinion Leaders (KOLs) and Data Monitoring Boards (DMBs). GCP is the fundamental required training for all team members conducting clinical trials. Training occurs throughout the lifecycle of the trial, and each member of the team must have records of adequate training and qualifications to conduct the study for their identified role. This chapter explains the Investigatorship members, the types of training conducted, and how training is documented.

Keywords

Documentation · Monitoring · Delegation · File · Quality system

Introduction

Training is an essential and required component of conducting successful clinical trials. The Investigatorship must be qualified and trained on Good Clinical Practice (GCP), the trial protocol under study, the use of the investigational product(s) (IP), standard operational procedures (SOPs), trial protocol design and operations, the local and regional regulations and guidelines for clinical research, and Clinical Trial Applications (CTAs). Training is a part of risk control, in that training activities provide systematic safeguards to ensure adherence to standard operating procedures, and training in processes and procedures.

The Investigatorship for executing the clinical trial consists of trial sponsor teams, GCP Contract Service Providers (CSPs), and Investigator site teams. The Investigatorship may also include Investigators such as Key Opinion Leaders (KOLs) and independent Data Monitoring Boards (DMBs) who provide specialized expertise.

Training occurs within each sector of the Investigatorship, and the foundation for all clinical trials training is GCP. The trial sponsor is responsible for ensuring that each Investigatorship team member is appropriately qualified and trained relevant to their function, and that training is documented. This chapter describes the Investigatorship team, types of training, and training records maintained during the trial lifecycle.

Trial Sponsor Team

The trial sponsor team is made up of individuals who based on their training and experience will submit the clinical trial application (CTA) for the investigational product (IP) under study and plan and implement the trial ensuring compliance with International Council for Harmonisation (ICH) GCP and regulatory requirements. The trial sponsor team includes qualified individuals in functional areas including clinical science, clinical operations, technical operations (also known as supply chain operations), information technology, biostatistics, data management, regulatory affairs, pharmacovigilance, and quality assurance. Since the trial sponsor team is responsible for the submission documents for the CTA, they are also accountable for the overall oversight of the clinical trial. It is therefore requisite that the trial sponsor team has adequate training and knowledge of global regulations and guidelines so the training can be implemented throughout the trial.

The Sponsor Quality Manual and Quality System

The trial sponsor develops and maintains a quality manual or equivalent document that describes the quality system in their organization. The manual explains the organizational structure and quality assurance of the sponsor team functions. The quality manual also refers to required trial sponsor team training requirements and types of procedural training for controlled documents. In addition, it is customary for the quality system to describe how issues are escalated and how continuous improvement areas are identified and addressed for managing the quality and training for implementing clinical trials.

The qualifications of the trial sponsor team are documented for each team member in curriculum vitae's (CVs) and licenses relevant to their job description. Each trial sponsor team member is required to have adequate training documentation to perform their duties that are identified in job descriptions.

The hierarchy for training of controlled documents in the trial sponsor quality system is described in Fig. 1, with the quality manual as the highest-level document, and policies, procedures, work instructions, and records that are lower levels in that order.

Training requirements are recorded in a training curriculum for each sponsor team member. An example training curriculum is described in Table 1.

Controlled document training can be performed in person as on-the-job training, group training, or read and understand training. The trainee signs training documentation confirming the date of the training and the documentation is maintained in a sponsor trial master file.

Fig. 1 Organization of quality system documents

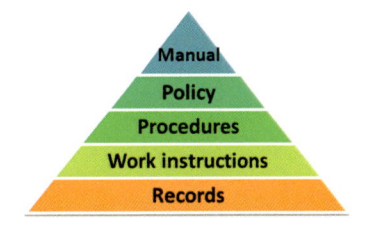

Table 1 Example of sponsor team training curriculum

Type/document number	Title	Biostatistics	Clinical research	Data management	Quality assurance	Regulatory affairs
SOP-00001	GCP training procedure	X	X	X	X	X
GCP training	GCP annual training session	X	X	X	X	X

External Training and Study-Specific Training

Sponsor teams may arrange trial-specific trainings and may attend courses such as seminars, webinars, or conferences to further their education and skills specific to their job duties. For these trainings, the trainee will print a certificate of attendance or the agenda/sign-in log for and maintain them in the sponsor trial master file.

GCP CSPs [(Including Contract Research Organizations (CROs)]

GCP CSPs are another important part of the Investigatorship. GCP CSPs are providers who perform trial development and execution services such as data management, statistical analysis, Randomization and Trial Supply Management (RTSM), and laboratory analysis. Clinical Research Organizations (CROs) are one type GCP CSP specific for study monitoring.

Clinical Research Organizations (CROs) are defined as:

> A person or an organization (commercial, academic, or other) contracted by the sponsor to perform one or more of a sponsor's trial-related duties and functions. (ICH E6 (R2) Glossary Section 1.20)

Each GCP CSP team member is also qualified by training and experience to perform their job duties.

Each GCP CSP will maintain a quality system, training curricula, and documentation in a similar way to the trial sponsor team. The trial sponsor team maintains adequate oversight of the GCP CSPs to ensure that the GCP CSP staff are qualified and have a training system and documented training records. For US Investigational New Drug (IND) trials, the transfer of regulatory obligations from the trial sponsor team to the GCP CSP for important functions identified in the Code of Federal Regulations (CFR) are documented by the trial sponsor on the FDA 1571 New Drug Application form (Section 15). and forwarded to FDA.

The trial sponsor team provides specialized training (e.g., detailed IP and trial-specific training) to the GCPs CSPs throughout the trial, and this training is documented and maintained in the trial master file. It is important to note that the trial sponsor team and GCP CSP team partner on many aspects to implement the clinical trial, and training development and management of training records is an essential part of this collaboration.

Investigator Site Team

The Investigator site team is made up of lead Investigators [(also known as principal investigators (PIs)], subinvestigators, and other site study personnel who are responsible for executing the trial according to GCP, health authority, institutional review board(IRB)/Ethical Committee (EC), and local regulations and guidelines. The PI is defined as:

> A person responsible for the conduct of the clinical trial at a trial site. If a trial is conducted by a team of individuals at a trial site, the investigator is the responsible leader of the team and may be called the principal investigator (ICH E6 (R2) Glossary Section 1.34).

A subinvestigator is defined as:

> Any individual member of the clinical trial team designated and supervised by the investigator at a trial site to perform critical trial-related procedures and/or to make important trial-related decisions (e.g., associates, residents, research fellows) (ICH E6 (R2) Glossary Section 1.56).

The PI and subinvestigators who are responsible for the conduct of the study under a US IND are documented on the FDA 1572 form or equivalent. The PI supervises the investigation at the Investigator site, and other members of the Investigator team may include subinvestigators, study coordinators, pharmacists, and laboratory personnel.

Each Investigator site team member must be qualified by education and experience to perform their functions at the study site and the PI has overall responsibility for delegating tasks to other qualified team members. The site/institution will also have a quality system and procedures requiring training.

PI Delegation of Authority

The delegation by the PI is documented in a Delegation of Authority Log that is updated as applicable during the trial. An example of a delegation of authority log is as follows:

Delegation of Authority Log

[STUDY NAME]

Site Number:_____

The purpose of this form is to: a) serve as the Delegation of Authority Log and b) ensure that the individuals performing study-related tasks/procedures are appropriately trained and authorized by the investigator to perform the tasks/procedures. This form should be completed prior to the initiation of any study-related tasks/procedures. The original form should be maintained at your site in the study regulatory/study binder. This form should be updated during the course of the study as needed.

Please Print	Obtain Informed Consent	Source Document Completion	Case Report Form (CRF) Completion	Assess Inclusion and -Exclusion Criteria	Physical Examination	Medical History	Medication History / Concomitant Medication	Collect Vital Signs	Review Vital Signs and Labs for Clinical Significance	Laboratory Specimen Collection/Shipping	AE Inquiry and Reporting	AE/SAE interpretation (severity/relationship to IP)	Administration of Investigational Product (IP)	IP Accountability	Regulatory Document Maintenance	Administrative	
NAME:	☐	☐	☐	☐	☐	☐	☐	☐	☐	☐	☐	☐	☐	☐	☐	☐	OTHER (specify):
STUDY ROLE:	SIGNATURE:														INITIALS:		DATES OF STUDY INVOLVEMENT:
NAME:	☐	☐	☐	☐	☐	☐	☐	☐	☐	☐	☐	☐	☐	☐	☐	☐	OTHER (specify):
STUDY ROLE:	SIGNATURE:														INITIALS:		DATES OF STUDY INVOLVEMENT:

I certify that the above individuals are appropriately trained, have read the Protocol and pertinent sections of 21CFR 50 and 56 and ICH GCPs, and are authorized to perform the above study-related tasks/procedures. Although I have delegated significant trial-related duties, as the principal investigator, I still maintain full responsibility for this trial.

Investigator Signature:_____   Date:_____

Source National Institute of Health (NIH) Delegation of Authority Log Version 2.0 24 April 2014

The trial sponsor team and/or the GCP CSP team collect training qualification documentation from the Investigator site team members (e.g., CVs, licenses, documentation of GCP training, etc.). They also provide the Investigator site team with specialized trial-specific trainings at site monitoring visits, Investigator group meetings, and other trial meetings. Each of these trainings are documented and forwarded to the trial master file and maintained in the Investigator site files.

Site Monitoring Visits

A site monitor identified by the trial sponsor team and/or the CSP has the responsibility of monitoring the Investigator site. Monitoring is defined as:

> The act of overseeing the progress of a clinical trial, and of ensuring that it is conducted, recorded, and reported in accordance with the protocol, standard operating procedures (SOPs), GCP, and the applicable regulatory requirement(s). (ICH E6 (R2) Glossary Section 1.38).

The site monitor performs monitoring as part of a monitoring plan according to the site sponsor and/or GCP CSP standard operating procedures. The site monitor conducts a pre-qualification visit prior to selecting the site, which includes an assessment that the Investigator site team are qualified by training and experience. After selection, the site monitor performs a site initiation visit ensuring that the Investigator site team is properly trained to conduct the study, including review of the Delegation of Authority Log, team member qualifications, startup recruitment, enrollment, IP administration and accountability, study protocol procedures, file maintenance, electronic systems such as electronic data capture (EDC), and RTSM, and any other operational requirements for the trial.

The monitoring visits are documented in monitoring visit reports and a follow-up letter is sent to the PI confirming the activities performed at each monitoring visit. These reports and letters are filed in the sponsor trial master file. The visit report is defined as:

> A written report from the monitor to the sponsor after each site visit and/or other trial related communication according to the sponsors SOPs. (ICH E6 R2 Glossary Section 1.39)

To document initial training prior to the commencement of the trial, the site initiation monitoring visit report is required to be filed at the at the Investigator site:

> To document that trial procedures were reviewed with the investigator and the investigator's trial staff. (ICH E6 R2, Section 8.2.20)

During the study, the site monitor conducts monitoring visits at regular intervals, and at the end of the study, the site monitor conducts a close-out visit. Each interim visit may include training as applicable, and further reviews of the Delegation of Authority Log to ensure the Investigator site team continues to be trained and qualified. The close-out visit includes specific training about final trial documentation and closure.

Other Training Meetings

Investigator meetings and communications between the trial sponsor team, GCP CSP team, and Investigator site team throughout the study are held to ensure adequate study training for new and existing team members as applicable.

Other External Teams

Other external team members such as KOLs and DMBs are qualified by education and experience to provide their expertise for the study. Training and communications with these external teams are documented according to the site sponsor required training procedures and filed in the sponsor trial master file.

Training Documentation and Files

Training documentation can be summarized as follows:

- Quality system and controlled document trainings (e.g., procedures, policies, etc.)
- GCP training certifications
- Professional training certifications
- Continuing education unit (CEU) accreditations
- CVs, job descriptions, and relevant licenses documenting qualifications
- Electronic system training including granting and revoking system access to systems (e.g., EDC, RTSM, pharmacovigilance system, etc.)
- Trial-specific training including agendas and attendance at Investigator meetings and other communications
- Site pre-qualification visits, initiation visits, interim visits, and close-out visits
- Monitoring visit reports and follow-up letters to Investigators

Training files for the entire Investigatorship are maintained as part of the sponsor trial master file and Investigator site files and must be made available to regulatory authorities upon request.

Summary and Conclusion

The Investigatorship is made up of the trial sponsor team, GCP CSPs, and Investigator site teams which may include Investigator external experts. Each team member must be adequately qualified and trained to perform their duties to conduct the clinical trial, and Investigators must adequately delegate authority to appropriate team members. GCP training is the foundation of all training for clinical trials. Training documentation is an important aspect of the trial and is maintained throughout the trial by the sponsor in the sponsor trial master file, and by the Investigators in the Investigator site file.

Key Facts

The facts covered in this chapter include: definitions of the Investigatorship team, their roles duties and requirements, and the overall guiding principles of ICH GCP for ensuring training and maintenance of the Investigatorship site files.

Cross-References

- ▶ Investigator Responsibilities
- ▶ Selection of Study Centers and Investigators
- ▶ Trial Organization and Governance

References

Code of Federal Regulations, Title 21, Part 312

Department of Health and Human Services, Food and Drug Administration, Investigational New Drug Application (IND) (Title 21 Code of Federal Regulations (CFR) Part 312) FDA 1572 (21 CFR 312.53(c))

Department of Health and Human Services, Food and Drug Administration, Investigational New Drug Application (IND) (Title 21 Code of Federal Regulations (CFR) Part 312) Form 1571 03/19

ICH E6 (R2) International Council for Harmonisation Guideline for Good Clinical Practice, Section 8.2.20

ICH E6 (R2) International Council for Harmonisation Guideline for Good Clinical Practice, Glossary Section 1.20

ICH E6 (R2) International Council for Harmonisation Guideline for Good Clinical Practice, Glossary Section 1.56

ICH E6 (R2) International Council for Harmonisation Guideline for Good Clinical Practice, Glossary Section 1.38

ICH E6 (R2) International Council for Harmonisation Guideline for Good Clinical Practice, Glossary Section 1.34

ICH E6 (R2) International Council for Harmonisation Guideline for Good Clinical Practice, Glossary Section 1.39

National Institute of Health (NIH) Delegation of Authority Log Version 2.0 24 April 2014

Responsibilities and Management of the Clinical Coordinating Center

32

Trinidad Ajazi

Contents

T. Ajazi (✉)
Alliance for Clinical Trials in Oncology, University of Chicago, Chicago, IL, USA
e-mail: tajazi@uchicago.edu

© Springer Nature Switzerland AG 2022
S. Piantadosi, C. L. Meinert (eds.), *Principles and Practice of Clinical Trials*,
https://doi.org/10.1007/978-3-319-52636-2_274

Abstract

Clinical coordinating centers of investigator-initiated multi-site clinical trials have a myriad of responsibilities throughout the life cycle of clinical trials from trial concept development to completion. At the core of all clinical research is the dual mandate to protect human subjects and ensure trial data integrity. National regulations and international guidelines are designed to enable regulatory compliance and achievement of these mandates. Integrated within clinical coordinating center activities are quality management mechanisms designed to monitor, control, and assure patient safety and data integrity.

This chapter summarizes the responsibilities of the clinical coordinating center with emphasis on efficient trial development and site selection, presents regulatory compliance requirements, focuses on practices for quality management, and describes clinical coordinating center management and network groups.

Keywords

Multi-site · Investigator-initiated · Clinical coordinating center · Clinical trial operations · Site management · Quality management · Regulatory compliance · Sponsor oversight · Research administration

Introduction

Clinical trials are often initiated by investigators in collaboration with their colleagues across multiple institutions. These multi-site investigator-initiated trials require coordinating centers to lead the implementation of the trial. The primary types of multi-site coordinating centers are the clinical coordinating center (CCC) and the data coordinating center (DCC). The clinical coordinating center is responsible for clinical trial operations, and the data coordinating center is responsible for statistics and data management functions. Some of the functions performed by the CCC and DCC may be combined under one coordinating center. The clinical and data coordinating centers may be integrated under one organization or reside in separate organizations. Collectively the CCC and DCC are responsible for implementation of multi-site clinical trials.

The clinical coordinating center of a multicenter research network provides the infrastructure for operationalizing clinical trials across participating centers. The primary responsibilities of the clinical coordinating centers include clinical trial operations and site management, quality management, regulatory compliance, communications, administration, and study results publication. The CCC is broadly responsible for oversight of all trial-related activities, inclusive of applicable clinical trial sponsor responsibilities.

In general, investigators seek to advance scientific discovery and positively impact healthcare practices. Clinical research in a global environment has grown increasingly complex. Regulatory oversight is paramount in all aspects of clinical trials. At the core of all operational activities is the dual mandate to protect the rights and well-being of human subjects and to ensure research data integrity. Management of the CCC requires strong leadership and clinical research expertise. This chapter focuses on the responsibilities and management of the clinical coordinating center and written from the perspective of nonprofit, academic-based clinical trial centers.

Responsibilities of the Clinical Coordinating Center

The clinical coordinating center is responsible for administrative support of governance and leadership functions, clinical trial development, project management, site management, regulatory affairs and compliance, quality control and assurance, research administration, trial registration and reporting, publication, and other operational services. How functional units are organized within coordinating centers overlap. The statistical and data management functions of the DCC are critical to trial implementation and should be synchronized with clinical trial operations. These activities are represented in Table 1 (Clinical coordinating center areas of responsibility). Some of these activities are further described below; research administration is described in the Management of Clinical Coordinating Centers section of the chapter.

Clinical Trial Development and Operations

Clinical trial development begins with concept development by scientific investigators. The study design with its primary and secondary endpoints are subject to scientific review both at the coordinating centers level and at the level of the funding agency or program (e.g., National Institutes of Health (NIH)) sponsoring the research. In addition to scientific review, the concept should also undergo an operational review with preliminary assessment of feasibility for required resources, trial budget and funding, specialized procedures, competing trials, patient populations, accrual barriers, Medicare coverage analysis, and other potential logistical challenges.

Clinical trial development is a team effort. Central to development are the project managers or protocol coordinators, the multi-site principal investigator (study PI), and the study statistician. These roles are key to efficient study development. Tools that enable operational efficiency include an upfront project plan and timeline projections and accepted model protocol and informed consent document templates. Protocols may include several co-chairs, including co-chairs for translational research aspects of the study. Other key members of the protocol development team include the medical officer, data manager, statistical programmer, study electronic data capture (EDC) builder, biorepository and reference laboratory personnel, regulatory affairs manager, and liaisons from disciplines such as nursing and pharmacy, as applicable. Additional reviewers responsible for assessing logistical feasibility at clinical sites and patient engagement include clinical research professionals,

Table 1 Clinical coordinating center areas of responsibility

Clinical trial development and operations	Regulatory affairs and compliance	Quality management
Project management Study design/concept development Protocol development Trial activation Protocol revision/amendment Trial closure/termination Trial publication Committee support Medical and clinical oversight Research collaborations Investigational product management Trial-related reporting	Investigational new drug (IND) Investigational device exemption (IDE) Institutional review board/ethics committee Clinical trial registration Conflict of interest/financial disclosure Trial master file (TMF) maintenance/essential regulatory documents Data and safety monitoring board support	Policies and standard operating procedures Quality control/monitoring Centralized monitoring Key performance evaluation On-site clinical monitoring Quality assurance Audit Inspection readiness Corrective and preventive action Good clinical practice (GCP) training
Site selection and management	Pharmacovigilance/drug safety management	**Communications and education**
Site selection Site start-up Site management Patient recruitment/accrual enhancement Site and personnel roster and credential management Site retention	Scientific misconduct/serious GCP breach Compliance: Code of Federal Regulations (Food and Drug Administration/Office of Human Research Protections) Compliance: International regulatory authorities Data privacy and security	Public relations Newsletters Education and training Meetings management Website content management Social media strategy Patient advocate relationships Other partnerships
Collaboration with statistics and data management in areas noted below	**Information technology/systems (shared with DCC)**	**Research administration and finance**
Statistical design Statistical analysis plan Patient enrollment and randomization Data collection Data management Data quality monitoring Data and statistical analysis Study reporting Publication Data privacy and security Data and safety monitoring board reporting	Patient enrollment and randomization Electronic data capture Clinical trial management system (CTMS) Trial master file (TMF) Reporting system Website Learning management system (LMS) Adverse event/safety management	Budgeting and finance Grants administration Legal, contracts, and trial agreements Fundraising Human resources Governance Steering/executive committee Publication committee/charter

community investigators, and patient advocates. The study PI is the primary author of the protocol.

The protocol document and related model informed consent document undergo several stages of authoring, review, and revision, based on the standard operating procedure (SOP) of the coordinating center. Case report forms are developed in parallel. Prior to release and activation of the study to participating sites for implementation, the relevant funding agency (e.g., NIH), regulatory authorities (e.g., Food and Drug Administration (FDA)), central institutional review board (CIRB), and other regulatory review bodies must review and approve the protocol. Prior to implementation at the site level, the institutional review board (IRB) or ethics committee of record must review and approve the protocol, according to relevant regulations. See Code of Federal Regulation (CFR) Title 21, Part 50 (Protection of Human Subjects) and Part 56 (Institutional Review Boards).

During the life cycle of a clinical trial, the protocol, clinical operations, and statistical teams are responsible for amending the protocol, when monitoring of the clinical trial signals the need to adjust trial parameters to improve safeguards for patient safety or mitigate logistical barriers in the conduct of the trial.

Site Selection

Selection of high-performing clinical trial sites is key to the successful initiation *and* completion of a clinical trial. Site personnel directly control trial participant recruitment, informed consent, visit schedules, trial procedures, data collection, and data submission. The CCC chooses sites with demonstrated ability to conduct clinical trials, in order to best ensure the integrity of research. High-performing sites have the structure, resources, and standard processes to recruit participants, enroll patients on study, adhere to protocol requirements, comply with applicable regulations, and submit date in a timely manner. Investigators at high-performing sites promote clinical trial participation, assess adverse events in real time, and provide necessary oversight of sub-investigators and research personnel.

Substandard sites are prone to GCP non-compliance, low accrual rates, protocol deviations, and delinquent and low-quality data submission. Such sites adversely consume CCC resources to monitor and manage the site for low returns. It is imperative to select qualified sites for successful clinical trial initiation, execution, and completion.

Depending on the complexity of trial requirements and the number of sites needed for successful trial completion, site selection could occur in multiple steps:

1. Identification of potential sites.
2. Site feasibility questionnaire and evaluation.
3. Site qualification visit, if applicable.
4. Final site selection.

During the site selection and startup process, coordinating center staff evaluate the following considerations:

1. Investigator credentials and research interests (curriculum vitae).
2. Investigator financial conflict of interest disclosure.
3. Patient population, registries.
4. Recruitment or outreach practices.
5. Previous history related to contracting and clinical trial startup timelines.
6. Institutional review board and site scientific committee review timelines.
7. Facilities and equipment, including specialized study-specific requirements.
8. Laboratory and biospecimen processing capabilities, as applicable.
9. Experience with clinical trial technologies, e.g., electronic data capture, electronic medical records, and interactive response technology.
10. Staff resources, experience and training (Good Clinical Practice (GCP) at minimum).
11. Site policies and standard operating procedures.
12. Quality reports, e.g., available quality assurance reports.
13. Regulatory inspection reports, e.g., FDA debarment and FDA inspection databases.
14. Satellite or affiliate management and oversight plan, if applicable.

Investigators in the FDA debarment database are not allowed to participate in clinical trials. The coordinating center staff need to assess the applicability of any FDA 483 that has been issued to the site. The FDA Form 483 is issued to firm management at the conclusion of an inspection when an investigator has observed any conditions that in their judgment may constitute violations of the Food Drug and Cosmetic (FD&C) Act and related acts. Coordinating center staff carefully consider the effectiveness of any applicable corrective and preventive action plan (CAPA) implemented by the site in response to an FDA 483.

Site Management

Following site selection, the CCC works with participating sites to prepare them for activation of the trial. Site startup activities may include conducting a site initiation visit (SIV) to confirm that sites have the appropriate facilities and equipment, provide study-specific training to investigators and site staff, review and collect regulatory documentation. Release of investigational product could be contingent on successful completion of an SIV, in addition to execution of the clinical trial agreement, IRB approval, access and training in the electronic data capture system, and other clinical trial management systems, as appropriate.

The CCC is responsible for tracking participating sites and active research personnel. A clinical trial management system (CTMS) is useful for maintaining site contacts and other relevant information. The CCC is responsible for maintaining a trial master file (TMF) of essential documents and ensuring that participating sites maintain essential documents in the investigator site file (ISF) or regulatory binder (electronic or hard copy). These documents must be maintained for continued enrollment of research subjects and clinical trial participation. ICH GCP sect. 8 provides guidance on required essential documents. Essential documents include the statement of investigator on FDA Form 1572, IRB approvals (initial, amendment, and continuing review) for research, and the delegation of authority log (DOA). The CCC and DCC should have checks in place to ensure that sites with expired or missing essential documents do not register research subjects to the trial. Upon submission of the DOA to the CCC and during monitoring visits, the CCC confirms that tasks delegated by the clinical investigator are appropriate and staff have received the proper training, prior to performance of research-related tasks.

Upon activation of a clinical site, coordinating center personnel maintain communication with sites to promote accrual of subjects to the clinical trial. In conjunction with the principal investigator, CCC staff develop a communication plan to educate sites regarding the clinical trial, development accrual enhancement materials such as trial websites, social media posts, brochures, newsletters, etc. It is a good idea to host meetings with participating site investigators and clinical research professionals to address questions and concerns, report on trial developments, share best practices and frequently asked questions.

It is important that the trial principal investigator is available to address site inquiries related to eligibility, patient and treatment management, disease status evaluation, adverse event reporting, and other inquiries that affect safety of research participants or the conduct of the clinical trial. Documentation of these inquiries and any related actions and decisions should be tracked by CCC personnel. During these interactions, the PI and CCC staff should monitor for potential protocol deviations. They should advise sites of any deviations that should be reported to the IRB and in the electronic data capture system. CCC personnel should be in close contact with the data managers of the trial to share concerns for site management and data management. Research nurses and clinical trial managers at the CCC assist the PI in addressing inquiries from participating sites. The regulatory manager is also available to respond to inquiries related to informed consents and IRB-related questions.

Regulatory Compliance

Compliance with regulatory requirements is required for all clinical trial activities. The CCC ensures that the clinical trial is conducted according to the regulations described below. In the United States, clinical trials are developed and implemented according to the Code of Federal Regulations (CFR). These regulations are codified to provide the rules for implementing laws enacted by the Congress.

All clinical trials funded in whole or in part by HHS agencies are required to follow Title 45 CFR Part 46 – Protection of Human Subjects. 45 CFR 46 includes the following subparts: A, Basic HHS Policy for Protection of Human Subjects; B, Additional Protections for Pregnant Women, Human Fetuses and Neonates Involved in Research; C, Additional Protections Pertaining to Biomedical and Behavioral

Research Involving Prisoners as Subjects; D, Additional Protections for Children Involved as Subjects in Research; and E, Registration of Institutional Review Boards. Subpart A, as adopted by multiple HHS agencies, including the National Institutes of Health (NIH), is also known as Federal Policy for the Protection of Human Subjects or the Common Rule.

The Food and Drug Administration (FDA) is responsible for regulating clinical trials of drugs, biological products, and medical devices. Clinical trials utilizing investigational products are under the jurisdiction of the FDA. Title 21 of the CFR contains the rules of the FDA. There are several key parts of Title 21 (Food and Drug Administration) that pertain to the clinical trials, including Part 50 – Protection of Human Subjects (Subpart A, General Provisions; Subpart B, Informed Consent of Human Subjects; Subpart D, Additional Safeguards for Children; Part 56, Institutional Review Boards; Part 312, Investigational New Drug Application; and Part 812, Investigational Device Exemptions). In addition, management of clinical trials involving investigational products that are submitted to the FDA for marketing approval needs to take into account 21 CFR Part 314 (Applications for FDA Approval to Market a New Drug). Other important parts of the CFR include Part 54 (Financial Disclosure by Clinical Investigators) and Part 11 (Electronic Records; Electronic Signatures). All trials involving investigational products or devices are conducted in accordance with CFR Title 21.

Clinical trials are conducted on a global basis. However, sponsors and investigators conducting clinical trials are required to abide by country-specific regulations. In order to address variations in country-specific requirements for developing pharmaceuticals in multiple countries, the International Council for Harmonisation of Technical Requirements for Pharmaceuticals for Human Use (ICH) developed guidelines to harmonize the conduct of clinical trials globally for participating countries. ICH guidelines cover multiple common topics including Quality (Q), Safety (S), Efficacy (E), and Multiple Disciplinary (M) Guidelines. E6 has become the international standard for Good Clinical Practice (GCP) and has been implemented in the United States. Compliance with ICH GCP ensures the protection of human subjects and clinical trial data integrity.

Per FDA regulations, an institutional review board is an appropriately constituted group that has been designated to review and monitor biomedical research involving human subjects. It has the authority to approve, require modification in, or disapprove research. The IRB assures the protection of the rights and welfare of humans participating as subjects in research. IRBs review research protocols and related materials, including the informed consent document.

Laws and regulations have been implemented to govern the conduct of clinical trials for the purposes of ensuring the protection of human subjects and clinical trial integrity. The policies and procedures implemented by clinical trial coordinating centers must comply with applicable regulations and related guidance documents. The federal laws and regulations, as well as related guidance documents and GCP principles, provide the foundation for all coordinating activities described in the following sections of this chapter.

Trial Sponsorship and Investigational New Drug Application

Clinical trials that include an intervention with an investigational drug or biological product require submission of an Investigational New Drug Application (IND) to the Food and Drug Administration (FDA). FDA approval of an IND provides the sponsor with the authorization to administer an investigational product to human subjects. These trials must be conducted according to 21 CFR Part 312 (Investigational New Drug Application). The IND is filed by the sponsor of the trial. According to 21CFR Part 312.3, a *sponsor* is a person who takes responsibility for and initiates a clinical investigation. The sponsor may be an individual or pharmaceutical company, governmental agency, academic institution, private organization, or other organizations.

If the IND is filed by the principal or lead investigator of a multi-site clinical trial when the site is also one of the clinical sites for the trial, the PI is considered the *sponsor-investigator* and is therefore responsible for initiating and conducting a clinical trial. The IND is cross-referenced with the IND filed by the pharmaceutical company. The coordinating center is responsible for working with the principal investigator to prepare the IND for submission. The CC also works with the pharmaceutical partner to secure the necessary documents required from the pharmaceutical company, including the Investigator Brochure (IB) and cross-reference or letter of authorization. The pharmaceutical company may file the IND and retain official sponsorship of the trial while transferring specified sponsor responsibilities to a coordinating center. In general, the coordinating center is responsible for ensuring that sponsor responsibilities according to 21 CFR Part 312, Subpart D (Responsibilities of Sponsors and Investigators) are met.

Sponsors are generally responsible for selecting qualified investigators, providing them with the information they need to conduct an investigation properly, ensuring proper monitoring of the investigation(s), ensuring that the investigation(s) is conducted in accordance with the general investigational plan and protocols contained in the IND, maintaining an effective IND with respect to the investigations, and ensuring that FDA and all participating investigators are promptly informed of significant new adverse effects or risks with respect to the drug (21 CFR 312.50).

General investigator responsibilities are described in sect. 312.60 and includes ensuring that an investigation is conducted according to the signed investigator statement (FDA Form 1572), the investigational plan (aka protocol), and applicable regulations; protecting the rights, safety, and welfare of subjects under the investigator's care; and controlling drugs under investigation. The investigator is responsible for informed consent of each human subject.

ICH GCP E6(R2) emphasizes the need for sponsor oversight and the sponsor's responsibilities for quality management including risk management, monitoring, quality control, and quality assurance. Quality management is discussed in later sections of this chapter.

Inspection Readiness

Coordinating centers (CCC and DCC) must be ready for inspection by a regulatory authority (RA), such as the FDA. Inspection readiness must be built into clinical trial operations, quality monitoring, and quality assurance activities. Good documentation practice is a basic requirement for inspection readiness, in *all* areas of research. Regulatory authorities will look for contemporaneous documentation showing sponsor oversight. Evidence that the coordinating center monitored the trial and maintained regulatory documentation in a *timely* manner is critical during an inspection. The FDA Bioresearch Monitoring Program (BIMO) provides a copy of the Compliance Program Guidance Manual (CPGM) utilized in FDA inspections. The CCC should utilize the BIMO as a guide for ensuring inspection readiness.

Quality Management

The CCC and DCC are responsible for quality management at multiple levels. Quality management should be conducted as a partnership between clinical operations, statistics and data management, as well as research collaborators. The principles and practice of quality management is evolving. The quality focus varies by the type of research organization and their aims, structure, and resources. In all cases, the coordinating centers seek compliance with regulations, integrity of safety and efficacy data, and the protection and well-being of subjects. The following is only a slice of the discussions surrounding quality management with a focus of the aspects of quality management conducted by the CCC and DCC.

Standard Operating Procedures

At a basic level, the coordinating center is responsible for developing and maintaining standard operating procedures. Responsible staff need to periodically review SOPs to ensure that they are in line with regulatory changes, as well as changes in systems or structure. The SOPs should cover all aspects of clinical trial development, management, oversight, conduct, and completion. In some cases, institutional policies and SOPs may determine how the CCC functions. The SOPs should provide consistency across the institution, but they need to account for variations in trial designs and circumstances. A good practice is to have levels of policies, SOPs, and working instructions as controlled documents that have increasing levels of detail. The working instructions could be more detailed and provide step-by-step instructions. These could be changed and tweaked as needed. Study-specific plans could augment SOPs but must remain consistent with the SOPs. This creates a balance and flexibility while retaining structure. One point to remember is that SOPs are only as good as training on SOPs. Staff training must be prescribed and maintained in a timely fashion.

Quality Control

The CCC is responsible for quality control (QC) and trial monitoring activities, as well as quality assurance (QA) activities. The latter is usually conducted in the form of systematic audits to ensure compliance. In November 2016, the International Council for Harmonisation (ICH) Integrated Addendum to ICH E6(R1) Guideline for Good Clinical Practice, E6(R2), was released. The FDA released its related Guidance for Industry for E6(R2) in March 2018. The addendum to ICH GCP E6 sect. 5 promotes implementation of a system to manage quality throughout all stages of the trial. According to ICH GCP E6(R2), a risk-based approach should define the quality management system. This includes provisions for critical processes and data identification of processes and data critical to ensure human subject protection and reliability of trial results. Risk management includes risk identification, evaluation, control, communication, review, and risk reporting.

Since the addendum was released, research organizations have developed strategies and processes for risk-based centralized monitoring. There are varying applications of this approach. At the core of these activities is the development of analytical reports and metrics that can be reviewed centrally and/or remotely. Evaluation of key performance indicators (KPIs), also known as key risk indicators (KRIs), such as data quality, data timeliness, query rates, protocol deviation rates, serious adverse event rates, and subject enrollment levels, assist the coordinating center in identifying sites that might be at risk. The determination leads to decisions regarding increased monitoring, auditing, and/or other corrective or preventive actions. Central review of monitoring KPIs is a joint activity between the CCC and DCC.

With the use of electronic systems, source data review and verification can be conducted remotely. The electronic tools for central monitoring are integrated with the electronic data capture system (EDC) maintained by the DCC. A central monitor assigned either by the DCC or CCC can review certified copies of source documents uploaded into the EDC system or a source document portal. A central monitor can remotely access a site's electronic medical record (EMR) system. Electronic source data documentation is reviewed against data recorded into the EDC. The success of central monitoring is dependent on careful planning. The critical data points for eligibility, trial intervention or treatment, adverse event/safety monitoring, and trial endpoint evaluation should be identified to focus the central monitoring activity. Central review of data, coupled with KPI metric reviews, enables the CCC and DCC to identify sites that require intervention, follow-up, increased on-site monitoring, auditing, or other forms of remediation.

Medical oversight by a designated medical officer or medical monitor is key to quality management activities. The medical officer provides clinical expertise and judgment. The medical officer is a point of escalation for other members of the study team. The medical officer is also responsible for considering potential impact on patient safety and recommending changes to the protocol based on trends analysis reports. Such recommendations are discussed with the trial statistician and other members of the study team.

The monitoring plan for a clinical trial should account for both centralized or remote monitoring and on-site monitoring. Routine on-site monitoring may be planned at a decreased frequency in combination with centralized monitoring. A level of source data verification conducted through on-site monitoring should be documented in the clinical monitoring plan. At-risk sites, identified through central monitoring, are given priority for on-site monitoring.

Quality Assurance

Quality assurance is an independent and recommended activity, usually conducted in the form of audits. Audits include site, TPO/CRO, system, and internal audits. The scope of the audit is identified in the audit plan. Auditor assessments include a review of compliance with regulations, GCP guidelines, SOPs, and trial plans. The auditor should be reviewing clinical trial management by the CCC. The audit should not be confused with monitoring, an ongoing quality control activity. In fact, audits assess the effectiveness of monitoring activities, clinical trial operations, and data center activities. An investigator site audit could reveal not only non-compliance by the investigator but also failures in other aspects of trial conduct at the sponsor-investigator CCC or CRO level. For example, investigator non-compliance could be coupled with monitoring observations if the monitors did not detect the non-compliance. Audit observations need to be conveyed to the affected parties in a timely manner followed by implementation of a corrective and preventive action (CAPA) plan with a root cause analysis, timelines, and measures for success. The coordinating center is responsible for quality assurance and evaluating the effectiveness of any CAPA implemented, according to SOPs.

Oversight of CROs

If the multicenter trial is large enough (e.g., 1000 research subjects and 50 sites), it might be necessary to outsource monitoring functions to a Clinical Research Organization (CRO). The ICH EG(R2) addendum also emphasized the need for sponsors to provide oversight to third parties contracted to perform responsibilities on their behalf. A few tips regarding oversight include review of CRO qualification and staff training, as well as frequent communication with CROs to share information on changes to the trial, provide instruction, and address inquiries. If the CRO is responsible for monitoring, review the monitoring reports and set and review metrics for trip report completion, site follow-up, and compliance with the monitoring plan. If the CRO is responsible for the trial master file, generate reports on timely completion and check accuracy of the TMF. Implement a pathway for the CRO to escalate issues to the coordinating center staff. Establish guidelines for how critical and major non-compliance need to be addressed and the SOP for CAPAs to follow. Be clear on what SOPs are applicable. Develop a quality management plan with the CRO. Document all continuous oversight activities.

Adverse Event and Safety Monitoring

The multi-site principal investigator and responsible personnel at the CCC and DCC are required to continuously review expedited or serious adverse events, as they are reported by participating sites. Following the FDA Guidance for Industry and Investigators for Safety Reporting Requirements for INDs and BA/BE Studies, investigators must assess if a reported adverse event meets the requirement for expedited reporting to the FDA of a Serious and Unexpected Suspected Adverse Reaction (SUSAR), in accordance with 21 CFR 312.32. The principal investigator is also responsible for reporting the SUSAR to the pharmaceutical partner. The CCC notifies participating sites of SUSARs (IND safety reports) and provides guidance on any related changes to risks associated with an investigational product and the informed consent document.

Management of Clinical Coordinating Centers

Management of the clinical coordinating center involves oversight by both the CCC leadership and research administration at the institutional level. Research administration provides the infrastructure and determines the policies that govern the responsibilities and management of a CCC.

Research Administration

Research administration at an institution may be comprised of several offices that administer various areas of sponsored research management and compliance including grants and contracts, financial administration, research integrity and compliance, core facilities, research computing, and legal counsel. An institutional review board (IRB) is part of research administration and must approve clinical research activities, prior to clinical trial initiation. A multi-site coordinating center trial requires approval from research administration of the multi-site principal investigator's institution. The multi-site PI may also be referred to as a sponsor-investigator, especially for clinical trials that involve investigational products requiring submission of sponsor-investigator IND. The PI serves as both the multi-site PI and PI at their site.

There are several avenues for funding multi-site investigator-initiated clinical trials. The coordinating center administration is responsible for raising funds and fiscal management. Sources of funding include nonprofit foundations, federal government agency grants, cooperative agreements or contracts, as well as public-private partnerships with pharmaceutical and biotechnology companies. The National Institutes of Health (NIH) and other federal agencies have a multitude of funding opportunities. Research proposals are usually submitted in response to a request for proposal (RFP) or funding opportunity announcement (FOA) from a funding agency. The multicenter research proposal is prepared by the principal investigator and co-investigators with assistance from coordinating center staff. These proposals contain the research plan, a description of the clinical coordinating center capabilities, and the budget. Research proposals to a funding agency are submitted through research administration and must have the approval of an authorized institutional official.

In addition to pre-award assistance, research administration provides post-award services including financial administration and financial reporting. The institution may also issue sub-award agreements or subcontracts to external investigators, or vendor service agreements to third-party organizations (e.g., central laboratories). In case the data coordinating center is not at the same institution, funding and collaboration agreements with the data coordinating center would be issued. Research administration will assist with negotiation of contracts and budgets with funding sponsors, participating sites, and subcontractors, enforcing legal and regulatory requirements for research administration, as necessary. The multi-site PI and their team are responsible for monitoring deliverables and ensuring that applicable terms of award are met. At specified time points, a progress report for the research plan and financial utilization is submitted to the funding agency by research administration. Another important function for research administration is overseeing potential financial conflicts of interest by investigator. When potential conflicts of interest arise, institutional policies for conflict management or elimination are implemented.

Industry Collaborations

In addition to grants management of federally funded clinical trials, research administration will work with a multi-site PI for an investigator-initiated trial and CCC in managing collaborations with industry. A common example of such a collaboration is a pharmaceutical company providing access to an investigational product for use in a trial. The collaboration could include additional funding support from the company for other aspects of the trial. The deliverables, including data sharing requirements, are addressed in the investigator-initiated clinical trial agreement (CTA). The CTA may include the following:

1. Clinical trial agreement components: conduct of the study; human subject enrollment requirement; participating site requirements; quality assurance and regulatory inspection readiness; vendor and subcontractor compliance; study data ownership and data sharing; record keeping; confidentiality; publication; safety reporting; inventions; compliance with law; term and termination; indemnification and insurance; payment and payment schedule.
2. Budget (exhibit).
3. Statement of work (exhibit).

Finance and contracts staff, in conjunction with project management personnel, negotiates the budget and agreement and ensures that all trial activities are funded appropriately. The budget staff works closely with study team members to determine research tests and procedures that are not covered by insurance. This could be part of a Medicare coverage analysis review. The study team also determines if funding requests are needed for correlative science. The CCC and research administration teams are responsible for tracking the terms and milestones of all agreements. This is a shared administrative and finance function. The scientific and resource benefits that translate into successful trial completion are well-worth the time and effort to negotiate the collaborations.

Institutional Approval of Clinical Coordinating Center

Prior to initiation of the clinical trial and CCC activities, the multi-site PI's institution may require approval of the CCC, per institutional policies. Research administration and the IRB will review the CCC to ensure compliance with regulatory requirements for the protection of human subjects. Institutional requirements include review of the clinical trial protocol and informed consent, the data and safety monitoring plan, as appropriate for a multi-site trial. The institution may request feasibility questionnaire for external sites. Institutional evaluation includes review of coordinating center responsibilities, qualifications and training of research staff, site selection, site management, data management procedures, statistical analysis plan, investigational product distribution and accountability, pharmacovigilance and safety reporting, protocol deviation monitoring, central and on-site monitoring, accrual plan, project management, and multi-site communication plans, as applicable. The relevant information may be contained in the protocol and other study plan documents. If applicable for interventional trials, the institution may require the implementation of an independent data and safety monitoring board.

The requirements for approval of a CCC may be obtained from research administration. For reference, a good example of CCC institutional requirements can be found on the website of Dana Farber/Harvard Cancer Center (DF/HCC).

Management

The coordinating center, multi-site PI, and participating site PIs are collectively responsible for meeting the criteria for grant awards and contracts. This requires collaborative management practices by the leadership and management team. The management team of the coordinating center is responsible for efficient and effective management of all centralized clinical trial activities. Continuous monitoring, documentation, and progress evaluations are necessary.

The multi-site principal investigator is responsible for fulfilling the obligations of the sponsor-investigator, including the initiation and management of the clinical trial at *all* clinical trial sites. The CCC may already be established within a program at the institution with a medical director who regularly oversees the activities of the CCC, or it may be newly established under the direction of the multi-site PI. The structure of the CCC management and staff may differ slightly between institutions. However, directors or senior managers who oversee clinical trial operations, administration, project management, and regulatory affairs are key to managing a clinical coordinating center. Research nurses, regulatory managers, clinical trial or project managers, and research coordinators are important staff members for a fully functional CCC.

Resource Management

Successful completion of a multi-site clinical trial is heavily dependent on the personnel staffing the clinical and data coordinating centers, as well as third-party service providers. CCC managers need to review the staffing plan periodically to ensure that sufficient staff are available to manage the trial. Staff planning is closely tied to the budget planning. Balancing anticipated resource needs and financial resources is a challenging and shared function between operations, administration, and finance managers. The CC cannot afford the mistake of understaffing and consequently risking trial timelines, resulting in regulatory non-compliance, oversight gaps, or other unmet trial obligations.

Initially hiring qualified personnel followed by an ongoing training and education program is necessary for the any health organization. Staff engagement, open feedback, and communication loops are keys to optimal CCC management and quality improvements.

Operational Efficiency and Project Management

In conjunction with the DCC, the clinical coordinating center is responsible for timely trial development to keep pace with scientific advancements and meet the requirements of the funding agency. Taking too long to launch a clinical trial may affect the relevancy of the scientific question and the impact of the results on clinical practice. In partnerships with industry, inefficient and slow timelines affect the ability of the industry partner to submit marketing applications for investigational products. In a competitive environment, delays place the CCC and its partner at a disadvantage.

Operational efficiency is achieved and monitored in part through careful project planning and management. The coordinating center needs to develop target timelines and milestones for protocol development. The CCC utilizes tools and computer applications for careful and constant monitoring deadlines with the goal of meeting target timelines. Project managers are accountable to CCC leadership for ensuring trial activation, progress, and completion. Project managers coordinate the activities of internal and external personnel and coordinate execution of many processes. During the study, project managers work closely with data analysis staff to generate reports for trends analysis reporting to oversee the conduct of the study. Contingency and escalation plans are part of the CCC SOPs and may be incorporated into the project plan or other study-specific plans.

Risk Management

Ultimately, the multi-site PI is responsible for the conduct of a clinical trial at all participating sites. Beyond the study design and compliance with clinical trial regulations, successful completion of a clinical trial starts with careful planning by CCC management. This includes ensuring that adequate human and financial resources are available throughout the life cycle of the trial. The management team needs to budget for personnel at the CCC and participating sites and personnel and resources for data coordinating center activities. There are a multitude of costs that must be included in the budget calculations, including clinical trial management systems, electronic data capture system, data and record storage, trial supply distribution, training, travel, site recruitment, patient recruitment, monitoring, project management, special equipment, laboratory services, site payments, and other costs related to subcontracts and vendor management. Throughout the life of the clinical trial, the management team is responsible for tracking expenses and ensuring that the trial remains within budget.

At the beginning of the project, the CCC management team is primarily responsible for risk assessment and risk management while the clinical trial is ongoing. Recent developments in clinical research, exemplified by changes to ICH GCP guidelines and FDA guidance, place a major emphasis on risk management. For example, a 2019 funding opportunity (PAR-19-329) posted by the National Heart, Lung and Blood Institute (NHLBI) titled Clinical Coordinating Center for Multi-Site Investigator-Initiated Clinical Trials emphasizes the focus on both risk management and operational efficiency, as well as the role of project management to proactively mitigate risks. The NHLBI requires a trial management plan that describes the strategy of the CCC to "ensure that management activities of the clinical trial are met including directly supporting the needs of scientific leadership to identify barriers, make timely responses, and optimize the allocation of limited resources" with a risk assessment and management plan that identifies a range of contingencies and solutions.

Identification of potential risks at the beginning of the trial is key to successful risk management. Monitoring of key risk indicators (KRIs), as part of quality management, ensures corrective and preventative action in a continuous improvement manner. Key risk considerations and indicators often depend on the type and complexity of the trial. CCCs often consider the patient population, competing clinical trial opportunities, accrual rate projections, expected screen failure rate, investigational new drug or device status, data timeliness and quality, adverse event rates, and protocol deviations rates. An example of a risk assessment tool is the Risk Assessment and Categorization Tool (RACT) developed by TransCelerate to assist with risk-based monitoring implementation.

Clinical Coordinating Center and Trial Governance

The multi-site clinical trial and the CCC may be governed by a steering committee or executive committee, chaired by the multi-site PI. Members of the executive committee may include multi-PIs of participating sites and statistical center representation. At the beginning of the trial, the executive committee is concerned about trial design, funding, and site selection. Upon trial initiation, this committee is charged with monitoring the progress of the trial and making decisions regarding issues escalated by CCC management. These issues often fall along the lines of key risk indicators described above. The multi-site PI and members of the executive committee serve as champions of the trial with other investigators and other research collaborators. Upon analysis of trial results, they are responsible for overseeing implementation of DSMB recommendation and publication of study results. The governance responsibilities of the executive committee may be documented in a charter.

Clinical and Data Coordinating Center Integrated Functions

The coordinating center may include the CCC and the DCC within the same institution, or the DCC may be part of a separate institution. The primary responsibilities of the DCC include statistical design, data management, data analysis, and publication of study results. Collectively the functions of the CCC and DCC encompass the breadth of centralized clinical trial management activities.

The functions of the DCC must be integrated with clinical operations throughout the life cycle of a clinical trial: development and activation, accrual phase, follow-up/data maturation, data analysis and reporting, and close-out. The DCC and CCC leaders are part of the multi-site management team and included in all levels of management discussion, planning, and review. DCC personnel including statisticians and data managers are members of the study team and key to both protocol development and trial management. The SOPs and workflow between the CCC and DCC are developed to dovetail and support all units. Frequent and open communications happen on a day-to-day basis for ongoing study management.

Alignment of CCC and DCC resources is important in multi-site coordinating center obligations for timely trial activation and completion, as well as ongoing trial management. The DCC is crucial not only for data analysis and results reporting but also in ongoing quality management analyses. Figure 1 depicts examples of integration between the clinical and data coordinating centers, over the life cycle of a clinical trial.

Clinical Trial Network Group Coordinating Center

This chapter focused on responsibilities of the clinical coordinating center for a multi-site clinical trial. Coordinating centers could be established to manage one or several trials. The number and type of participating clinical sites are configured based on trial needs. These participating sites could evolve into an established clinical trial network. Clinical trial networks that conduct large-scale clinical trials with a portfolio of clinical trials may be referred to as network groups or cooperative research groups. The operation centers of these network groups have all of the components of an investigator-initiated coordinating center with some advantages

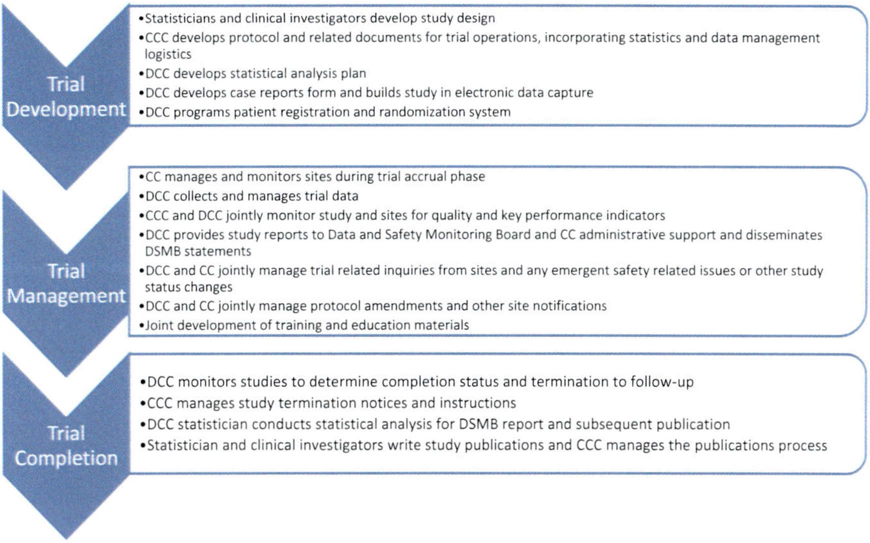

Fig. 1 Clinical coordinating center (CCC) and Data coordinating center (DCC) integrated function examples

and disadvantages. An example of established network groups is the National Clinical Trials Network (NCTN) groups, funded by the National Cancer Institute (NCI). The groups include the Alliance for Clinical Trials in Oncology, ECOG-ACRIN, NRG Oncology, SWOG, Children's Oncology Group, and Canadian Cancer Trials Group. The coordinating centers of these groups are a paired set of an operations center (i.e., clinical coordinating center) and statistics and data management center (i.e., data coordinating center).

The advantages to these types of networks include a membership model for participating sites. These participating sites are required to adhere to membership performance requirements, in order to participate in network trials. Site selection and qualification is streamlined for sites interested in clinical trial participation. The established nature of the group's policies and procedures and centralized infrastructure provided by the NCI itself offer an opportunity to launch peer-reviewed clinical trials in a uniform fashion. These networks offer consistency in how trials are managed, monitored, and audited. They can leverage the utilization of a standard electronic data capture system and data management procedures across multiple clinical trials. These large networks enjoy the scientific participation and expertise of investigators across the country, as members of both scientific and administrative committees. Clinical trial development procedures have been standardized with the aim of optimizing operational efficiency. They are able to monitor institutional performance across multiple trials and sites, offering education and training opportunities for improvement of clinical trial conduct. Nevertheless, these groups face challenges related to resource and funding constraints inherent in managing a large portfolio of clinical trials. As with all multi-site coordinating centers, these network coordinating centers face similar challenges for completing trial accrual, managing quality and ensuring regulatory compliance for the protection of human subjects, trial integrity, and data quality. Research collaborations with other research groups, including international partners, as well as industry partnerships are important to the success of collaborative clinical research. Within the academic research and the investigator-initiated clinical research community, the choice for multicenter clinical trials includes implementation through a network group or an institution-based coordinating center.

Summary

The clinical coordinating center is responsible for managing all stages of a clinical trial life cycle: trial development, activation, accrual, follow-up, results reporting, and closure. Multi-site clinical trial management functions include risk management, project management, protocol development, site selection and management,

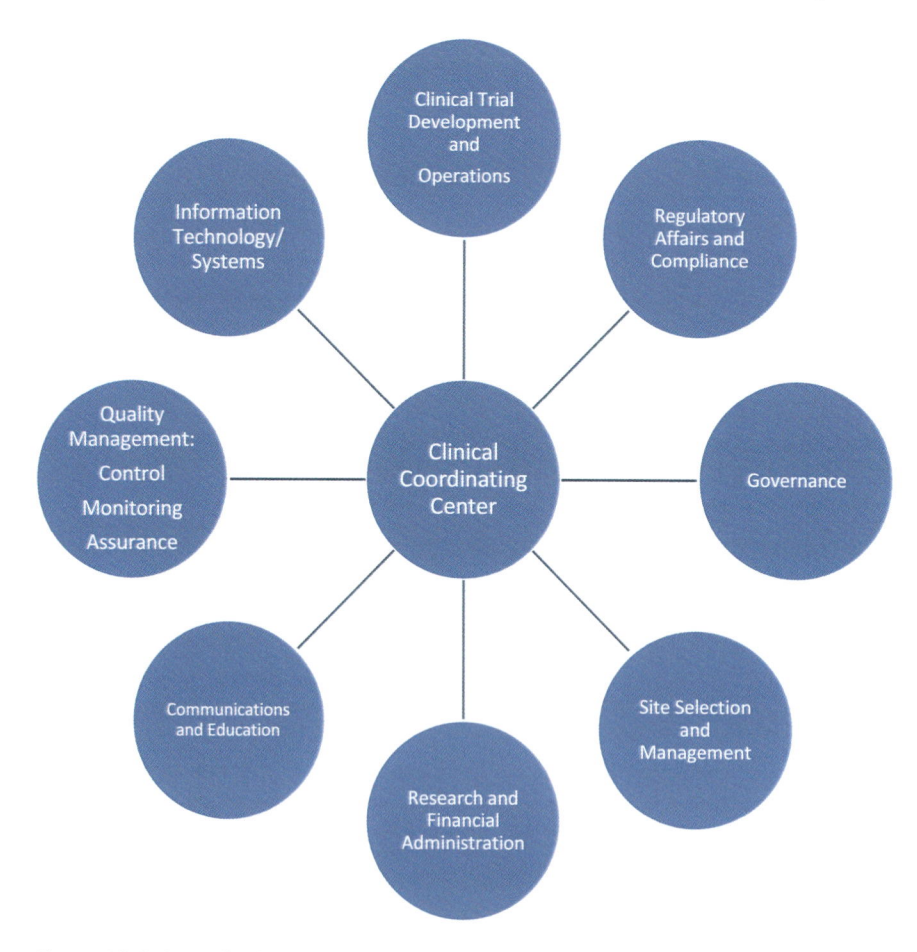

Fig. 2 Clinical coordinating center responsibilities

reporting to regulatory authorities, data and safety monitoring, centralized and remote monitoring, quality control and assurance, pharmacovigilance and safety reporting, regulatory affairs, communications, grants and contracts management, and financial and research administration. The purpose of the coordinating center is to enable and facilitate clinical research operations. A summary of the clinical coordinating center responsibilities is shown in Fig. 2.

Quality management processes, integrating both ongoing quality control and assurance mechanisms, protect against the risk of non-compliance with applicable regulations. Documented sponsor oversight, accountability, and inspection readiness are not optional. Clinical coordinating centers must strive for inspection readiness at all times. Clinical coordinating center management is responsible for ensuring regulatory compliance. They need to obtain sufficient resources for efficient clinical trial operations and implement risk and quality management policies and procedures.

Key Facts

1. Coordinating centers are responsible for clinical operations, site management, regulatory compliance, communications, administration, information systems, and quality management.
2. At the core of all clinical trial operations is the protection of human subjects and data integrity.
3. Selection of high-performing sites is important for successful trial initiation *and* completion.
4. Site management requires constant communication with participating sites.
5. Project management, planning, and execution ensure that trial timelines and milestones are met.
6. Quality management includes both quality control and quality assurance.
7. Risk-based monitoring and risk management processes aid in meeting GCP guidelines.
8. Inspection readiness must be ongoing and constant with documented sponsor oversight.
9. Clinical coordinating centers and data coordinating centers collectively manage clinical trials.
10. Coordinating centers of network groups coordinate a portfolio of clinical trials for a large site network.

Cross-References

▶ Good Clinical Practice
▶ Multicenter and Network Trials
▶ Selection of Study Centers and Investigators
▶ Trial Organization and Governance

References

FDA Site Investigational New Drug Application Resources. Available online. Accessed 07 Sep 2020. https://www.fda.gov/drugs/types-applications/investigational-new-drug-ind-application

E6(R2) Good Clinical Practice: Integrated Addendum to ICH E6(R1). Available online. Accessed 07 Sep 2020. https://www.fda.gov/regulatory-information/search-fda-guidance-documents/e6r2-good-clinical-practice-integrated-addendum-ich-e6r1

Food and Drug Administration (2017) Compliance Program 7348.810 Bioresearch Monitoring, Sponsors, Contract Research Organizations and Monitors. Available online. Accessed 07 SEP 2020. https://www.fda.gov/inspections-compliance-enforcement-and-criminal-investigations/fda-bioresearch-monitoring-information/compliance-program-7348810-bioresearch-monitoring

Dana Farber/Harvard Cancer Center, Investigator-Sponsored Multi-center Clinical Trials. Available online. Accessed 07 Sep 2020. https://www.dfhcc.harvard.edu/research/clinical-research-support/office-of-data-quality/services-support/dfhcc-multi-center-trials/

NHLBI Funding Opportunity, PAR-19-329, Clinical Coordinating Center for Multi-Site Investigator – Initiated Clinical Trials. Available online. Accessed 07 Sep 2020. https://grants.nih.gov/grants/guide/pa-files/par-19-329.html

TransCelerate Risk-Assessment and Categorization Tool. Available online. Accessed 07 Sep 2020. https://www.transceleratebiopharmainc.com/initiatives/risk-based-monitoring/

Efficient Management of a Publicly Funded Cancer Clinical Trials Portfolio

33

Catherine Tangen and Michael LeBlanc

Contents

C. Tangen (✉) · M. LeBlanc
SWOG Statistical Center, Fred Hutchinson Cancer Research Center, Seattle, WA, USA
e-mail: ctangen@fredhutch.org; mleblanc@fredhutch.org

© Springer Nature Switzerland AG 2022
S. Piantadosi, C. L. Meinert (eds.), *Principles and Practice of Clinical Trials*,
https://doi.org/10.1007/978-3-319-52636-2_61

Abstract

The implementation, management, and reporting of any single well-designed cancer clinical trial is an extremely complex and expensive undertaking. However, within our group, there is the opportunity to simultaneously design, implement, monitor, and analyze up to approximately 100 publicly funded clinical trials across the development spectrum. Operationally, we aggressively seek to optimize and standardize processes and software that are common across studies, increase efficiency, and focus on the quality and reliability of study results. Implementing novel software applications increases the quality and efficiency of data evaluation, monitoring, and statistical analysis across multiple disease and study types. Conventions and cross-study tools are the key to quality monitoring and analysis of complex portfolio of studies. A strategy of fully utilizing the commonalities across the trials leads to better quality results of any given study in the portfolio as well as more efficient utilization of public funds to conduct the studies.

In this chapter the structure and processes are described in the context of SWOG Cancer Research Network, one of the four National Clinical Trial Network (NCTN) adult cancer clinical trial groups funded by the US National Institutes of Health (NIH) under a cooperative agreement with the US National Cancer Institute (NCI).

Keywords

Clinical trial · Cancer · Statistics · Portfolio · Data management · Protocol development · Statistical design · Translational medicine · Software · Data safety monitoring committee · Database

Introduction: SWOG Statistics and Data Management Within the NCTN

The mission of the SWOG Cancer Research Network, as a partner in the NCTN (see references for website link), is to significantly improve lives through cancer clinical trials and translational research. The SWOG Network Operations Center, which includes the office of the Group Chair, the contracts and legal team, and communications, is located in Portland, Oregon, and the SWOG Operations Center which oversees protocol development and audit functions is located in San Antonio, Texas. We will focus on trial portfolio strategies at the SWOG Statistics and Data Management Center (Statistical Center) located in Seattle, WA, where all trial and ancillary study data reside. The Statistical Center is led by the Director, referred to as the Group Statistician. There are currently 12 statistical faculty who receive some fraction of funding from SWOG. The faculty typically have other non-SWOG research interests and receive additional funding from other grant activities outside of SWOG. An additional 15 SRAs (MS degree statisticians) and 2 additional Statistical Unit Assistants (BS degree statisticians), who are fully funded by SWOG activities, round out the statistical team. The goal of the Statistical Center is to provide leadership in the statistical design and data management of oncology clinical trials for SWOG and to safely and efficiently monitor and report on clinical investigations over a portfolio of clinical trials. Critically, the Group must analyze the clinical outcomes in a consistent and reproducible way. The portfolio of managed trials includes both trials to evaluate new cancer treatments (both single and multi-arm Phase II and randomized Phase II, Phase II/III, and Phase III trials) and other studies involving cancer prevention, supportive care and symptom management, palliative care, as well as trials of comparative effectiveness of treatments. These nontreatment studies include both randomized and cohort studies and are conducted in collaboration with the NCI Community Oncology Research Program (NCORP) program (see references for website link).

The SWOG Statistical Center designs, implements, and manages their trial portfolio through (A) the SWOG disease committee structure, interactions, and protocol development; (B) use of expert teams, strategic meetings, and standardized policies; (C) use of standardized data collection, coding, and a comprehensive portfolio database; (D) development of in-house tools for design, monitoring, and analysis of clinical trials; (E) utilization of a portfolio-wide Data and Safety Monitoring Committee; and (F) standardization of our interactions with outside groups including biospecimen and data sharing. Expanded descriptions follow.

Disease Committee Structure, Interactions, and Study Development

Disease Committee Structure Within the Statistical Center

The Statistical Center structure, and the primary work of SWOG, is accomplished through anatomic disease committees. Each committee is assigned at least one Ph.D. statistician (faculty), one or more master's level statistician(s) referred to as Statistical Research Associates (SRA), and one or more data coordinator(s) who work as part of a larger team with the clinical and translational medicine members of the disease committee. Within the Statistical Center, these committees function under the direction of the faculty statistician(s), with priorities set in consultation with the respective clinical disease committee chair and the Group Statistician.

During study development, statisticians work with the study chair to develop the trial design and help lead the protocol through the SWOG and NCI approval processes and protocol implementation. Assessments of feasibility, experimental design, sample size, randomization schemes, data analysis plans, and key elements of data collection are further refined by the statisticians and the study team during the development process. Statisticians and the protocol coordinators work with the study chair to launch the proposed trial. Several statisticians have responsibilities and methodological skills that address general needs across diseases, which facilitates standardization within the Statistical Center (see the "Using Expert Cross-Disease Teams (Cores), Strategic Meetings, and Standardized Policies" section).

Communications Within and Between the Statistical Center

Communications are critical for integrating the work of the statisticians with data management staff. Important in-person meetings at the Statistical Center include chief meetings with senior faculty, senior SRA, and data management and applications development management. Chief meetings are used to set priorities within the Statistical Center and to discuss how to respond to new initiatives, regulatory changes, and other challenges. Other important meetings that primarily include Statistical Center faculty and staff are twice-monthly meeting of all Statistical Center statisticians to discuss policy issues, programming and software needs, standards and guidelines, and statistical issues. One of these twice-monthly meetings includes a statistical analysis or methodology presentation and discussion. There is a monthly meeting of the SRAs, where they discuss study implementation issues, evaluate workloads and priorities, and share ideas. This also serves as a forum for continued training. Monthly disease committee meetings are led by a faculty statistician with attendance by the respective disease committee statisticians and data coordinators. This meeting serves to set analysis and data evaluation priorities, to summarize accrual and adverse event issues, and to discuss any concerns for ongoing trials. In addition, electronic case report form (CRF) development ideas, design concerns, study structure setup in the database, and evaluation requirements are discussed for studies in development. There is also a weekly statistical capsule review meeting and protocol review meeting. These meetings are concept- or protocol-specific (see Protocol Development below for more details). Finally, the biannual Statistical Center all-staff meeting is a format to showcase scientific accomplishments over the past 6 months, to introduce new staff, and to discuss performance goals for the upcoming 6 months.

Strong links exist between the Operations Center and the Statistical Center. Importantly, the Group Statistician and Group Chair have a scheduled weekly one-on-one teleconference, and they are in almost daily email contact to promote the efficient scientific and administrative functioning of SWOG. Senior statistical faculty also have close contact with the Director of Operations, who works with the Group Chair to oversee and direct the operational and administrative activities of SWOG in support of its scientific missions.

Statistical and other data-related issues are fundamental to any new study's approval. The Group Statistician and Statistical Center Deputy Director are members of the SWOG Executive Committee ("triage"), along with the Group Chair, executive officers, Director of Operations, and Director of Protocols. The statistical design review by the Group Statistician and Deputy Director at this meeting is an integral component of each study evaluation. The committee meets weekly and reviews capsules for scientific soundness, feasibility, appropriateness to SWOG's mission, priorities, and resources. Approved studies are assigned a SWOG study number and sent for approval at the NCI prior to protocol development. Concepts often need to go through several reviews prior to approval by triage. This senior level of review provides strong scientific feedback and consistency and typically results in a high rate of approval at the NCI.

Protocol Development Process

As described in the Disease Committee section above ("Disease Committee Structure, Interactions, and Study Development"), for new studies there are initial conferences with the committee statistician to discuss appropriate study design options, eligibility criteria, endpoints, accrual estimates (and hence feasibility), preliminary statistical plans, and proposed sample sizes. In addition, preliminary discussions of eligibility, translational medicine questions, and details of treatment are also considered at this time.

As the first review step in our protocol development process, the short study proposal (capsule) is discussed at an internal statistical review meeting at the Statistical Center to assess the proposed study design and analysis plans. At this meeting, translational medicine, patient-reported outcome concepts, and trial design are discussed. This review is performed by the Group Statistician and Deputy Director, a designated rotating faculty statistician, and the SRAs, who are usually divided into two teams to share the workload. Once a capsule has been reviewed, it goes on to Triage review by the SWOG Executive Committee (Fig. 1).

During protocol development there is a high level of interaction among the study's scientific study leadership, statisticians, data management staff, and application development (Rave) staff. After trial activation, interactions rest more strongly on statistics and data management staff. External involvement with the protocol coordinator is very high during protocol development and diminishes but still carries on through management as amendments and other protocol issues arise.

Reengineering Protocol Implementation and Development (RaPID) Review: Once there is a working version of the protocol, an in-person meeting (typically for Phase III trials) or an extended conference call (for Phase II trials) is scheduled to carefully review all sections of the protocol; this is known as the RaPID review meeting. This meeting includes the study chair(s), the protocol coordinator, Director of Protocols, Statistical Center statisticians, and data coordinators from the respective disease committee. In a subsequent conference call with the study statisticians and study chairs, data elements to be captured on the study case report forms are finalized. This is the first step in the study build process. Having all study personnel focused together for 4–5 h on the protocol development is an extremely efficient way to identify and address key logistical and scientific issues for the trial, and it leads to faster finalization of the document.

Protocol Review Committee: After the RaPID meeting and an additional review for compliance to standards are conducted by the SWOG Operations Center, the protocol is submitted to the Protocol Review Committee (PRC) at the Statistical

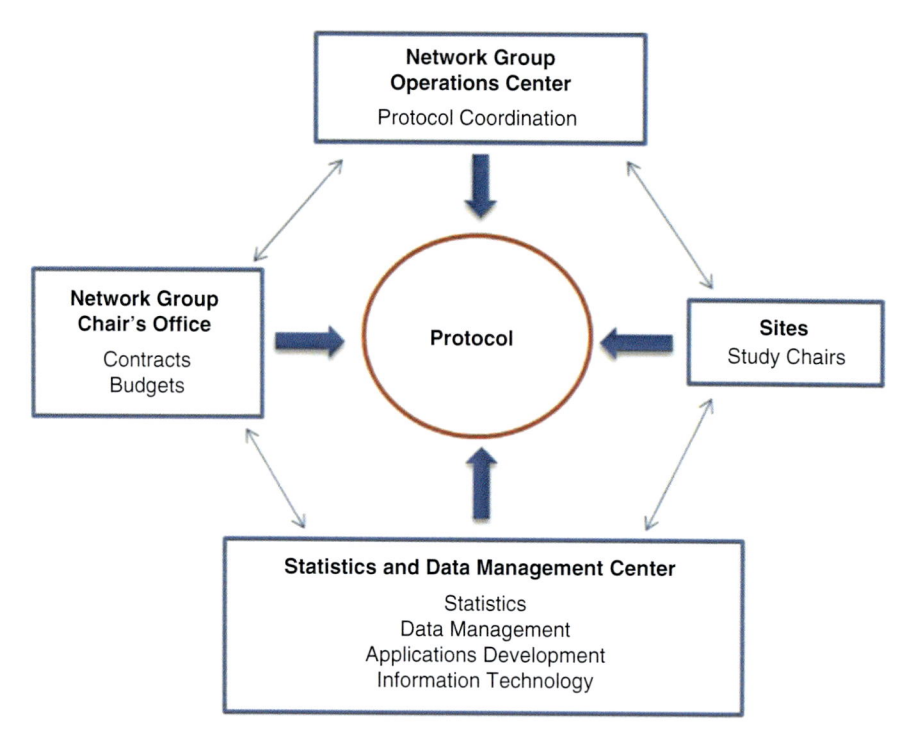

Fig. 1 Protocol standardized workflow

Center. The PRC meets weekly or as needed; committee members receive a copy of the protocol, draft data collection forms, and a copy of the NCI Protocol Submission Worksheet. This committee is chaired by one of the faculty statisticians and consists of at least one other faculty statistician, the Deputy Director, and 5–6 master's degree level statisticians, with the goal of having multiple independent reviewers for each study. The study team, the Director of Protocols, and the protocol coordinator from the SWOG Operations Center attend by teleconference. Study chairs are encouraged to participate and do so as their schedules permits.

The review provides critiques and recommendations to eliminate internal inconsistencies and provide clarification in the protocol document, especially for eligibility, data and specimen collection, and other implementation issues. Moreover, this review ensures consistency across studies and disease committees for our approach to the design and conduct of trials.

Using Expert Cross-Disease Teams (Cores), Strategic Meetings, and Standardized Policies

There are many commonalities among trials conducted across diseases within our group. Trials are becoming more complex due to the addition of extensive biospecimen collection and high dimensional lab assessments, the emerging importance of quality of life or other patient-reported outcomes (PROs), the intent for sponsoring companies pursue regulatory registration of their drug, and the wide variety of clinical trial designs that may be applicable for a given study. To avoid the need to develop this type of expertise within each disease committee and to bring the best processes, statistical methods and data collection strategies, expert teams, or "cores" have been developed that can be accessed by all committees when designing, conducting, and analyzing clinical trials. These cores include recruitment and retention, patient-reported outcomes, FDA application intent, clinical trial design, and translational medicine. These cores include members from both statistics and data management.

Recruitment and Retention Core

This group provides enhanced statistical input for accruing minority and medically underserved populations. We have a committed Statistical Center team of staff and faculty with expertise in these populations to support the activity of SWOG. The SWOG Statistical Center directly serves trial recruitment goals with a full-time staff expert (Recruitment and Retention Coordinator) for accrual-related issues on trials and a faculty statistician with research interests in design analysis of studies involving accrual and representativeness. The Recruitment and Retention Coordinator works closely with study leadership, study teams, and the SWOG Recruitment and Retention Committee to provide expertise and support in the development of study-specific recruitment and retention strategies and materials. This coordinator also participates in NCI working groups related to this mission.

Patient-Reported Outcomes (PRO) Core

This core team oversees the scientific review and conduct of PRO sub-studies for treatment trials. The PRO core administers the review process for new PRO proposals, including assessing scientific merit, feasibility, and resource allocation within the Symptom Control and Quality of Life Committee. For approved sub-studies, the PRO core provides the statistical design, monitoring, and analysis resources for the conduct of the PRO study, guided by a set of key design and analysis principles developed for PRO studies. The staff, funded primarily through NCORP, includes a faculty statistician, master's level statisticians, and PRO expert data coordinators.

FDA Application Core

The goal of this core team is to ensure efficiency in process and procedures for FDA registration trials across disease committees. This is accomplished by reviewing of case report forms with extended data requirements and validated data systems, including biomarker-driven treatment assignment. The team provides training with emphasis on regulations and additional documentation appropriate for study management at the Statistical Center and study sites. Core team members function as resources to ensure patient safety and data integrity checks across these trials. The team includes members from both statistics and data management, including senior statisticians, a CDISC expert, a SAS programmer, a statistician experienced with prior FDA submissions, and a senior data management consultant. Funding for activities in this core beyond NCI requirements and expectations comes from non-NIH sources.

Clinical Trial Methods Core and Translational Medicine Methods Core

These cores have been introduced with the goal of introducing new designs and analysis strategies, enhancing consistency across disease committees, and providing a sounding board for ideas. Members of these groups include SWOG statistical faculty as well as non-SWOG faculty who may not be directly supported by our grants but who have methodological interests in clinical trials or translational medicine. A goal of the cores is to assess solutions for trial design and TM analyses that may be appropriate across committees. Each core identifies and facilitates short topics of discussion and relevant journal papers for the broader group to review during statistics meetings, thereby aiding the dissemination of new approaches and methods. These cores are also responsible for maintaining guideline documentation for best practices within SWOG. These cores ensure that state-of-the-art solutions are used and help identify new statistical methodologies that are needed for the best conduct of clinical trial activities.

Data science skills are supplemented by leveraging unique expertise located outside of the Statistical Center but within the parent institution. These individuals are included as necessary for special projects and funding flows from appropriate grant sources for a finite amount of time to address special topics such as biomarker treatment designs, tumor heterogeneity, genomics, mobile data, computational linguistics, and natural language processing.

Rave® Study Build Core

Medidata Rave® is a configurable electronic data capture (EDC) system that includes data capture, management, and monitoring. Patient data received through Rave® are accessible by Clinical Research Associates (CRAs), data coordinators, study chairs, statisticians, monitors, and auditors, with appropriate permission controls for access in place. The Rave® application facilitates a collaborative and uniform environment for data capture and review at multiple levels. For trials that are double-blinded, Rave® and all the systems and tools outlined in this section blind all users to treatment assignment to avoid any potential bias in the review of the patient's data. The Statistical Center has developed expertise in Rave® in the areas of custom functions, calendaring, case report form presentation, and edit checks, all of which help to personalize the user experience to the specific patient and study while at the same time providing consistent quality processes across studies. Our philosophy is to maximize data accuracy and to create case report forms that are easy to understand and personalized to the patient and that include comprehensive and informative edit checks. Our approach is consistently rigorous, whether the trial has FDA registration potential or not.

Training Opportunities

To ensure quality, consistency, and reliability in SWOG's numerous clinical trials, effective training is critical for all personnel involved in the design, conduct, and analysis of the studies. That includes data coordinators, statisticians, clinical research associates, and medical study leadership. The Statistical Center is actively involved in developing these training programs which cover topics such as protocol development, data monitoring, ethics, statistical design, and trial management for clinical investigators. This training takes place in person at our biannual group meetings and via web-based technology which tracks completion of courses.

Standardized Publication Policy

Authorship for SWOG also follows standards, including statistical representation. For primary results of the primary endpoint either in abstract or manuscript, SWOG policy dictates that the first/lead author is the study chair. The lead, contributing biostatistician is listed as second author followed by the study co-chairs involved in study management and evaluation as listed in the protocol. The policy also provides guidance on other types of publications and presentations

Standardized Data Collection, Coding, and a Comprehensive Portfolio Database

The first steps of quality and statistical standardization are derived from (1) development of protocols that are clearly stated and inclusive of all criteria and procedures and (2) data collection necessary to address the key objectives of the trial.

The SWOG data capture system has evolved over time starting with CRF-scanned data into the database via an optical character recognition system and then to an in-house EDC system which allowed users to enter and amend data from a web-based portal as well as upload source documentation. This was used until acquisition and implementation of Rave® mandated by the NCI in 2014 for all network trial groups. Medidata Rave® is a configurable EDC system that includes data capture, management, and monitoring.

Rave® has excellent features for single studies. However, to best utilize cross-portfolio strategies, dynamic integration of data across trials is chosen, and CRF data from Rave® is uploaded to the SWOG database. The variables are then mapped into standardized coding across studies. As described in the "Comprehensive Statistical Reporting Tool" section below, this allows for cross-study reporting, improved umbrella trial support, more extensive patient follow-up, and further exploratory analysis opportunities. A key feature of the SWOG Statistical Center study design processes is the mapping of data elements to a standard set of domains and codes, which facilitates efficient analysis. Where possible, many of the coding conventions are standardized across types and stages of cancer.

Unlike some other NCTN groups that leave their data stored at a remote, central location, the Statistical Center, in cooperation with Medidata, uses Rave® Web Services to create a process for downloading data from Rave® into the SWOG database on a nightly basis. An important advantage of our approach is that it allows for unified monitoring and reporting across SWOG coordinated studies. Having the data from Rave® CRFs stored in the SWOG database is critical to the Statistical Center data management and statistical analysis processes. It allows continued use of our suite of custom-built applications, such as patient evaluation tools, and the Statisticians' Report Worksheet (SRW, described in a later section) and other reports that are informed by data in the SWOG database. Having Rave® data in the SWOG database also allows us to combine both Rave® and clinical trials data collected on earlier pre-Rave® EDC for further analysis. This facilitates our ability to conduct SWOG database analyses that combine multiple SWOG trials over a long period of time.

Having an organization that manages a portfolio of trials also allows for a unified approach with respect to network security, information exchange security, access controls, and disaster recovery and contingency plans. The Statistical Center approaches data security and confidentiality with a focus on the confidentiality, integrity, and availability of data. Processes and procedures involving network services and data management applications are influenced by federal requirements for computer, network, and data security. Network security is based on best practices for electronic computing and networking and regulatory compliance. Security is addressed through a defense-in-depth approach. Multiple layers of defense are utilized to address potential security vulnerabilities. Policies and procedures for disaster recovery are modified as needed and reviewed annually. Outside professional consultation, review, and auditing provide additional feedback and result in updates to policies, procedures, and training as appropriate. All web application traffic is secured and protected from tampering or eavesdropping by use of industry standard cryptographic protocols. Operating system and database controls restrict inappropriate access privileges to data, files, and other objects that require protection from modification.

In-House Tools for Design, Study Monitoring, and Analysis of Clinical Trials

The Statistical Center is successful in creating custom software applications specifically designed for the needs of a group running a wide array of clinical studies. To maintain the necessary control of those applications, enhancements are applied as needed. These tools leverage the standardized data collection and comprehensive database structure previously described. Key tools to manage the SWOG portfolio are described below:

Comprehensive Statistical Reporting Tool

SWOG has conducted hundreds of clinical trials, making standardization of reports critical. However, working in a wide variety of cancer settings, being able to customize reports is necessary. To help achieve this balance, the Statistical Center uses a custom-built statistical analysis reporting software application. This trial platform-based reproducible research tool (Statisticians' Report Worksheet, SRW) epitomizes our statistical philosophy: While there is flexibility across diseases and studies, common coding conventions and cross-study tools are the key to quality monitoring and analysis of a portfolio of studies as numerous and complex as those in the NCTN. SRW is the primary tool used by statisticians across disease committees to construct standardized reports, tables, and graphs for all studies. SRW incorporates a web-based interface and the data from our SWOG database to create ready-to-print reports.

   SRW extracts data from the database to create SAS datasets, i.e., a "snapshot" of the patient data, and then automatically archives the resultant dataset. SRW outputs summaries in common formats such as Word, HTML, and PDF. SRW is used for reporting SWOG studies in the semiannual Report of Studies (ROS) and Data and Safety Monitoring Committee (DSMC) reports. This application is facilitated by having the Rave$^{®}$ data from every study directly incorporated into the SWOG database together with data from our pre-Rave$^{®}$ electronic data capture system as previously described. The SRW application uses standardized modules to compose study reports featuring standardized charts, tables, graphs, and descriptive information. Statisticians can customize the tables to adapt to their study requirements. Examples of customizable features are label definitions, table format information, and selected text such as objectives, patient population, accrual goals, and study summaries. The use of SRW provides a consistent approach to testing and verifying analysis code for commonly required analyses rather than having all analyses based on individual SAS programs. This standard for reproducible research (e.g., Gentleman and Temple Lang 2007; Iqbal et al. 2016) mechanism is feasible because the Statistical Center implements standardized coding choices of primary data elements including eligibility, treatment status, adverse events, and outcome, across disease committees. Our primary time-to-event outcomes are uniformly defined and

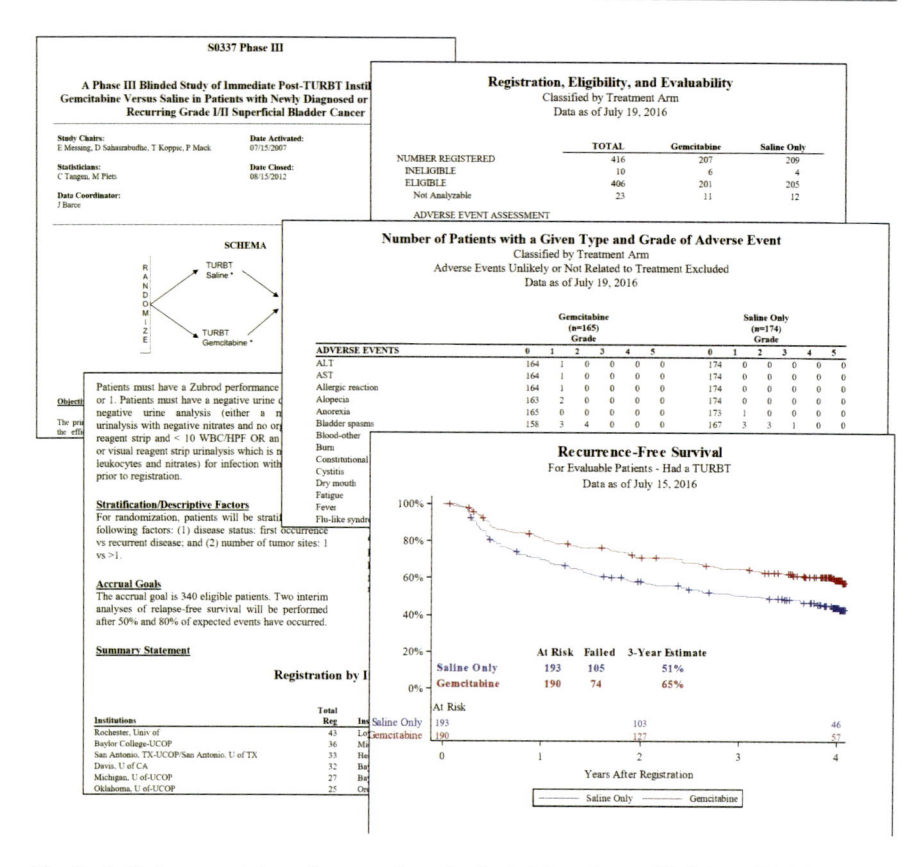

Fig. 2 A tiled representation of a report from the Statisticians Report Worksheet (SRW) program

named across studies. The reporting mechanism normalizes how Phase II and Phase III study data are presented but with study-specific flexibility with respect to tables. A collage representation of a study report is presented in Fig. 2.

Specimen Tracking Application

SWOG has developed a sophisticated system for tracking shipment of biological specimens from the point of collection to arrival at laboratories for analysis and/or to the specimen biorepository for banking for future use. All banked specimens have been consolidated in a single bank, the Nationwide Children's Hospital Biopathology Center in Columbus, Ohio. During the last 5 years, it tracked specimen submission for over 100 SWOG studies, representing approximately 59,000 submissions. The Specimen Tracking System is fully metadata-driven and generic enough for any study but allows for customization as needed. A new study can be set up in less than an hour.

For all SWOG studies, CRAs use the application to log specimens and indicate when those specimens are shipped to the appropriate biorepository or laboratory. Specimen-specific questions can be configured to gather information about the specimens for use by the laboratory processing the sample (e.g., when slides were cut, how long a sample was frozen). Laboratory staff use the application to indicate when those shipments are received and in what condition and to indicate if the specimens were aliquoted and/or shipped to another destination. Laboratory staff can also enter assay test results which are communicated in real time to CRAs at the institutions or the Statistical Center for eligibility, stratification, and/or treatment decisions.

Every patient registered to a SWOG study is assigned a pseudo patient ID that can be used when transmitting data to a laboratory. Only Statistical Center staff can link these pseudo patient IDs to the clinical data. Thus, a laboratory performing an assay with specimens received from the bank will not have treatment assignment or clinical outcome access when performing the assay. Prior to merging clinical data with lab data, the Statistical Center requires that the lab send us their data so that it can be stored in our database for future use.

Public Use Statistical Design Calculators

Every year, a large number of prospective clinical trial and translational medicine statistical design specifications must be evaluated in order to identify the optimal design. To facilitate this statistical development and encouraging standards across the portfolio, SWOG has designed a suite of trial power and sample size calculators. Clearly, efficient methods are needed to facilitate evaluation of the potential design and underlying model scenarios. While many sample size and power calculators are available for simple trial designs, continued development of improved tools for design and analyses involving multiple subgroups and complex trial monitoring are needed. Re-implementation and expansion of existing tools to be mobile accessible are ongoing to move them to a cloud-based setting using OpenCPU, a system for embedded scientific computing and reproducible research (Ooms 2014). Integration of both JavaScript-based and R-based calculations can be accomplished while retaining a common look and feel in the mobile environment. As an example, Fig. 3 shows a statistical calculator that provides an interaction test for a predictive marker and randomized treatment assignment in terms of survival outcome data. While each type of calculator requires different input parameters, there is a relatively standard presentation of input and output parameters across the set of power and sample-size calculators.

Automatic Monthly Study Reports

The comprehensive SWOG database also facilitates the generation of ongoing study monitoring data summaries which are reviewed by statisticians, data coordinators,

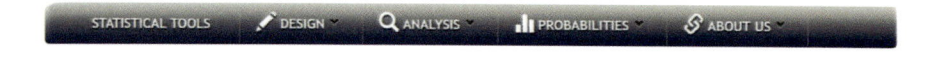

Survival Interaction

Interaction Survival is a program to calculate either estimates of sample size or power for tests of interaction. Exponential distributions are assumed and are specified as a ratio of the hazard ratio for the treatment effect in stratum 1 to the hazard ratio for the treatment effect in stratum 2. The program allows for unequal sample size allocation in the four cells defined by the two treatment groups and two strata. An exponentially distributed competing risk is also permitted.

User Input	Program Output

• Sample size ○ Power	• 1 Sided ○ 2 Sided	Alpha .05
Accrual	Follow	Comp Risk 0.00

Cell Freq Treat1/Strat1 .25	Cell Freq Treat1/Strat2 .25	Hazard Rate Treat1/Strat1	Hazard Rate Treat1/Strat2
Cell Freq Treat2/Strat1 .25	Cell Freq Treat2/Strat2 .25	Haz Ratio T1/T2 Strat1	Haz Ratio T1/T2 Strat2

Power .90	Sample size

Calculate

Fig. 3 An example of one of the web-based calculators used in the design of clinical and translation medicine studies for SWOG. Each calculator uses standard coloring for input and output parameters and includes a linked help file

and in some cases study chairs. For instance, summary reports of adverse events, SAE, and treatment data are generated monthly and emailed to study team members for careful monitoring of trial data.

Site Performance Metrics Reports

SWOG Institutional Performance Report (IPR) measures the timeliness of data and specimen submission across all SWOG studies. Additional metrics are in development including assessment of responsiveness to queries, serious adverse event (SAE) reporting timeliness, patient eligibility rates, and specimen quality indicators. Site principal investigators and their staff as well as SWOG leadership receive these reports on a regular basis, monitor progress of concerning sites, and provide intervention and support as appropriate and disciplinary action as a last resort.

Portfolio-Wide Data Safety Monitoring Committee

General Structure

A single Data Safety Monitoring Committee (DSMC) monitors all SWOG-coordinated Phase III and randomized Phase II clinical trials. Occasionally, single-arm trials are also monitored by the DSMC. For very large prevention trials, a separate DSMC is formed where some members are chosen due to their expertise outside of cancer. Typically, there are approximately 30 trials that are being monitored at any given time, representing diverse cancers, stages, and treatment modalities. There are numerous benefits of having one DSMC for all trials. There is consistency in communication and decision-making and a greater efficiency to reviewing all the trials at the same time. There is also an understanding of the National Cancer Trial Network (NCTN) structure, as well as trust and respect among members with diverse expertise who become quite familiar with each other. However, to lessen the review burden by the members, it is important to standardize reports so that the look and feel is similar across trials to aid in the scientific review.

The membership of the DSMC follows the National Cancer Institute (NCI) DSMC policy. The SWOG DSMC policy can be found on the public side of the SWOG website (SWOG.org) under policies and procedures. Members are appointed for 3-year terms (renewable once). The committee includes physicians and statisticians from within and outside SWOG who are selected based on their experience, reputation for objectivity, absence of conflicts of interest, and knowledge of good clinical trial methodology. The committee includes a patient advocate and a voting statistician from outside SWOG. Three nonvoting members of the DSMC come from the NCI – two physicians and an NCI statistician. The SWOG Group Statistician is also a non-voting member of the DSMC. The majority of voting DSMC members are not affiliated with SWOG, and voting quorums for a DSMC meeting require that the majority of voting members do not belong to SWOG.

The primary responsibility of the DSMC is to review interim analyses of outcome data (prepared by the study statistician) and to recommend whether the study needs to be changed or terminated based on these analyses. The committee also determines whether and to whom confidential outcome results should be released for planning purposes prior to the public reporting of study results. The DSMC reviews reports of related external studies as needed to evaluate whether a SWOG study needs to be changed or terminated or if communication is needed with participating patients. The DSMC reviews interim toxicity data, although that is primarily the responsibility of the study committee on a more ongoing basis. The DSMC reviews major modifications to the study proposed by the study committee prior to their implementation (e.g., termination, dropping an arm based on toxicity results or other trials reported, increasing or decreasing target sample size or duration). The DSMC meets twice yearly at a minimum. Each year, one meeting is held face-to-face in conjunction with the SWOG meeting, and the other biannual meeting is conducted as a conference call at the SWOG meeting. There are attendance requirements.

Standard Report Formatting

Standardized reporting of DSMC reports and communications are critical to efficiently oversee so many different trials. As previously described, SWOG follows common statistical principles in terms of interim monitoring for both futility and efficacy, so the specifications and reporting in the DSMC reports have a similar presentation across studies. Every 6 months the status of each trial being monitored is developed into a report by the study statistician, and each study report is reviewed by the Group Statistician and Deputy Director for accuracy and consistency. Each report contains two parts, a cover letter and the study report generated by SRW. The cover letter provides an overview of the study including current accrual status, any notable issues related to safety or feasibility, concerns about design assumptions, or external information. A table showing the number of planned interim analyses and their expected schedule is included. Although each trial has its own unique features, the table structure looks similar to the following (Table 1).

Also included in the cover memo are results of any conducted interim analysis and interpretation with respect to prespecified statistical boundaries. In the memo, the DSMC is also reminded when prior interim analyses were conducted and when the next analysis is projected to occur and any prior permissions the DSMC has allowed for the trial. The overall format of these memos is kept similar across studies, so the DSMC members know where to look to find specific pieces of information.

The second part of the DSMC report is prepared using our Statisticians' Report Worksheet (SRW), a tool that was described previously. Each report has a similar look and feel. The face sheet includes information about study title, study phase, activation date and date of accrual closure if applicable, study leaders, and a schema of the study design. Following that header, there is text about primary and secondary objectives, the eligible study population, accrual goals, and a summary of the ineligibility, toxicity assessment and most frequent or severe adverse events, major treatment deviations, and other notable aspects of the trial. Standardized tables about accrual, eligibility, patient characteristics, treatment status, and detailed adverse events are also included. Response rates and time to event data are included as appropriate for formal interim analyses.

A compiled notebook of all the reports is carefully reviewed by the Group Statistician and Deputy Director of the Statistical Center before it is finalized. The DSMC receives the notebook at least 3 weeks prior to the biannual DSMC meeting along with a suggested draft agenda for the meeting. The DSMC members are invited to add to the agenda as they see fit. The study chair may also prepare a report for the DSMC addressing specific toxicity concerns or other concerns about the conduct of the study. However, the study chair does not have access to the DSMC study report prepared by the statistician. The statistician's report may contain recommendations on whether to close the study, whether to report the results, whether the design assumptions should be adjusted, whether to continue accrual or follow-up, and/or whether a DSMC discussion is needed. Unless a DSMC discussion is requested by a DSMC member, the study report is accepted without discussion.

Table 1 Example interim analysis table provided to DSMC for an ongoing monitored trial. Phase III two-armed trial testing superiority of an experimental agent

Interim analysis	Expected time since start of trial	# of expected events		% of expected death information	Interim testing	
		Standard arm	Experimental arm (assuming Ha: HR = 0.75)		Superiority one-sided α (Ho: HR = 1.0)	Futility one-sided α (Ho: HR = 0.75)
1	3.2 years	107	88	38%	N/A	0.01
2	4 years	190	158	67%	0.005	0.01
3	5 years	246	207	86%	0.005	0.01
Final	5.75 years	283	240	100%	0.022	N/A

The DSMC meeting includes three parts. The first part is an open session in which members of the study team and respective disease committee leadership may be invited by the DSMC to answer questions or present their requests. Following the open session, there is a closed session limited to DSMC members and possibly the study statistician in which outcome results will be presented either by a member of the DSMC, the designated SWOG Statistician, or the study statistician. A fully closed executive session follows in which the DSMC discusses outcome results and then votes. At the fully closed executive session, those present are limited to DSMC members.

The DSMC provides written recommendations to the SWOG Group Chair. If he agrees, he will forward the DSMC recommendations to the National Cancer Institute for their evaluation. Details of this process of communication and required actions are covered in our DSMC policy.

Individuals invited to serve on the DSMC (voting and nonvoting) disclose to the Group Chair any potential, real, or perceived conflicts of interest. The Statistical Center representative to the DSMC is also a member of SWOG's Conflict Management Committee, serving as a liaison between the two committees.

General Interim Analysis Strategies

While there is some study flexibility, the SWOG Statistical Center sets standards with respect to interim analysis strategies. Stopping rules are based on group sequential designs to preserve overall error rates but allow for early stopping if extreme results are observed. In addition to the specification of Type I and Type II errors, a typical design for a Phase III study would call for the specification of a small number of interim analyses, between two and five, with a small probability of concluding that treatment is efficacious under the null hypothesis. The timing of interim analyses is based on overall information or event calculation for time-to-event studies. SWOG statisticians also typically define a one-sided test of "futility" using a similar early stopping rule based on testing the alternative hypothesis, rather than performing a test based on conditional power. For many studies, critical p-values are chosen for interim stopping at a small number of conservative early assessments that test the alternative hypothesis (e.g., Green et al. 2016; Fleming et al. 1984). Some plans also include an assessment at 50% information time and stop if an estimated hazard ratio is not favoring the experimental treatment. This guideline is easy to describe and can be less conservative than testing the alternative hypothesis. With respect to a time scale of interim analyses, a study by Freidlin et al. (2016) is supported using combined-arm event information in most instances. However, there is flexibility depending on the specific trial features. Regardless of the interim analysis strategy, the design properties such as power, Type 1 error, and stopping probabilities must be assessed and presented in the statistical section of the protocol.

Most Phase III trials involve two treatment arms. Trials with more than two arms or biomarker-based subgroups are fully addressed in the interim analysis plans. To facilitate interpretation by the SWOG DSMC, the report includes a table of estimates/p-values and actions defined by the statistical analysis plan in the protocol.

Statistical Center External Interactions

SWOG's Statistical Center staff need to effectively interact with external entities to carry out their clinical trial mission. Interested investigators approach SWOG to access biospecimens, trial data, or both. Standard, transparent processes need to be in place to handle and evaluate these queries.

Data Sharing

There are two paths for obtaining trial data from the group's studies: through the NCTN/NCORP Data Archive and by direct application to SWOG to request data. The Statistical Center follows established procedures for archiving SWOG data with the official NCTN/NCORP Data Archive. Data from qualifying studies must be archived at the NCI within 6 months of publication. Qualifying datasets include data from recently reported Phase III trials. The scope of required data sharing has also increased to include data used in many secondary analyses of NCTN and NCORP trial data. Standard operating procedures (SOPs) are developed at the Statistical Center to document detailed steps of the processes. A statistician creates the files required to be archived with the NCI that are sufficient to reproduce all results reported in the primary manuscript. The Statistical Center administrator assists with creating the data dictionary and reviews the datasets to ensure compliance with the guidelines. For trial data that are not stored in the NCTN/NCORP Data Archive, a second path is used to obtain data. Investigators submit a brief proposal to SWOG that includes some background for their proposed data analysis, objectives, statistical analysis methods to be used, and data elements requested. After evaluating for feasibility and ensuring no overlap with ongoing work, the SWOG Executive Committee approves the proposal, and a data usage agreement is executed between the investigator and SWOG. Requested data are then shared with the investigator. A pseudo-patient ID is used to link records. Data are shared in the preferred format of the investigator which typically involves Excel spreadsheets or SAS datasets.

Biospecimen Sharing

Requests for SWOG specimens are common and may arise from SWOG, other NCTN groups, or nonaffiliated investigators. For SWOG-led intergroup studies, the specimens are usually housed in the SWOG biorepository at Nationwide Children's Hospital. Appropriate permissions are required, usually from the NCI Correlative Sciences Steering Committee. Once a material usage agreement (MUA) and data usage agreement (DUA) (if applicable) are executed and communicated to the biobank and Statistical Center, statisticians use our linked biospecimen inventory at the Statistical Center to produce pull lists that have the proper required consent for the translational study, which is then communicated to the biorepository. With the introduction of the NCI Navigator system, there will be increased opportunities and effort for Statistical Center statisticians to both support assessing the feasibility of proposed translational medicine studies and, where appropriate, collaborate on the design and analysis of the resulting studies.

Most trial specimens can be requested via a new resource recently launched by the NCI: NCTN Navigator. Cancer researchers interested in conducting studies using biological specimens and clinical data collected from cancer treatment trials in the NCTN can use this resource. It includes information about specimens, such as tumor and blood samples, donated by patients in NCI-sponsored clinical trials. The clinical trials included in Navigator are published Phase III studies that evaluated cancer treatments. Investigators can use the NCTN Navigator website to search the inventory for specimens with specific characteristics. Investigators who develop proposals and get approval can use the specimens, along with the trial participants' clinical information, in their research. SWOG has a full specimen inventory database from our unified biobank at Nationwide Children's Hospital. Specimen data are linked to SWOG clinical trial data elements to enable efficient overall specimen data management. This simplifies specimen utilization for patients meeting various clinical criteria as well as the creation of reports or datasets that combine data from the clinical and biorepository databases. It also enhances the efficiency of interactions with the NCI Navigator system. Our enhanced database includes coding for projects for which specimens are requested and indicates the disbursement of specimens, project completion, and the return of unused specimens to the SWOG biorepository.

Summary and Conclusion

Our approach to designing, monitoring, and analyzing of a diverse portfolio of trials is to use standardized processes and software tools. In addition to the software tools and reports described, a set of NCI/NCTN tools are used which work across the NCTN groups and then employ standardized software applications to increase the quality and efficiency of study implementation, data evaluation, monitoring, and reporting across SWOG's portfolio of clinical trials. The structure of the SWOG comprehensive database of clinical and biorepository inventory enhances our efficiencies. In addition, it facilitates data sharing and the use of archived biospecimens by outside researchers. Recognizing the specifics of software and procedures for efficient trial portfolio management in the NCTN setting may not directly be applicable to single institutions or organizations external to the NCI; the goal of standardization of the trial design, protocol development, standardized trial data elements, and expert teams to support the group are good practices for most groups overseeing multiple simultaneously running clinical trials.

Key Facts

To provide statistical design and data management and efficiently monitor and report over a portfolio of clinical trials, communications need to be facilitated between statisticians and data management staff including regularly scheduled meetings between senior faculty, senior statistical research associates, data management, and applications development management.

A standardized, multidisciplinary process for development and review of commonly structured protocols results in clear, scientifically sound documents that result in quality and efficiency in the conduct of our trials and provide enrolling sites with a format in which they are familiar.

Portfolio-wide processes are developed to avoid the need to develop expertise (e.g., recruitment and retention, patient-reported outcomes, FDA application intent, trial design, study build, translational medicine) within each disease committee. We form expert teams (or cores) that can be accessed by all committees when designing, conducting, and analyzing clinical trials.

A key feature of our study design processes is the mapping of data elements to a standard set of domains and codes, which facilitates efficient analysis and enables our ability to conduct analyses that combine multiple trials over a long period of time.

Creation of custom software applications helps to address the needs of a group running a wide array of clinical trials. Because of standardized data collection and a comprehensive database structure, applications such as a standardized yet flexible statistical report writing tool, a specimen tracking system, and site performance metrics reports can be developed.

Having an organization that manages a portfolio of trials allows for a unified approach with respect to network security, information exchange security, confidentiality, access controls, and disaster recovery and contingency plans. Additionally, cross-portfolio training can be applied to address common features and issues, recognizing that study-specific training also is necessary. A portfolio-wide Data Safety Monitoring Committee can also be utilized.

Standard, transparent processes need to be in place to handle and evaluate queries from external entities wishing to access biospecimens, trial data, or both.

References

Fleming TR, Harrington DP, O'Brien PC (1984) Designs for group sequential tests. Control Clin Trials 5(4):348–361

Freidlin B, Othus M, Korn EL (2016) Information time scales for interim analyses of randomized clinical trials. Clin Trials 13(4):391–399. https://doi.org/10.1177/1740774516644752. PMID 27136947

Gentleman R, Temple Lang D (2007) Statistical analyses and reproducible research. J Comput Graph Stat 16:1–23. https://doi.org/10.1198/106186007X178663

Green S, Benedetti J, Smith A, Crowley J (2016) Clinical trials in oncology, 3rd edn. CRC Press, Boca Raton

Iqbal SA, Wallach JD, Khoury MJ, Schully SD, Ioannidis J (2016) Reproducible research practices and transparency across the biomedical literature. PLoS Biol 14(1):e1002333. https://doi.org/10.1371/journal.pbio.1002333. PMID: 26726926. PMCID: PMC4699702

NCI Community Oncology Research Program (NCORP). www.cancer.gov/research/areas/clinical-trials/ncorp

NCI's National Clinical Trials Network (NCTN). www.cancer.gov/research/areas/clinical-trials/nctn

Ooms J (2014) The OpenCPU system: towards a universal interface for scientific computing through separation of concerns. https://arxiv.org/abs/1406.4806

Archiving Records and Materials

34

Winifred Werther and Curtis L. Meinert

Contents

W. Werther (✉)
Center for Observational Research, Amgen Inc, South San Francisco, CA, USA
e-mail: wwerther@amgen.com

C. L. Meinert
Department of Epidemiology, School of Public Health, Johns Hopkins University, Baltimore, MD, USA
e-mail: cmeiner1@jhu.edu

Abstract

An archive, in the context of a trial, is a collection of documents and records relevant to the design and conduct of the trial maintained as a historical repository. Archiving is a process that starts before the first person is enrolled and continues to the end of the trial when all analyses are complete and the investigator group disbands.

So, when a trial is finished, money has run out, and investigators have dispersed, what do you have archived and where? The answer to the first question is "everything you may need later," and the answer to the second is "someplace readily accessible far into the foreseeable future." Both answers are correct but not helpful because the first question requires a crystal ball of what might be needed and the second requires a place like the Smithsonian and there are no Smithsonians for archiving records of clinical trials.

This chapter is about the process of archiving and about what to archive.

Keywords

Trial master file · Archiving · Electronic

Introduction

An archive is a place where records or historical materials are stored and preserved. The place may be a physical location, like the National Archives where records can be accessed and viewed, or an electronic address serving the same purpose, the latter usually the case for clinical trials. The International Council for Harmonisation (ICH) good clinical practice (GCP) guidelines are foundational for guidelines on archiving. These guidelines are as set forth by the European Medicines Agency (EMA 2018).

But even if there were no legal requirements for documentation and archiving, investigators would document on their own. They need documentation should they need to retrace steps or check on what they did. They need documentation if questions arise from outside the trial regarding what they did or how they did it.

Archiving can be a safeguard for questions that might occur during and after conduct of the trial. A few examples of questions follow. First, investigators in VIGOR (Vioxx Gastrointestinal Outcomes Research) published their results in November 2000 in the NEJM (Bombardier et al. 2000). The NEJM expressions of concern regarding counts in VIGOR came 5 years later (Curfman et al. 2005, 2006). Second, troubles in the National Surgical Adjuvant Breast and Bowel Project (NSABP) came from falsified data in breast cancer trials (Crewdson 1994). Third, the University Group Diabetes Program (UGDP) was a randomized multicenter secondary prevention trial designed to test whether commonly used treatments for type 2 diabetes were useful in delaying the cardiovascular and neurological sequelae of the disease (UGDP 1970a). The trial started in 1960 and finished in 1978. About mid-way through investigators stopped the use of one of the treatments, tolbutamide (an oral drug widely regarded as safe and effective in the diabetic community), because there were concerns regarding safety (UGDP 1970b). The decision brought an avalanche of criticisms from diabetologists and ultimately led to a review of the trial by a special committee commissioned by the International Biometric Society. The committee met several times from 1972 thru 1974 and published its report in JAMA in 1975 (Gilbert et al. 1975). The first meeting of the committee was at the coordinating center for the trial in the fall of 1972. The first thing the committee wanted to see was a description of the randomization procedure used in the trial, written in 1960, before the trial started. The problem was that, somehow, after all those years in a dark filing cabinet, various sentences, "crystal clear" when written, had morphed into puzzling statements.

Lesson: Foundational documents, like the system for randomization, should be read and reviewed by multiple members of the investigational team before archiving. As exemplified in these historical examples of clinical trial archive use, investigators and sponsors can and should expect many different reasons for needing and using the archive for clinical trial activities.

Trial Master File (TMF)

The TMF, broadly, is a collection of documents and files created over the course of a trial that enables sponsors, monitors, agencies, authorities, or persons to check and reconstruct what was done. The TMF is discussed in the European Medicines Agency Guideline on the content, management, and archiving of the clinical trial master file (paper and/or electronic) (EMA 2018). The TMF is often managed and maintained electronically and is referred to as the electronic TMF or eTMF.

The executive summary of the Guideline on the content, management, and archiving of the clinical trial master file provides an overview of the intention of the TMF and is quoted here:

Trial master file (TMF) plays a key role in the successful management of a trial by the investigator/institutions and sponsors. The essential documents and data records stored in the TMF enable the operational staff as well as monitors, auditors and inspectors to evaluate compliance with the protocol, the trial's safe conduct and the quality of the data obtained. This guideline is intended to assist the sponsors and investigators/institutions in complying with the requirements of the current legislation (Directive 2001/20/EC and Directive 2005/28/EC), as well as ICH E6 Good Clinical Practice (GCP) Guideline ('ICH GCP guideline'), regarding the structure, content, management and archiving of the clinical trial master file (TMF). The guidance also applies to the legal representatives and contract research organisation (CROs), which according to the ICH GCP guideline includes any third party such as vendors and service providers to the extent of their assumed sponsor trial-related duties and functions. The ICH GCP guideline provides information in relation to essential documents to be collected during the conduct of a clinical trial. The risk-based approach to quality management also has an impact on the content of the TMF. To ensure continued guidance once the Clinical Trials Regulation (EU) No. 536/2014 ('Regulation') comes into application, this guidance already prospectively considers the specific requirements of the Regulation with respect to the TMF.

The table of contents of the Guideline on the content, management, and archiving of the clinical trial master file is a good reference point when planning a TMF and is provided below:

1. Executive summary
2. Introduction
3. Trial master file structure and contents
    3.1. Sponsor and investigator trial master file
    3.2. Contract research organisations
    3.3. Third parties-contracted by investigator/institution
    3.4. Trial master file structure
    3.5. Trial master file contents
        3.5.1. Essential documents
        3.5.2. Superseded documents
        3.5.3. Correspondence
        3.5.4. Contemporariness of trial master file
4. Security and control of trial master file
    4.1. Access to trial master file
        4.1.1. Storage areas for trial master file
        4.1.2. Sponsor/CRO electronic trial master file
        4.1.3. Investigator electronic trial master file
    4.2. Quality of trial master file
5. Scanning or transfers to other media
    5.1. Certified copies
    5.2. Other copies
    5.3. Scanning or transfer to other media
    5.4. Validation of the digitisation and transfer process
    5.5. Destruction of original documents after digitisation and transfer
6. Archiving and retention of trial master file
    6.1. Archiving of sponsor trial master file
    6.2. Archiving of investigator/institution trial master file
    6.3. Retention times of trial master file
    6.4. Archiving, retention and change of ownership/responsibility
7. References

Prerequisites

The study team needs to document in real time for the TMF to be sufficient to allow people or authorities to reconstruct how the trial was conducted after it is finished. To accomplish this there must be understanding prior to starting the trial of what gets documented and by whom. Also, required are understandings as to where documents will be stored and whether in hard or electronic form. To accomplish timely archiving, the roles and responsibilities of the trial team will be defined by the coordinating center.

The quality and extent of documentation can be expected to vary by who funds the trial, its size, and location. Small single-center, investigator-initiated, trials may not be as well documented as multicenter international trials. Sponsors subject to oversight by regulatory agencies can be expected to be quite compulsive about maintaining the TMF. Indeed typically, in those cases, it will be the sponsor who maintains the majority of documenting either themselves or through a contract research organization (CRO).

Clearly, if there are two or more administrative parties in a trial who are responsible for archiving, then there must be agreement on division of labor as to who maintains the archive that produces archived copies of documents. Duplicate documents, produced by different parties, are not virtues when it comes to documentation because, invariably, they will differ.

Experience teaches that documenting is a not a favorite activity of trialists. More likely than not, investigators assume it will be done by "somebody else," and their eyes glaze when protocols and procedures for documentation are discussed at investigator meetings.

Key Study Documents

The study protocol, consent forms, and data collection forms are at the heart of the trial. All three should be open to the public, except for details that have the potential of biasing results, for example, details regarding masking and randomization schemes. The Investigator's Brochure is another key study document that is necessary when the clinical trial involves an investigational drug.

Study Protocol

The protocol is roughly akin to a blueprint for a building but far less detailed than blueprints. The protocol, unlike blueprints, allows room for clinical judgment. To facilitate inclusion of the proper details for the trial conduct, SPIRIT (Standard Protocol Items: Recommendations for Interventional Trials) is a published document with a 33-item list of information to be included in protocols (Chan et al. 2013).

Protocols should be open to the public. One way to accomplish this is by posting on registration sites, such as ClinicalTrials.gov. ClinicalTrials.gov has a field to include protocols, but it is only sparingly used: 5,721 postings out of 145,844 completed trials, 3.9% of completed trials, as of 3 April 2020 (US NLM 2020).

Publishing protocols as standalone manuscripts in a clinical trial journal is one way to make them public, but perhaps the best way is as supplemental material in results publications, but even if done for every results publication the practice would cover only a fraction of trials since the majority of trials are never published. A stumbling block in publicizing protocols is the desires of proprietary sponsors to keep competitors from knowing what they are doing. Posting protocols may give away business secrets.

The reality is that protocols are subject to change over the course of a trial through the documentation of protocol amendments. The study archive postings need to be updated if they are to retain their informative value. Some of the changes may be minor, but some can be substantive changes to enrollment criteria, changes in dosages schedules, or addition or deletion of treatments in the trial.

The study protocol and all subsequent amendments are archived in the TMF.

Consent Forms

Consents are necessary prerequisites to enrolling persons into clinical trials. All transactions concerning consents must be archived should questions arise later regarding content in each version of the informed consent and when they were used at the trial sites and signed by the trial participant.

Consents may be oral or written depending on settings and circumstance. The language and content of the informed consent document are controlled by local IRBs, even if the trial is done with a central IRB (NIH 2016; FDA 2006).

Clinics in multicenter trials may be provided with prototype consent statements prepared by the coordinating center or some other leadership center in the trial, but individual clinics and local IRBs are free to change language or add statements to the prototype, provided the primary information transmitted remains unaltered. Individual clinics are responsible for archiving their own consent statements, as approved by local IRBs. The trial leadership is responsible for archiving master consent statement and changes thereto in the TMF.

Data Collection Forms

The data collection schedule is outlined in the protocol. Copies of data collection forms (electronic or paper) and changes thereto during the trial should be documented in sufficient detail to permit reconstruction of the data collection effort, if necessary, after the trial is finished. Electronic data collection systems need to have audit trail functions to track changes to data collection during the conduct of the trial.

Investigator's Brochure

An Investigator's Brochure exists only if the trial involves an investigational product under the control of the FDA or other regulatory agencies. The brochure serves to summarize information about the product, recommended doses, and likely side effects. The holder of the investigational new drug (IND) application is responsible for updates to the brochure and distribution to IRBs and study centers involved in studying the product. Changes to the Investigator's Brochure over time should be archived in the TMF.

Key Communications

Communications and correspondences regarding clinical trials are archived in the TMF, and requirements are described in the EMA Guideline (EMA 2018). There are many types of correspondences to consider when organizing them for the archive.

IRB Transmissions and Communications

Individual study centers are responsible for communications to and from their respective IRBs and for archiving same. The study coordinating center, office of the chair, sponsor, or some other party in multicenter trials is responsible for archiving communications to and from the study parent IRB, including communications concerning the study protocol and changes to it, prototype consent forms, and data collection forms.

Reports of Adverse Events

Adverse events must be reported to IRBs and all clinics in the trial. Typically, the clinic in which the event occurred reports the event to the study coordinating center or like leadership center in multicenter trials, and it in turn reports the event to all study centers and sponsors. Sponsors have an obligation to maintain an adverse event database for the investigational or marketed product and an obligation to report adverse events to regulatory authorities with specific timelines. Regulatory authorities may place clinical trials on hold based on adverse event reporting. Communications on adverse event reporting should be included in the study archive.

Directives from Sponsors and Regulatory Agencies

Directives from sponsors and regulatory agencies concerning the trial must be communicated to study IRBs and study centers and implemented as indicated. Archiving is the responsibility of study coordinating center or like leadership center in the trial.

Inquiries from Persons or Journalists Concerning the Trial

Queries from persons or the press concerning the trial should be logged with details as to resolution. Questions from patients in trials usually are addressed at the clinic level. Multicenter trials will have structures for dealing with questions from the press or others not involved in the trial. The usual course is to refer those queries to the study chair or some other responsible person in the organization structure of the trial. Correspondence should be logged and archived.

The Trial Data System and Database

The trial data system, including the database, is the soul of the trial. In this electronic age, it will likely be comprised of dozens of programs to construct and manage the data system and as many to monitor and analyze data during and after completion of the trial, many of which will be updated or changed over the course of the trial. The developer and operator of the data system are responsible for archiving data system programs. Data analysts are responsible for archiving analysis programs.

The prize possession of a trial is its data. Obviously, the finished, identified, dataset must be archived but must be edited and cleaned of outstanding edits and checks before archiving. Once the dataset is frozen for archiving, changes or updates are nuisances, especially if the changes impact on counts or results in published papers.

The archive must be secure, password protected, and in a location likely to allow access for a minimum of 20 years after deposit.

But nothing is forever, and, hence, eventually files maybe unreadable because technologies change. When the UGDP ended, the dataset was deposited at the National Technical Information Service (NTIS) on magnetic tape. Even if it still exists there, it would be hard to find anyone capable of reading magnetic tapes.

Dataset can have value long after trials are finished. The Coronary Drug Project (CDP) ran from 1966 to 1985 (CDP 1973). Just recently a person requested the dataset to do a follow-up study of enrollees. The dataset disappeared when the institution housing the coordinating center for the trial ceased to exist in 2010.

Investigators must decide if they produce a deidentified dataset for use by people outside the research group. Increasingly, the expectation is that there will be a deidentified dataset available, but deidentifying data is no mean task. It takes time, costs money, and requires skilled people to do the deidentifying. Clinical research teams can hire experts on deidentification to ensure proper procedures are followed. If done, the set may be available on request or may be deposited at a commercial enterprise specialized in such services.

Another use of deidentified data may be participation in meta-analyses or pooling of placebo-treated patients across trials to better understand the underlying patient population. Cooperative groups and groups led by medical associations are leading some efforts to pool deidentified patient level data.

Registration

Registration on websites for trials, such as ClinicalTrials.gov, is a form of archiving, though not mentioned in the EMA guidelines for archiving. However, the EMA does maintain EudraCT (European Union Drug Regulating Authorities Clinical Trials Database), which is the European database for all interventional clinical trials on medicinal products authorized in the European Union and outside the EU if they are part of the Pediatric Investigation Plan from 1 May 2004 onwards. It has been established in accordance with Directive 2001/20/EC. Protocol and results information on interventional clinical trials are made publicly available through the European Union Clinical Trials Register since September 2011 (EMA 2020).

Trials are to be registered prior to start of enrollment and registrations are to be updated to completion of the trial. The ClinicalTrials.gov website has a field for posting protocols and logging updates to it over the course of the trial and for listing citations to publications from the investigator group.

Results, without written comments, are to be posted to the website within 1 year after completion of the trial. The bad news is that only a small fraction of the registrations contains posted results. For example, for trials completed in 2018, only 13% had posted results, as of 9 April 2020 (US NLM 2020).

Other Study Documents

Trials, like people, need curriculum vitae (CV) to list key facts, activities, and accomplishments. An example is the CV for the National Emphysema Treatment Trial (NETT 1999) posted at trialsmeinertsway.com (Meinert 2020). Its content is as below:

1. Background and rationale   1
2. Design summary   3
3. Summary of pulmonary rehabilitation program   8
4. Consent, data collection, and telephone contact schedule through Dec   9
    2002
5. Substudies   10
6. Landmark events   11
7. Participating centers, groups, and committees   12
8. Publications   13
9. Presentations   23
10. Meetings   26
11. Site visits   37
12. Meetings/conference calls and site visits by year of study   38
13. Support statement   39
14. Contract numbers, funding period, and ClinicalTrials.gov number   40
15. Repositories   41
16. Items on file at the National Technical Information Service   42
17. NETT website   43
18. Accessing the NETT Limited Access Dataset   44

Other documents that should be archived:

• Manuals of operations and study handbooks, data collection forms, and revision histories

- Policy and procedures memoranda (memos having force of protocol distributed to study centers)
- Funding history
- Photographs and digital media images

Access to the Archive

Trials, especially multicenter trials, have a website built specifically for use by investigators in the trial. Typical study websites will include the Investigator's Brochure, current version of the study protocol, study handbooks and manuals, copies of data collection forms, and other information of importance to investigators in the trial. Access must be password protected. If public access to the protocol, consent forms, and data collection forms is provided, it will be provided on a public website.

Access to the TMF or eTMF is controlled by the coordinating center, and staff working on the trial will be given access according to roles; for example, an editor can upload documents, while staff who need to access files only will be given read-only access.

TMF Retention Time

For trials conducted under Directive 2001/20 of the European Union, the sponsor and investigator must ensure that the documents in the TMF are retained for at least 5 years after the conclusion of the trial or in accordance with national regulations; for example, Germany requires a 10-year period of retention (de Mey 2018). Some countries require 20 years or longer.

Summary and Conclusions

Archiving records and materials is a critical activity during the conduct of clinical trials. The repository for the archive is referred to as the TMF. The most used guideline on creating and maintaining the TMF is published by the EMA. Successful archiving includes specified roles and responsibilities of the staff charged with archiving for the trial. Special attention should be made to key documents of the trial including the protocol and consent forms and the various versions used during the trial. Correspondence and communications with trial sponsors, press, and others are included in the archive. The database system and database demand special considerations when locking for archiving. One method for archiving publicly is to include the trial protocol and results in a clinical trial registry, such as ClinicalTrials.gov. Access to the archive is controlled by the leadership of the trial. Retention for archives varies by country and region and needs to be taken into consideration when planning the archive.

Key Facts

- The trial master file (TMF) serves as the archive for a clinical trial and can be paper and/or electronic.
- Guidelines on the TMF have been published by the EMA.
- Many considerations go into creating and maintaining the TMF including key documents, communications, data systems, and other documents. All versions of documents used during the trial are included in the archive.
- Registration of the trial offers an opportunity to provide documents from the archive to the public.
- Access to the TMF is controlled by the clinical trial leadership.
- Retention time is a consideration when choosing where to house the TMF.

Cross-References

- ▶ Good Clinical Practice
- ▶ Regulatory Requirements in Clinical Trials
- ▶ Responsibilities and Management of the Clinical Coordinating Center
- ▶ Trial Organization and Governance

References

Bombardier C, Laine L, Reicin A, Shapiro D, Burgos-Vargas R, Davis B, Day R, Ferraz MB, Hawkey CJ, Hochberg MC, Kvien TK, Schnitzer TJ for the VIGOR Study Group (2000) Comparison of upper gastrointestinal toxicity of rofecoxib and naproxen in patients with rheumatoid arthritis. N Engl J Med 343:1520–1528
Chan A-W, Tetzlaff JM, Altman DG, Laupacis A, Gøtzsche PC, Krleža-Jeric K, Hróbjartsson A, Mann H, Dickersin K, Berlin J, Doré C, Parulekar W, Summerskill W, Groves T, Schulz K, Sox H, Rockhold FW, Rennie D, Moher D (2013) SPIRIT 2013 statement: defining standard protocol items for clinical trials. Ann Intern Med 158:200–207
Coronary Drug Project Research Group (1973) The coronary drug project: design, methods, and baseline results. Circulation 47(Suppl I):I-1–I-50
Crewdson J Fraud in breast cancer study, Chicago tribune, 13 March 1994
Curfman GD, Morrissey S, Drazen JM (2005) Expression of concern: Bombardier et al., comparison of upper gastrointestinal toxicity of Rofecoxib and naproxen in patients with rheumatoid arthritis. N Engl J Med 343:1520–1528. N Engl J Med 2005;353:2813–2814
Curfman GD, Morrissey S, Drazen JM (2006) Expression of concern reaffirmed. N Engl J Med 354: 1193
De Mey C (2018) Archiving – how long? https://wwwacps-networkcom/2018/11/08/ct-lost-in-delegation-2/. Accessed 23 Dec 2020
European Medicines Agency (EMA) Good Clinical Practice Inspectors Working Group (2018) Guideline on the content, management and archiving of the clinical trial master file (paper and/or electronic) https://www.ema.europa.eu/en/documents/scientific-guideline/guideline-content-management-archiving-clinical-trial-master-file-paper/electronic_en.pdf. Accessed 23 Dec 2020
European Medicines Agency (EMA) (2020) EudraCT public home page. https://eudracte maeuropaeu/. Accessed 23 Dec 2020

Gilbert JP, Meier P, Rümke CL, Saracci R, Zelen M, White C (1975) Report of the Committee for the Assessment of biometric aspects of controlled trials of hypoglycemic agents. JAMA 231: 583–608

Meinert CL (2020) Trials Meinerts Way. https://jhuccs1us/clm/defaultasp. Accessed 9 Apr 2020

National Emphysema Treatment Trial Research Group (1999) Rationale and design of the National Emphysema Treatment Trial (NETT): a prospective randomized trial of lung volume reduction surgery. Chest 116:1,750–1,761

United States Food and Drug Administration (FDA) (2006) Using a Centralized IRB Review Process in Multicenter Clinical Trials Guidance for Industry. https://www.fda.gov/regulatory-information/search-fda-guidance-documents/using-centralized-irb-review-process-multicenter-clinical-trials. Accessed 23 Dec 2020

United States National Institutes of Health (NIH) (2016) Final NIH policy on the use of a single institutional review Board for Multi-Site Research. https://grantsnihgov/grants/guide/notice-files/not-od-16-094html. Accessed 23 Dec 2020

United States National Library of Medicine (US NLM) (2020) ClinicalTrials.gov https://www.clinicaltrials.gov/. Accessed 3 Apr 2020

University Group Diabetes Program Research Group (1970a) A study of the effects of hypoglycemic agents on vascular complications in patients with adult-onset diabetes: I. Design, methods, and baseline characteristics. Diabetes 19(suppl 2):747–783

University Group Diabetes Program Research Group (1970b) A study of the effects of hypoglycemic agents on vascular complications in patients with adult-onset diabetes: II. Mortality results. Diabetes 19(Suppl 2):785–830

Good Clinical Practice

35

Claire Weber

Contents

Abstract

Good clinical practice (GCP) is an international quality standard that is provided by the International Council on Harmonization (ICH), an international body that defines standards, which governments can transpose into regulations for all phases of clinical trials involving human subjects. GCP applies to the trial sponsor team, the institutional review boards (IRB)/ethics committees (EC) and the investigator site teams. This chapter describes the GCP concepts, a GCP historical timeline, and how GCP in all phases of clinical trials and drug development through regulatory approval is the standard for clinical research.

Keywords

ICH · GCP · Ethical · Consent · Privacy · Regulations · Guidelines · Sponsor · IRB/EC · Investigator

C. Weber (⊠)
Excellence Consulting, LLC, Moraga, CA, USA
e-mail: cweber@excellence-llc.com

© Springer Nature Switzerland AG 2022
S. Piantadosi, C. L. Meinert (eds.), *Principles and Practice of Clinical Trials*,
https://doi.org/10.1007/978-3-319-52636-2_64

Introduction

Clinical research is conducted according to a set of standards which has been formalized in many international guidelines and regulations. GCP must be instituted in all clinical research and is the standard for designing, conducting, recording, and reporting trials that involve the participation of human subjects. The primary goals of GCP are to protect all research participants and assure that only worthy treatments are approved for use for future patients. If the clinical study follows GCP, the data generated from the trial will be mutually accepted by many of the regulatory agencies around the world in support of an approval to market the drug. GCP encompasses local and regional laws, directives, regulations, guidance documents, and standard operating procedures (SOPs) for use by the trial sponsor, the IRB/EC, and the investigator site team.

GCP Definition

Good clinical practice is defined as:

> An international ethical and scientific quality standard for designing, conducting, recording, and reporting trials that involve the participation of human subjects. Compliance with this standard provides public assurance that the rights, safety, and well-being of trial subjects are protected, consistent with the principles that have origin in the Declaration of Helsinki, and that the clinical trial data are credible (ICH E6 [R2] Introduction Page 1).

And it is further defined as:

> A standard for the design, conduct, performance, monitoring, auditing, recording, analyses, and reporting of clinical trials that provide assurance that the data and reported results are credible and accurate, and that the rights, integrity, and confidentiality of trial subjects are protected (ICH E6 [R2] Glossary Section 1.24).

GCP, combined with good manufacturing practice (GMP) standards, good laboratory practice (GLP) standards, good pharmacovigilance practice (GPVP), good distribution practice (GDP), and good documentation practice (GDoP) are referred to as GxP. GxP applies to all aspects of drug development. This chapter only pertains to GCP, but it should be noted that GCP shares some common elements with definitions of other areas of GxP, since they each are standards to ensure drug products are safe, pure and not adulterated, and effective. Although GCP was developed for clinical investigational drug studies, the principles are also used in medical device studies, and other social/behavioral studies.

ICH and GCP

The International Council on Harmonization of Technical Requirements for registration of Pharmaceuticals for Human Use (ICH) is a joint effort by the regulatory authorities and pharmaceutical industry representatives of Europe, Japan, and the USA. Beginning in 1990, the ICH has published many guidelines. Informed by a lengthy list of predicate documents (e.g., the Nuremberg Code, Declaration of Helsinki, European Community and Nordic Guidelines, and various local regional laws and regulations), GCP is codified in principles called ICH GCP (ICH E6 (R2) Pages 8–10) that is widely recognized as authoritative in defining the obligations of sponsors, investigators, and institutional review boards and ethics committees (IRBs/ECs). ICH E6 is the primary GCP guideline, however there are other important ICH guidelines for clinical research that also address GCP including (but not limited to):

- ICH E2A-E2F: Pharmacovigilance
- ICH E7 Studies in support of special populations: Geriatrics
- ICH E8: General considerations for clinical studies
- ICH E11: Clinical investigation of medicinal products in the pediatric population
- ICH E19: Safety data collection

GCP Historical Timeline

The following key events were instrumental for the development of GCP:
   The Nuremberg Code of 1947:

- On August 20, 1947, the judges delivered their verdict in the "Doctors Trial" against Karl Brandt and 22 others. These trials focused on doctors involved in the human experiments in concentration camps. The suspects were involved in over 3,500,000 sterilizations of German citizens.
- Instituted informed consent and absence of coercion, and voluntary participation.

The Declaration of Geneva of 1948:

- One of the first and most important actions of the World Medical Association (WMA), regarding a physicians' dedication to the humanitarian goals of medicine
- Physician's oath, to be sworn at the time a person enters the Medical profession, was added to the Declaration of Geneva and adopted by the General Assembly of the World Medical Association
- Pledge in view of the medical crimes that been committed in Nazi Germany and includes "I will maintain the utmost respect for human life; even under threat, I will not use my medical knowledge contrary to the laws of humanity"

The Declaration of Helsinki of 1964:

- Well-being of subjects takes precedence.
- Respect for persons.
- Protection of subject's health and rights.

- Special protection for vulnerable populations.
- Safeguarding research subjects.

Informed consent.

- Adhering to an approved research plan/protocol which is reviewed by an independent committee (IRB/EC).
- Autonomy – subjects must be able to quit at any time.
- Scientifically valid – study design and study conduct.
- Minimize the risk – harm, injury, and suffering.
- Biomedical research on human subjects must conform to scientific principles.
- Be based on valid laboratory and animal experimentation.
- Required studies to be conducted only by scientifically qualified persons and supervised by a clinical competent medical authority.

1962 Kefauver Amendment to Food Drug and Cosmetic Act:

- FDA officials began to lobby members of Congress and draft legislation in the late 1950s to address gaps in oversight in drug manufacturing and marketing.
- Drug manufacturers are required to prove to the FDA the effectiveness and safety of the product before marketing.
- These efforts coincided with how an FDA official refused to give a positive opinion on a drug called thalidomide, used to treat morning sickness and nausea and found to have caused hundreds of birth defects, in Western Europe.
- Raised the issue of the importance of keeping good records and documentations.
- FDA had veto power over new drugs entering the market.
- Drugs now had to demonstrate evidence of effectiveness as well as safety, dramatically increasing the amount of time, resources, and scientific expertise required to develop a new drug. The Modern Clinical Trial System was implemented, the 1962 Amendment required interpretation of effectiveness to include "substantial evidence" in "adequate and well-controlled investigations."

The Medicines Act of 1968 from the Department of Health and Social Services (DHSS):

- Merged a number of previous medical regulations to provide broad legal standards on the manufacture and supply of medicines which related to general practice.
- Introduced three categories of medicine: prescription-only drugs, which are available only from a pharmacist if prescribed by a doctor; pharmacy medicines, available only from a pharmacist but without a prescription; and general sales medicine which may be bought from any shop without a prescription. It made possession of prescription drugs without a prescription an offence.

Table 1 The Belmont Report Summary of Ethical Principles

Ethical principles for research	Applications of ethical principles for research
Respect for persons Individuals should be treated as autonomous agents Persons with diminished autonomy are entitled to protection	**Informed consent** Volunteer research participants, to the degree that they are capable, must be given the opportunity to choose what shall or shall not happen to them The consent process must include three elements: Information Comprehension Voluntary participation
Beneficence Human participants should not be harmed Research should maximize possible benefits and minimize possible risks	**Assessment of risks and benefits** The nature and scope of risks and benefits must be assessed in a systematic way
Justice The benefits and risks of research must be distributed fairly	**Selection of participants** There must be fair procedures and outcomes in the selection of research participants

The Belmont Report, 1979, ethical principles, and applications summarized in Table 1:

The timeline of these events, culminating with the Belmont Report, led to ultimate framework for the ICH, and GCP.

Key Aspects of ICH GCP

Consent
Consent is a critical aspect of GCP and is defined as:

A process by which a subject voluntarily confirms his or her willingness to participate in a particular trial, after having been informed of all aspects of the trial that are relevant to the subject's decision to participate. Informed consent is documented by means of a written, signed, and dated informed consent (ICH E6 (R2) Glossary Section 1.28).

In addition to consent, trials with children and with impaired individuals may need to include an assent signed by the subject, in addition to the consent signed by the legal representative.

GCP requires that all elements of consent/assent are appropriately obtained and documented.

IRB/EC
The IRB/EC is defined as:

An independent body constituted of medical, scientific, and nonscientific members whose responsibility is to ensure the protection of the rights, safety, and well-being of human subjects involved in a trial by, among other things, reviewing, approving, and providing continuing review of trial protocol and amendments and of the methods and material to be used in obtaining and documenting informed consent of the trial subjects (ICH E6 [R2] Glossary Section 1.31).

GCP requires that all studies are reviewed and overseen by IRB/ECs.

Privacy

The US Health Insurance Portability Accountability Act (HIPAA) of 1996 Privacy Rule and the European Union (EU) General Data Protection Regulation (GDPR), and other similar international regulations are important aspects of GCP as safeguards to protect the privacy of personal health information and rights to examine and obtain a copy of health records.

GCP requires that the subject's privacy is protected.

International, Local, and Regional Laws, Directives, and Regulations

Regulatory authority documents (e.g., US FDA code of Federal Regulations [CFR], EU Clinical Trial Directive, etc.) include the ICH GCP principles for the conduct of clinical trials. Other international and local regional laws, directives, and regulations also include ICH GCP principles. Sponsors, IRB/EC, and the investigator site team document the operational details for incorporating GCP in standard operating procedures. Thus, regulations/guidelines and standard operating procedures reinforce GCP as described in Fig. 1.

GCP Documents Also Known as Essential Documents

Essential documents are defined as:

Fig. 1 ICH/GCP overlap with SOPs, Laws, Regulations and Guidelines

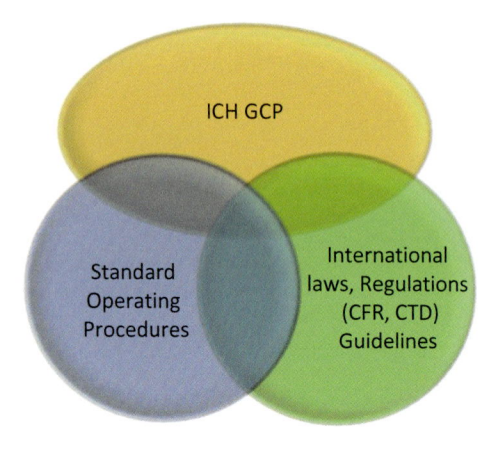

Documents which individually and collectively permit evaluation of the conduct of a study and the quality of the data produced (ICH E6 [R2] Glossary Section 1.23).

Examples of GCP documents for clinical trials include:

- Protocol
- Consent form
- Regulatory authority approvals (Country, IRB/IEC)
- Investigator's brochure
- Plans – e.g., monitoring, medical oversight, risk management, statistical analysis plan (SAP), blinding/masking, pharmacovigilance, etc.
- Investigator site source documents
- Investigator statement – FDA form 1572 and financial disclosure
- Electronic or paper case report form (CRF)
- Clinical study report (CSR)
- Standard operating procedures and training
- Trial master file (sponsor and investigator site)

Essential documents demonstrate that GCP is followed, and the trial master file is the master archive of the essential documents.

Summary and Conclusion

GCP is an international quality standard that is provided by the ICH for all phases of clinical trials, and drug development through regulatory approval. The goals of GCP are to protect all research participants and assure that only worthy treatments are approved for use for future patients. ICH E6 (R2) includes GCP principles (referred to as ICH GCP) that are widely recognized as authoritative in defining obligations of sponsors, investigator site teams, and IRB/ECs. The IRB/EC and implementation of consent and privacy are critical aspects of GCP. ICH GCP principles are included in standard operating procedures, as well as international, local, and regional laws, directives, and regulations. Essential documents demonstrate that GCP is followed. The trial sponsor team, the investigator site team, and IRB/EC are all responsible for protecting human subjects who volunteer to participate and must be trained on and follow GCP. If the clinical study follows GCP, the data generated from the trial will be mutually accepted by many of the regulatory agencies around the world in support of an approval to market the drug.

Key Facts

The facts covered in this chapter include: Goals and definitions of GCP and ICH, historical timeline of key events leading to GCP, key aspects of GCP, clinical research teams responsible for following GCP, and GCP essential documents.

Cross-References

▶ Archiving Records and Materials
▶ Clinical Trials, Ethics, and Human Protections Policies
▶ Consent Forms and Procedures
▶ Documentation: Essential Documents and Standard Operating Procedures
▶ Institutional Review Boards and Ethics Committees
▶ Investigator Responsibilities
▶ Regulatory Requirements in Clinical Trials
▶ Training the Investigatorship

References

Act of October 10, 1962 (Drug Amendments Act of 1962), Public Law 87-781, 76 STAT 780, which amended the Federal Food, Drug, and Cosmetic Act to assure the safety, effectiveness, and reliability of drugs, authorize standardization of drug names, and clarify and strengthen existing inspection authority
Clinical Trial Directive: Directive 2001/20/EC of the European Parliament and of the Council of 4 April 2001 on the approximation of the laws, regulations and administrative provisions of the Member States relating to the implementation of good clinical practice in the conduct of clinical trials on medicinal products for human use
Declaration of Helsinki of 1964
EMA GCP Directive 2005/28/EC
FDA Code of Federal Regulations (CFR), Title 21, Part 312
Health Insurance Portability and Accountability Act of 1996 (HIPAA)
ICH E6 (R2) International Council for Harmonisation Guideline for Good Clinical Practice Guideline for Good Clinical Practice (Introduction, p 1, Glossary Section 1.24, pp 8–10, Glossary Section 1.28, Glossary Section 1.31, Glossary Section 1.23)
Medicines Act 1968 c.67
Regulation (EU) 2016/679 (General Data Protection Regulation), and Directive 95/46/EC
The Belmont report: ethical principles and guidelines for the protection of human subjects of research (1978). The Commission, Bethesda
The Nazi doctors and the Nuremberg Code: human rights in human experimentation (1995). Oxford University Press, New York
World Medical Association (2001) World Medical Association declaration of Helsinki. Ethical principles for medical research involving human subjects. Bull World Health Organ 79(4): 373–374. World Health Organization

Institutional Review Boards and Ethics Committees

36

Keren R. Dunn

Contents

Abstract

Institutional review boards (IRBs) are committees established in accordance with US federal regulations to review and monitor clinical trials and other research with human subjects. IRBs evolved from a history of egregious ethical violations in research with human subjects and the ethics codes and declarations that ensued, and were first mandated by US law in 1974, with the passing of the National Research Act. IRBs help to ensure the protection of the rights and welfare of

K. R. Dunn (✉)
Office of Research Compliance and Quality Improvement, Cedars-Sinai Medical Center, Los Angeles, CA, USA
e-mail: keren.dunn@cshs.org

© Springer Nature Switzerland AG 2022
S. Piantadosi, C. L. Meinert (eds.), *Principles and Practice of Clinical Trials*,
https://doi.org/10.1007/978-3-319-52636-2_65

human subjects by applying the ethical principles of the Belmont Report, respect for persons, beneficence, and justice, in their review of research projects. They have the authority to approve, require modifications to, or disapprove proposed research. IRBs review plans to obtain and document informed consent from research participants and can waive the requirements for informed consent in certain circumstances. IRBs may exist within the institution where research is being conducted or institutions can rely on an external IRB with a written agreement. While the term IRB is unique to the USA, clinical trials internationally adhere to the ethical principles of the Declaration of Helsinki, which requires independent review by an ethics committee.

Keywords

Institutional review board · IRB · Ethics committee · Belmont Report · Common Rule · Informed consent

Introduction

IRBs in the United States and ethics committees around the world conduct independent review of research with human subjects and provide a core protection for the rights and welfare of participants in clinical research. IRB or ethics committee review is also critical in gaining and maintaining public trust of clinical research due to a history of egregious ethical violations in the conduct of clinical research. This chapter provides an overview of the history of ethical violations in clinical research and emergence of IRBs and ethics committees, a summary of IRB functions and operations, an outline of the requirements for informed consent, and an overview of recent changes to the system of IRB review and oversight. A timeline of key milestones in research ethics and the establishment of IRBs in shown in Fig. 3.

History of Research Ethics and Emergence of IRBs

The foundation of modern-day research ethics in the USA and around the world begins with the Nuremberg Code, which emerged in 1947 from the Nuremberg trials, in which Nazi physicians were tried for their conduct of atrocious medical and scientific experiments on prisoners in concentration camps (White 2020). The Nuremberg Code includes ten basic principles for the conduct of ethical research with human subjects, covering voluntary and informed consent, risk/benefit assessment that is favorable, subject right to withdraw, and research expertise and responsibility (U.S. Government Printing Office 1949; Rice 2008). In 1964, the World Medical Association created the Declaration of Helsinki, an ethical code of conduct that built upon the principles outlined in the Nuremberg Code, but added the tenets that the interests of subjects must be placed above the interests of society and that every subject should be given the best known treatment (Rice 2008). Additionally, the Declaration of Helsinki expanded upon the requirement for voluntary and informed consent from the Nuremberg Code to address the ethical participation of children and compromised adults in research (White 2020). Despite US involvement in the development of both the Nuremberg Code and Declaration of Helsinki, there are multiple documented cases of serious research ethical violations in the US throughout the 1950s and 1960s (White 2020).

In 1966, a well-respected anesthesiologist from Massachusetts General Hospital, Henry Beecher, published an article in the New England Journal of Medicine outlining multiple examples of ethical violations he had garnered from a review of publications in an "excellent journal" (Harkness et al. 2001). Beecher's examples included, among other violations, studies where known effective treatment was withheld from subjects and studies where subjects were exposed to excessive and unjustified risk of harm (Beecher 1966). In conclusion, Beecher advocated that "it is absolutely essential to strive for (informed consent) for moral, sociologic and legal reasons" (Beecher 1966). Additionally, he concluded, "there is the more reliable safeguard provided by the presence of an intelligent, informed, conscientious, compassionate, responsible investigator" (Beecher 1966). Notably, Beecher was not an advocate for independent review and oversight, despite the influence his work had on the emergence of the system of institutional review boards (IRBs) (Harkness et al. 2001).

Perhaps the most infamous research ethics violation in the USA in the twentieth century, "Tuskegee Study of Untreated Syphilis in the Negro Male," was exposed in an article published in the Washington Star by Jean Heller in 1972 (White 2020). The study began in 1932, when there were no safe and effective treatments available for syphilis and enrolled 600 African American men from the community around Tuskegee, Alabama (White 2020). Although penicillin was proven to be an effective treatment for syphilis by 1945 and was widely used, the men in the study were not informed and not offered treatment so that the researchers could continue to learn about the natural course of the disease (White 2020). The study continued for 40 years until it was publicly exposed in 1972 (White 2020).

Public outcry about the Tuskegee Study and other ethics violations, as well as concern from the medical community following Beecher's article, led congress to pass the National Research Act in 1974, which established federal regulations for the protection of human subjects (45 CFR 46) and paved the way for the modern system of institutional review boards (IRBs) for the oversight of research with human subjects (Rice 2008). The National Research Act mandated that any entity applying for an NIH grant or contract must provide assurances that it has established an IRB to protect the rights of human subjects in biomedical and behavioral research (US Congress Senate 1974).

The National Commission and the Belmont Report

The National Research Act also established the National Commission for the Protection of Human Subjects of Biomedical and Behavioral Research (the Commission). The

Fig. 1 Transcribed excerpt from the Commission's report: *Institutional Review Boards*

duties of the Commission were: 1) to identify the basic ethical principles which should guide the conduct of research with human subjects; 2) develop guidelines for the conduct of research with human subjects in accordance with those ethical principles; and 3) advise the secretary on administrative actions to apply the guidelines and on any other matters related to the protection of human research subjects (US Congress Senate 1974).

The Commission published multiple reports between 1975 and 1979. On September 1, 1978, the Commission published a report entitled *Institutional Review Boards*, which outlined recommendations for the IRB review mechanism and evaluation of IRB performance, as well as steps to improve the ethical review process (National Commission 1978). Figure 1 includes an excerpt from this report on IRBs.

The Belmont Report, named for the location of the Commission's four-day intensive meetings at the Belmont Conference Center in 1976, was issued September 30, 1978 and published in the Federal Register April 18, 1979 (National Commission 1979). The Belmont Report described the boundaries between the practice of medicine and research, outlined the basic ethical principles to guide research with human subjects, and delineated the application of these ethical principles (National Commission 1979). Figure 2 includes a summary of the ethical principles and their applications outlined in the Belmont Report.

In 1981, revised regulations for the protection of human subjects (45 CFR 46) incorporating most of the recommendations of the Belmont Report were signed by the secretary of the Department of Health and Human Services (DHHS) and the Food and Drug Administration (FDA) adopted similar regulations covering

The Belmont Report Ethical Principles and Applications

Ethical Principles	Applications
Respect for Persons • Respect the autonomy of individuals • Protect individuals with diminished autonomy (e.g., prisoners)	Informed Consent • Consent process includes information, comprehension, and voluntariness. • Incomplete disclosure of information must be justified by its necessity to accomplish the research goals, that there are no significant risks omitted from the disclosure, and when appropriate, there is a debriefing plan.
Beneficence • Do not harm • Maximize possible benefits and minimize possible harms • Consider both individual and societal benefits	Assessment of Risks and Benefits • Appropriate study design • Risks must be justified, and benefit/risk ratio must be favorable. • Consider both the probability and magnitude of any harm. • Consider risks of psychological, physical, legal, social and economic harm.
Justice • Fair distribution of benefits and burdens of research	Selection of Subjects • Opportunities to participate in potentially beneficial research must be distributed fairly. • Burdens of research should not be borne unfairly by disadvantaged populations.

Fig. 2 Summary of the Belmont Report's ethical principles and their applications

requirements for IRBs (21 CFR 56) and informed consent (21 CFR 50) in FDA regulated clinical investigations (White 2020). In an effort to harmonize regulations across the federal government, the Federal Policy for the Protection of Human Subjects (45 CFR 46) was adopted in 1991 by 15 federal departments and agencies to become known as the "Common Rule" (White 2020). The FDA has not signed on to the Common Rule, but has committed to amending its own regulations at 21 CFR parts 50 and 56 to align with the Common Rule to the extent possible (White 2020).

Ethics Violations and Calls for Reform at the Turn of the Century

In 1999 and 2001, there were two highly publicized tragic deaths of research subjects participating in studies at separate renowned institutions (White 2020). Jesse Gelsinger was born with a mild form of ornithine transcarbamylase (OTC) deficiency that was well managed with diet and medication and had just turned 18 when he volunteered to participate a phase 1 gene therapy study for the treatment of OTC deficiency (White 2020). Shortly after receiving the experimental gene therapy, Gelsinger experienced an acute inflammatory response leading to multiorgan failure and died just 4 days later (White 2020). This led to an investigation, which raised questions about significant ethics and regulatory violations, including, among others, whether Gelsinger was enrolled in violation of the eligibility criteria in the IRB-approved protocol and a conflict of interest for the director of the gene studies program that was not disclosed (White 2020). Ellen Roche was a healthy 24-year-old lab technician when she volunteered in 2001 to participate in a physiology study in which subjects were administered inhaled hexamethonium (White 2020). Within 24 h Roche developed significant pulmonary abnormalities, which progressed to multiorgan failure, and ultimately, she died within a month (White 2020). Concerns raised from the investigation of this case included lack of identification of reported complications associated with hexamethonium in the literature, failure to apply for an investigational new drug application (IND) or to inquire with the FDA about the need for an IND, lack of information in the consent form about the regulatory status of hexamethonium, missing reports of complications in prior publications, and use of a chemical grade agent, rather than pharmaceutical grade (White 2020).

In September 2000, in response to the Gelsinger tragedy (and before the tragedy of Roche's death), Donna Shalala, secretary of Health and Human Services, published a plan and urgent call to action to strengthen protections for human research subjects in the New England Journal of Medicine (Shalala 2000). Shalala outlined several steps taken by the government, including expansion of the role of the Office for Protection from Research Risks (OPRR) and renaming it the Office for Human Research Protections (OHRP), along with the appointment of new leadership (Shalala 2000). However, Shalala made the case that ultimate responsibility to protect human subjects lies with the institutions performing research (Shalala 2000). With respect to IRBs, Shalala stated:

> IRBs, the key element of the system to protect research subjects, are under increasing strain. In June 1998, the Office of Inspector General of the Department of Health and Human Services issued four investigative reports, which indicated that IRBs have excessive workloads and inadequate resources. At a number of institutions, IRB oversight was inadequate, and on occasion, researchers were not providing the boards with sufficient information for them to evaluate clinical trials fully.

During this time period, serious discussions about accreditation emerged as a solution to ensuring the quality of IRBs and institutional systems for the protection of human research subjects (Steinbrook 2002). The Association of American Medical Colleges, along with six other partnering organizations, founded the Association for the Accreditation of Human Research Protection Programs (AAHRPP) in 2001 (Steinbrook 2002). Calls for reform continued in the years that followed. Proposed reforms included mandatory accreditation of IRBs and institutional human research protections, credentialing of IRB personnel, and centralized IRBs for review of multisite studies (Emanuel et al. 2004).

Revision of the Common Rule

A path to revise the Common Rule began in 2011, when the federal government sought input from the public with the release of an advance notice of proposed rulemaking (ANPRM). The ANPRM described shortcomings of the current regulations, citing changes to the research enterprise since the Common Rule was first enacted 20 years earlier, including "the proliferation of multi-site clinical trials and

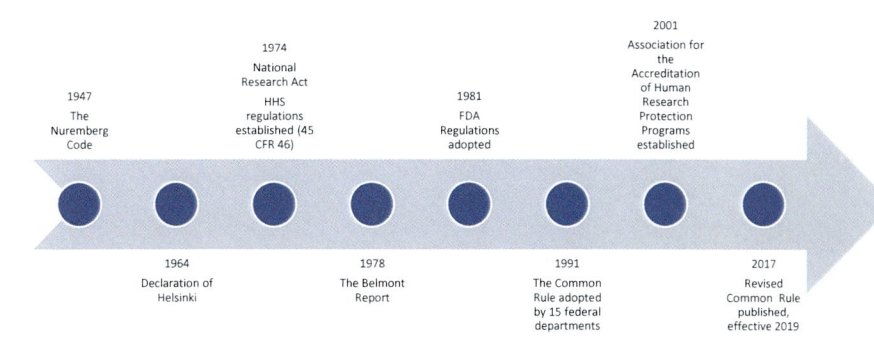

Fig. 3 Timeline of key milestones in research ethics and establishment of IRBs

observational studies, the expansion of health services research, research in the social and behavioral sciences, and research involving databases, the Internet, and biological specimen repositories, and the use of advanced technologies, such as genomics" (DHHS 2011). The ANPRM sought public input with respect to the protection of human subjects in research, while reducing burden, delay, and ambiguity for investigators (DHHS 2011).

The final revised Common Rule was published in the Federal Register in January 2017 and became effective in January 2019. Significant revisions in the final rule incorporated standards for the language and organization of informed consent forms, including the required use of a concise and focused presentation of the key information most likely to facilitate understanding and decision-making about whether or not to participate in the research (Menikoff et al. 2017). Additional revisions reduced burden on IRBs and researchers for the management and review of low-risk studies, including elimination of the requirement for annual progress reports and IRB continuing review for many of these studies and additional allowances for researchers to screen potential research subjects based on review of medical records or other information available to them (Menikoff et al. 2017). Additionally, the revised Common Rule included provisions for broad informed consent, whereby participants can agree to the secondary unspecified future research use of their private identifiable information that was originally collected for clinical care or other specific research studies (Menikoff ct al. 2017). Lastly, the revised Common Rule included a requirement for single-IRB review of multisite studies in most cases, aiming to avoid the burden for study sponsors, researchers, and IRBs associated with multiple IRB reviews of the same protocol (Menikoff et al. 2017).

IRB Functions and Operations

The Common Rule requires that institutions conducting or otherwise engaged in research with human subjects supported by a federal department or agency provide an assurance that it will comply with the Common Rule (45 CFR 46.103). This assurance of compliance, submitted to the federal Office for Human Research

Protections, is called a Federalwide Assurance (FWA) and must be signed by an institutional official authorized to act on behalf of the institution and to take responsibility for the institution's compliance with the Common Rule requirements (45 CFR 46.103).

While the Common Rule only applies to research conducted or supported by a federal department or agency, institutions submitting an FWA are required to provide an assurance that all of its human subjects research activities will be guided by an appropriate code, declaration, or statement of ethical principles such as the Declaration of Helsinki by the World Medical Association or the Belmont Report. In addition to a general assurance of compliance the FWA provides assurances regarding the institution's written procedures for its IRB operations, that the institution will provide copies of its written procedures to OHRP upon request, that the institution ensures adequate resources for each of its IRBs, and that when the institution relies on an external IRB, the reliance arrangement is documented in a written agreement. Institutions must renew their FWA every 5 years and are required to submit updates within 90 days of certain significant changes (OHRP 2021).

Since 2009, both the Common Rule and FDA regulations require that IRBs must be registered before the IRB can be designated under an institution's FWA and before the IRB can review research involving FDA-regulated products (45 CFR 46 Subpart E, 21 CFR 56.106). Registration of IRBs requires the name and contact information for the institution running the IRB, the name and contact information for the IRB and IRB chairperson, approximate number of active protocols involving FDA-regulated products reviewed by the IRB, and a description of the types of FDA-regulated products used in research reviewed by the IRB. IRB registration must be renewed every 3 years and updated within 90 days or 30 days of certain significant changes (45 CFR 46 Subpart E, 21 CFR 56.106).

According to federal regulations, an IRB must have at least five members, including at least one scientist, at least one nonscientist, and at least one member who is not affiliated with the institution themselves or through an immediate family member. IRB membership must be qualified through experience, expertise, and diversity to promote respect for its recommendations and determinations. The IRB should include members knowledgeable about institutional commitments, regulations and applicable laws, and standards of professional conduct to facilitate effective review of proposed research. IRBs routinely reviewing research with potentially vulnerable subject populations, including children, prisoners, cognitively impaired individuals, or socioeconomically disadvantaged individuals, should include members familiar and experienced with these populations (45 CFR 46.107 and 21 CFR 56.107). IRBs must be allocated resources, including sufficient staff and adequate meeting space (45 CFR 46.108).

IRB Review of Research and Definitions

All research involving human subjects (see definitions in Table 1) that is conducted or supported by a federal department or agency is subject to the regulations in the Common Rule (45 CFR 46), including the requirements for IRB review and

Table 1 Selected definitions transcribed from the Common Rule (45 CFR 46.102) and FDA regulations (21 CFR 56.102)

Term	Definition
Human subject	Common Rule: A living individual about whom an investigator (whether professional or student) conducting research (i) Obtains information or biospecimens through intervention or interaction with the individual, and uses, studies, or analyzes the information or biospecimens (ii) Obtains, uses, studies, analyzes, or generates identifiable private information or identifiable biospecimens FDA: An individual who is or becomes a participant in research, either as a recipient of the test article or as a control. A subject may be either a healthy human or a patient
Intervention	Includes both physical procedures by which information or biospecimens are gathered (e.g., venipuncture) and manipulations of the subject or the subject's environment that are performed for research purposes
Interaction	Includes communication or interpersonal contact between investigator and subject
Private information	Includes information about behavior that occurs in a context in which an individual can reasonably expect that no observation or recording is taking place, and information that has been provided for specific purposes by an individual and that the individual can reasonably expect will not be made public (e.g., a medical record)
Identifiable private information	Private information for which the identity of the subject is or may readily be ascertained by the investigator or associated with the information
Identifiable biospecimen	A biospecimen for which the identity of the subject is or may readily be ascertained by the investigator or associated with the biospecimen
Research	A systematic investigation, including research development, testing, and evaluation, designed to develop or contribute to generalizable knowledge
Clinical trial (Common Rule only)	A research study in which one or more human subjects are prospectively assigned to one or more interventions (which may include placebo or other control) to evaluate the effects of the interventions on biomedical or behavioral health-related outcomes
Clinical investigation (FDA only)	Any experiment that involves a test article and one or more human subjects and that either is subject to requirements for prior submission to the Food and Drug Administration under section 505(i) or 520 (g) of the act, or is not subject to requirements for prior submission to the Food and Drug Administration under these sections of the act, but the results of which are intended to be submitted later to, or held for inspection by, the Food and Drug Administration as part of an application for a research or marketing permit
Test article (FDA only)	Any drug for human use, biological product for human use, medical device for human use, human food additive, color additive, electronic product, or any other article subject to regulation under the act or under sections 351 or 354-360F of the Public Health Service Act
Minimal risk	The probability and magnitude of harm or discomfort anticipated in the research are not greater in and of themselves than those ordinarily encountered in daily life or during the performance of routine physical or psychological examinations or tests

approval and informed consent. Although these regulations only apply to federally conducted or supported research, institutions with an FWA are required to apply similar protections to all their research involving human subjects (OHRP 2021). Additionally, the International Committee of Medical Journal Editors (ICMJE) notes that authors should seek approval to conduct research from an independent review body such as an IRB or ethics committee (ICMJE 2019), additional incentive for researchers to seek and for institutions to require IRB approval of all research with human subjects. Since FDA oversight is focused on drugs, biologics, and medical devices, different terminology is used to define the research subject to IRB review. The FDA regulations at 21 CFR Parts 50 and 56 (informed consent and IRB review) apply to clinical investigations, as defined in Table 1.

IRBs have the authority to approve, require modifications to, or disapprove research and are required to conduct continuing review of research at least annually, except that most minimal risk research and ongoing research that remains open only for long-term data collection and analysis does not require continuing review in accordance with the revised Common Rule (45 CFR 46.109 and 21 CFR 56.109). IRBs are required to notify investigators and the institution in writing of its decisions to approve or disapprove research activities. The reason for disapproval must be explained in writing and the investigator must be given an opportunity to respond in writing (45 CFR 46.109 and 21 CFR 56.109).

IRB Review Levels

When research is required to be reviewed at a convened IRB meeting, a quorum must be met, meaning a majority of members must be present, including at least one nonscientist. A majority of members present must vote to approve research for the research to be approved (45 CFR 46.108 and 21 CFR 56.108). IRB meetings can be held via audio or video conference, but each member must have received review materials prior to the meeting and must be able to participate in the discussion of protocols actively and equally (DHHS OHRP & FDA 2017). Members who have a conflict of interest related to research under review by the IRB may not participate in the review of that research except to provide information requested by the IRB. The IRB can invite consultants with expertise to assist with the review of research, but the consultant cannot vote (45 CFR 46.107 and 21 CFR 56.107).

Although many research submissions require review by the IRB at a convened meeting, most minimal risk research is eligible for an expedited review procedure by an IRB chairperson or other experienced designated member of the IRB. The following categories of research are eligible for expedited review if they are determined to pose minimal risk and meet other specified conditions:

- Studies of drugs or medical devices where an IND or IDE is not required
- Research involving blood draws (depending on the subject population, volume, and frequency of collection)
- Noninvasive collection of biological specimens such as saliva or nail clippings

- Noninvasive procedures such as MRI or ultrasound
- Secondary research use of data or specimens collected for other purposes (if not exempt)
- Collection of voice, video, digital, or image recordings, and surveys, interviews, or focus groups
- Continuing review of research that originally required review by the convened IRB, but remains active for long-term follow-up of subjects or data analysis only, or where no subjects have been enrolled and no additional risks have been identified

A complete list of the categories of research eligible for expedited IRB review is posted in the Federal Register (DHHS NIH 1998). Minor changes to previously approved research can also be reviewed by expedited IRB review. While the IRB chairperson or designated member has the authority to approve or require modifications to research activities eligible for expedited review, only the convened IRB has the authority to disapprove research (45 CFR 46.110 and 21 CFR 56.110).

Certain categories of research with human subjects are exempt from the requirements for IRB review and informed consent under the Common Rule (45 CFR 46.104). Exempt research includes the following categories of research under specified circumstances for each category:

- Education research
- Surveys, interviews, educational assessments, and observation of public behavior
- Benign behavioral interventions
- Research with information or biospecimens collected for other purposes (e.g., clinical)
- Federal research and demonstration projects
- Taste and food quality evaluation
- Storage of information or biospecimens for secondary research with broad consent
- Secondary research with information or biospecimens under broad consent

Certain exempt research categories require that the IRB conduct "limited IRB review," a form of expedited review focused on protections of privacy and confidentiality (45 CFR 46.104).

IRB Records

Both the Common Rule and FDA regulations require that IRBs prepare and maintain records in paper or electronic form, documenting their activities (45 CFR 46.115 and 21 CFR 56.115). IRB records must be maintained for at least 3 years after completion of the research and they must be made available to applicable federal oversight agencies for inspection and copying upon request. Both the Common Rule and FDA regulations note that IRB records must include the following:

- Research proposals for review
- Scientific evaluations associated with the proposals, if applicable
- Correspondence between the IRB and researchers
- Approved consent forms
- Progress reports submitted by the researchers
- Records of continuing review activities
- Reports of any injuries to subjects
- Statements of significant new findings provided to subjects
- Detailed IRB meeting minutes, which must include the following:
  - Meeting attendance
  - Actions taken by the IRB
  - The vote on actions taken, including numbers voting for, against, and abstaining
  - Basis for required changes to research or disapprovals
  - Summary of discussion of controverted issues and their resolution
- IRB membership rosters with details to show name, expertise, and affiliation of each member
- Written procedures for IRB operations, including:
  - Conducting initial and continuing review of research
  - Reporting its review findings and actions to the investigator and institution
  - Determining which research projects require continuing review more frequently and which projects need verification from independent sources that no material changes have occurred since last IRB review
  - Ensuring prompt reporting to the IRB of proposed changes in research and that investigators will not implement changes until they have been reviewed and approved by the IRB except when necessary for immediate subject safety
  - Ensuring prompt reporting to the IRB, institutional officials, and applicable regulatory agencies of any unanticipated problems involving risks to subjects or others, any serious or continuing noncompliance, and any suspension or termination of IRB approval
- Additionally, the Common Rule requires additional records, which are not generally applicable to FDA-regulated research. The following records were added in the revised Common Rule, and are intended to discourage unnecessary time and effort being spent on the review and oversight of low-risk studies:
  - Rationale for conducting continuing review of minimal risk research that would not normally require continuing review
  - Rationale for an expedited reviewer determining that research with procedures generally considered minimal risk is more than minimal risk and, therefore, not eligible for expedited review

Criteria for IRB Approval

Whether research is reviewed by expedited review or at a convened IRB meeting, regulations outline criteria for IRB approval of research. The IRB is required to obtain and review information sufficient to determine whether the proposed research meets criteria for IRB approval. Table 2 outlines the general criteria for IRB approval of research. In addition to the general criteria for IRB approval, regulations outline additional protections for pregnant women, fetuses, and neonates, prisoners, and children in research, including additional requirements for IRB membership, criteria for inclusion of these potentially vulnerable populations, and additional considerations for informed consent and child assent (45 CFR 46 Subparts B, C, and D and 21 CFR 50 Subpart D).

Informed Consent

One of the key assertions outlined in the Nuremberg Code, the Declaration of Helsinki, and the Belmont Report is that informed consent is critical to the ethical conduct of research with human subjects. Therefore, it is not surprising that the process and plans for documentation of informed consent are a significant focus of the IRB review process. The informed consent of the subject or their legally authorized representative is required for all research subject to IRB review unless the IRB determines the research is eligible for a waiver or alteration of the requirements for informed consent. Researchers are required to provide information in language that is understandable to the subject and subjects must be given sufficient opportunity to discuss and consider their decision to participate in a setting and manner that minimizes any possibility of coercion or undue influence. Additionally, regulations specify that the informed consent cannot include any exculpatory language where subjects appear to give up any legal rights (45 CFR 46.116 and 21 CFR 50.20). The revised Common Rule also specifies that subjects should be given information that a "reasonable person" would want to make a decision about participation in the research, that the consent must begin with a concise summary of key information, and that the informed consent must be organized in a manner that facilitates understanding of reasons why one may not want to participate (45 CFR 46.116).

Documentation of Informed Consent

Generally, informed consent must be documented using an IRB-approved consent form that contains all the basic and applicable additional elements of informed consent. Table 3 includes a listing of the basic and additional elements of informed consent. The subject or their legally authorized representative must be given sufficient time to read the consent form or have it read to them before they sign it. A copy of the consent form is required to be given to the person signing. Both the Common Rule and FDA regulations allow for the use of a short form written consent document stating that the required elements of informed consent have been presented to the subject orally, along with an IRB-approved written summary of the oral presentation (45 CFR 46.117 and 21 CFR 50.27). The short form option is often

Table 2 Criteria for IRB approval transcribed from 45 CFR 46.111 and 21 CFR 56.111

Topic	Regulatory criteria for IRB approval
Minimizing risks	Risks to subjects are minimized (i) by using procedures that are consistent with sound research design and that do not unnecessarily expose subjects to risk, and (ii) whenever appropriate, by using procedures already being performed on the subjects for diagnostic or treatment purposes
Favorable benefit/risk ratio	Risks to subjects are reasonable in relation to anticipated benefits, if any, to subjects, and the importance of the knowledge that may reasonably be expected to result. In evaluating risks and benefits, the IRB should consider only those risks and benefits that may result from the research (as distinguished from risks and benefits of therapies subjects would receive even if not participating in the research). The IRB should not consider possible long-range effects of applying knowledge gained in the research (e.g., the possible effects of the research on public policy) as among those research risks that fall within the purview of its responsibility
Equitable selection of subjects	Selection of subjects is equitable. In making this assessment the IRB should take into account the purposes of the research and the setting in which the research will be conducted. The IRB should be particularly cognizant of the special problems of research that involves a category of subjects who are vulnerable to coercion or undue influence, such as children, prisoners, individuals with impaired decision-making capacity, or economically or educationally disadvantaged persons *Note: The language describing potentially vulnerable populations was updated in the revised Common Rule. FDA regulations still contain original language, which also includes specific reference to pregnant women, handicapped, or mentally disabled persons*
Informed consent	Informed consent will be sought from each prospective subject or the subject's legally authorized representative
Documentation of informed consent	Informed consent will be appropriately documented or appropriately waived *Note: FDA regulations do not include provisions for IRBs to waive consent; however, there has been FDA guidance issued on this topic, which is described in the informed consent section of this chapter*
Data and safety monitoring	When appropriate, the research plan makes adequate provision for monitoring the data collected to ensure the safety of subjects
Privacy and confidentiality	When appropriate, there are adequate provisions to protect the privacy of subjects and to maintain the confidentiality of data
Vulnerable subjects	When some or all of the subjects are likely to be vulnerable to coercion or undue influence, such as children, prisoners, individuals with impaired decision-making capacity, or economically or educationally disadvantaged persons, additional safeguards have been included in the study to protect the rights and welfare of these subjects *Note: Like the section on equitable selection of subjects, the language in this section was updated in the revised Common Rule. FDA regulations still contain original language to describe potentially vulnerable populations*

Table 3 Elements of informed consent transcribed from 45 CFR 46.116 and 21 CFR 50.25

Category	Required elements of consent
Basic elements of informed consent (45 CFR 46.116(b) and 21 CFR 50.25(a))	1. A statement that the study involves research, an explanation of the purposes of the research and the expected duration of the subject's participation, a description of the procedures to be followed, and identification of any procedures that are experimental. 2. A description of any reasonably foreseeable risks or discomforts to the subject. 3. A description of any benefits to the subject or to others that may reasonably be expected from the research. 4. A disclosure of appropriate alternative procedures or courses of treatment, if any, that might be advantageous to the subject. 5. A statement describing the extent, if any, to which confidentiality of records identifying the subject will be maintained. 6. For research involving more than minimal risk, an explanation as to whether any compensation and an explanation as to whether any medical treatments are available if injury occurs and, if so, what they consist of, or where further information may be obtained. 7. An explanation of whom to contact for answers to pertinent questions about the research and research subjects' rights, and whom to contact in the event of a research-related injury to the subject. 8. A statement that participation is voluntary, refusal to participate will involve no penalty or loss of benefits to which the subject is otherwise entitled, and the subject may discontinue participation at any time without penalty or loss of benefits to which the subject is otherwise entitled. 9. One of the following statements about any research that involves the collection of identifiable private information or identifiable biospecimens: a. A statement that identifiers might be removed from the identifiable private information or identifiable biospecimens and that, after such removal, the information or biospecimens could be used for future research studies or distributed to another investigator for future research studies without additional informed consent from the subject or the legally authorized representative, if this might be a possibility, or b. A statement that the subject's information or biospecimens collected as part of the

(continued)

Table 3 (continued)

Category	Required elements of consent
	research, even if identifiers are removed, will not be used or distributed for future research studies. *Notes:* *Item number 9 was added in the revised Common Rule and is not included in FDA regulations.* *There is one additional basic element of consent required under FDA regulations: the possibility that the FDA may inspect the records.*
Additional elements of informed consent, to be included when appropriate (45 CFR 46.116 (c) and 21 CFR 50.25(b))	1. A statement that the particular treatment or procedure may involve risks to the subject (or to the embryo or fetus, if the subject is or may become pregnant) that are currently unforeseeable. 2. Anticipated circumstances under which the subject's participation may be terminated by the investigator without regard to the subject's or the legally authorized representative's consent. 3. Any additional costs to the subject that may result from participation in the research. 4. The consequences of a subject's decision to withdraw from the research and procedures for orderly termination of participation by the subject. 5. A statement that significant new findings developed during the course of the research that may relate to the subject's willingness to continue participation will be provided to the subject. 6. The approximate number of subjects involved in the study. 7. A statement that the subject's biospecimens (even if identifiers are removed) may be used for commercial profit and whether the subject will or will not share in this commercial profit. 8. A statement regarding whether clinically relevant research results, including individual research results, will be disclosed to subjects, and if so, under what conditions. 9. For research involving biospecimens, whether the research will (if known) or might include whole genome sequencing (i.e., sequencing of a human germline or somatic specimen with the intent to generate the genome or exome sequence of that specimen).

(continued)

Table 3 (continued)

Category	Required elements of consent
	Notes:
	Item numbers 7, 8, and 9 were added in the revised Common Rule and are not included in FDA regulations.
	There is one additional element of consent required under FDA regulations for applicable clinical trials (21 CFR 50.25(c)): a statement and brief description about registration of the clinical trial on ClinicalTrials.gov, a clinical trial registry.
	There are separate requirements for "broad consent" for storage, maintenance, and secondary research use of identifiable private information or identifiable biospecimens defined at 45 CFR 46.116(d). These requirements have been omitted from this table for brevity.

approved by IRBs as an option for documenting informed consent, along with the use of an interpreter, for subjects who require an informed consent process in a non-English language where the need for a written translation of the full informed consent form had not been anticipated. The Common Rule also allows the IRB to waive the requirement for obtaining a signed informed consent form for certain minimal risk research or where a breach of confidentiality is the primary risk and the signed consent form would be the only record identifying the subject (45 CFR 46.117).

Waivers of Informed Consent

For general research to be eligible for a waiver or alteration of informed consent under the Common Rule (45 CFR 46.116(f)), the IRB must find that all the following criteria are met:

- The research involves no more than minimal risk to the subjects
- The research could not practicably be carried out without the requested waiver or alteration
- If the research involves using identifiable private information or identifiable biospecimens, the research could not practicably be carried out without using such information or biospecimens in an identifiable format
- The waiver or alteration will not adversely affect the rights and welfare of the subjects
- Whenever appropriate, the subjects or legally authorized representatives will be provided with additional pertinent information after participation

While the Common Rule allows an IRB to waive or alter requirements for informed consent, FDA regulations do not. However, FDA issued guidance in 2017 noting an intent to update its regulations to allow waivers and alterations of informed consent for certain minimal risk clinical investigations, which will align with waivers allowed under the Common Rule. In the meantime, the FDA notes it will not object to IRBs allowing such waivers (DHHS, FDA 2017). FDA regulations do allow for an exception from the requirement for informed consent to treat a patient/subject with an investigational drug or device in a life-threatening emergency situation. When this exception from the requirement for informed consent is used, a report must be submitted to the IRB within 5 business days (21 CFR 50.23).

Both DHHS and the FDA also allow the IRB to approve a waiver of the requirements for informed consent in research involving human subjects in emergency medical situations (e.g., heart attack, stroke, and trauma) where it may not be possible to obtain consent from the subject or their legally authorized representative. Application of this exception requires significant consideration, time, effort, and planning by the researchers and the IRB. Additional required steps and protections necessary for the IRB to grant a waiver of consent for emergency research include community consultation, public disclosure about the research, and procedures to inform subjects or their representative about the research and their right to discontinue participation at the earliest opportunity (21 CFR 50.24).

Single IRB Review and IRB Reliance

The NIH released a policy that became effective in January 2018, requiring the use of a single IRB for the review of multisite human subjects research funded by the NIH (2016). Subsequently, the revised Common Rule required the use of a single IRB for multisite research that became effective in January 2020. In a single IRB review model, institutions are required to document reliance on an IRB it does not operate and the delineation of responsibilities for each entity, the relying institution and reviewing IRB (45 CFR 46.103(e)). FDA regulations allow single IRB review of multisite clinical investigations, but it is not required.

The purpose of single IRB review was summarized in the NIH notice as follows (NIH 2016):

> The goal of this policy is to enhance and streamline the IRB review process in the context of multi-site research so that research can proceed as effectively and expeditiously as possible. Eliminating duplicative IRB review is expected to reduce unnecessary administrative burdens and systemic inefficiencies without diminishing human subjects protections. The shift in workload away from conducting redundant reviews is also expected to allow IRBs to concentrate more time and attention on the review of single site protocols, thereby enhancing research oversight.

In preparation for the federal mandates and to support and facilitate single IRB review, beginning in 2014, the NIH funded an initiative to develop a standard national master IRB reliance agreement (Cobb et al.). This evolved into the

Streamlined, Multisite, Accelerated, Resources for Trials (SMART) IRB Platform, the foundation of which is the SMART IRB Master Common Reciprocal IRB Authorization Agreement (SMART IRB Agreement), an umbrella agreement among the participating institutions (Cobb et al.). Eligible institutions can join the SMART IRB Agreement, which eliminates the need for participating institutions to negotiate a new IRB reliance agreement for each study reviewed under the single IRB review model (Cobb et al.). Once joining, an institution can decide on a study-by-study basis whether to use the Smart IRB Agreement (Cobb et al. 2019).

Ethics Committees

While the operation of IRBs in the USA is established by federal regulations, research ethics committees (RECs) internationally evolved from the Declaration of Helsinki, which has included independent committee review and oversight of biomedical research with human subjects since 1975 (WMA 2013). An excerpt from the Declaration of Helsinki is included in Fig. 4.

While regulations governing the requirements for ethics committee review and operation of ethics committees vary around the world, significant efforts toward harmonization were realized with the publication of the *International Ethical Guidelines for Biomedical Research Involving Human Subjects* in 1993 by the Council for International Organizations of Medical Sciences (CIOMS) (White 2020). These guidelines aimed to provide direction in the application of ethical principles from the Declaration of Helsinki, particularly in developing countries, and included a section on the constitution and responsibilities of ethical review committees (White 2020).

Excerpt on Ethics Committees from the Declaration of Helsinki (WMA 2013)

The research protocol must be submitted for consideration, comment, guidance and approval to the concerned research ethics committee before the study begins. This committee must be transparent in its functioning, must be independent of the researcher, the sponsor and any other undue influence and must be duly qualified. It must take into consideration the laws and regulations of the country or countries in which the research is to be performed as well as applicable international norms and standards but these must not be allowed to reduce or eliminate any of the protections for research subjects set forth in this Declaration.

The committee must have the right to monitor ongoing studies. The researcher must provide monitoring information to the committee, especially information about any serious adverse events. No amendment to the protocol may be made without consideration and approval by the committee. After the end of the study, the researchers must submit a final report to the committee containing a summary of the study's findings and conclusions.

Fig. 4 Excerpt on ethics committees from the Declaration of Helsinki (WMA 2013)

Summary and Conclusion

IRBs in the USA and ethics committees internationally have been a cornerstone in the review and oversight of clinical trials and other research involving human subjects since the 1970s, with the passing of the National Research Act in 1974 and amendment of the Declaration of Helsinki in 1975. IRBs are guided by the ethical principles of the Belmont Code and they carry out their responsibilities for the protection of the rights and welfare of human research subjects in accordance with the Common Rule (45 CFR 46) and/or FDA regulations at 21 CFR parts 50 and 56, depending on the scope and funding source of the research they are reviewing. In order to approve research, IRBs are required to ensure that risks are minimized and there is a favorable risk/benefit ratio, there is an adequate plan for data and safety monitoring and protection of privacy and confidentiality, that selection of subjects is equitable, and there is a plan to obtain and document informed consent from subjects. Additionally, IRBs give special consideration to the protection of potentially vulnerable subject populations. The changing research landscape and some highly publicized tragedies led to calls for reform around the turn of the 21st century, which resulted in development of programs for the accreditation of IRBs and institutional human research protection programs, a revised Common Rule that became effective in 2019, and the trend toward single IRB review of multisite studies. While responsibility for the protection of human subjects is shared among multiple parties, IRBs and ethics committees play a critical role in the review and oversight of clinical trials and research with human subjects.

Key Facts

- IRBs, first mandated by US law in 1974, are established in accordance with federal regulations to review and monitor clinical trials and other research with human subjects.
- IRBs help to ensure protection of the rights and welfare of human subjects by applying the ethical principles of the Belmont Code, respect for persons, beneficence, and justice.
- IRBs consider the regulatory criteria for approval of research, including plans to obtain and document informed consent from research participants.
- IRBs may exist within the institution where research is being conducted or institutions can rely on an external IRB with a written agreement. Single IRB review of multisite studies is mandated by NIH policy and the Common Rule.
- Outside the USA, independent review of research with human subjects is conducted by ethics committees.

Cross-References

▶ Clinical Trials, Ethics, and Human Protections Policies
▶ Consent Forms and Procedures

References

Beecher HK (1966) Ethics and clinical research. N Engl J Med 274(24):1354–1360. https://doi.org/10.1056/NEJM196606162742405

Cobb N, Witte E, Cervone M, Kirby A, MacFadden D, Nadler L, Bierer BE (2019) The SMART IRB platform: a national resource for IRB review for multisite studies. J Clin Transl Sci 3(4):129–139. https://doi.org/10.1017/cts.2019.394

Department of Health and Human Services (2011) Human subjects research protections: enhancing protections for research subjects and reducing burden, delay, and ambiguity for investigators. Fed Register 76(143):44512–44531. https://www.federalregister.gov/documents/2011/07/26/2011-18792/human-subjects-research-protections-enhancing-protections-for-research-subjects-and-reducing-burden. Accessed 26 Jun 2021

Department of Health and Human Services, FDA (2017) IRB Waiver or alteration of informed consent for clinical investigations involving no more than minimal risk to human subjects guidance for sponsors, investigators, and institutional review boards. https://www.fda.gov/media/106587/download. Accessed 26 Jun 2021

Department of Health and Human Services, NIH (1998) Protection of human subjects: categories of research that may be reviewed by the Institutional Review Board (IRB) through an expedited review procedure. Fed Register 63(216):60364–60367. https://www.hhs.gov/ohrp/regulations-and-policy/guidance/categories-of-research-expedited-review-procedure-1998/index.html. Accessed 4 Jun 2021

Department of Health and Human Services OHRP and FDA (2017) Minutes of Institutional Review Board (IRB) meetings guidance for institutions and IRBs. https://www.hhs.gov/ohrp/minutes-institutional-review-board-irb-meetings-guidance-institutions-and-irbs.html-0. Accessed 26 Jun 2021

Emanuel EJ, Wood A, Fleischman A, Bowen A, Getz KA, Grady C, Levine C, Hammerschmidt DE, Faden R, Eckenwiler L, Muse CT, Sugarman J (2004) Oversight of human participants research: identifying problems to evaluate reform proposals. Ann Intern Med 141(4):282–291. https://doi.org/10.7326/0003-4819-141-4-200408170-00008

Harkness J, Lederer SE, Wikler D (2001) Laying ethical foundations for clinical research. Bull World Health Organ 79(4):365–366

International Committee of Medical Journal Editors (2019) Recommendations for the conduct, reporting, editing, and Publication of scholarly work in Medical Journals. http://www.icmje.org/icmje-recommendations.pdf. Accessed 1 Jul 2021

Menikoff J, Kaneshiro J, Pritchard I (2017) The common rule, updated. N Engl J Med 375:613–615. https://doi.org/10.1056/NEJMp1700736

National Commission for the Protection of Human Subjects of Biomedical and Behavioral Research (1978) Reports and recommendations institutional review boards. https://www.hhs.gov/ohrp/regulations-and-policy/belmont-report/access-other-reports-by-the-national-commission/index.html. Accessed 30 Jun 2021

National Commission for the Protection of Human Subjects of Biomedical and Behavioral Research (1979) The Belmont report. https://www.hhs.gov/ohrp/sites/default/files/the-belmont-report-508c_FINAL.pdf. Accessed 4 Jun 2021

National Institutes of Health (2016) Final NIH policy on the use of a single institutional review board for multi-site research. NOT-OD-16-094. https://grants.nih.gov/grants/guide/notice-files/NOT-OD-16-094.html. Accessed 1 Jul 2021

Office for Human Research Protections (OHRP) (2021) Assurance process frequently asked questions. https://www.hhs.gov/ohrp/register-irbs-and-obtain-fwas/fwas/assurance-process-faq/index.html. Accessed 1 Jul 2021

Rice TW (2008) The historical, ethical, and legal background of human-subjects research. Respir Care 53(10):1325–1329

Shalala D (2000) Protecting research subjects – what must be done. N Engl J Med 343(11):808–810. https://doi.org/10.1056/NEJM200009143431112

Steinbrook R (2002) Improving protection for research subjects. N Engl J Med 346(18):1425–1430. https://doi.org/10.1056/NEJM200205023461828

US Congress Senate (1974) (Reprint of) National Research Act. https://www.govinfo.gov/content/pkg/STATUTE-88/pdf/STATUTE-88-Pg342.pdf. Accessed 4 Jun 2021

U.S. Government Printing Office (1949) The Nuremberg Code: Trials of war criminals before the Nuremberg military tribunals under control council law No. 10, vol 2. pp. 181–182. https://history.nih.gov/display/history/Nuremberg+Code. Accessed 4 Jun 2021

White MG (2020) Why human subjects research protection is important. Ochsner J 20(1):16–33. https://doi.org/10.31486/toj.20.5012

World Medical Association (2013) WMA Declaration of Helsinki – ethical principles for medical research involving human subjects as amended by the 64th WMA General Assembly, Fortaleza, Brazil. https://www.wma.net/policies-post/wma-declaration-of-helsinki-ethical-principles-for-medical-research-involving-human-subjects/. Accessed 4 Jun 2021

Data and Safety Monitoring and Reporting 37

Sheriza Baksh and Lijuan Zeng

Contents

Abstract

Data safety and monitoring boards (DSMB) are comprised of a group of clinical experts, statisticians, and other representatives with pertinent experience, who collectively monitor the data and conduct of ongoing clinical trials to ensure the safety of trial participants and the integrity of the trial. Over the years, the frequency of the use of a DSMB has increased; its mandate has been expanded to evaluate interim efficacy results, make recommendations for early termination of a trial, conduct sample size reassessments, and support the technical aspects of

S. Baksh (✉)
Johns Hopkins Bloomberg School of Public Health, Baltimore, MD, USA
e-mail: sbaksh4@jhu.edu

L. Zeng
Statistics Collaborative, Inc., Washington, DC, USA

© Springer Nature Switzerland AG 2022
S. Piantadosi, C. L. Meinert (eds.), *Principles and Practice of Clinical Trials*,
https://doi.org/10.1007/978-3-319-52636-2_209

a trial through other recommendations. Given the complex issues a DSMB may face, it is important for a DSMB to gain the support the members need from relevant parties in order to function effectively and independently and to make informed judgments. This chapter starts by introducing when a DSMB is warranted, and provides guidance on the formation of a DSMB, highlighting approaches to ensuring adherence to data confidentiality and principles of independence. The chapter then provides an overview of different types of DSMB meetings, templates for a DSMB charter, and considerations for open and closed reports. Lastly, a listing of guidance documents on DSMB from regulatory agencies and others is provided for reference.

Keywords

Data Monitoring Committee · Data Safety Monitoring Board · Interim data sharing

Introduction

A data and safety monitoring board (DSMB), also known as a data monitoring committee (DMC), or an independent data and safety monitoring committee (IDMC), serves an integral part of many trials in ensuring study participant safety, assessing data integrity, and monitoring study progress. In this chapter, we will use DSMB as an umbrella term to refer to data and safety monitoring boards, data monitoring committees, and independent data and safety monitoring committee.

A study's DSMB serves as an independent resource for study investigators and sponsors to ensure the integrity of the data, the ethical conduct of the study, and the safety of study participants. DSMBs are often formed as part of large, phase 3, multicenter clinical trials, but they may be also used in smaller, phase 1 and 2 clinical trials, where study participants are considered to comprise a vulnerable population or when interventions are high risk. Additionally, DSMBs may be needed in emergency trials, when consent might be waived (Eckstein 2015). The independence of a DSMB enables study recommendations to be made in the best interests of the study population and for the maximum benefit for the intended target population. Note that not all trials need DSMB. For example, having a DSMB may not be practical for trials with fast enrollment or short duration, nor would it be necessary for trials for non-critical indications or low-risk investigational drugs.

The DSMB can have a variety of duties based upon the needs of a particular study or request from the study Sponsor. These are often outlined in a DSMB charter or a data and safety monitoring plan (DSMP) that the DSMB, study investigators, and study Sponsor agree upon at the beginning of the study. Depending on the timing of the formation of the DSMB, the DSMB may have varying input on the development of the study protocol. Among their duties are reviewing study protocols, statistical analysis plans, consent documents, and other participant facing documents, advising the trial's Steering Committee, evaluating data for stopping the trial, and reviewing interim analyses (Clemens et al. 2005). Through the course of the study, the DSMB periodically meets to review and discuss the emerging data and the study performance so as to provide recommendations in line with the jurisdiction outlined in the charter. Recommendations may stem from the discussions in these meetings. A summary of the recommendations from the meeting may also be shared with the institutional review boards and other regulatory bodies to keep them abreast of any potential safety concerns for study participants.

While not explicitly required for all clinical trials, the jurisdiction for DSMBs has been spelled out by various regulatory and governmental agencies across the world. While there might be slight variations in what each agency requires, each of these governing bodies outlined the following as integral to a functional and effective DSMB: primacy of patient safety, ensuring data integrity, and continual oversight of study performance metrics. Table 1 lists key guidance documents that outline the purview of DSMBs from various regulatory agencies across the world. Investigators undertaking clinical trials in specific countries should seek to abide by requirements outlined in the guidance documents pertinent to the countries in which their trials are being conducted. While this list is not exhaustive, it provides a sample of what one can expect when organizing a DSMB across countries.

Table 1 Guideline documents for DSMBs by country/multi-governmental organizations

Country/Multi-Governmental Organizations	Governing body	Document
United States	National Institutes of Health Food and Drug Administration	NIH Policy for Data and Safety Monitoring (National Institutes of Health 1998) Guidance for clinical trial sponsors: establishment and operation of clinical trial data monitoring committees (FDA 2006)
European Union	European Medicines Agency	Guideline on Data Monitoring Committee (European Medicines Agency 2005)
Japan	Pharmaceuticals and Medical Devices Agency	Guideline on Data Monitoring Committee (PFSB/ELD notification No.0404-1) (Pharmaceutical and Food Safety Bureau 2013)
Australia	National Health and Medical Research Council	Data Safety Monitoring Boards (DSMBs) (National Health and Medical Research Council 2018)
Brazil	Agência Nacional de Vigilância Sanitária, Ministry of Health	Resolution of the Board of Directors – RDC No. 9 (ANVISA 2015)
Tanzania	Tanzania Food and Drugs Authority	Guidelines for Application to Conduct Clinical Trials in Tanzania (Tanzania Food and Drugs Authority 2017)

DSMB Organization

Formation

Once a study has been funded and initial planning is underway, Sponsors may elect to appoint a DSMB to assist with study oversight. One goal in forming an effective DSMB is to ensure the expertise necessary for monitoring the risks and benefits to study participants with a limited number of individuals. In some instances, an ethicist or patient advocate, or both, as part of the DSMB might be prudent. Members with this perspective can be especially helpful when the study involves participants for whom consent is waived or for whom their condition or the studied intervention is of a sensitive or controversial nature. While the optimal number of DSMB members is often up for debate, the expertise of the members should be balanced for discussion of trial issues and consensus formation.

The independence of a DSMB is essential in order that members consider both the safety of trial participants as well as the potential risk and benefits to the intended target patient population for the intervention under study. This holistic approach to trial integrity depends on the DSMB's independence from competing interests, research activities, and financial incentives. Without these assurances, both those charged with study oversight, as well as the general public, cannot be assured that the recommendations stemming from the DSMB are in the best interest of patient safety and their corresponding benefit-risk profile. There are many ways to protect against potential or perceived bias. Among these strategies is a disclosure of conflict of interests (COI) at the time of DSMB formation and at the beginning of each data review.

In some situations, DSMB may choose to designate voting and non-voting members. In these situations, both voting and non-voting members participate in discussions of study data; however, the voting members are tasked with deciding upon study recommendations, including determination of continuation with recruitment. Best practices typically recommend against this however, and instead advocate for recommendations stemming from consensus views in the closed session (Fleming et al. 2017). While compositions may vary from trial to trial, DSMBs may have a clinical expert, statistician, clinical trialist, patient advocate or representative, and/or a Sponsor representative (Fig. 1). Non-voting members of the DSMB tend to be those from the investigative team, and the voting members are generally those who remain independent from the study activities. Including sponsor representatives in the closed sessions of a DSMB is more common in government-sponsored trials than in industry-sponsored trials, where industry sponsors usually hire an Independent Statistical Reporting Group (ISRG) for preparing and presenting closed and/or open reports to DSMB (Fig. 2). Given that the principal investigator is steeped in the clinical area, he/she may recommend individuals best suited to adjudicate patient safety and interests for a disease area, but the Sponsor ultimately signs off on the members for the DSMB. Members of the clinical study team are not typically present in either the open or closed session of the DSMB meeting; however, the principal investigator may attend the open portion of the meeting to provide a scientific and operational update of the study, and answer questions from the DSMB. Study

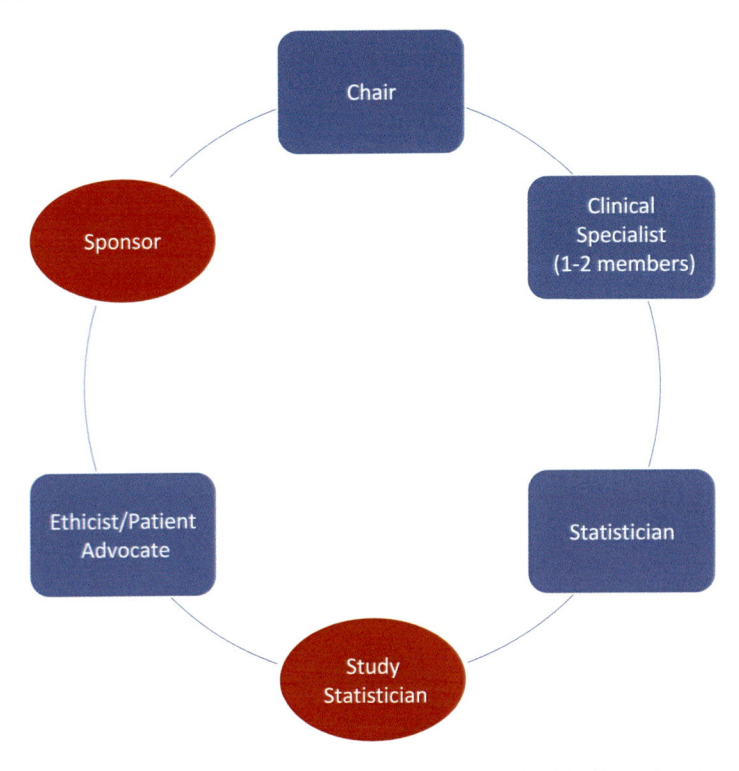

Fig. 1 Example of DSMB composition in government-sponsored trials. *Typical voting members are shown in blue rectangles, and typical non-voting members are shown in red ovals*

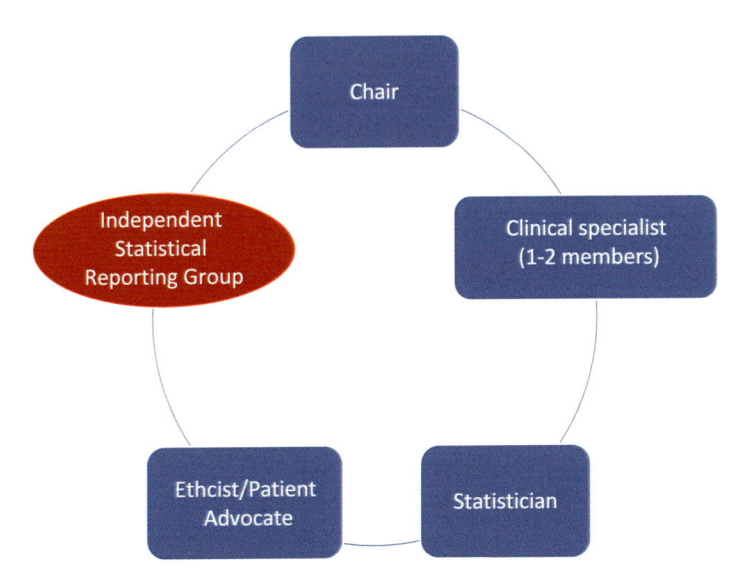

Fig. 2 Example of DSMB composition in industry-sponsored trials. *Voting members are shown in blue rectangles, and non-voting members are shown in red ovals*

statisticians (in government-sponsored trials) and members of ISRG (in industry-sponsored trials) may present or orient the DSMB to the study materials, explain the analyses that were conducted as well as any assumptions around those analyses.

The study Sponsor will appoint a chair for the DSMB. This individual is usually either an expert in the clinical area under study or a statistician. The chair will be tasked with running the flow of the meeting, coordinating with other DSMB members for consensus on recommendations, and providing a central voice for any clinical concerns with study conduct. The chair will communicate with the Sponsor to relay the DSMB's recommendations on continuance of the study. This recommendation is often also shared with the IRBs for studies. Because of the influential nature of this role, it is imperative that the DSMB chair is able to lead the group, encourage all members to express their views, and forge a consensus.

Charter

The DSMB charter serves as a guideline for DSMB operations, outlining DSMB responsibilities, providing principles for guiding DSMB decisions, and describing procedures and workflow for the DSMB (Herson 2017; Fleming et al. 2017). The trial sponsor usually prepares a draft charter which is later reviewed collectively by the sponsor, DSMB, ISRG, and any other key parties involved. Table 2 provides an outline of the organization of a typical DSMB charter.

Although the DSMB may vary in composition and practices depending on the study, core elements of the DSMB charter remain similar across studies. Templates for DSMB charters have been proposed in reference books (e.g., Ellenberg et al. 2019; Herson 2017). DAMOCLES, (Data Monitoring Committees: Lessons, Ethics, Statistics) Study Group (DAMOCLES Study Group, 2005) also provides templates for DSMB charters.

Meeting Types

The types of DSMB meetings that are held during the trial should be described in the DSMB Charter. The objectives, frequency, and schedule of meetings are generally decided upon during the formation of the DSMB in conjunction with the investigators and Sponsor. The main meeting types are as follows:

Initial/Organizational/Kick-Off Meeting

The initial DSMB meeting, also known as the *organizational* or *kick-off* meeting, should ideally be held prior to the first patient first visit. During this meeting, DSMB members can get acquainted with each other and the sponsor's study team, exchange thoughts on the study design, and share their own experiences and insights. The sponsor or investigator usually presents the current version of the protocol and DSMB charter, and the independent reporting statistician may present the draft

Table 2 Example of Charter contents	1. Introduction *(A brief description of trial information; purpose and key parties involved)*
	2. Committee members/organization
	3. Confidentiality, independence, conflict of interest disclosure
	4. Committees related to safety or trial conduct
	5. Responsibilities of the parties involved
	a. DSMB (Chair, Statistician, other members)
	b. Sponsor or its designee
	c. Independent Statistical Reporting Group
	d. Contract Research Organization
	e. Executive Committee/Steering Committee
	6. DSMB meetings
	a. Types of meeting: Kick-off/Initial/Organizational meeting; safety review; interim analysis; final closure meeting; ad-hoc meeting
	b. Meeting frequencies and format (in-person or teleconference)
	c. Quorum
	d. Voting or reaching consensus
	7. Meeting documentation
	a. Open session minutes/notes
	b. Closed session minutes/notes
	c. Executive session minutes/notes
	d. DSMB recommendation
	8. Data review plan
	a. Safety review contents
	b. Efficacy review contents
	9. Interim analysis plan
	a. Statistical guidelines
	10. Organization diagram and data flow
	11. Communication flow related to
	a. Safety concerns
	b. Pre-specified interim analysis results
	c. Regular safety review meeting recommendation
	12. Duration, disbandment of DSMB
	13. Appendix
	a. Recommendation form format
	b. DSMB contact information
	c. Sponsor key personnel contact information
	d. Independent statistical group contact information

report templates to solicit any feedback from the DSMB during the early stages of interaction. This is a valuable opportunity for study investigators to gather input from other leaders in the clinical field.

To have a productive meeting, the study materials such as protocols, important forms, patient-facing materials, the draft DSMB charter, and other relevant materials should be made available to the DSMB *prior* to the initial meeting. Shortly after the meeting, the Sponsor or DSMB, or both will approve and sign the charter, according to the Sponsor's SOPs.

Meetings Following First Patient First Visit

The DSMB Charter should outline how frequently the DSMB will be meeting. Soon after the initial meeting, a representative of the ISRG will schedule the first data review meeting, which usually takes place after a specified number of patients are enrolled, or at a pre-specified timeframe, whichever occurs first. Because of the inherent uncertainty of rate of enrollment, it is operationally easier to meet at a pre-specified time, in that the meeting can be scheduled ahead of time.

In cases where enrollment is slow, having the first data review meeting at a pre-specified timeframe (e.g., at 6 months after first patient first visit) ensures that the DSMB have an opportunity to review available data from patients already enrolled, monitor performance metrics, and assess safety profiles on the study drug. In scenarios where enrollment is much faster than expected, the first data review meeting can be held on a date earlier than originally planned.

Safety Review Meetings

The frequency of safety review meetings specified in the charter depends on the study's disease areas, study design, expected accrual, and expected safety profile from previous studies (when applicable). For example, oncology trials commonly hold safety review meetings every three or four months, biannually, or annually. On the other hand, in trials of orphan diseases trials where sample size is inherently small, the DSMB may meet once data from a threshold number of new patients become available to review data from newly enrolled patients, as well as cumulative data from all enrolled.

Interim Analysis Review Meetings

To control the overall type-I error rate of the trial, the criteria, statistical analyses, and actions taken toward each potential outcome for interim analyses should be pre-specified in the protocols, DSMB charters, statistical analysis plan (SAP), and/or additional interim analysis plan documents. Refer to ▶ Chap. 59, "Interim Analysis in Clinical Trials" for more details on interim analysis.

Ad-hoc Meetings

Between pre-specified safety and efficacy review meetings, the DSMB and Sponsor may request ad-hoc meetings to review ad-hoc analyses, address emerging safety issues from monthly safety reports (or SAE narratives), or discuss important new information external to trials. When the DSMB requests an ad-hoc meeting, the details of the meetings should not be communicated to the Sponsor until the conclusion of the trial unless the DSMB issues a recommendation to modify or terminate the trial in response to findings from the meetings. The documentation for the ad-hoc meetings should still follow the same process as the periodic data review meetings. Note that the implications of additional analyses should be considered and factored into the alpha-spending as specified in the SAP *a priori*.

Final Results/End-of-Trial Meeting

As the trial results become available after the final database lock, Sponsors may plan a meeting (also known as the End-of-Trial Meeting) to share with the DSMB the final analysis results and interpretation. Some sponsors may choose to present a press release of the study results; some sponsors may release a publication draft with the DSMB directly. Holding a Final Results meeting is a valuable opportunity for the sponsors to solicit any feedback from the DSMB regarding their experience during the course of the trial.

Meeting Settings: In-person vs Remote

The actual format of various DSMB meeting will depend on the scheduling, DSMB preferences, and complexity of issues to be discussed at the meeting. In-person DSMB meetings, which often allow for more effective interactions and communication, are preferred at the initial meeting, interim efficacy/futility analysis meeting, final meeting and/or other pre-specified review meeting.

For example, it is generally preferable to have an in-person meeting for the study kick-off. This allows DSMB members to get familiarized with each other and share their experiences. When an important decision is made regarding whether the DSMB is recommending early termination of a study due to safety, efficacy, or futility, it is valuable to have DSMB members in the same room, if possible, in order to assess the benefit and risk profiles of study drugs carefully, thoughtfully exchange their opinions and concerns, and finally come to a consensus had there been conflicting feedback. Moreover, having the DSMB meet in-person on a regular basis (e.g., annually) is recommended. However, meeting in-person may not always be necessary or efficient. Once the DSMB becomes very familiar with the trial or has observed no major safety issue after numerous meetings, it may be sufficient to meet by teleconference or videoconference. Meeting in-person may not be possible for ad-hoc discussions on emerging trial issues given the short notice and not practically feasible if the DSMB needs to closely monitor the trial population and meet frequently (i.e., every other week) to review new information.

Quorum

DSMB members should make every attempt to attend each meeting either in-person or by teleconference. However, in cases where not all members can be present, the DSMB Chair, or designee, should contact any absent individual before or after the meeting, or both, to obtain their opinion in writing after their review of all materials discussed during the meeting. The inclusion of opinions from absent members is at the discretion of the DSMB, as outlined and pre-specified in the charter.

Usually, at a minimum, the DSMB Chair and the DSMB Statistician should be present to hold a meeting. However, many charters require that all voting members be present, unless there are extenuating circumstances, for making a recommendation to the Sponsor related to early termination or any other modification of study protocol.

Independence

To provide an objective assessment of the benefit and risk profile of study drugs and make recommendations on the studies, members of the DSMB must remain independent and avoid all COIs that could affect their decision making. COIs can arise in many situations – some are easier to ascertain (for example, financial or research interests), while others can be harder to avoid or cannot be fully eliminated. For example, owning shares or investing in the sponsor's company stocks are obvious financial COIs, which preclude one's eligibility from serving on the committee.

DSMB members usually receive some honorarium (financial compensation) from the sponsors for their time serving on the boards; however, the amount of the honorarium should not be so high that it might potentially bias the DSMB's decision making. For more details on financial COIs, refer to ▶ Chap. 28, "Financial Conflicts of Interest in Clinical Trials."

Other than financial incentives, potential research-driven or intellectual COIs are also common among clinical and statistical experts who are usually involved in or serve as consultants for multiple research projects. In general, the investigators in a trial may not serve on a DSMB for a competing trial. One may not even serve as the DSMB for competing trials at the same time to avoid inadvertently sharing confidential information across trials.

It is not, however, uncommon for a single DSMB to monitor multiple ongoing trials in the same or related programs as this allows the DSMB to more efficiently make informed recommendation based on information from the associated trials. Requiring members to be completely free from any COIs is difficult to achieve given the varying subject matter expertise required on each board. As such, full disclosure of any potential COI is critical to avoid compromising the DSMB's recommendations as the trial proceeds. If, through the course of the study, any of these tenets of independence have changed, the members should disclose their status to the chair of the DSMB and the study Sponsor who will decide whether the member is still sufficiently independent to remain on the Board.

Confidentiality

Maintaining confidentiality of all interim information (data, analyses, meeting discussions, documentations, etc.) from an ongoing trial is one of the most crucial principles to protect the integrity and credibility of the trial.

In general, limited trial data by aggregated treatment groups can be presented in the open session to facilitate an informative discussion between sponsors and the DSMB to address issues related to trial conduct or management (e.g., enrollment, dropout, protocol deviations, or timeliness of data from different sources).

Unblinded comparative safety and efficacy data should be accessible only to the DSMB and ISRG. The FDA Guidance (2006) states: "Even for trials not conducted in a double-blind fashion, where investigators and patients are aware of individual treatment assignment and outcome at their sites, the summary evaluations of comparative unblinded treatment results across all participating centers would usually not be available to anyone other than the DSMB."

Although it may be tempting to use positive trial data from interim analyses to inform subsequent planning of product development, caution needs to be taken for interpretating and relying on the immature trial results from interim analyses as studies (Woloshin et al. 2018; Wayant and Vassar 2018) have shown inconsistent results in magnitude and even direction between interim assessments and final analyses at the end of the trials. The spread of unreliable interim comparative efficacy data may adversely affect patient adherence to study drugs, recruitment, and long-term follow-up (Ellenberg et al. 2019). Inappropriate release of interim data could even lead to early termination due to breach of confidentiality (see example below regarding the LIGHT trial, Nissen et al. 2016). The FDA Guidance on Establishment and Operation of Clinical Trials Data Monitoring Committees (2006) states the following:

> Knowledge of unblinded interim comparisons from a clinical trial is generally not necessary for those conducting or sponsoring the trial; further, such knowledge can bias the outcome of the study by inappropriately including its continuing conduct or the plan of analyses. Unblinded interim data and the results of comparative interim analysis, therefore, should generally not be accessible by anyone other than DSMB members or the statistician(s) performing these analyses and presenting to the DSMB.

In some cases, the DSMB needs to notify the Sponsor and release safety data to Sponsors who will inform regulatory agencies. When DSMBs observe an increased risk in certain safety events, the committee may raise the concern to the Sponsor and recommend informing investigators and patients. The DSMB may recommend collecting additional information to support further safety reviews, or on some occasions, modifying the trial procedures to protect patients in the trial. DSMBs, in this case, may share relevant safety data with limited individuals from the Sponsor to support subsequent procedures.

In anticipating the need to release unblinded data and meeting materials from the DSMB, a data access plan or other relevant SOPs is important to limit the spread of confidential information by specifying when the data could be shared, who will have access, and how unblinded materials and results will be communicated or transferred. Often, the Sponsor may appoint a 'firewalled' group, internally or externally (e.g., members from Executive Committees or Steering Committees), to receive these data if the DSMB recommendation warrants this.

The following example shows the detrimental impact of inappropriate handling of confidential interim trial data and highlights the importance of maintaining confidentiality of data from the ongoing trials to preserve the integrity of the ongoing trial.

Example *of early termination due to inappropriate public release of confidential interim data by the sponsor – the LIGHT trial* (Nissen et al. 2016)

The LIGHT trial compared the effect of naltrexone-bupropion to placebo on major adverse cardiovascular events (MACE) in overweight and obese patients with cardiovascular risk factors. The study used a two-stage noninferiority design, with an interim-analysis at 25% information time to rule out an upper bound of the 95% confidence internal of the hazard ratio (HR) exceeding 2.0 for regulatory approval, followed by a HR at the study completion to exclude 1.4 post-approval. After approximately 25% of the expected events, the first interim analysis was conducted; the data ruled out the null hypothesis as the HR did not exceed the 2.0 risk margin. The DSMB released the initial noninferiority analysis results to a core team from the sponsor, according to the data access plan, for regulatory filing while the blinded trial continued as planned. However, the Sponsor disseminated the unblinded results far beyond the intended core team. Even worse, the Sponsor publicly released the 25% interim analysis by applying for a patent. Subsequently, while the trial was ongoing, the Sponsor reported to the SEC that the HR was 0.59 (95% CI, 0.39–0.90) (SEC 2015). Around the same time, the 50% interim analysis time results became available, showing a HR of 0.88 (99.7% CI, 0.57–1.34), which was less favorable than the HR released in the SEC document. The study was terminated early because of the release of confidential trial data. Had the sponsors properly handled the confidential information from the IA, the study would have continued to completion so that information on the long-term safety profile of the study drug would have been learned.

DSMB Meetings

Structure of Meetings

DSMB meetings, much like many other types of study meetings, are often a dance between study investigators, experts in the field, and other vested parties, such as the study Sponsor. As such, the meeting structure reflects this power dynamic and enables important information to reach the DSMB members in the closed session, while offering others from the investigative team an opportunity to weigh in during the open session. Additionally, any interpretation of the recommendations, summaries, or subsequent actions taken must be done in light of these interpersonal dynamics. A typical data review meeting consists of an open session, a closed session, and optional executive and closed sessions (described below) afterwards. Each session has a predetermined roster, agreed upon and outlined in the DSMB charter. Adhering to these agreements maintains data integrity while allowing for recommendations and decision-making in light of study data presented by treatment group. Both the open and closed sessions may have an accompanying report with the data to be reviewed and discussed. We have provided a sample table of contents in Table 3. While not exhaustive, this list contains elements one might consider presenting in a meeting following the first patient, first visit.

Table 3 Components of a DSMB Report	*Open Session Report*
	1. Study overview
	2. Scientific updates
	3. Recent protocol amendment(s)
	4. Statistical analysis plan
	5. Performance metrics
	a. Screenings over time
	b. Randomizations over time
	c. Data currency
	d. Protocol deviations
	e. Withdrawals over time
	6. Baseline characteristics, aggregated
	7. Safety outcomes
	a. Adverse events, aggregated
	b. Serious adverse events, aggregated
	Closed Session Report
	All the following data are presented by treatment group
	1. Baseline characteristics
	2. Study disposition and treatment status
	3. Protocol deviations
	4. Efficacy outcomes
	5. Safety outcomes
	a. Adverse events
	b. Serious adverse events
	c. Unanticipated events
	d. Safety laboratory assessments

Open Session

The open session, attended by representatives from sponsors or investigators, the DSMB, and the ISRG, provides the DSMB opportunities to discuss with the Sponsor issues related to data quality, trial conduct, and trial management in a blinded manner. Topics include but are not limited to enrollment, dropouts, timeliness of data from different sources, protocol deviations, and inclusion/exclusion questions. The Sponsor can use this opportunity to seek advice from the DSMB on emerging trial issues.

The open sessions usually start by checking with the DSMB to assess if any new conflict of interest has arisen. The study team or Sponsor representative then may take the lead in presenting their perspectives on the trial progress and new information from relevant clinical programs or literature external to the trial that may have an impact on the study.

The Sponsor representatives should also provide updates regarding action items from the Sponsor from previous meetings if they were not resolved soon after the meetings. In general, the open session for a periodic safety data review should be concise to ensure that the DSMB has enough time to discuss contents by treatment group in the closed session. The open session is usually accompanied by a corresponding, confidential open session report which may contain a brief overview of the study with any protocol changes that have been made since the last DSMB meeting. There may also be a discussion of any proposed changes for the DSMB to provide input; however, the input from the DSMB should not be based on unblinded trial data. The Sponsor might include a copy of the DSMB charter and the statistical analysis plan as a quick reference for all in attendance. In addition to these study documents, the open report may contain performance metrics, baseline characteristics of the study population, and aggregated safety data. It is generally not advised to present efficacy data in the open session; however, if such data must be discussed in this forum, efficacy data should be presented in aggregate.

Some sponsors and study teams may choose to blind themselves from certain data domains even for open-label trials. For example, certain laboratory endpoints can be used to make tentative inference about statistical evidence concerning the safety or efficacy of the study drug. The DSMB needs to be cautious during the open session discussion to avoid inadvertently disclosing any unblinding information to the sponsors.

Closed Session

In the closed session, attended by DSMB and ISRG only, the DSMB reviews data on such issues as enrollment, trial status, safety, and efficacy presented by treatment group, and discusses overall benefit and risk profile of the study drugs. Variations abound as to how to approach a closed session: some DSMB Chairs may lead the discussions; others may assign members with different expertise to lead topics related to different issues; others may designate the high-level review to an ISRG statistician who is most familiar with data and reports and is able to highlight new information from the previous reviews, answer questions related to data, and interpret the presentations included in the closed session report. Regardless of the meeting styles, all DSMB members should have thoroughly reviewed the reports prior to the meetings.

To facilitate a productive data review and discussion during the closed session, the closed report should contain comprehensive data that are presented in a comprehensible manner (Buhr et al. 2018). Depending on the study objective and the focus of the review, the structure and contents of the reports may vary. Typically, the closed report starts with an executive summary table of the study, highlighting high-level study status, safety, and/or efficacy events by treatment group, followed by more detailed summaries presented in tables and figures. When detailed information on patients and events is needed, listings of event of interest are provided to supplement the review. The presentations in the closed reports should be presented by unblinded treatment groups to inform assessments on the relative benefit-to-risk profiles. In general, the closed reports should cover pre-specified efficacy assessments, adverse events with corresponding clinical details by treatment group, protocol deviations and subsequent actions, and any unanticipated events that may have occurred. These data are also discussed in light of the information presented in the scientific updates from the open session. The DSMB may discuss areas where they may like to request additional analyses or subgroup analyses to better understand the patterns that are emerging.

At the end of the closed session, the DSMB should strive to come to a consensus with respect to recommendations for the trial continuation, instead of using a majority vote approach. In situations where consensus cannot be met, a supermajority may be recorded with discussions and rationale for the decision-making documented in the closed session minutes. In addition, the DSMB can discuss and request ad-hoc analyses for the ISRG or Sponsor to address in follow-up meetings or correspondences.

Executive session

After the closed session, there may be an optional executive session limited to the actual members of the DSMB, where the DSMB has the opportunity to escalate action items to the Sponsor and communicate the meeting recommendations verbally. Whether an executive session is warranted is at the discretion of the DSMB. There is typically no data prepared specifically for discussion during the executive session. The outcome of this executive session, however, is recorded into the meeting minutes and might be shared with the IRB or other regulatory authorities.

Recommendations and Follow-up

A DSMB meeting can result in a variety of outcomes implicating the trajectory of the study. Typically, the DSMB can recommend one of four things: 1) continuation of the study without modification, 2) continuation of the study with recommended modifications, 3) termination of the study, or 4) suspension of enrollment pending resolution of issues or concerns. Each of these options carries considerable risks and benefits to the final interpretation of trial results and overall conclusions for the patient population. In addition to these overarching recommendations, the DSMB may also recommend that the investigative team amend the current protocol, change enrollment strategies, improve the speed and accuracy of data entry, open or close clinical sites, audit clinical sites, as well as other changes to trial activities. These suggested changes may emanate from changes in trial data or other external factors discussed during the meeting. After the conclusion of the meeting, the DSMB chair, in consultation with the other members of the DSMB, typically prepare a letter recommending continuation or termination of the trial along with any other suggested changes or additional analyses. This letter is then submitted to all the IRBs involved in the trial. Below, we highlight a few real-world examples of DSMB recommendations for consideration.

Example of external regulatory authorities intervening in trial conduct – the ATMOSPHERE trial (Swedberg et al. 2016)

The Aliskiren Trial to Minimize Outcomes in Patients with Heart Failure (ATMOSPHERE) trial provides an example of several external factors determining the trajectory of a clinical trial. In this study, participants were randomized to enalapril, aliskiren, or a combination of both drugs for the prevention of death from cardiovascular causes or hospitalization for heart failure. Aliskiren had previously been approved for patients with hypertension in the United States and European Union. Concurrent with ATMOSPHERE, aliskiren was also used in two similar trials, ASTRONAUT and ALTITUDE for slightly different populations. The DSMB for ATMOSPHERE also served as the DSMB for ASTRONAUT and they were aware of the accumulating data from ALTITUDE. ASTRONAUT, which had closed recruitment, showed a higher proportion of participants with renal dysfunction on aliskiren than on placebo (14.1% vs. 10.2%). ALTITUDE had accumulated 69% of projected events and reported increased adverse events associated with aliskiren. After reviewing the data from ALTITUDE and ASTRONAUT, but not ATMOSPHERE, the Clinical Trials Facilitation Group of the European Union requested to the sponsor Novartis discontinuing aliskiren in all patients with diabetes in ATMOSPHERE. Despite the assurance from the DSMB for ATMOSPHERE that they had carefully considered the data from ALTITUDE and ASTRONAUT in their recommendation to proceed, Novartis complied with the request of the Clinical Trials Facilitation Group to pause the treatment among diabetic patients. Because of the censoring of follow-up time during the treatment pause, the study had to extend for an additional year to meet the targeted number of events.

Example *of DSMB stopping trial based on primary outcome – the EOLIA trial* (Harrington and Drazen 2018)

In the ECMO to Rescue Lung Injury for Severe ARDS (EOLIA) trial, investigators studied the use of extracorporeal membrane oxygenation (ECMO) compared to standard of care in the treatment of severe acute respiratory distress syndrome (ARDS) (Combes et al. 2018). Because of the nature of the intervention, treating clinicians were unmasked to the treatment groups. Consequently, following the protocol those randomized to standard of care could, theoretically, be switched to ECMO during the course of treatment for rescue use. By the end of the trial, 28% of those randomized to the standard of care had switched to ECMO, with 57% of these crossover participants dying. The investigators noted that the high proportion of crossover inhibited their ability to draw conclusions about the use of ECMO for the primary outcome of mortality at 60 days. They did, however, see a significant effect of ECMO on the secondary outcome of treatment failure, defined as death in the ECMO group versus death or crossover in the standard of care group. After roughly three-quarters of the projected participants were enrolled, the DSMB stopped the trial for futility at the fourth interim analysis. Critics of this decision contend that had the trial continued, investigators might have had greater evidence for the secondary outcomes, some of which were trending toward favoring ECMO as a treatment. These critics encourage future DSMB members to treat the stopping guidelines as true guidelines and consider the impact of these decisions on other outcomes, both safety and efficacy, in the trial (Harrington and Drazen 2018).

Example *of emerging evidence influencing DSMB – the MOXCON trial* (Pocock et al. 2004)

The MOXonidine CONgestive Heart Failure (MOXCON) trial provides a classic example of a trial that was halted for safety concerns. The study was designed to investigate the use of moxonidine for the prevention of all-cause mortality in patients with NYHA class II–IV heart failure (Cohn et al. 2003). Initially powered to detect a 20% reduction in all-cause mortality, the study required 724 deaths. Of note, a concurrent dose-finding trial of moxonidine was not completed at the time of the start of MOXCON. While concerns were raised, MOXCON was permitted to start, despite the fact it was studying the highest dose used in the dose-finding study. An interim analysis when roughly one-quarter of the expected enrollment had occurred began showing a trend of increased mortality with the use of moxonidine. Despite the early indicators of increased risk for mortality, the small numbers of deaths combined with the lack of safety concerns in the then completed dose-finding trial led the DSMB to recommend continuation with a planned teleconference before the next 6-month safety analysis. At this analysis, a nominal p-value of less than 0.05 was observed, with 37 deaths in the moxonidine group and 20 deaths in the placebo group. After an investigation of the potential causes of the deaths, time to death, dosing, other serious adverse events, and baseline characteristics, the DSMB was put in the discomforting position of recommending termination after less than 10% of the expected deaths had occurred.

The DSMB then discussed this concern with the MOXCON Executive Committee and came to a consensus to recommend stopping randomization and closing out participants currently enrolled and being treated in the trial. They ultimately left the final decisions up to the MOXCON Senior Management. In their published debrief of this experience, the DSMB also noted that they recognized the difficult position the Executive Committee faced: continuing to proceed with MOXCON despite a contrary recommendation from the DSMB could potentially raise serious concerns about the interpretation of the results at the completion of the trial. The importance of this power dynamic and delineation of roles is especially evident at the time of decision-making.

Each of these examples provides unique snapshots of how DSMB recommendations can be unpredictable and determinative of a study's direction. Regardless of how impactful or mundane the recommendations, they are recommendations. Ultimately, decision-making for the study rests with the study Sponsor, as do the consequences of those decisions.

Summary and Conclusions

A DSMB provides an integral role in the conduct of many multicenter clinical trials. It serves as a check on competing interests in the name of participant safety and a balance to the inherent biases trial investigators and Sponsors may hold regarding the outcome of the trial. While they are not an overarching governing body for a clinical trial, their recommendations do carry weight, and when presented to the outside scientific community, can influence the interpretation of trial results as illustrated in the examples in this chapter. What can sometimes seem like a rudimentary task at the outset of a trial, developing a DSMB charter and defining the purview of this group can impede or enhance the utility of a DSMB in the conduct of the trial. It is imperative that the members of the DSMB, trial investigators, and trial

Sponsors carefully consider the needs of the study, the independence of the DSMB, and the potential concerns of the patient group impacted by the study results when developing this document. Through this collaborative and intentional effort, the DSMB can best serve in its capacity to monitor the trial for study integrity, safety, and efficacy.

Key Facts

1. DSMBs best serve as an independent check on data integrity and patient safety and as a balance to the decision-making power of study leadership.
2. While DSMBs provide recommendations for the trajectory of a trial, their suggestions command respect from the broader scientific community, as the recommendations balance competing interests of other study stakeholders.
3. Investing in the development of a comprehensive DSMB Charter, with consideration for the needs of the study and the patient population, will not lead to anticipating every possible decision to be made, but rather will provide the parameters for effective decision-making when difficult situations arise.

Cross-References

► Financial Conflicts of Interest in Clinical Trials
► Interim Analysis in Clinical Trials
► Issues for Masked Data Monitoring

References

ANVISA (2015) Resolution of the board of directors – RDC no. 9. Ministry of Health. Retrieved from http://antigo.anvisa.gov.br/documents/10181/3503972/RDC_09_2015_COMP.pdf/e26e9a44-9cf4-4b30-95bc-feb39e1bacc6

Buhr KA, Downs M, Rhorer J, Bechhofer R, Wittes J (2018) Reports to independent data monitoring committees: an appeal for clarity, completeness, and comprehensibility. Ther Innov Regul Sci 52(4):459–468. https://doi.org/10.1177/2168479017739268. Epub 2017 Nov 13

Clemens F, Elbourne D, Darbyshire J, Pocock S (2005) Data monitoring in randomized controlled trials: surveys of recent practice and policies. Clin Trials 2(1):22–33. https://doi.org/10.1191/1740774505cn064oa

Cohn JN, Pfeffer MA, Rouleau J, Sharpe N, Swedberg K, Straub M, ... Wright TJ (2003) Adverse mortality effect of central sympathetic inhibition with sustained-release moxonidine in patients with heart failure (MOXCON). Eur J Heart Fail 5(5):659–667. https://doi.org/10.1016/s1388-9842(03)00163-6

Combes A, Hajage D, Capellier G, Demoule A, Lavoué S, Guervilly C, ... Mercat A (2018) Extracorporeal membrane oxygenation for severe acute respiratory distress syndrome. N Engl J Med 378(21):1965–1975. https://doi.org/10.1056/NEJMoa1800385

DAMOCLES Study Group (2005) A proposed charter for clinical trial data monitoring committees: helping them do their job well. Lancet 365:711–722

Eckstein L (2015) Building a more connected DSMB: better integrating ethics review and safety monitoring. Account Res 22(2):81–105. https://doi.org/10.1080/08989621.2014.919230

Ellenberg SS, Fleming TR, DeMets DL (2019) Data monitoring committees in clinical trials: a practical perspective, 2nd edn. Wiley, Hoboken, NJ

European Medicines Agency (2005) Guideline on data monitoring committees. (EMEA/CHMP/ EWP/5872/03 Corr). European Medicines Agency, London. Retrieved from https://www.ema. europa.eu/en/documents/scientific-guideline/guideline-data-monitoring-committees_en.pdf

Fleming TR, DeMets DL, Roe MT, Wittes J, Calis KA, Vora AN, Meisel A, Bain RP, Konstam MA, Pencina MJ, Gordon DJ, Mahaffey KW, Hennekens CH, Neaton JD, Pearson GD, Andersson TL, Pfeffer MA, Ellenberg SS (2017) Data monitoring committees: promoting best practices to address emerging challenges. Clin Trials 14(2):115–123. https://doi.org/10.1177/ 1740774516688915. Epub 2017 Feb 1. PMID: 28359194; PMCID: PMC5380168

Harrington D, Drazen JM (2018) Learning from a trial stopped by a data and safety monitoring board. N Engl J Med 378(21):2031–2032. https://doi.org/10.1056/NEJMe1805123

Herson J (2017) Data and safety monitoring committees in clinical trials, 2nd edn. Taylor & Francis, Boca Raton, FL

National Health and Medical Research Council (2018) Data safety monitoring boards (DSMBs). (978-1-86496-004-4). National Health and Medical Research Council. Retrieved from www. nhmrc.gov.au/guidelines-publications/EH59C

National Institutes of Health (1998) NIH policy for data and safety monitoring. National Institutes of Health. Retrieved from https://grants.nih.gov/grants/guide/notice-files/not98-084.html

Nissen SE, Wolski KE, Prcela L et al (2016) Effect of naltrexone-bupropion on major adverse cardiovascular events in overweight and obese patients with cardiovascular risk factors: a randomized clinical trial. JAMA 315(10):990–1004. https://doi.org/10.1001/jama.2016.1558

Pharmaceutical and Food Safety Bureau (2013) Guideline on data monitoring committee (PFSB/ ELD notification No.0404-1). Ministry of Health, Labour and Welfare, Japan. Retrieved from https://www.pmda.go.jp/files/000232300.pdf

Pocock S, Wilhelmsen L, Dickstein K, Francis G, Wittes J (2004) The data monitoring experience in the MOXCON trial. Eur Heart J 25(22):1974–1978. https://doi.org/10.1016/j.ehj.2004. 09.015

Swedberg K, Borer JS, Pitt B, Pocock S, Rouleau J (2016) Challenges to data monitoring committees when regulatory authorities intervene. N Engl J Med 374(16):1580–1584. https:// doi.org/10.1056/NEJMsb1601674

Tanzania Food and Drugs Authority (2017) Guidelines for application to conduct clinical trials in Tanzania, 3rd edn. Retrieved from https://www.tmda.go.tz/uploads/publications/ en1554368837-TANZANIA%20CLINICAL%20TRIAL%20GUIDELINES-%202017.pdf

U.S. Food and Drug Administration (2006) Guidance for clinical trial sponsors: establishment and operation of clinical trial data monitoring committees. March 2006. Available at: https://www. fda.gov/media/75398/download

U.S. Securities and Exchange Commission (2015) From 8-K. Orexigen Therapeutics, Inc. File number 001-33415. March 3, 2015. Available at: https://www.sec.gov/Archives/edgar/data/ 1382911/000119312515074251/d882841d8k.htm

Wayant C, Vassar M (2018) A comparison of matched interim analysis publications and final analysis publications in oncology clinical trials. Ann Oncol 29:2384–2390. https://doi.org/10. 1093/annonc/mdy447

Woloshin S, Schwartz LM, Bagley PJ, Blunt HB, White B (2018) Characteristics of interim publications of randomized clinical trials and comparison with final publications. JAMA 319 (4):404–406. https://doi.org/10.1001/jama.2017.20653

Post-Approval Regulatory Requirements

38

Winifred Werther and Anita M. Loughlin

Contents

Abstract

Health authorities throughout the world have regulations for requesting additional research in the post-approval setting. This chapter focuses on the regulations in the USA and European Union (EU). The history of post-approval studies can be traced through changing regulations enforced by the US Food and Drug Administration (FDA) and the EU European Medicines Agency (EMA).

W. Werther (✉)
Center for Observational Research, Amgen Inc, South San Francisco, CA, USA
e-mail: wwerther@amgen.com

A. M. Loughlin
Corrona LLC, Waltham, MA, USA
e-mail: aloughlin@corrona.org

© Springer Nature Switzerland AG 2022
S. Piantadosi, C. L. Meinert (eds.), *Principles and Practice of Clinical Trials*,
https://doi.org/10.1007/978-3-319-52636-2_256

Post-approval studies are either clinical trials (interventional) or observational (non-interventional) studies. Choosing a study design may be influenced by the strengths and weaknesses of the design options and available data sources.

Imposed post-approval studies are reviewed for compliance by the regulatory agencies. For clinical trials that are ongoing at the time of approval, often these are classified as post-marketing commitment (PMC) in the USA or post-authorization measure (PAM) in the EU. Findings of these trials can be submitted to the health authorities for addition to the prescribing information. The FDA and EMA both track progress on PMC/PMRs and PAMs, respectively.

Post-approval studies are necessary to continually gather data on the safety and effectiveness of approved drugs. These studies are regulated by health authorities, included in registries (e.g., ClinicalTrials.gov, ENCePP), and tracked to completion. This chapter reviews the history of the regulations, terminology, study designs, and systematic reviews of the published post-approval studies.

Keywords

Post approval · Post marketing · Post authorization · Pharmacovigilance · Pharmacoepidemiologic

List of Abbreviations

CFR	Code of Federal Regulations
EMA	European Medicines Agency
EU	European Union
FDA	Food and Drug Administration
FDAAA	Food and drug Administration Amendments Act
MAH	Market authorization holder
PAES	Post-authorization efficacy study
PAM	Post-authorization measure
PAS	Post-authorization study
PASS	Post-authorization safety study
PMC	Post-marketing commitment
PMR	Post-marketing requirement
PREA	Pediatric Research Equity Act
REMS	Risk evaluation and mitigation strategy
USA	United States

Introduction

The collection of information on safety and efficacy of medical treatments often does not end with the approval of medical products. Health authorities throughout the world have regulations for requesting additional research in the post-approval setting. Post-approval research can include clinical trial methodologies, as well as observational studies.

The data included in regulatory submissions for approval of medical inventions, specifically drugs and devices, are limited by the scope of the pre-approval clinical trials. There may be limitations in safety and efficacy based on patient characteristics, duration of therapy, size of patient population, and the ability to identify rare outcomes. A few examples of when additional trials and studies may be requested by the regulatory agencies are as follows. First, if pre-approval or registrational studies were limited to specific age groups, additional studies in unstudied age groups likely to receive the treatment may be required. Second, if the outcome required for approval in a clinical trial is defined as event-free survival or progression-free survival, additional data collection to provide estimates for overall survival may be required in the post-approval setting. Lastly, rare safety outcomes are difficult to estimate in pre-approval trials, and for treatments for chronic diseases, large observational studies may be required to further quantify known safety events and to identify new safety events.

Some high-profile drug withdrawals, where risks outweighed the benefits to patients in the post-approval setting, have provided additional motivation in support of required post-approval safety studies. The following are two high-profile drug withdrawals. In 2004, the post-approval trials for rofecoxib (Vioxx) identified an increased risk of heart attack and stroke, which lead to its removal from the US market (Krumholtz 2007; Prakash and Valentine 2007). In 2005, the occurrence of progressive multifocal leukoencephalopathy leads to the issuance of a Food and Drug Administration (FDA) Drug Safety Communication and voluntary withdrawal from the market for natalizumab (Tysabri) (FDA 2018; Kappos et al. 2011). In the case of natalizumab, the drug was reintroduced to the market when its benefit-risk profile for the difficult-to-treat relapsing-remitting form of multiple sclerosis was maintained by minimizing the risk through patient selection, detailed safety monitoring recommendations for the early detection of PML, and management of PML recommendations. In addition, post-approval studies were conducted.

In this chapter, we will focus on the post-approval regulatory requirements in the USA and the European Union (EU). For terminology, in the USA, the term post marketing is used for drugs and post approval is used for medical devices, while in Europe, the term post authorization is used for both drugs and devices. In this chapter, we will use the term post approval to refer to post marketing and post authorization for drugs and devices. Regulatory agencies can require additional studies, or they may enter an agreement with a sponsor or market authorization holder (MAH) for additional studies that are deemed voluntary, and therefore not required. The history of required and voluntary post-approval studies can be traced through changes in regulations. This chapter will not address the conduct of clinical trials for new indications of approved drugs, as those trials while conducted in the post-approval setting are required to follow the same regulations for approval of a new drug.

History of US and EU Regulations

History of Post-Approval Studies in the USA

First, in the USA, the 1997 FDA Modernization Act introduced the requirement for the FDA regarding post-approval studies, as referred to in the US regulations as post-marketing studies or post-marketing requirements (PMRs). In 1999, the FDA published the rule regarding post-marketing commitment (PMC), which was defined as studies, including clinical trials, conducted by an applicant after FDA has approved a drug for marketing or licensing that were intended to further refine the safety, efficacy, or optimal use of a product or to ensure consistency and reliability of product quality. In 2006, as a complement to the final rule from 1999, the FDA issued a guidance for industry on PMCs. In 2007, the FDA Amendments Act (FDAAA), which clarified reasons for post-marketing studies, was signed into law by the US president. FDAAA included the new provision that gave the FDA the authority to require risk evaluation and mitigation strategy (REMS), in addition to PMR and PMC. In 2011, a new guidance for industry was released on post-marketing studies and clinical trials with implementation into Section 505(o)(3) of the Federal Food, Drug, and Cosmetic Act which stated that the FDA can require post-approval clinical trials and studies (FDA 2011). In this guidance, clinical trials were defined as any prospective investigation in which the applicant or investigator determines the method of assigning the drug product or other interventions to one or more human subjects, and studies were defined as all other investigations.

In the USA, with the 2007 FDAAA, there was a change in the rationale for requesting a post-approval study from a sponsor. Before 2007, the following three reasons were used when requiring post-marketing studies:

- Post-marketing studies or clinical trials to demonstrate clinical benefit for drugs approved under the Accelerated Approval requirements in 21 Code of Federal Regulations (CFR) 314.510 and 21 CFR 601.41
- Deferred pediatric studies (21 CFR 314.55(b) and 601.27(b)), where studies are required under the Pediatric Research Equity Act (PREA)
- Studies or clinical trials to demonstrate safety and efficacy in humans that must be conducted at the time of use of products approved under the Animal Rule (21 CFR 314.610(b)(1) and 601.91(b)(1))

After FDAAA in 2007, the reasons for a post-marketing study were broadened to:

- Assess a known serious risk related to the use of the drug
- Assess signals of serious risk related to the use of the drug
- Identify an unexpected serious risk when available data indicate the potential for a serious risk

There are four mechanisms that provide the FDA with the authority to require PMR. They are through Accelerated Approval, the Animal Rule, the Pediatric Research Equity Act, and FDAAA. These authorities are described in Table 1.

Table 1 Post-marketing requirement authorities of the US Food and Drug Administration. (Adapted from Wallach et al. 2018)

Authority	Year implemented	Purpose	Requirement
Accelerated Approval pathway	1992	To expedite the approval of novel drugs that treat serious diseases and fill unmet medical needs, on the basis of surrogate or intermediate endpoints "reasonably likely" to predict clinical benefit	FDA has the authority to require post-market studies or clinical trials to confirm efficacy
Animal Rule	2002	To allow for the approval of novel drugs when human efficacy studies and field trials are not ethical and feasible	When feasible and ethical, FDA can require post-market studies in humans
Pediatric Research Equity Act (PREA)	2003	To provide pediatric use information in drug product labeling for drugs and biological products developed for indications that occur in both adult and pediatric populations. FDA can approve novel drugs for use in adults without corresponding studies for the same indication in the relevant pediatric population	FDA can include deferred pediatric studies or clinical trials as post-marketing requirements
Food and Drug Administration Amendments Act (FDAAA), Section 505(o)(3)	2007; effective March 2008	To provide additional information for novel treatments approved under Section 505 of FDAAA or Section 351 of the Public Health Services Act	FDA can require post-market studies that assess known serious risks, signs of serious risks, or unexpected serious risks related to the use of a novel drug

History and Legal Framework of Post-Approval Studies in Europe

The European Medicines Agency (EMA), the EU Member States, and the European Commission are responsible for implementing and operating the legislation that deals with post-approval studies, as referred to in EMA legislation as post-authorization studies, including pharmacovigilance studies. Pharmacovigilance studies are research studies with the objective of studying drug safety. The EMA plays a key role in coordinating activities relating to post-approval studies by working with a wide range of stakeholders including the European Commission, pharmaceutical companies, national medicines regulatory authorities, patients, and healthcare professionals to ensure effective implementation and operation of the pharmacovigilance legislation, which includes post-authorization safety studies (PASS). Post-authorization efficacy studies (PAES) are another type of study conducted in the post-approval setting. However, PAES are not part of the pharmacovigilance legislation.

Post-Authorization Safety Study (PASS)

The 2010 European Pharmacovigilance Legislation created the legal framework for post-authorization studies (PAS), including PASS. This was the biggest change in EU regulations since 1995 and was implemented in 2012 (EMA 2012).

Based on Directive 2001/83/EC and Regulation (EC) No 726/2004, the EMA may require PAS (Goedecke 2017). The pharmacovigilance legislation includes directives and legislations that can be found at the EMA website (EMA 2012). The following text on the rationale for the directive and regulation is directly from the EMA website:

The development of the pharmacovigilance legislation was based on the observation that adverse drug reactions (ADRs), 'noxious and unintended' responses to a medicine, caused around 197,000 deaths per year in the EU.
Because of this, in 2005 the European Commission began a review of the European system of safety monitoring including sponsoring an independent study, as well as extensive public consultation through 2006 and 2007.
This process resulted in the adoption of a Directive and Regulation by the European Parliament and Council of Ministers in December 2010, bringing about significant changes in the safety monitoring of medicines across the EU.

Per the directive and regulation implemented in 2012 and the EMA website (EMA 2020a), a PASS is a study that is carried out after a drug has been authorized. The purpose of the PASS is to evaluate the safety and benefit-risk profile of a drug and support regulatory decision-making. A PASS aims to (1) identify, characterize, or quantify a safety hazard; (2) confirm the safety profile of a drug; or (3) measure the effectiveness of risk management measures. Risk management measures are activities carried out by the sponsor to assess the risks associated with drugs. Risk management measures are tracked in risk management plans (RMP). Sponsors are required to submit an RMP to the EMA when applying for a marketing authorization.

A PAS design is either clinical trial or observational. A PAS is either imposed or voluntary. The EMA's Pharmacovigilance Risk Assessment Committee (PRAC) is responsible for assessing the protocols of imposed PASS and for assessing their results. A voluntary PASS is conducted by sponsors on their own initiative. Non-imposed PAS that are requested by the EMA in RMPs are deemed voluntary PASS. An RMP includes activities agreed upon by EMA and sponsors to continually study the risks of a drug.

EMA has published guidance on the format and content of study protocols and final study reports for non-interventional studies, together with the PRAC assessment report templates. The guidance is based on Commission Implementing Regulation No 520/2012 of 19 June 2012, which was implemented in January 2013. For clinical trials, sponsors should follow the instructions in volume 10 of the rules governing medicinal products in the European Union (EU). Further guidance for PASS is available in the following document: Guideline on good pharmacovigilance practices: Module VIII – Post-authorisation safety studies (EMA 2017).

Post-Authorization Efficacy Studies (PAES)

In the EU, similar to PASS, PAES may be voluntary or imposed. However, the legislation behind the PAES is not the same as the pharmacovigilance regulations (EMA 2016). The PAES can be imposed by a competent authority, either centrally or nationally. One way that PAES can be imposed is within the scope of Delegated Regulation (EU) No 357/20141; it states:

- At the time of granting the initial marketing authorization (MA) where concerns relating to some aspects of the efficacy of the medicinal product are identified and can be resolved only after the medicinal product has been marketed [Art 9(4)(cc) of REG/Art 21a(f) of DIR]
- After granting of a MA where the understanding of the disease or the clinical methodology or the use of the medicinal product under real-life conditions indicates that previous efficacy evaluations might have to be revised significantly [Art 10a(1)(b) of REG/Art 22a(1)(b) of DIR]

Also, PAES can be imposed outside of the scope of Delegated Regulation (EU) No 357/2014. PAES may be imposed in the following specific situations:

- A conditional MA granted in accordance with Article 14(7) of Regulation (EC) No 726/2004
- A MA granted in exceptional circumstances and subject to certain conditions in accordance with Article 14(8) of Regulation (EC) No 726/2004 or Article 22 of Directive 2001/83/EC
- A MA granted to an advanced therapy medicinal product in accordance with Article 14 of Regulation (EC) No 1394/2007
- The pediatric use of a medicinal product in accordance with Article 34(2) of Regulation (EC) No 1901/2006
- A referral procedure such as initiated in accordance with Articles 31 or 107i of Directive 2001/83/EC or Article 20 of Regulation (EC) No 726/2004

The recommended study designs for PAES include randomized and non-randomized designs. Consideration for clinical trial and observational study methodologies is described in the PAES guidance document (EMA 2016) as follows:

Clinical trial design options for the design of PAES could include explanatory and pragmatic trials. Explanatory trials generally measure the benefit of a treatment under ideal conditions to establish whether the treatment works. Pragmatic trials examine interventions under circumstances that approach real-world practice, with more heterogeneous patient populations, possibly less-standardized treatment protocols and delivery in routine clinical settings as opposed to a research environment. Minimal or no restrictions may be placed on modifying dose, dosing regimens, co-therapies or comorbidities or treatment switching.

Non-randomized (for treatment) studies may be considered for investigating post-authorization benefits where one or more of the following situations apply: randomization is unethical or unfeasible, outcomes are infrequent, the generalizability of randomized trials is particularly limited, outcomes are highly predictable, or effect sizes are very large. Observational PAES may additionally be useful to identify effect modifiers, namely factors that result in important differences in the level of efficacy of the drug between patients within the authorized indication and which may not have been detectable in the pivotal trials conducted prior to authorization.

Post-Approval Terminology and Definitions

Terminology used by the FDA and EMA is described in the table below and includes term, definition, terminology usage, examples, timing, reporting, and registration. Briefly, the FDA uses the term risk evaluation and mitigation strategy (REMS) to track post-approval safety studies that can be either post-marketing requirement (PMR) or post-marketing commitment (PMC). However, PMR and PMC can be conducted outside of REMS. Timing and reporting are described in the table. The EMA uses post-authorization measures (PAMs) to track post-authorization safety studies (PASS) and post-authorization efficacy studies (PAES) (Tables 2 and 3).

Post-Approval Study Designs

Post-approval studies are either clinical trials (interventional) or observational (non-interventional) studies. Choosing a study design may be influenced by the strengths and weaknesses of the design options. The Table 4 below provides points to consider including for each study design: strengths, weaknesses, and usefulness in the post-approval setting.

Clinical Trials

Providing results from clinical trials in the post-approval setting can be necessary under many conditions. To name a few, confirmatory efficacy findings are required, patients with unique characteristics are studied, patients with new indications are studied, and efficacy measures have changed significantly during the conduct of the registrational trials.

Clinical trial designs may include pragmatic trials, as well as synthetic trials. Large pragmatic trials are trials where simple designs are used to study large numbers of patients with high external validity (Patsopoulous 2011). Synthetic trials are clinical trials that use real-world data or pooled clinical trial data to recreate

Table 2 Terminology for post-approval studies for the USA

Term	Definition	Terminology usage	Examples/components	Timing	Reporting	Registration
Risk evaluation and mitigation strategy (REMS)	A required risk management strategy that can include one or more elements to ensure that the benefits of a drug outweigh its risks	Describes the elements required in the risk management strategy	Elements of REMS: Medication guide; Patient package insert; Communication plan; Elements to assure safe use (ETASU); Implementation system	Before or at approval or after approval if FDA becomes aware of new safety information	Must include PMR and PMC updates	
Post-marketing requirement (PMR)	Clinical trials and studies required for any or all of three purposes: To assess a known serious risk related to the use of the drug; To assess signals of serious risk related to the use of the drug; To identify an unexpected serious risk when available data indicates the potential for serious risk	Describes all required post-marketing studies or clinical trials, including those required by four authorities: FDAAA, Pediatric Research, Accelerated Approval, Animal Rule	Observational pharmacoepidemiologic studies; Meta-analyses; Clinical trials with safety endpoint evaluated; Safety studies in animals; In vitro laboratory safety studies; Pharmacokinetic studies or clinical trials; Studies or clinical trials to evaluate drug interactions or bioavailability	At time of approval or after approval if FDA becomes aware of new safety information	Annual to FDA	Voluntary registration at ClinicalTrials.gov for clinical trials and studies

(continued)

Table 2 (continued)

Term	Definition	Terminology usage	Examples/components	Timing	Reporting	Registration
Post-marketing commitment (PMC)	Studies (including clinical trials), conducted by an applicant after FDA has approved a drug for marketing or licensing, that were intended to further refine the safety, efficacy, or optimal use of a product or to ensure consistency and reliability of product quality	Describes studies and clinical trials that applicants have agreed to conduct, but that will generally not be considered as meeting a statutory purpose and so will not be required	Drug and biologic quality studies Pharmacoepidemiologic studies on natural history of disease or background rates for adverse events in a population not treated with the drug Studies and clinical trials for non-serious risk or safety signals Clinical trials with primary endpoint related to further defining efficacy	At time of approval	Annual to FDA	Voluntary registration at ClinicalTrials.gov for clinical trials and studies

Reference: FDA REMS Overview_121110-cln.pdf from FDA website https://www.fda.gov/aboutfda/transparency/basics/ucm325201.htm

Table 3 Terminology for post-approval studies for the European Union

Term	Definition	Terminology usage	Examples/components	Timing	Reporting	Registration
Post-authorization measures (PAM)	Additional data post authorization, as it is necessary from a public health perspective to complement the available data with additional data about the safety and, in certain cases, the efficacy or quality of authorized medicinal products		PAMs fall within one of the following categories [EMA codes]: Specific obligation [SOB] Annex II condition [ANX] Additional pharmacovigilance activity in the risk management plan (RMP) [MEA] (e. g., interim results of imposed/non-imposed interventional/non-interventional clinical or nonclinical studies) Legally binding measure [LEG] (e. g., cumulative review following a request originating from a PSUR or a signal evaluation [SDA], Corrective Action/Preventive			

(continued)

Table 3 (continued)

Term	Definition	Terminology usage	Examples/components	Timing	Reporting	Registration
			Action (CAPA), pediatric [P46] submissions, MAH's justification for not submitting a requested variation) Recommendation [REC], e.g., quality improvement			
Post-authorization safety study (PASS)	Any study relating to an authorized medicinal product conducted with the aim of identifying, characterizing, or quantifying a safety hazard, of confirming the safety profile of the medicinal product, or of measuring the effectiveness of risk management measures	Includes clinical trials and non-interventional studies May be imposed (required) or voluntary (not required)	PASS categories in RMP for clinical trials or non-interventional: Category 1: imposed PASS Category 2: specific obligation Category 3: required as part of RMP Note: Categorization is from GVP V.B.6.3	As a condition of granting marketing authorization or after granting market authorization if there are concerns about risks of the authorized medicinal product	Imposed, non-interventional PASS reporting to PRAC within 12 months of end of data collection Abstract of results posted to EU PAS Register (www.encepp.eu)	Clinical trials must be registered at European Union Clinical Trials Portal and Database (www.clinicaltrialsregister.eu) Non-interventional studies must be registered at European Union Post-Authorization Study (EU PAS) Register (www.encepp.eu)

Post-authorization efficacy study (PAES)	Post-authorization efficacy studies (PAES) of medicinal products are studies conducted within the authorized therapeutic indication to complement available efficacy data in the light of well-reasoned scientific uncertainties on aspects of the evidence of benefits that should be, or can only be, addressed post-authorization Note: Not a legal definition, it is a working definition from EMA/PDCO/CAT/ CMDh/PRAC/ CHMP/261500/2015 Draft-scientic-guidance-post-authorisation-efficacy-studies-first-version_en.pdf	Clinical trials and non-interventional studies imposed for conditional marketing authorization or marketing authorization under exceptional circumstance and other conditions	From 2014 to 2017, all PAES have been clinical trials			Clinical trials must be registered at European Union Clinical Trials Portal and Database

Table 4 Strengths and weaknesses of common post-approval study designs

Design	Strengths	Weaknesses	Usefulness in post-approval setting
Clinical trial: randomized	Specify safety and/or efficacy outcomes Specify exposure For comparative trials, use randomization and masking to reduce bias	Operationally complex Size of study has limitations, and follow-up may result in long duration to answer question Limited generalizability	Answer specific safety/efficacy question identified in pre-approval setting
Clinical trial: pragmatic	Minimal criteria for exposure to mimic real-world use of approved product Simplified protocol compared to pre-approval trial protocols	Size of study can be large to compensate for diverse patient exposure data	Expected wide use of drug quickly to foster enrollment and faster study conduct
Clinical trial: synthetic	Data are already collected Comparative safety and efficacy possible	Not yet accepted by regulatory agencies	Conducted for exploratory or confirmative results
Observational: prospective cohort study	Identify incidence of safety event Accurate measurement of exposure	If outcome is rare, large sample size and long duration may be necessary Size and duration of study may drive up cost	Randomization is not ethical Studying exposed patients only; no need for control group
Observational: retrospective cohort study	Data are collected and available from administrative healthcare data or patient registries Identify incidence of safety event	Relies on previous documentation of exposures and outcomes Delay from approval until the data are available for retrospective review	When exposure period is short and data will accumulate quickly for timely analysis

clinical trial arms with the intent to provide comparative analyses within the data source or as comparators to external clinical trials. Synthetic trials provide comparative effectiveness results by analyzing existing data sources without collecting new information (Berry et al. 2017; Zauderer et al. 2019).

There are operational concerns when conducting trials in the post-approval setting including the need to maintain equipoise. In the accelerated/expedited approval setting, ongoing trials are typically listed as required post-approval trials so that the trials continue to completion. This is especially important if approvals are granted on surrogate outcomes. The ongoing trials will often provide hard outcomes, such as survival, as compared to disease progression.

Clinical trials in special populations, such as pediatric patients, may be conducted in the post-approval setting as part of a pediatric investigation plan. For diseases that occur rarely in pediatric populations, these trials are not typically completed at the time of filing for regulatory approval and thus continue in the post-approval setting.

Observational Studies

Observational studies complement interventional studies and are peculiarly suited for studies where randomization is not ethical, or for studying broader populations, specifically populations not well represented in clinical trials, and for understanding actual results (e.g., safety and effectiveness) in real-world practice. Pharmacoepidemiologic safety studies are designed to assess the risk associated with drug exposure and to test prespecified hypotheses (ISPE 2015; Berger et al. 2012). Guidance for the design and conduct of post-approval safety studies in the USA and EU has been developed. Table 5 provides some suggested sources for these guidance documents and guidelines for pharmacoepidemiologic research (Berger et al. 2012, 2017; Dreyer et al. 2010; ENCePP 2010, 2017; FDA 2013; ISPE 2015).

Table 5 Sources for guidance for observational studies for drug safety research

Guidance for safety studies
European Network of Centers for Pharmacoepidemiology and Pharmacovigilance (ENCePP), Guidelines on Good Pharmacovigilance (GVP) – Module VIII – Post-authorization safety studies (Revision 3). 2017. Online: https://www.ema.europa.eu/en/documents/scientific-guideline/ guideline-good-pharmacovigilance-practices-gvp-module-viii-post-authorisation-safety-studies-rev-3_en.pdf. Accessed 12 Jun 2020.
FDA. Best Practices for Conducting and Reporting Pharmacoepidemiology Safety Studies Using Electronic Healthcare Data Sets. May 2013. Online: https://www.fda.gov/regulatory-information/search-fda-guidance-documents/best-practices-conducting-and-reporting-pharmacoepidemiologic-safety-studies-using-electronic. Accessed 12 Jun 2020.
Guidelines for pharmacoepidemiologic studies
ENCePP, Guidelines on Methodological Standards in Pharmacoepidemiology (Revision 7), 2010. Online: http://www.encepp.eu/standards_and_guidances/documents/ ENCePPGuideonMethStandardsinPE_Rev7.pdf, Accessed 12 Jun 2020.
International Society for Pharmacoepidemiology (ISPE), Guidelines for Good Pharmacoepidemiology Practice (Revision 3), 2015. Online:https://www.pharmacoepi.org/ resources/policies/guidelines-08027/#1. Accessed 12 Jun 2020.
Berger ML, Sox H, Willke RJ, et al. Good practices for real-world data studies of treatment and/ or comparative effectiveness: Recommendations from the joint ISPOR-ISPE Special Task Force on real-world evidence in health care decision making. *Pharmacoepidemiol Drug Saf.* 2017;26 (9):1033–1039.
Berger ML, Dreyer N, Anderson F, Towse A, Sedrakyan A, Normand SL. Prospective observational studies to assess comparative effectiveness: the ISPOR good research practices task force report. *Value Health.* 2012;15(2):217–230.
Dreyer NA, Schneeweiss S, McNeil B, et al.; on behalf of the GRACE Initiative. GRACE principles: recognizing high-quality observationalstudies of comparative effectiveness. Am J Manag Care 2010;16:467–71.

The design of the observational study should be guided by the research question, the availability of data to answer the question, and an understanding of the limitations of the study to be conducted. This section will describe study designs commonly used for post-authorization studies but is not intended to replace textbooks on epidemiologic study design.

A thorough study protocol provides the parameters of the observational study including the following sections that define the design and conduct of the study (FDA 2013; ENCEPP 2010; ICPE 2015; Dreyer et al. 2010).

- **Research Question and Objectives** – this section defines both the issue that which leads to the study and specified hypotheses or outcomes that will be measured. This should include both primary and secondary objectives.
- **Study Design** – this section provides the overall research design (e.g., cohort, case-control) that will be used to answer the research question.
- **Study Population** – this section describes the source population and the comparison groups. In defining the source population, the protocol will outline the inclusion and exclusion criteria for the study population. For example, the study population may restrict to patients with a specific diagnosis likely to receive the drug or may include a subset of this population (e.g., pregnant women and their infants). Within the source population, the comparison groups in post-approval studies are defined by either exposure to a specific drug(s) of interest or by the presence of specific safety outcome of interest.
- **Data Source** – this section describes the data used to assess the research question. Data source includes primary data collection, patient-based or exposure-based registries, and secondary data sources (e.g., administrative claims data and electronic health records).
- **Data Collection and Covariates** – these sections describe both how drug exposures of interest and safety outcomes are operationally defined and measured, as well as how other risk factors, comorbidity, co-medication, potential confounders, and effect modifying variables are defined and measured.
- **Analysis Plan** – this section both describes how confounding or other biases are assessed and/or controlled and the statistical methods used to describe and compare the comparison groups, including the occurrence of outcome (e.g., incidence) and measure of association (e.g., relative risk, odds ratios, mean differences) and its confidence interval. It may describe additional planned such as intention-to-treat analysis, as treated analysis, subgroup analyses, sensitivity analyses and meta-analytic techniques to combine findings across data sources.
- **Limitations of Research Methods** – this section describes any potential limitations of study design, data sources, and analytic methods, including issues of confounding, bias, generalizability, and random error, as well as efforts made to reduce limitations with the proposed research plan.

Changes to study protocol should be documented in final report and the impact of changes on interpretation of study discussed (FDA 2013).

Observational Study Data Sources

The choice and effectiveness of treatment may be affected by practice setting (academic vs. community hospital), healthcare environment (e.g., commercial insurer, or single-payer system, or fee for service), the experience of healthcare providers (specialist vs. general practice), as well as availability of medical history of patient. Therefore, careful consideration must be made when choosing the appropriate data source.

Sources with Primary Data Collection

Post-approval observational studies can recruit patients by specific disease or by specific drug exposures, follow these patients over time, and collect pertinent data, prospectively, to assess the safety and effectiveness of a medical product of interest. Primary data collection may include patient-reported data, physician-reported data, and data abstracted from the patients' medical records. In addition, data can be collected to supplement patient data obtained in a secondary data source. The types of data not well documented in secondary data sources are duration of disease, behavioral factors (e.g., smoking, alcohol consumption, exercise), drug adherence, and patient quality of life. These data can be collected directly from patient via survey- or interview-based data collection. Medical record abstract may be used to collect additional patient information (e.g., potential confounding factors), or reason for discontinuation of a drug, and can be used to collect data to validate a diagnosis identified in secondary data (ENCEPP 2010).

Registries, specifically patient disease registries and pregnancy registries, are examples where patients are recruited, and data is collected prospectively during follow-up (Blumenthal 2017; Gliklich et al. 2014). Patient disease registries collect clinical data related to the disease onset, progression, and treatment course. At registry enrollment patient details are collected, including demographics, lifestyle and behavioral characteristics, patients' medical history, past and current drug utilization, and comorbidities. At regular intervals, prospectively, these data are updated. Important to post-approval study data is the identification of an initiation of new medications, or the onset of new symptoms or disease diagnosis. Patient disease registries are common for difficult-to-treat chronic diseases (e.g., multiple sclerosis and rheumatoid arthritis) and rare diseases (e.g., cystic fibrosis and Pompe disease (lysosomal storage disorder)) (NIH 2019). Patient registries are a useful source of patients for recruitment into clinical trials, as well as to identify patients for observational studies.

Because clinical trials conducted to assess the safety and efficacy of a new medical product often do not include pregnant women, a post-approval requirement may include the establishment of a pregnancy exposure registry. A pregnancy exposure registry enrolls women who have taken a drug of interest when they are pregnant. The registry will prospectively collect information on maternal events and delivery outcomes (e.g., spontaneous abortion) through the end of pregnancy and will collect data on infant events (e.g., infant death or major congenital malformations) usually in the first year of life (FDA 2020a).

One strength of primary data collection, such as in registries, is that patients are well characterized over time, and needed information on patient exposure, outcomes, and potentially confounding factors can be captured. A second strength for registries is the ability to collect information on patient using survey tools and validated instruments. Patient-reported health data may include quality of life, symptoms (e.g., pain scores or fatigue), use of over-the-counter medications, patient preferences, behavioral data, family history, and biological specimens. Yet, there are limitations; following many patients for a long time and the collection of prospective data are both time-consuming and very expensive. As in clinical trials, protocol-specified inclusion and exclusion criteria help to limit systematic selection bias in registries, and the use of validated and standardized assessments can reduce misclassification of disease and outcomes; yet while patient-reported events are essential to registry data, these data are subjective and certain forms of bias, such as recall bias, may influence the data.

Sources with Secondary Data Collection

The use of large, longitudinal, healthcare databases, such as electronic health record (EHR) databases, or health administrative claims databases has improved the efficiencies of observational studies. However, observational studies conducted using these sources must be performed within the limitations of data. A primary limitation of both data sources is that EHR and claims data are gathered for the purpose of patient care and billing, respectively, and not for research. Therefore, the fitness of the database to define exposure, outcomes, and potential confounding variable needs to be considered carefully. Hall et al. published a guidance and a checklist for selection of appropriate healthcare database for observational studies (Hall et al. 2012).

Electronic Health Records

An electronic health record (EHR) is a digital version of individual patient's medical chart, captured in real time, and is intended to provide a broad view of a patient's characteristics, medical history and comorbidity, drug utilization and treatment history, and the documentation of new onset of diagnoses. When using different EHR data sources, investigators must understand if the patient records include the entire record of patient care, or just a portion of it. For example, patients receiving treatment from multiple physicians, offices, or hospitals might have their care data captured in several different medical record data sources. Therefore, investigators using an EHR data source should describe the steps taken to ensure complete capture of patient care over time to facilitate the likelihood that all exposures and safety outcomes of interest will be captured. An example of an EHR source in Europe is the Clinical Practice Research Datalink (CPRD) that includes all people attending general practitioners in the UK. Other databases that link both electronic medical records with administrative health data are found in Italy (regional), the Netherlands (national), and other Nordic countries (e.g., Sweden (national healthcare database and disease registries) and Denmark (national)). Canada has a national EHR system, and data that are available from three provinces are available for pharmacoepidemiologic research. In the USA EHR data is available from large healthcare networks with shared electronic medical record system (e.g., Kaiser Permanente) and EHR systems (e.g., Optum EHR Research Database, Flatiron) that integrate electronic medical records across different systems into a common data platform, inclusive of data from a generalizable national sample of private practices, hospitals, and integrated health networks.

Health Administrative Claims Data

Health administrative claims data are a comprehensive source of longitudinal medical care data, including patient enrollment data (demographics), outpatient and inpatient medical claims (diagnoses, procedures, and laboratory claims), pharmacy claims (medications dispensed), and associated costs. These data are captured by health insurers, across all healthcare providers caring for patient, for the purpose of billing. Investigators using administrative claims data sources should address continuity of coverage (enrollment and disenrollment), particularly for claims data sources in the USA, because patients often enroll and disenroll in different health plans in relation to changes in employment or other life circumstances. Such documentation allows only periods of enrollment during which data are available on the patients of interest to be included in the study, and periods of disenrollment when data are not available on patients can be appropriately excluded. Definitions of *enrollment* or *continuous coverage* should be developed and documented, particularly in studies using more than one data source. While generally used as de-identified data (patient private information is redacted), in instances and with the right approvals, claims data can be linked to other sources, including EHR systems, registry data (e.g., cancer registries), and vital records (e.g., National Death Index) that improve the capture of long-term outcomes such as cancer and death.

In Europe and Canada, administrative data is captured as part of national and regional healthcare data sources, as described above. Examples of US sources of administrative claims data include Medicare, Medicaid, Veterans Administration System, as well as data available from commercial insurers (e.g., UnitedHealthcare, HealthCore, and MarketScan). Certain differences affect whether a non-US data source can be used to address specific drug safety hypotheses in a way that is relevant to the US population. Various factors in non-US healthcare systems, such as medication tiering (e.g., first-line, second-line) and patient coverage selection, influence the degree to which patients on a given therapy in other countries might differ in disease severity from patients on the same therapy.

Other Data Sources

Other secondary sources of health data that are useful tools in safety assessments are pharmacy claims data, national vital status records (e.g., the National Death Index, or Birth Registry), cancer registry data, and telehealth data.

Observational Study Designs

Cohort Studies

The efficiencies gained by using large healthcare databases make cohort studies a viable alternative to clinical trials, for large comparative effectiveness and safety studies. Cohort studies identify a population at risk and an exposure to medical products of interest and follow patients over time for the occurrence of events. In cohort studies, the comparison cohorts are selected from the same population at risk yet are unexposed at time of enrollment into the cohort and are similarly followed over time for the occurrence of events. Cohort studies provide the opportunity to determine the incidence rate of adverse events in addition to the relative risk of an adverse event. They are useful for identification of multiple events in the same study. In addition, cohort studies are useful for examining safety concerns in special populations, such as the children, the elderly, pregnant women, or patients with comorbid conditions that are often underrepresented in clinical trials (EMA 2017; FDA 2013).

Prospective and retrospective cohort studies serve different purposes in the post-approval setting. Prospective cohort studies are used for safety studies early after approval and release of a drug into the market. Retrospective cohort studies are conducted in secondary data sources when a drug has been on the market for some time and there is a new safety concern. See Table 4 for the strengths and weaknesses of prospective and retrospective cohort study designs.

Other Observation Designs

Other designs have been proposed to assess the associations between intermittent exposure (e.g., vaccination) and short-term events. These designs include case-control, self-controlled case-series, case-crossover, and case-time control studies. In these designs, only cases are used, and the control information is obtained as unexposed person-time experience of the cases themselves. One important strength of these designs is that confounding variables that do not change over time with individuals are automatically matched (EMA 2017).

Meta-analyses are common in observational research. These analyses involve statistical techniques that integrate and summarize the results across several studies with the same or similar research objectives can extend the understanding of the research question. They are important in identifying how both differences in research design and data source affect results, as well as to obtain an overall risk estimate (Chou and Helfand 2005; ENCePP 2010).

Bias in Observational Studies

Threats to validity of observational studies to assess drug safety include selection bias, misclassification, immortal time bias, channeling, and confounding by indication (Berger et al. 2017; FDA 2013). Selection bias occurs when there is selective recruitment of study populations such that populations are not representative of the populations you are trying to compare. Misclassification occurs when there is incorrect information about either the exposure, outcome, or covariates that describe the underlying populations. Immortal time refers to a period of cohort follow-up time during which an outcome of interest could not have occurred. Immortal time bias arises when the period between cohort entry and date of first exposure to a drug, during which the event of interest has not occurred, is either misclassified or simply excluded and not accounted for in the analysis (Berger et al. 2017; Suissa 2007, 2008). Channeling and confounding by indication occur when the estimate of the effect (exposure → outcome) results from imbalance of determinants of disease (or their proxies) across compared groups (FDA 2013). Channeling refers to the situation where drugs are prescribed to patients differently based on the presence or absence of factors prognostic of patient outcomes. Confounding by indication is a type of channeling bias that occurs when the indication, which is associated with drug exposure, is an independent risk factor for the outcome. Biases that threaten pharmacoepidemiologic safety studies conducted in secondary data sources, and methods to handle these biases, need to be taken into consideration when planning these studies.

Study designs with new users, with active comparators, or that are matched by disease risk score are methods that reduce these biases, in that a comparison is made between patients with the same indication initiating different treatments (ENCePP 2010).

Study design choices that make the study groups more similar are important tools for controlling for confounding and biases. The goal of the study design is to facilitate comparisons of people with similar chance of benefiting from the treatment or experiencing harm. There are few epidemiology and statistical method used to handle confounding in pharmacoepidemiologic studies (e.g., restriction, matching, adjustment, and weighting). Methods, such as propensity score (PS) matching and inverse probability treatment weighting (IPTW) using the PS, are two common ways to reduce bias in comparative safety studies using real-world large secondary data sources (Austin 2011; Austin and Stuart 2015; Rosenbaum and Rubin 2007/1983). PS is defined as the conditional probability of being treated with drug of interest given observed set of pretreatment characteristics. PS is estimated using logistic regression, where treatment group is the dependent variable. Potential independent variables in the logistic regression will include a priori specified characteristics, potential confounding factors, and effect modifying factors. Exposed and unexposed treatment groups are matched based on PS score, using a greedy matching algorithm. Treatment groups matched by PS should be well balanced with respect to known (and possibly unknown) confounders; therefore, the outcomes observed across treatment groups can be directly compared.

Enforcement of Post-Approval Studies by Regulatory Agencies

When they are imposed, post-approval studies are reviewed for compliance by the regulatory agencies. For clinical trials that are ongoing at the time of approval, often these are classified as PMC in the USA or PAM in the EU. Findings of these trials can be submitted to the health authorities for addition to the prescribing information, including expansion of the indications and/or update of the efficacy data. On the contrary, imposed observational studies for safety concerns can lead to changes in prescribing information and add to list of potential adverse effects. The FDA and EMA both track progress on PMC/PMRs and PAMs, respectively.

In the USA, PMC and PMR studies are registered at ClinicalTrials.gov, whether they are clinical trials or observational studies. In Europe, the EMA publishes the protocols, abstracts, and final study reports of PAS in the EU PAS register hosted on the European Network of Centres in Pharmacoepidemiology and Pharmacovigilance (ENCePP) website.

US PMC and PMR Enforcement

The FDA publishes an annual report that provides a summary of the progress of PMC and PMR that were agreed upon at the time of medicinal product approval. This annual report is required according to the FDA Modernization Act of 1997 and is published to the Federal Register. The report includes data from the PMR/PMC database maintained by the FDA (2020b). The PMR/PMC database is searchable and available to the public at the FDA website https://www.accessdata.fda.gov/scripts/cder/pmc/.

The most recent FDA annual report includes fiscal year 2018. PMC/PMRs are categorized as pending, ongoing, delayed, terminated, submitted, fulfilled, and released. In addition, PMRs/PMCs may be characterized as open or closed. Open PMRs/PMCs comprise those that are pending, ongoing, delayed, submitted, or terminated, whereas closed PMRs/PMCs are either fulfilled or released. Open PMRs are described as on- or off-schedule. On-schedule PMRs/PMCs are those that are pending, ongoing, or submitted. Off-schedule PMRs/PMCs are those that have missed one of the milestone dates in the original schedule and are categorized as either delayed or terminated.

The fiscal year 2018 annual report shows that 69% of PMR/PMC annual status reports were received on time. For those that were open but not due, 79% for new drug application and 86% for biologics license application PMRs were progressing on schedule, and most open PMCs – 76% for new drug applications and 84% of biologics license applications – were also on schedule (FDA 2019).

EU PAM Enforcement

The EMA assesses compliance to specific obligations specified in PAMs through the analysis of their database including due dates. The assessment is conducted annually, for both the annual renewal (for conditional marketing authorizations) and annual reassessment (for marketing authorizations under exceptional circumstances) (EMA 2020b).

When issues of non-compliance with PAM are identified, the relevant EMA committees can take one or more of the following actions:

- Letter to the MAH by the chair of the committee
- Oral explanation by MAH to the committee
- Initiation of a referral procedure with a view to vary/suspend/revoke the Market Authorization in light of Article 116 of Directive 2001/83/EC
- Inspection to be performed upon request of the committee(s)

Also, if the medicinal product has conditional approval, the marketing authorization can be varied, suspended, or revoked.

Such regulatory action regarding non-compliance of a PAM may be made public by the Agency on the Agency website, e.g., in the European public assessment report (EPAR) of the affected products.

Systematic Reviews of Post-Approval Studies in the USA and EU

Several analyses of post-approval study conducted in the USA and EU have been published. A summary of these analyses is described below.

Reviews of Post-Approval Studies in the USA

In the USA, following accelerated or expedited approval, the FDA may require additional confirmatory clinical trials. These required trials and their results have been the subject of several systematic review studies (Beaver et al. 2018; Naci et al. 2017; Wallach et al. 2018).

Naci et al. studied characteristics of pre- and post-approval clinical trials reviewed at the US FDA from 2009 to 2013 (Naci et al. 2017). They reported on trials for 22 drugs with 24 indications examined. Of these post-approval trials, 42% (10 of 24 indications studied) confirmed the efficacy of a previously analyzed surrogate endpoint within 3 years of Accelerated Approval. Among the 58% of post-approval trials that had not confirmed the indication for trial at time of review, half of the trials were still ongoing and the other half either were terminated, failed to confirm results, or were delayed by more than a year. There were two indications where the post-approval trial failed to confirm clinical benefit, yet these findings did not result in reversal of the approval, and no additional trials were imposed.

Wallach et al. studied post-approval studies required by the US FDA between 2009 and 2012 and allowed for at least 4 years of follow-up (Wallach et al. 2018). Among the 134 prospective cohort studies, registries, and clinical trials, 102 (76%) were registered on ClinicalTrials.gov. There were 65 completed studies, and 47 (72%) of these had reported results in ClinicalTrials.gov or in a publication. However, most (32 of 47, 68%) did not report results in the timeframe stated in the post-marketing requirement.

Beaver et al. reviewed the accelerated US FDA approvals of oncology and malignant hematology medicinal products from 1992 to 2017 (Beaver et al. 2018). They identified 93 products with Accelerated Approvals for new indications. Of these, 51 (55%) completed their post-approval studies and confirmed benefit within a median of 3.4 years, while 5 (5%) post-approval studies concerned indications that were withdrawn from the market. The remainder have ongoing confirmatory studies.

Reviews of Post-Approval Studies in the EU

In the EU, several studies have been conducted to measure compliance with the EU regulation and registration of PAS.

Blake et al. conducted the first review of the PAS register maintained by ENCePP (Blake et al. 2011). This analysis included PAS required by EMA between 2007 and 2009. As assessed in 2009, 60 PAS had been registered for 32 medicinal products and 52 had progressed to data collection, 7 were deemed no longer necessary by the Committee for Medicinal Products for Humans (CHMP), and the final study did not have a final decision. Of the 47 studies being "carried out" at the time of publication, 14 were randomized controlled trials; the remainder were either non-controlled trials or observational (non-interventional) studies.

Engel et al. specifically studied PASS protocols reviewed under the EU pharmacovigilance legislation (Engel et al. 2017). During 2012 to 2015, PRAC reviewed 189 PASS protocols, of which 58 (31%) were imposed and 131 were voluntary but required in the RMP for the medicinal product. Of 57 studies with protocols available in ENCePP, 67% were primary data collection and 33% used secondary data; in addition, the authors report that 65% did not include a comparator population. Only 2 of the 57 protocols explicitly stated hypothesis testing analyses were planned; therefore, we expect very few PASS used a clinical trial design. The authors did not report results on interventional vs. non-interventional study design.

Summary and Conclusions

Health authorities throughout the world have regulations for requesting additional research in the post-approval setting. This chapter focuses on the regulations in the USA and EU. The history of post-approval studies can be traced through changing regulations enforced by the FDA and EMA.

Specific terminology for post-approval studies is used by the FDA and EMA. Briefly, the FDA uses the term risk evaluation and mitigation strategy (REMS) to track post-approval safety studies that can be either post-marketing requirements (PMRs) or post-marketing commitments (PMCs). However, PMR and PMC can be conducted outside of REMS. The EMA uses post-authorization measures (PAM) to track post-authorization safety studies (PASS) and post-authorization efficacy studies (PAES).

Post-approval studies are either clinical trials (interventional) or observational (non-interventional) studies. Choosing a study design may be influenced by the strengths and weaknesses of the design options, as described in Table 4.

Imposed post-approval studies are reviewed for compliance by the regulatory agencies. For clinical trials that are ongoing at the time of approval, often these are classified as PMC in the USA or PAM in the EU. Findings of these trials can be submitted to the health authorities for addition to the prescribing information. The FDA and EMA both track progress on PMC/PMRs and PAMs, respectively.

In conclusion, post-approval studies are necessary to continually gather data on the safety and effectiveness of approved drugs. These studies are regulated by health authorities, included in registries (e.g., ClinicalTrials.gov, ENCePP), and tracked to completion. Given the inclusion of post-approval studies in public databases, they are the subject of systematic reviews.

Key Facts

- Post-approval studies can be required by regulatory agencies or voluntarily conducted by sponsors and market authorization holders.
- Post-approval studies use clinical trial or observational methodologies.
- Post-approval studies that are post-authorization safety studies (PASS) are registered in the ENCePP PAS study registry.
- Required post-approval studies are tracked by regulatory authorities for completion and compliance to timelines.

Cross-References

► Introduction to Meta-Analysis
► Pragmatic Randomized Trials Using Claims or Electronic Health Record Data
► Regulatory Requirements in Clinical Trials

References

Austin PC (2011) An introduction to propensity score methods for reducing the effects of confounding in observational studies. Multivariate Behav Res 46(3):399–424

Austin PC, Stuart EA (2015) Moving towards best practice when using inverse probability of treatment weighting (IPTW) using the propensity score to estimate causal treatment effects in observational studies. Stat Med 34(28):3661–3679

Beaver JA, Howie LN, Pelosof L, Kim T, Liu J, Goldberg KB, Sridhara R, Blumenthal GM, Farrell AT, Keegan P, Pazdur R, Kluetz PG (2018) A 25-year experience of US Food and Drug Administration approval of malignant hematology and oncology drugs and biologics. JAMA Oncol. https://doi.org/10.1001/jamaoncol.2017.5618. Published online March 1, 2018

Berger ML, Dreyer N, Anderson F, Towse A, Sedrakyan A, Normand SL (2012) Prospective observational studies to assess comparative effectiveness: the ISPOR good research practices task force report. Value Health 15(2):217–230

Berger ML, Sox H, Willke RJ, Brixner DL, Eichler HG, Goettsch W, Madigan D, Makady A, Schneeweiss S, Tarricone R, Wang SV, Watkins J, Mullins CD (2017) Good practices for real-world data studies of treatment and/or comparative effectiveness: recommendations from the joint ISPOR-ISPE Special Task Force on real-world evidence in health care decision making. Pharmacoepidemiol Drug Saf 26(9):1033–1039

Berry DA, Elanshoff M, Blotner S, Davi R, Beineke P, Chandler M, Lee DS, Chen LC, Sarkar S (2017) Creating a synthetic control arm from previous clinical trials: Application to establishing early end points as indicators of overall survival in acute myeloid leukemia (AML). ASCO abstract. J Clin Oncol 35(15_Suppl):7021. https://doi.org/10.1200/JCO.2017.35.15_suppl. 7021. Published online May 30, 2017. https://ascopubs.org/doi/full/10.1200/CCI.19.00037

Blake KV, Prilla S, Accadebled S, Guimier M, Biscaro M, Persson I, Arlett P, Blackburn S, Fitt H (2011) European Medicines Agency review of post-authorisation studies with implications for the European Network of Centres for Pharmacoepidemiology and Pharmacovigilance. Pharmacoepidemiol Drug Saf 20:1021–1029

Blumenthal S (2017) The use of clinical registries in the United States: a landscape survey. EGEMS (Wash DC) 5(1):26. https://doi.org/10.5334/egems.248. Published 2017 Dec 7

Chou R, Helfand M (2005) Challenges in systematic reviews that assess treatment harms. Ann Intern Med 142(12 Pt 2):1090–1099

Dreyer NA, Schneeweiss S, McNeil B, Berger ML, Walker AM, Ollendorf DA, Gliklich RE, on behalf of the GRACE Initiative (2010) GRACE principles: recognizing high-quality observational studies of comparative effectiveness. Am J Manag Care 16:467–471

Engel P, Almas MF, DeBruin ML, Starzyk K, Blackburn S, Dreyer NA (2017) Lessons learned on the design and the conduct of Post-Authorization Safety Studies: review of 3 years of PRAC oversight. Br J Clin Pharmacol 83:884–893

European Medicines Agency (2012) Legal framework: pharmacovigilance. Available at https://www.ema.europa.eu/en/human-regulatory/overview/pharmacovigilance/legal-framework-pharmacovigilance. Accessed 12 June 2020

European Medicines Agency (2016) Scientific guidance on post-authorisation efficacy studies. Available at https://www.ema.europa.eu/en/documents/scientific-guideline/scientific-guidance-post-authorisation-efficacy-studies-first-version_en.pdf. Accessed 12 June 2020

European Medicines Agency (2017) Guideline on good pharmacovigilance practice (GVP). Available at https://www.ema.europa.eu/en/documents/scientific-guideline/guideline-good-pharmacovigilance-practices-gvp-module-viii-post-authorisation-safety-studies-rev-3_en.pdf. Accessed 12 June 2020

European Medicines Agency (2020a) Post-authorisation safety studies (PASS). Available at https://www.ema.europa.eu/en/human-regulatory/post-authorisation/pharmacovigilance/post-authorisation-safety-studies-pass-0. Accessed 12 June 2020

European Medicines Agency (2020b) Post-authorisation measures: questions and answers. https://www.ema.europa.eu/en/human-regulatory/post-authorisation/post-authorisation-measures-questions-answers. Accessed 12 June 2020

European Network of Centers for Pharmacoepidemiology and Pharmacovigilance (ENCePP) (2010) Guidelines on methodological standards in Pharmacoepidemiology (Revision 7), 2010. Online: http://www.encepp.eu/standards_and_guidances/documents/ENCePPGuideonMethStandardsinPE_Rev7.pdf. Accessed 12 June 2020

European Network of Centers for Pharmacoepidemiology and Pharmacovigilance (ENCePP) (2017) Guidelines on Good Pharmacovigilance (GVP) – Module VIII – Post-authorization safety studies (Revision 3). Online: https://www.ema.europa.eu/en/documents/scientific-guideline/guideline-good-pharmacovigilance-practices-gvp-module-viii-post-authorisation-safety-studies-rev-3_en.pdf. Accessed 12 June 2020

Food and Drug Administration (2011) Guidance for industry postmarketing studies and clinical trials – implementation of section 505(o)(3) of the Federal Food, Drug, and Cosmetic Act. Available at https://www.fda.gov/downloads/Drugs/GuidanceComplianceRegulatoryInformation/Guidances/UCM172001.pdf or https://www.fda.gov/regulatory-information/search-fda-guidance-documents/postmarketing-studies-and-clinical-trials-implementation-section-505o3-federal-food-drug-and. Accessed 12 June 2020

Food and Drug Administration (2013) Best practices for conducting and reporting pharmacoepidemiology safety studies using electronic healthcare data sets. May 2013. Online: https://www.fda.gov/regulatory-information/search-fda-guidance-documents/best-practices-conducting-and-reporting-pharmacoepidemiologic-safety-studies-using-electronic. Accessed 12 June 2020

Food and Drug Administration (2018) FDA drug safety communication: new risk factor for Progressive Multifocal Leukoencephalopathy (PML) associated with Tysabri (natalizumab). Available at https://www.fda.gov/drugs/drug-safety-and-availability/fda-drug-safety-communication-new-risk-factor-progressive-multifocal-leukoencephalopathy-pml. Accessed 12 June 2020

Food and Drug Administration (2019) FDA in brief: FDA issues annual report on efforts to hold industry accountable for fulfilling critical post-marketing studies of the benefits, safety of new drugs. https://www.fda.gov/news-events/fda-brief/fda-brief-fda-issues-annual-report-efforts-hold-industry-accountable-fulfilling-critical-post. Accessed 12 June 2020

Food and Drug Administration (2020a) List of pregnancy exposure registries updated 17 Jan 2020. Online: https://www.fda.gov/science-research/womens-health-research/list-pregnancy-exposure-registries. Accessed 20 Feb 2020

Food and Drug Administration (2020b) Postmarketing requirements and commitments: reports. https://www.fda.gov/drugs/postmarket-requirements-and-commitments/postmarketing-require ments-and-commitments-reports. Accessed 12 June 2020

Gliklich R, Dreyer N, Leavy M (eds) (2014) Registries for evaluating patient outcomes: a user's guide, 3rd edn. Two volumes. (Prepared by the Outcome DEcIDE Center [Outcome Sciences, Inc., a Quintiles company] under Contract No. 290 2005 00351 TO7.) AHRQ Publication No. 13(14)-EHC111. Agency for Healthcare Research and Quality, Rockville. http://www.effectivehealthcare.ahrq.gov/registries-guide-3.cfm

Goedecke T (2017) EU PASS/PAES Requirements for Disclosure. Available at https://www.ema.europa.eu/en/documents/presentation/presentation-eu-pass/paes-requirements-disclosure-thomas-goedecke_en.pdf. Accessed 12 June 2020

Hall GC, Sauer B, Bourke A, Brown JS, Reynolds MW, LoCasale R (2012) Guidelines for good database selection and use in pharmacoepidemiology research [published correction appears in Pharmacoepidemiol Drug Saf. 2012;21(11):1249. Casale, Robert Lo [corrected to LoCasale, Robert]]. Pharmacoepidemiol Drug Saf 21(1):1–10. https://doi.org/10.1002/pds.2229

International Society for Pharmacoepidemiology (2015) Guidelines for good pharmacoepidemiology practice (Revision 3), 2015. Online: https://www.pharmacoepi.org/resources/policies/guidelines-08027/#1. Accessed 12 June 2020

Kappos L, Bates D, Edan G, Eraksoy M, Garcia-Merino A, Grigoriadis N, Hartung HP, Havrdová E, Hillert J, Hohlfeld R, Kremenchutzky M, Lyon-Caen O, Miller A, Pozzilli C, Ravnborg M, Saida T, Sindic C, Vass K, Clifford DB, Hauser S, Major EO, O'Connor PW, Weiner HL, Clanet M, Gold R, Hirsch HH, Radü EW, Sørensen PS, King J (2011) Natalizumab treatment for multiple sclerosis: updated recommendations for patient selection and monitoring. Lancet Neurol 10(8):745–758

Krumholz HM, Ross JS, Presler AH, Egilman DS (2007) What have we learnt from Vioxx? BMJ 334(7585):120–123. https://doi.org/10.1136/bmj.39024.487720.68

Naci H, Smalley KR, Kesselheim AS (2017) Characteristics of preapproval and postapproval studies for drugs granted accelerated approval by the US Food and Drug Administration. JAMA 318(7):626–636. https://doi.org/10.1001/jama.2017.9415

National Institutes of Health (2019) List of registries, last reviewed 18 Nov 2019. Available at: https://www.nih.gov/health-information/nih-clinical-research-trials-you/list-registries. Accessed 12 June 2020

Patsopoulous NA (2011) A pragmatic view on pragmatic trials. Dialogues Clin Neurosci 13:217–224

Prakash S, Valentine V (2007) Timeline: the rise and fall of Vioxx November 10, 2007. https://www.npr.org/2007/11/10/5470430/timeline-the-rise-and-fall-of-vioxx

Rosenbaum PR, Rubin DB (2007) The central role of the propensity score in observational studies for causal effects. Biometrika 70(1 (Apr, 1983)):41–55

Suissa S (2007) Immortal time bias in observational studies of drug effects. Pharmacoepidemiol Drug Saf 16(3):241–249

Suissa S (2008) Immortal time bias in pharmaco-epidemiology. Am J Epidemiol 167(4):492–499

Wallach JD, Egilman AC, Dhruva SS, McCarthy ME, Miller JE, Woloshin S, Schwartz LM, Ross JS (2018) Postmarket studies required by the US Food and Drug Administration for new drugs and biologics approved between 2009 and 2012: cross sectional analysis. BMJ 361:k2031

Zauderer MG, Grigorenko A, May P, Kastango N, Wagner I, Caroline A (2019) Creating a synthetic clinical trial: comparative effectiveness analyses using electronic medical record. JCO Clin Cancer Inform. https://doi.org/10.1200/CCI.19.00037. Published online June 21, 2019